D1453238

CONTEMPORARY CONCEPTS IN CARDIOLOGY

Pathophysiology and Clinical Management

198. Antoine Lafont, Eric Topol (eds.): *Arterial Remodeling: A Critical Factor in Restenosis.* 1997   ISBN 0-7923-8008-8

199. Michele Mercuri, David D. McPherson, Hisham Bassiouny, Seymour Glagov (eds.):*Non-Invasive Imaging of Atherosclerosis*   ISBN 0-7923-8036-3

200. Walmor C. DeMello, Michiel J. Janse(eds.): *Heart Cell Communication in Health and Disease*   ISBN 0-7923-8052-5

201. P.E. Vardas (ed.): *Cardiac Arrhythmias Pacing and Electrophysiology.* The Expert View. 1998   ISBN 0-7923-4908-3

202. E.E. van der Wall, P.K. Blanksma, M.G. Niemeyer, W. Vaalburg and H.J.G.M. Crijns (eds.) *Advanced Imaging in Coronary Artery Disease, PET, SPECT, MRI, I VUS, EBCT. 1998*   ISBN 0-7923-5083-9

203. R.L. Wilensky (ed.) *Unstable Coronary Artery Syndromes, Pathophysiology, Diagnosis and Treatment. 1998.*   ISBN 0-7923-8201-3

204. J.H.C. Reiber, E.E. van der Wall (eds.): *What's New in Cardiovascular Imaging?* 1998   ISBN 0-7923-5121-5

205. Juan Carlos Kaski, David W. Holt (eds.): *Myocardial Damage Early Detection by Novel Biochemical Markers. 1998.*   ISBN 0-7923-5140-1

207. Gary F. Baxter, Derek M. Yellon, *Delayed Preconditioning and Adaptive Cardioprotection. 1998.*   ISBN 0-7923-5259-9

208. Bernard Swynghedauw, *Molecular Cardiology for the Cardiologist, Second Edition* 1998.   ISBN 0-7923-8323-0

209. Geoffrey Burnstock, James G.Dobson, Jr., Bruce T. Liang, Joel Linden (eds): *Cardiovascular Biology of Purines. 1998.*   ISBN: 0-7923-8334-6

210. Brian D. Hoit, Richard A. Walsh (eds): *Cardiovascular Physiology in the Genetically Engineered Mouse. 1998.*   ISBN: 0-7923-8356-7

211. Peter Whittaker, George S. Abela (eds.): *Direct Myocardial Revascularization: History, Methodology, Technology* 1998.   ISBN: 0-7923-8398-2

212. C.A. Nienaber, R. Fattori (eds.): Diagnosis and Treatment of Aortic Diseases. 1999.   ISBN: 0-7923-5517-2

213. Juan Carlos Kaski (ed.): *Chest Pain with Normal Coronary Angiograms: Pathogenesis, Diagnosis and Management.* 1999.   ISBN: 0-7923-8421-0

214. P.A. Doevendans, R.S. Reneman and M. Van Bilsen (eds): *Cardiovascular Specific Gene Expression.* 1999   ISBN:0-7923-5633-0

215. G. Pons-Lladó, F. Carreras, X. Borrás, Subirana and L.J. Jiménez-Borreguero (eds.): *Atlas of Practical Cardiac Applications of MRI.* 1999   ISBN: 0-7923-5636-5

216. L.W. Klein, J.E. Calvin, *Resource Utilization in Cardiac Disease.* 1999.   ISBN:0-7923-8509-8

217. R. Gorlin, G. Dangas, P. K. Toutouzas, M.M Konstadoulakis, *Contemporary Concepts in Cardiology, Pathophysiology and Clinical Management.*1999   ISBN:0-7923-8514-4

previous volumes are still available

KLUWER ACADEMIC PUBLISHERS - DORDRECHT/BOSTON/LONDON

CONTEMPORARY CONCEPTS IN CARDIOLOGY
Pathophysiology and Clinical Management

Richard Gorlin
George Dangas
*Mount Sinai School
of Medicine, New York*

Pavlos K. Toutouzas
M.M. Konstadoulakis
*National University of Athens
School of Medicine*

Foreword by
J. Willis Hurst

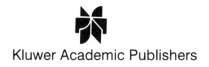

Kluwer Academic Publishers

Distributors for North, Central and South America:
Kluwer Academic Publishers
101 Philip Drive
Assinippi Park
Norwell, Massachusetts 02061 USA
Telephone (781) 871-6600
Fax (781) 871-6528
E-Mail <kluwer@wkap.com>

Distributors for all other countries:
Kluwer Academic Publishers Group
Distribution Centre
Post Office Box 322
3300 AH Dordrecht, THE NETHERLANDS
Telephone 31 78 6392 392
Fax 31 78 6546 474
E-Mail <orderdept@wkap.nl>

Electronic Services <http://www.wkap.nl>

 Library of Congress Cataloging-in-Publication Data

A C.I.P. Catalogue record for this book is available
from the Library of Congress.

Themata sygchrones kardiologias. English. Contemporary concepts in cardiology:
    Pathophysiology and clinical management/[edited by] Richard Gorlin...[et al.]
foreword by J. Willis Hurst.
    P. Cm. --(Developments in cardiovascular medicine: 217)
Includes index.
ISBN 0-7923-8514-4 (alk. Paper)
1. Cardiovascular system--Diseases--Treatment. I. Gorlin, Richard, 1926- . II.
Title. III Series: Developments in cardiovascular medicine : v. 217. [DNLM: 1.
Cardiovascular Diseases--diagnosis. 2. Cardiovascular Diseases--physiopathology.
3. Cardiovascular Diseases--therapy, WG 120 T383 1999]. RC671.T47 1999
616.1--dc21   DNLM/DLC   99-26059
for Library of Congress   CIP
Copyright © 1999 by Kluwer Academic Publishers.

Printed on acid-free paper.
Printed in the United States of America

To our students and colleagues
R.G., P.K.T

To my parents and my associates
G.D.

To my parents
M.M.K

CONTEMPORARY CONCEPTS IN CARDIOLOGY
Pathophysiology and Clinical Management

Section A
CORONARY ARTERY DISEASE

Section B
HYPERTENSION

Section C
CARDIOMYOPATHIES

Section D
CARDIAC GENETICS

Section E
NONINVASIVE CARDIOLOGY

Section F
INTERVENTIONAL CARDIOLOGY

Section G
ELECTROPHYSIOLOGY

FOREWORD

This book, "Contemporary Concepts in Cardiology", has been created by a superb group of editors including Richard Gorlin and George Dangas form New York, and Pavlos K. Toutouzas and M.M. Konstadoulakis from Athens.

Aside from its scientific merit, the book will serve as tribute to Professor Richard Gorlin, whose death occurred before the book reached the bookselves of the readers. Gorlin taught us all the importance of learning the pathophysiologic mechanisms that are responsible for clinical conditions. Simply stated, he believed the art of medicine was improved if one understood why things happened. The legendary Gene Stead wrote why he and his associates perceived his teacher Soma Weiss as a great man. One reason he gives was, "his forte was to elicit the symptoms and signs and to relate them to pathophysiology." (Essays by E.A. Stead Jr. A way of thinking: a primer on the art of being a doctor. Edited by B.F. Haynes. Durham: Carolina Academic Press 1995: 65).

This book deals with contemporary concepts, and it is not presented as a complete treatise on cardiovascular problems. Rather it deals with current issues in which considerable progress and new insights are being developed. The book has been divided into seven sections: Coronary Artery Disease, Hypertension, Cardiomyopathies, Cardiac Genetics, Non-invasive Cardiology, Interventional Cardiology, and Electrophysiology. Each of the chapters leads the reader into a deeper understanding of the subject. Soma Weiss would, I believe, enjoy this book.

The editors and authors have done an excellent job in selecting and discussing the subjects that are currently being investigated and in which a conceptual understanding will improve the function and wisdom of the physician who studies their words.

J. Willis Hurst, MD
Consultant to the Division of Cadiology
Professor and Chairman, Emeritus,
Department of Medicine
Emory University School of Medicine
Atlanta, Georgia, USA

PREFACE

In the era of instant global communication, medicine is an international discipline characterized by a wide range of patient referral systems, world-wide discussion of clinical and research findings, and an explosion in the medical literature. Perhaps no field has progressed more than cardiology in the past few years.

The present text has been conceived as a supplement to the classic cardiology textbooks for the use of practicing physicians, cardiologists-in-training, medical students, and research investigators. We focus on associations between refinements in the understanding of disease and clinical applications. The material is presented in a way that limns the latest advances and focuses thinking towards future developments in cardiology.

We assembled a respected international panel of contributors so that each chapter is authored by a well-known specialist in his or her field. Every attempt was made to avoid the fragmentation which often characterizes the digest approach. Because the constant flow of information makes it nearly impossible to construct a timely book on advances in cardiology, the included chapters that describe the current concepts in cardiology and their underlying rationale, rather than attempting a comprehensive review of the most recent papers in each discipline. As new work emerges, it should fit into the overall blueprint.

This book would not have been possible without the help of many people. First, we thank the editorial team of the University of Athens for their collaboration. Next, we recognize the authors for their willingness to participate in this task and for their concise contributions. Thanks are also due to Karen Sadock, A.B., M.Div., for expert editorial review, and to I. Tiernan and M. Healy from the New York team, as well as to V. Kalaitzi and S. Tapa from the Athens team for their assistance. Finally, we acknowledge Melissa Ramondetta and Margarita Papailiou on behalf of the publishers.

George Dangas, Richard Gorlin

Mount Sinai School of Medicine, New York

PROLOGUE

We live in an era that Cardiology is punctuated by the rapid expansion of its scientific base; new technology and an availability of diagnostic and therapeutic modalities have never previously benn encountered.

In this book we attempt to describe the important changes of the cardiology within the last couple of years. The advances made in cardiology are reviewed by the pioneers of this field. Thorough analyses of the results of national and international trials, on hypertension and hyperlipidemias are analyzed and evaluated.

Normal cardiovascular function are affected profoundly by a large number of processes at the molecular and genetic lever that are now being understood. It is becoming clear that these abnormalities are the basis of many cardiovascular diseases. Research in the genetics of many diseases has been given added impetus by the increasing likelihood tha gene therapy will become a realistic therapeutic option. For this reason, in this book, special emphasis is given on Molecular Cardiology and its potential application on prevention, diagnosis and therapy.

We dedicate this book to every physician and we believe that it comes to fill a gap in the current literature, emphasizing a possible victory of non-invasive cardiology, which seems to be ready for the challenge of the year 2000.

Pavlos K. Toutouzas, M.M. Konstadoulakis
National University of Athens School of Medicine
Athens, Greece

CONTRIBUTING AUTHORS

Todd J. Anderson, MD, F.R.C.P.(C)
Assistant Professor of Medicine
Alberta Heritage Foundation
for Medical Research
Foothills Hospital, University of Calgary
Calgary, CANADA

Thomas C. Andrews, MD
Assistant Professor of Medicine
University of Texas
Southwestern Medical Center
Dallas, TX, USA

Aris Antoniou, MD
Assistant Professor of Radiology
University of Athens School of Medicine
Aretaieion University Hospital
Athens, GREECE

Lina Badimon, PhD
Professor of Medicine and Cardiology
University of Barcelona
School of Medicine
Barcelona, SPAIN

Juan J. Badimon, PhD
Associate Professor of Medicine
Director, Cardiovascular Research
Laboratories
Cardiovascular Institute
Mount Sinai School of Medicine
New York, NY, USA

John A. Bittl, MD
Ocala Heart Institute
Florida, USA

Dr Margaret Brown
Department of Physiology
University of Birmingham
School of Medicine
Birmingham, UK

Christopher P. Cannon, MD
Assistant Professor of Medicine
Harvard Medical School
Cardiovascular Division
Brigham & Women's Hospital
Boston, MA, USA

François Charbonneau, MD, F.R.C.P.(C)
Assistant Professor of Medicine
Cardiovascular Division
Montreal Heart Institute
McGill University
Montreal, Quebec, CANADA

James H. Chesebro, MD
Professor of Medicine
Director of Clinical Research
Cardiovascular Institute
Mount Sinai School of Medicine
New York, NY, USA

Elena Citkowitz, MD, PhD
Director, Lipid Clinic and
Cardiac Rehabilitation
Hospital of St. Raphael
Assistant Clinical Professor of Medicine
Yale University School of Medicine
New Haven, NY, USA

James Coromilas, MD
Assosiate Professor of Clinical Medicine
Director, Electrophysiology Laboratory
Columbia University,
College of Physicians & Surgeons
New York, NY, USA

George Dangas, MD
Consultant Cardiovascular Institute
Mount Sinai Medical Center
Mount Sinai School of Medicine
New York, NY, USA

Richard B. Devereux, MD
Professor of Medicine,
Division of Cardiology
Director, Echocardiography Laboratory
The New York Hospital-
Cornell Medical Center
New York, NY, USA

David P. Dutka, DM, MRCP
Department of Medicine
(Clinical Cardiology)
Royal Postgraduate Medical School
Hammersmith Hospital,
London, UK

Antonio Fernandez - Ortiz, MD, PhD
Assistant Professor of Medicine
Hospital Universitario San Carlos
Madrid, SPAIN

Ronald S. Freudenberger, MD
Assistant Professor of Medicine
Director, Transplant Cardiology
University of Maryland
   School of Medicine
Baltimore USA

Valentin Fuster, MD, PhD
Richard Gorlin, MD/Heart Research
   Foundation Professor of Cardiology
Dean of Academic Affairs, Mount Sinai
   Medical School
Director, Cardiovascular Institute
Mount Sinai Medical Center
New York, NY, USA

Peter Ganz, MD
Assosiate Professor of Medicine
Harvard Medical School
Associate Director, Cardiac
   Catheterization Laboratory
Brigham & Women's Hospital
Boston, MA, USA

Alan Gass, MD
Assistant Professor of Medicine
Director, Transplant Cardiology Section
Cardiovascular Institute
Mount Sinai Medical Center
New York, NY, USA

J. Anthony Gomes, MD
Professor of Medicine
Director, Electrophysiology Section
Cardiovascular Institute
Mount Sinai Medical Center
New York, NY, USA

Richard Gorlin, MD (1925-1997)
Dr. George Baher Professor of Medicine
Senior Vice President
Mount Sinai Medical Center
New York, NY, USA

Rebecca T. Hahn, MD
Assistant Professor of Medicine
Assistant Director,
   Echocardiography Laboratory
The New York Hospital-
   Cornell Medical Center
New York, NY, USA

Peter N. Herbert, MD
Clinical Professor of Medicine
Yale University School of Medicine
Chairman, Department of Medicine
Hospital of Saint Raphael
New Haven, CT, USA

David R. Holmes, Jr., MD
Professor of Medicine
   Mayo Medical School
Director, Adult Cardiac Catheterization
   Laboratory
Mayo Clinic and Mayo Foundation
Rochester, MN, USA

Dr. Olga Hudlicka
Professor and Head,
   Department of Physiology
University of Birmingham
   School of Medicine
Birmingham, UK

Diwakar Jain, MD
Assistant Professor of Medicine
Division of Cardiovascular Medicine
Yale University School of Medicine
New Haven, CT, USA

John Kassotis, MD
Section of Electrophysiology,
   Division of Cardiology
Columbia University
   College of Pysicians & Surgeons
New York, NY, USA

Alan S. Katz, MD
Assistant Professor of Medicine
Brown University School of Medicine
Director of Echocardiography,
   The Miriam Hospital
Providence, RI, USA

Philip J. Keeling, MD, MRCP
Senior Registrar in Cardiology
St George's Hospital Medical School
London, UK

Annapoorna S. Kini, MD
Cardiovascular Institute
Mount Sinai Medical Center
New York, NY, USA

Manoussos M. Konstadoulakis, MD
Molecular Immunology Laboratory
Hippokrateion University Hopital
University of Athens School of Medicine
Athens, GREECE

Peter A. Kringstein, MD
Hypertension Section,
    Cardiovascular Institute
Mount Sinai Medical Center
New York, NY, USA

George D. Kymionis, MD
Molecular Immunology Laboratory
Hippokrateion University Hospital
University of Athens School of Medicine
Athens, GREECE

Gaetano A. Lanza, MD
Department of Cardiology
Catholic University of Rome
Rome, ITALY

Emanuel Leandros, MD
Assistant Professor
Department of Surgery
National University of Athens
Athens, GREECE

Martin B. Leon, MD
Director,
    Cardiology Research Foundation
Washington Hospital Center
Clinical Professor of Medicine
Georgetown University
Washington, DC, USA

Daniel K. Levy, MD
Cardiovascular Institute
Mount Sinai Medical Center
New York, NY, USA

Leslie J. Lipka, MD, PhD
Instructor in Clinical Medicine,
    Division of Cardiology
Columbia University,
    College of Physicians & Surgeons
New York, NY, USA

Ethan D. Loeb, MD
Hypertension Section,
    Cardiovascular Institute
Mount Sinai Medical Center
New York, NY, USA

Joseph Loscalzo, MD, PhD
Whitaker Professor of Medicine and
    Biochemistry
Boston University School of Medicine
Director, Whitaker Cardiovascular
    Institute
Vice-Chairman, Department of Medicine
Chief, Cardiology Section
Boston University Medical Center
Boston, MA, USA

Calum MacRae, MD
Department of Genetics
Harvard Medical School
Boston, MA, USA

Attilio Maseri, MD
Professor of Cardiology
Director, Department of Cardiology
Catholic University of Rome
Rome, ITALY

William J. McKenna, MD
Professor of Cardiac Medicine
Department of Cardiological Sciences
Saint George's Hospital Medical School
London, UK

Roxana Mehran, MD
Director, Clinical Research and Data
    Coordinating Center
Cardiology Research Foundation
Washington Hospital Center
Washington, DC, USA

Davendra Mehta, MD, PhD
Assistant Professor of Medicine
Mount Sinai School of Medicine
Director of Electrophysiology
Bronx VA Medical Center
New York, NY, USA

Ian T. Meredith, M.B.B.S., Ph.D.
Deputy Director, Vascular Medicine and
   Hypertension
Monash Medical Center
Melbourne, AUSTRALIA

Beat J. Meyer, MD
Assistant Professor of Medicine
Cardiac Catheterization Laboratory
University Hospital Inselspital
Bern, SWITZERLAND

Theodore D. Mountokalakis, MD
Professor and Chairman
Department of Internal Medicine
Sotiria Univeristy Hospital
National University of Athens
Athens, GREECE

David W.M. Muller, MBBS
Professor of Medicine
Director, Cardiac Catherization
   Laboratories
St. Vincent's Hospital Center
Sydney, AUSTRALIA

Celia M. Oakley, DM, FRCP
Professor of Cardiology
Hammersmith Hospital
Royal Postgraduate Medical School
London, UK

Robert A. Phillips, MD, PhD
Assosiate Professor of Medicine
Director, Hypertension Section
Cardiovascular Institute
Mount Sinai Medical Center
New York, NY, USA

Christos Pitsavos, MD
Assistant Professor of Cardiology
Department of Cardiology
Hippokrateion University Hospital
National University of Athens
Athens, GREECE

Roy Sauberman, MD
Section of Electrophysiology,
   Division of Cardiology
Columbia University,
   College of Pysicians & Surgeons
New York, NY, USA

Brian Schafer, MD
Cardiovascular Division
Wilford Hall Medical Center
San Antonio, TX, USA

Robert S. Schwartz, MD
Professor of Medicine,
   Mayo Medical School
Division of Cardiovascular Diseases
   and Internal Medicine
Mayo Clinic and Mayo Foundation
Rochester, MN, USA

Andrew P. Selwyn, MD
Professor of Medicine
Harvard Medical School
Director, Cardiac Catheterization
   Laboratory
Brigham & Women's Hospital
Boston, MA, USA

Samin K. Sharma, MD
Assistant Professor of Medicine
Director, Cardiac Catheterization
   Laboratory
Cardiovascular Institute
Mount Sinai Medical Center
New York, NY, USA

Ralph V. Shohet, MD
Assistant Professor of Medicine
Division of Cardiology
The University of Texas
Southwestern Medical Center at Dallas
Dallas, TX, USA

Fred Slogoff, MD
Hypertension Section,
   Cardiovascular Institute
Mount Sinai School of Medicine
New York, NY, USA

Donald A. Smith, MD, MPH
Assistant Professor of Medicine and
   Community Medicine
Director, Lipids and Metabolism Section
Cardiovascular Institute
Mount Sinai Medical Center
New York, NY, USA

Christodoulos I. Stefanadis, MD
Associate Professor of Cardiology
Department of Cardiology
Hippokrateion University Hospital
National University of Athens
Athens, GREECE

Peter H. Stone, MD
Assosiate Professor of Medicine
Harvard Medical School
Co-Director, Sammuel A. Levine
    Cardiac Unit
Director, Clinical Trials
Cardiovascular Division
Brigham & Women's Hospital
Boston, MA, USA

Farris K. Timimi, MD
Cardiovascular Division
Brigham and Women's Hospital
Harvard Medical School
Boston, MA, USA

Henry H. Ting, MD
Cardiovascular Division
Brigham and Women's Hospital
Harvard Medical School
Boston, MA, USA

Marina G. Toutouza, MD
Cardiovascular Research Laboratories
Hippokrateion University Hospital
Athens, GREECE

Pavlos K. Toutouzas, MD
Professor and Chairman
Department of Cardiology
Hippokrateion University Hospital
National University of Athens
Athens, GREECE

Lampros Vlahos, MD
Professor and Chairman
Department of Radiology
Aretaieion University Hospital
University of Athens National
Athens, GREECE

Eric Wasserman, MD
Hypertension Section,
    Cardiovascular Institute
Mount Sinai School of Medicine
New York, NY, USA

R. Sanders Williams, MD
Distinguished Professor,
Chair in Cardiovascular Diseases
Chief, Division of Cardiology
The University of Texas
Southwestern Medical Center at Dallas
Dallas, TX, USA

Paul G. Yock, MD
Associate Professor of Medicine
Stanford University School of Medicine
Director, Center for Rersearch in
    Cardiovascular Interventions
Stanford University Medical Center
Palo Alto, CA, USA

Barry L. Zaret, MD
Robert B. Berliner Professor of Medicine
Professor of Diagnostic Radiology
Chief, Section of Cardiovascular
    Medicine
Yale University School of Medicine
New Haven, CT, USA

Section A
CORONARY ARTERY DISEASE

1 PATHOGENESIS OF ATHEROSCLEROSIS

Antonio Fernandez-Ortiz, Juan J Badimon, Valentin Fuster

Atherosclerosis is the result of a complex interaction between blood elements, disturbed flow, and vessel wall abnormality. In the prevalent view, atherosclerosis is considered a specialized type of chronic, inflammatory, fibroproliferative response of the arterial wall to various sources of injury.[1] Several pathologic processes are involved in atherosclerotic plaque evolution: chronic endothelial injury, with increased permeability, endothelial activation, and monocyte recruitment; cellular growth, with smooth muscle cell migration, proliferation, and extracellular matrix synthesis; degeneration, with lipid accumulation, necrosis, and calcification; inflammation, with leukocyte activation and extracellular matrix degradation; and thrombosis, with platelet recruitment and fibrin formation. In addition, biologic processes may be involved in lesion stabilization or even regression. This chapter will review pivotal cellular and mollecular events in the processes of initiation, progression, stabilization and regression of atherosclerotic lesions.

Atherosclerotic plaque initiation and progression

Endothelial Injury

The endothelium is intimatelly involved in the pathogenesis of atherosclerosis. Non-adaptive changes in the functional properties of the vascular endothelium, provoked by various pathologic stimuli, can result in localized alterations in the interaction of cellular and macromolecular components of circulating blood with the arterial wall. These include: altered permeability to plasma lipoproteins, increased cytokine and growth factor production, imbalances in procoagulant and fibrinolytic activity, and hiperadhesiveness for blood leukocytes. These manifestations, collectively termed *"endothelial dysfunction"*, play an important role in the initiation of atherosclerosis.

Among endothelial injury sources, hypercholesterolemia has been extensively investigated. There is accumulating evidence to suggest a direct injurious effect of elevated levels of LDL cholesterol, in particular its oxidative derivative, on the endothelium.[2] Lysolecithin, a product formed as a consequence of lipid peroxidation of LDL particles, has been related to abnormal endothelium-dependent vasomotion.[3] In addition, hypercholesterolemia by itself is a stimulus to augmented generation of superoxide radicals by the endothelium which directly inactivates nitric oxide and increases the subsequent oxidation of LDL particles.[4] More importantly, a recent randomized study has shown that coronary artery endothelial dysfunction in patients with hypercholesterolemia can be significantly improved by a combination of LDL-lowering and antioxidant therapy.[5] Others forms of endothelial injury such as those that can be induced by advanced glycosilated end-products in diabetes (particularly insulin dependent), chemical irritants in tobacco smoke, circulating vasoactive amines, immunocomplexes, and certain viral infections may potentiate chronic endothelial injury favoring further accumulation of lipids and monocytes into the intima.

In addition to biochemical injury, biomechanical forces are involved in the process of atherogenesis by determining the location where lesions form earlier and more rapidly than elsewhere. Endothelial dysfunction appears to occur first at sites of decreased shear, where there are back currents and eddy currents, such as at branches and bifurcations in the arterial tree.[6] It has been shown that endothelial cells undergo morphological alterations in response to change in the degree and orientation of shear forces. Elongated endothelial cells are located in regions of high shear stress, whereas poligonal endothelial cells are located in low shear stress regions [7], and these alterations may contribute to change endothelial cell permeability for atherogenic lipoprotein particles.

Lipid accumulation into the vessel wall

The peculiar properties of atherosclerotic intima that lead to accumulation of lipids have not been identified. Most lipids deposited in atherosclerotic lesions are derived from plasma LDL. The LDL receptor, discovered by Goldstein and Brown [8], tightly regulates the cholesterol content of cells. Under normal conditions, vascular cells cannot increase their cholesterol content beyond a certain point even in the presence of very high concentration of native LDL in the medium. However, it has been shown that chemical acetylation of LDL modified it to a form that is taken up rapidly by macrophages via a specific, saturable receptor -the acetyl LDL receptor or scavenger receptor-.[9] Unlike the LDL receptor, this receptor did not down-regulate when the cholesterol content of the cell increased. Later, it was shown that any of the major cell types characterizing an atherosclerotic lesion -endothelial cells, smooth muscle cells, and monocyte/macrophages- could carry out LDL modification and, interestingly, this modification could be strongly inhibited by the addition of antioxidants to the medium.[10] Altough, to this day, we cannot describe with great detail the conditions in which LDL undergoes oxidative modification in

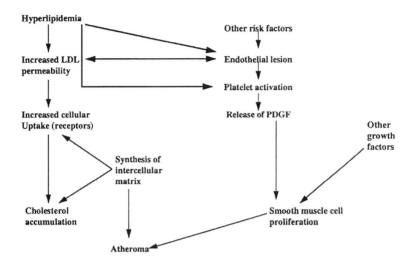

Figure 1.1 Multifactorial theory on the origin of atherosclerosis

vivo, we are sure that oxidative modification of LDL particles play a major role in the pathogenesis of lipid accumulation into atherosclerotic vessel wall. In addition, recent observation have shown that lipids may also accumulate gradually in the extracellular matrix of the deep intima as a result of direct binding between insudating LDL and specific glycosaminoglycans related to chondroitin sulfate [11], collagen, and/or fibrinogen.[12]

Monocyte recruitment and macrophage formation

It is likely that the focal accumulation of monocytes/macrophages in atherogenesis involves the local expression of specific adhesive glycoproteins on the endothelial surface and the generation of chemotactic factors by altered endothelium, its adherent leukocytes, and possibly underlying smooth muscle cells. Oxidized LDL may have an initial role in monocyte recruitment by inducing the expresion of adhesive cell-surface glycoproteins in the endothelium, the most important being E-Selectin, VCAM-1 (athero-ELAM), ICAM-1 and a recently characterized leukocyte-binding molecule.[1,13,14] Later on, several specific molecules may be relevant in attracting monocytes to the subendothelial space, such as specific chemotacting protein synthetized by vascular cells (monocyte chemotactic protein-1, MCP-1), colony stimulating factors (CSFs) and transforming growth factor- β(TGF-β). In more advanced stages, during which there is significant connective tissue production and tissue necrosis, peptides fragments from fibrin, fibronectin, elastin, collagen degradation, and thrombin may be the predominat monocyte chemoattractans elaborated. After entering the vessel wall, monocytes undergo a remarkable series of changes in their biological properties to become tissue macrophages. Among various receptors expressed by cultured macrophages, the acetyl-LDL or scavenger receptor increases dramatically being responsible for much of the uptake of lipoprotein that converts the macrophage into a foam cell. Such lipid-laden cells constitute the hallmark component of fatty streaks, the initiate visible phase of atherosclerotic lesions. It has been shown that some of the lipid-laden cells in fatty streaks are derived from smooth muscle cells, but the number of such cells is small compared to the number of macrophages-derived foam cells. Certainly, smooth muscle cells play their major role in the progression of atherosclerotic lesions by their replication and synthesis of connective tissue matrix as we discuss below.

Smooth muscle cell proliferation

The only actual evidence that smooth muscle proliferation occurs in atherosclerotic plaques depends on evidence that the lesions are monoclonal or oligoclonal. Monoclonality implies that smooth muscle cell proliferation must occur during the formation of the lesion and that the initial group of cells giving rise to the lesion must be very small.[15] It is uncertain if smooth muscle cell replication occurs at a very low rate over several years or replication occurs at a high rate in an episodic fashion. Moreover, plaque smooth muscle cells, at least in vitro, have a very high rate of spontaneous cell death, and this high levels of apoptosis may account for the apparent short replicative life span of these cells suggesting that plaque cells undergone some as-yet-undefined injury in vivo.[16] The smooth muscle proliferative response depens on a series of complex signals based upon cellular interaction in the local microenvironment of the artery. Several growth-regulatory molecules may play critical roles in this process, including platelet-derived growth factor (PDGF), TGF-β, fibroblast growth factor (FGF), tumor necrosis factor alfa (TNF-α), interleukines-1 and -2 (IL-1. IL-2), oxidized LDL, and thrombin. Interestingly, recent lineage studies of vascular smooth muscle origins in the avian and mammalian embryo have shown that the tunica media of large elastic arteries is composed of cells arising differently from the ectoderm and mesoderm embryonic lineages.[17] These two smooth muscle cell populations may respond differently to local stimuli for growth and morphogenesis, adaptive remodeling, repair of arterial injury and vascular disease later in life. The finding that smooth muscle cells in different vessels (aorta, coronary artery, femoral artery) are derived from different lineages in development may suggest a basis for vessel type-specific differences in rates of primary atherosclerotic lesion formation.[17]

Extracellular matrix synthesis

"Modulation" from a contractile to a synthetic phenotype of smooth muscle cells into the subendothelial space has been stablished as a key event in the evolution of atherosclerosis. The term synthetic is used because cultured cells lose much of their microfilaments and, as seen by transmission electron microscopy, acquire an exten-

sive rough endoplasmic reticulum. The synthetic phenotype of smooth muscle cells are capable of expressing genes for a number of growth-regulatory molecule and cytokine receptors, and they can response to those mediators by proliferation and synthesis of extracellular matrix.[1] Extracellular matrix is made up of collagen, elastin, and proteglycans. Both chemical and mechanical factors stimulate smooth muscle cells to make connective tissue. TGF-β is one of the most potent chemical factors involved in matrix formation [18], and chronic pulsatile distension in the arterial wall also favors the synthesis of collagen by smooth muscle cells.[19] Interestingly, accelerated smooth muscle cell proliferation and matrix synthesis driven by superficial inflamation, endothelial denudation, platelet adhesion/degranulation, thrombin generation, and other blood-derived growth factors, has been related to episodic atherosclerotic plaque growth.[20]

Lipid-rich core formation

If excess influx of lipids predominates over its efflux and over the proliferative response, the atherosclerotic process progresses into the more clinically relevant lipid-rich core formation. The atheromatous core within a plaque is devoid of supporting collagen, avascular, hypocellular (except at the periphery of the core), rich in extracellular lipids, and soft like gruel.[21] The relative contribution of direct lipids trapping versus foam cell necrosis in the formation of the atheromatous core and its growth is unknown. Foam cell necrosis has been widely belived to be more important, and the soft lipid-rich core within a plaque is also called a "necrotic core" and "atheronecrosis".[22] However, recent observations suggest that the core does not originate primarily from dead foam cells in the superficial intima (fatty streaks) but rathers arises from lipids accumulating gradually in the extracellular matrix of the deep intima as a result of complex binding between insudating LDL and glycosaminoglycans, collagen, and/or fibrinogen.[12,23] Characteristically, initial deposits of extracellular cholesterol esters are water insoluble and form an oil-lipid crystalline phase; however, as lesions progress, additional extracellular accumulation of free cholesterol results in the formation of cholesterol crystals into the lipid core.[21,24]

Mature atherosclerotic plaque evolution

As the name atherosclerosis implies, mature plaques tipically consist of two main componets: soft, lipid-rich atheromatous "gruel" and hard, collagen-rich sclerotic tissue. The sclerotic component (fibrous tissue) usually is by far the more voluminous component of the plaque, constituting >70% of an average stenotic coronary plaque.[25] Sclerosis, however is relatively innocuous because fibrous tissue appears to stabilize plaques, protecting them against disruption.[24] In contrast, the ususally less voluminous atheromatous component is the more dangerous component, because the soft atheromatous gruel destabilizes plaques, making them vulnerable to rupture, whereby the highly thrombogenic gruel is exposed to the flowing blood, leading to thrombosis, a potentially life-threatening event.[24,26]

Dramatic differences in the incidence, composition, and severity of primary atherosclerotic lesions are commonly found in different vessel of the same individual or in different segments of the same vessel. Atherogenic risk factors correlate with the coronary plaque burden (extent of plaquing) found at autopsy[27], but apart from an increase in calcification with age and possibly male sex [28] , a relation of specific risk factors to segment-specific differences in lesion susceptibility within the artery remains to be identified.

Unstable plaque evolution

Mature plaques containing a soft atheromatous core are unstable and may rupture; i.e. the fibrous cap separating the core from the lumen may disintegrate, tear, or break, whereby the highly thrombogenic gruel is suddenly exposed to the flowing blood.[24,26,29] The risk of plaque disruption is related to intrinsic properties of individual plaques (their vulnerability) and extrinsic forces acting on plaques (rupture triggers). The former predispose plaques to rupture, whereas the latter may precipitate disruption if vulnerable plaques are present.

Plaque vulnerability to rupture

Plaque vulnerability to rupture depens mainly on: size and consistency of the atheromatous core, thickness and collagen content of the fibrous cap, inflammation within the fibrous cap, and cap "fatigue".

Postmortem studies of infarct-related arteries have shown larger atheromatous cores in segments with plaque disruption than in segments with intact surface[30] , and computer modeling analysis of tensile stress across the vessel wall has shown high concentrations of stress at the ends of plaque caps overlaying an area of lipid pool, particularly if lipid pool exceeds ´45% of the vessel wall circumference[31]. In addition, the consistency (composition) of the gruel may be also important for stability. Cholesterol esters soften plaques whereas crystalline cholesterol has the opposite effect.[32] On the basis of animal experiments, lipid-lowering therapy in humans is expected to deplete plaque lipid, with an overall reduction in cholesteryl esters (liquid and mobile) and a relative increase in crystalline cholesterol (solid and inert), theoretically resulting in a stiffer and more stable atheromatous core.[32,33] Cap thickness and collagen content are also important. Compared with intact caps, ruptured ones contain less collagen and their tensile stress is reduced [25]. Furthermore, the site of ruptured atherosclerotic plaques is usually heavily infiltrated by macrophages and T cells, suggesting that a localized inflammatory process contributes to instability and rupture [34]. Macrophage-derived foam cells may release toxic products (free radicals and products of lipid oxidation) and proteolytic enzymes (metalloproteinases) leading to degradation of the connective tissue matrix and thinning of the fibrous cap overlying the lipid core.[35] Experiments showing an increase in collagen breakdown when monocyte-derived macrophage are incubated with human atherosclerotic plaques, clearly indicate that macrophages could be responsible for plaque disruption.[36] In addition, mast cells, a powerful neutral protease-containing effector cell, have been also localized at the shoulder regions of the atheromatous plaques suggesting that they may also play a part in triggering matrix degradation and ensuing rupture of coronary plaques.[37] Finally, in the coronary tree, marked oscillations in shear stress, acute change in coronary pressure or tone, and bending and twisting of an artery during each heart contraction may fatigue and weaken a fibrous cap that ultimately may rupture spontaneously, ie, unprovoked or untriggered.[38]

Triggers of plaque rupture

Coronary plaques are constantly stressed by a variety of mechanical and hemodynamic forces that may precipitate or trigger disruption of vulnerable plaques.[38,39] According to Laplace's law, the higher the blood pressure and the larger the luminal diameter, the more tension (tensile stress) develops in the wall.[39] If components within the wall (sof gruel, for example) are unable to bear the imposed load, the stress is redistributed to adjacent structures (fibrous cap over gruel, for example), where it may be concentrated at critical points.[40] The consistency of the gruel may be important for this stress redistribution because the stiffer the gruel, the more stress it can bear, and correspondingly less stress is redistributed to the adjacent fibrous cap.[40] Theoretically, the tension created in fibrous caps of mildly or moderately stenotic plaques may be greater than that created in caps of severely stenotic plaques (smaller lumen) with the same cap thickness and exposed to the same blood pressure. Consequently, mildly or moderately stenostic plaques are generally stressed more than severely stenotic plaques and could therefore be more prone to rupture. However, high grade stenoses may also be subjected to strong compressive forces due to the accelerated velocities in the throat. The local Bernoulli's static pressure in the throat of the stenosis may become less than the external surrounding pressure of the artery, causing a negative transmural pressure around the stenotic region.[41] Colapse of severe but compliant stenoses due to negative transmural pressures may produce highly concentrated compressive stresses from buckling of the wall with bending deformation, preferentially involving plaque edges, and theoretically, this could contribute to plaque disruption.[41] Finally, circumferential bending may also contribute to plaque rupture. For normal compliant arteries, the cyclic diastolic-systolic change in lumen diameter is about 10%, but it becomes smaller with age and during atherogenesis because of the increased in stiffness.[42] Eccentric plaques typically bends at their edges , ie, at the junction between the stiff plaque and the more compliant plaque-free vessel wall. Cyclic bending may, in the long-term, weaken these points, leading to unprovoked "spontaneous" fatigue disruption, whereas a sudden acentuated bending may trigger rupture of a weakened cap.

Thrombotic response

Probably, most ruptured plaques are resealed by a small mural thrombus which becomes organized contributing to an episodic, clinically silent, growth of the lesion.[43] However, when thrombi are large, they can impair coronary blood flow leading to acute syndromes of myocardial ischemia.[29,43] It is likely that many variables determine whether a ruptured plaque proceeds rapidly to an occlusive thrombus or persists as a mural non-oclussive thrombus. Local factors such as quantity (fissure size) and quality of thrombogenic substrate exposed after plaque rupture (plaque composition), and rheology of blood flow at the site of rupture together with systemic factors inducing hypercoagulable or thrombogenic states [chatecolamines, lipoprotein(a), fibrinolytic system] may modulate thrombosis at the time of plaque rupture.

Experimentally, the thrombotic response is influenced by the various components of the atherosclerotic plaque exposed following rupture. Exposure of macrophage-rich or collagen-rich matrix, which might be present in small plaque fissures, is associated with less platelet deposition than that seen after exposure of the lipid-rich core of the plaque.[26] Consequently, atheromatous plaques containing lipid-rich "gruel" are not only the most vulnerable plaque to rupture, they are also the most thrombogenic when their content is exposed to flowing blood after rupture. The component(s) responsible for such high thrombogenicity found in the gruel is unknown. Tissue factor protein (derived from disintegrated macrophages?) has been identified immunohistochemically in a scattered pattern within the atheromatous core of human carotid plaques.[44] The time course for the appearance of tissue factor in plaque is not known. Tissue factor mRNA expression and tissue factor activity have been shown to be elevated after balloon injury in rats, implying that a procoagulant response is part of the proliferative response of the vessel wall to injury.[45]

Acute thrombotic response to plaque disruption depends also in part on the degree of stenosis and sudden geometric changes following the rupture. High shear rates at the site of a significant stenosis will predispose to increased platelet and fibrin(ogen) deposition by forcing both to the periphery where they may be deposited at the site of plaque rupture.[46] A small geometric change with only mild stenosis may result in a small mural thrombus, whereas a larger geometric change with severe stenosis may result in a transient or persistent thrombotic occlusion. Furthermore, the disruption of a plaque at the apex of an stenosis may result in a thrombus that is richer in platelets and, therefore, less amenable to fibrinolytic agents than a thrombus formed in a zone distal to the apex.

Besides local factors, clinical and experimental evidence have suggested that systemic factors inducing a primary hypercoagulable or thrombogenic state may be responsible for formation of a large thrombus after plaque disruption. Platelet activation and the generation of thrombin may be enhanced by high levels of sympathetic activity, hypercholesterolemia, increased level of Lp(a), and other metabolic abnormalities, such as diabetes mellitus.[29,43] Hemostatic proteins, specifically fibrinogen and factor VII, have been also implicated as major thrombogenic risk factors. Several prospective studies have shown a high plasma fibrinogen concentration to be highly significant independent risk factor for coronary artery disease, specifically associated with myocardial infarction.[47] High levels of factor VII coag-

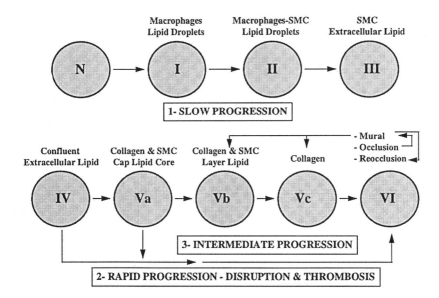

Figure 1.2 *Evolution of coronary atherosclerosis*

ulant activity are also associated with an increased risk of coronary events.[47] Both proteins are elevated in relation to age, obesity, hyperlipidemia, diabetes, smoking and emotional stress [48], thus they may also explain partially the effect of other risk factors associated with the disease.

Stable plaque evolution

Alternatively to plaque rupture and thrombus formation, if at early stages of atherosclerotic plaque evolution, smooth muscle cell proliferation and extracellular matrix synthesis predominates over lipid and macrophage accumulation into the vessel wall, lesions may grow giving rise to an advanced sclerotic plaque.[49] Such lesions consist entirely or almost entirely of scar collagen, and lipid may have regressed or it may never have been in the lesion. Collagen formation is the major contributor to the volume of atherosclerotic plaques, and collagen-rich lesions constitute frequently the pathophysiologic basis for stable coronary syndromes. Interestingly, human vessels can undergo massive accumulations of atherosclerotic mass without lumen narrowing. The vessel compensates for the new mass by undergoing a compensatory redistribution of vessel wall mass so that lumen size is maintained.[50] This remodeling permits a normal level of blood flow until an adaptational limit is exceeded. This limit appears to occur when approximately 40% or more of the area bounded by the external elastic lamina is occupied by atherosclerotic mass.

Clinical consequences of coronary plaque evolution

Clinical ischemic consequences of coronary lesions depend on many factors such as the degree and acuteness of blood flow obstruction, the duration of decreased perfusion and the relative myocardial oxygen demand at the time of blood flow obstruction. Plaque disruption by itself is asymptomatic, and the associated rapid plaque growth is usually clinically silent. Autopsy data indicate that 9% of "normal" healthy persons have asymptomatic disrupted plaques in their coronary arteries, increasing to 22% in persons with diabetes or hypertension.[51] Ischemic syndromes may develop if a lesion ruptures inducing significant intraluminal thrombus formation (unstable lesions) or if a lesion directly provokes a significant narrowing of the arterial lumen (stable lesions).

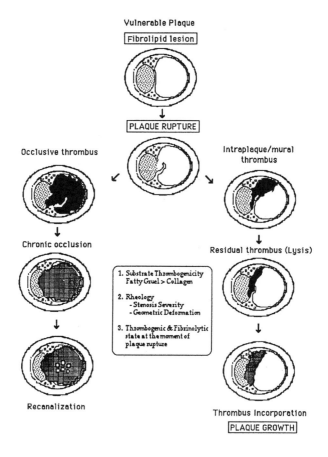

Figure 1.3 The fate of the "vulnerable" plaque.

Unstable coronary syndromes

In unstable angina, a relatively small fissuring or disruption of an atherosclerotic plaque may lead to an acute change in plaque structure and a reduction in coronary blood flow, resulting in exacerbation of angina. Transient episodes of thrombotic vessel occlusion at the site of plaque rupture may occur, leading to angina at rest. This thrombus is usually labile and results in temporary vascular occlusion, perhaps lasting only 10-20 min. In addition, vasoconstriction may contribute to a reduction in coronary flow. In non-Q wave infarction, more severe plaque damage would result in more persistent thrombotic occlusion, perhaps lasting up to 1 hour. About one fourth of patients with non-Q wave infarction may have an infarct-related vessel occluded for more than one hour, but the distal myocardial territory is usually supplied by collaterals. In Q wave infarction, larger plaque fissures may result in the formation of a large, fixed and persistent thrombus. This leads to an abrupt cessation of myocardial perfusion for more than 1 hour resulting in transmural necrosis of the involved myocardium. The coronary lesion responsible for the infarction is frequently only mildly to moderately stenotic, wich supports that plaque rupture with superimposed thrombus rather than the severity of the lesion is the primary determinat of acute occlusion. For out-of-hospital cardiac arrest or sudden death, the lesion responsible is often similar to that of unstable angina: a disrupted plaque with superimposed nonocclusive thrombosis.

In summary, the natural history of acute coronary syndromes probably mirrors that of the underlying plaque rupture and thrombus formation. Stabilization would correspond to resealing of a rupture, accentuation of symptoms to development of labile thrombosis, non-Q wave infarction to development of transient occlusion, and transmural Q-wave infarction to establishment of a persistent occlusive thrombus. Furthermore, this natural history may be modified by vascular tone and presence of collateral circulation.

Stable coronary syndromes

In patients with stable angina, mature atherosclerotic lesions consisting either on advanced fibrolipid plaques (60%) or predominantly pure fibrotic lesions (40%) may lead to a significant coronary blood flow obstruction (usually more than 75% cross-sectional area luminal narrowing equivalent to 50% diameter reduction). There is usually no plaque ulceration or thrombosis, however, intraplaque hemorrhage and rest from thrombus organization may be observed. Generally, the pattern of angina does not correlate with the extent or severity of the atherosclerotic disease. Mild or infrequent angina does not imply mild or insignificant disease. At the present time it appears that prognosis in stable angina is most accurately predicted by the number and severity of indivudual obstructions of the three major coronary arteries and by left ventricular function.

Atherosclerotic plaque stabilization and regression

In approaching the concept of reversibility or arrest of the coronary atherosclerotic process, it is esential to keep in mind that atherosclerosis disease starts at a young age and takes many years to progress into the symptomatic stage. By the time the first symptoms of coronary atherosclerosis appear, the disease is usualy advanced to two- or three-vessel involvement. Overall, the term "nonsignificant" when applied to atherosclerotic lesions with less than 50% luminal stenosis at coronary angiography may be often misleading and should be revisited. It is now quite evident that a fissure may develope in an atherosclerotic plaque that occupies less than 50% of the diameter of a coronary artery and such plaque may become a nidus for thombosis. Although angiography is helpful as a determinant of the severity of coronary disease, and the number of diseased vessels are known markers of cardiac morbidity and mortality, it cannot accurately predict the site of future coronary occlusion. Overall, angiography may understimate the extent and severity of atherosclerotic involvement of coronary arteries. It is of value to consider, however, that the more severe the coronary disease is at angiography, the higher is the likelihood of the presence of small plaques prone to disruption. This highlights the need for a practical method to identify vulnerable lesions before the first symptoms appear. In this field, noninvasive imaging of plaques with a high content of lipids is emerging as an important research tool, given the susceptibility of these plaques to rupture. In addition to intravascular ultrasound and coronary angioscopy, it may soon be possible to detect fatty plaques within the vascular system by high-resolution biochemical imaging techniques such as nuclear magnetic resonance.[52,53] Once vulnerable plaque is identified, approaches may be taken toward retardation in the progression or even reversibility of plaque, reduction in the susceptibility of plaque rupture, and/or prevention of thrombosis after plaque rupture.

Approaches that has been taken toward retardation or even reversibility of atherosclerotic lesions include: better control of atherogenic risk factors, specially by reducing plasma cholesterol levels; enhancement of lipid-removal pathways from the vessel wall, particularly by increasing plasma HDL levels; and reduction of LDL oxidation by using antioxidant agents. Each of these approaches, by acting on the lipid-rich plaque more prone to rupture, might prevent progression and even induce removal of fat and regression of atherosclerotic plaques. However, the clinical improvement seen with cholesterol lowering therapy seems to be disproportionate to the small degree of anatomical regression of atherosclerotic stenoses that can be achieved by these therapies.[54,55] It is likely that in plaques with large cholesterol pools, the resortion of cholesterol may diminish the propensity of the plaque to rupture, and an increase in the relative collagen content of the plaque may account for increasing plaque stability without significant reduction in plaque size.

Other approaches, besides hypolipidemic therapy, that may possibly reduce the incidence of plaque rupture include angiotensin-converting enzyme inhibitors and beta-blockers. Recent evidence from three large placebo-controlled trials of angiotensin-converting enzyme inhibitors in patients with ischemic heart disease and/or mild left ventricular dysfunction points to a reduction of 14% to 28% in the incidence of myocardial infarction and other ischemic cardiac events.[56-58] The mechanism of such reduction in infarction is uncertain. Experimentally, angiotensin-converting enzyme inhibitors have shown to reduce intimal hyperplasia following endothelial injury, however there is no convincing clinical evidence that the prevention of infarction by these agents could be related to the prevention of preceding atherogenesis. Alternatively, enhanced fibrinolysis by angiotensin-converting enzyme inhibitors [59], and microcirculatory vasodilating properties of these agents [60] may be the clue to the benefit of these agents in preventing myocardial infarction. Meta-analysis of secondary prevention trials with β-blockers has shown a 20% reduction in cardiac mortality, an additional 25% reduction in the incidence of reinfarction and a 30% reduction in the incidence of sudden death.[61] β-blockers reduce the circumferential plaque stress, and therefore the possibility of plaque rupture, by reducing blood pressure and blunting hypertensive pressure surges, and may also, by reducing heart rate, increase plaque tensile strength.

Because thrombus formation appears to be an important factor in the progression of atherosclerotic lesions and in the conversion of chronic to acute events after plaque rupture, a promising approach in the prevention of this process would be the use of antithrombotic therapy. The most beneficial effect of antiplatelet and anticoagulant agents has been observed in the prevention of acute coronary syndromes. Aspirin has shown to be effective in unstable angina and acute myocardial infarction, during and after coronary revascularization, in the secondary prevention of chronic coronary and cerebrovascular disease, and in primary prevention particularly in high-risk groups [62]. Combination therapy with low doses of aspirin and anticoagualnt agents may have additive effect. The rationale behind this combination is to block to some extent both platelet activation and the generation of thrombin by the intrinsic and extrinsinc coagulation systems. The hope is to achieve this objective without enhancing bleeding. Finally, newer antithrombotic approaches which act directly by blocking the platelet membrane receptor glycoprotein IIb/IIIa, or by direct inhibition of thrombin, are under active clinical investigation. The monoclonal antibody 7E3 is currently the most advanced antiglycoprotein IIb/IIIa agent in clinical development. It has been preliminary tested in patients with unstable angina and postfibrinolysis in acute myocardial infarction with very promising results.[63,64] Specific thrombin inhibitors, such as hirudin, a 65-residue polypeptide derived from the salivary gland of the medicinal leech, and now available by recombinant laboratory synthesis, have some adventages over heparin in patients with unstable angina and acute myocardial infarction. However, the increased risk of bleeding associated with these new antithrombotic strategies remains a concern.[65]

REFERENCES

1. Ross R. The pathogenesis of atherosclerosis: a perspective for the 1990s. Nature 1993:362:801.

2. Seiler C, et al. Influence of serum cholesterol and other coronary risk factors on vasomotion of angiographically normal coronary arteries. Circulation, 1993: 88:2139.

3. Mangin EL Jr, et al. Effects of lysolipids and oxidatively modified low density lipoprotein on endothelium-dependent relaxation of rabbit aorta. Cir Res, 1993: 72:161.

4. Ohara Y, Peterson TE, Harrison DG: Hypercholesterolemia increases endothelial superoxide anion production. J Clin Invest, 1993: 91:2546.

5. Anderson TJ, et al. The effect of cholesterol-lowering and antioxidant therapy on endothelium-dependent coronary vasomotion. N Eng J Med, 1995: 332:488.

6. Gibson CM, et al. Relation of vessel wall shear stress to atherosclerosis progression in human coronary arteries. Atherosc Thromb, 1993: 13:310.

7. Levesque MJ, et al. Correlation of endothelial cell shape and wall shear stress in a stenosed dog aorta. Arteriosclerosis, 1986: 6:220.

8. Goldstein JL, Brown MS: The low density lipoprotein pathway and its relation to atherosclerosis. Annu Rev Biochem, 1977 46:897.

9. Goldstein JL, et al. Binding site on macrophages that mediates uptake and degradation of acetylated low density lipoprotein, producing massive cholesterol deposition. Proc Natl Acad Sci USA, 1979: 76:333.

10. Steinbrecher UP, et al. Modification of low density lipoprotein by endothelial cells involves lipid peroxidation and degradation of low density lipoprotein phospholipids. Proc Natl Acad Sci USA, 1984: 83:3883.

11. Camejo G, et al. Identification of apoB-100 segments mediating the interaction of low-density lipoproteins with arterial proteoglycans. Arteriosclerosis, 1988: 8:368.

12. Guyton JR, Klemp KF. Development of the atherosclerotic core region: chemical and ultrastructural analysis of microdissected atherosclerotic lesions from human aorta. Arterioscler Thromb, 1994: 14:1305.

13. Valente AJ, et al. Mechanism in intimal monocyte-macrophage recruitment. a special role for monocyte chemotactic protein-1. Circulation, 1992: 86:III20.

14. Kim JA, et al. Partial characterization of leukocyte binding molecules on endothelial cells induced by minimally oxidized LDL. Arterio Thromb, 1994: 24:427.

15. Schwartz SM, deBlois D, O'Brien ERM. The intima: soil for atherosclerosis and restenosis. Circulation Res, 1995: 77:445.

16. Bennett MR, Evan GI, Schwartz SM. Apoptosis of human vascualr smooth muscle cells derived fron normal vessels and coronary atherosclerotic plaques. J Clin Invest, 1995: 95:2266.

17. Majesky MW. Smooth muscle cell subtypes: a lineage model. Restenosis Summit VII. The Cleveland Clinic Fundation, 1995 :176.

18. Sporn MB, et al. Some recent advances in the chemistry and biology of transforming growth factor-beta. J Cell Biol, 1987: 105:1039.

19. Ross R: Atherosclerosis: a problem of the biology of the arterial wall cells and their interactions with blood components. Atherosclerosis, 1981: 1:293.

20. Flugelman MY, et al. Smooth muscle cell abundance and fibroblast growth factors in coronary lesions of patients with nonfatal unstable angina: a clue to the mechanism of transformation from the stable to the unstable clinical state. Circulation, 1993: 88:2493.

21. Lundberg B. Chemical composition and physical state of lipids deposits in atherosclerosis. Atherosclerosis, 1985: 56:93.

22. Witztum JL. The oxidation hypothesis in atherosclerosis. Lancet, 1994; 344:793.

23. Wight TN. The cell biology of arterial proteoglycans. Arteriosclerosis, 1989: 9:1.

24. Falk E, Shah PK, Fuster V. Coronary plaque disruption. Circulation, 1995:; 92:657.

25. Kragel AH, et al. Morphometric analysis of the composition of atherosclerotic plaques in the four major epicardial coronaries in acute myocardial infarction and sudden coronary death. Circulation, 1989: 80:1747.

26. Fernández-Ortiz A, et al. Characterization of the relative thrombogenicity of atherosclerotic plaque components: Implications for consequences of plaque rupture. J Am Coll Cardiol,

1994: 23:1562.

27. Pathobiological Determinants of Atherosclerosis in Youth (PDAY) Research Group. Natural history of aortic and coronary atherosclerotic lesions in youth: findings from the PDAY study. Arterioscler Thromb, 1993: 13:1291.

28. Devries S, et al. Influence of age and gender on the presence of coronary calcium detected by ultrafast computed tomography. J Am Coll Cardiol, 1995:; 25:76.

29. Fuster V. Lewis A Conner Memorial Lecture. Mechanisms leading to myocardial infarction: Insights from studies of vascular biology. Circulation, 1994: 90:2126.

30. Gertz SD, Roberts WC. Hemodynamic shear force in rupture of coronary arterial atherosclerotic plaques. Am J Cardiol, 1990: 66:1368.

31. Richardson RD, Davies MJ, Born GVR: Influence of plaque configuration and stress distribution on fissuring of coronary atherosclerotic plaques. Lancet, 1989:; 2:941.

32. Small DM. Progression and regression of atherosclerotic lesions: insights from lipid physical biochemistry. Arteriosclerosis, 1988: 8:103.

33. Loree HM, et al. Mechanical properties of model atherosclerotic lesion lipid pools. Arterioscler Thromb, 1994: 14:230.

34. van der Wall AC, et al. Site of intimal rupture or erosion of thrombosed coronary atherosclerotic plaques is characterized by an inflammatory process irrespective of the dominant plaque morphology, Circulation, 1994: 89:36.

35. Galis ZS, et al. Increased expression of matrix metalloproteinases and matrix degrading activity in vulnerable regions of human atherosclerotic plaques. J Clin Invest, 1994: 94:2493.

36. Shah PK, et al. Human monocyte-derived macrophages induce collagen breakdown in fibrous caps of atherosclerotic plaques. Potential role of metrix-degrading metalloproteinases and implications fros plaque rupture. Circulation, 1995: 92:1565.

37. Kaartinen M, Penttild A, Kovanen PT. Accumulation of activated mast cells in the shoulder region of human coronary atheroma, the predilection site of atheromatous rupture. Circulation, 1994: 90:1669.

38. MacIsaac AI, Thomas JD, Topol EJ. Toward the quiescent coronary plaque. J Am Coll Cardiol, 1993: 22:1228.

39. Lee RT, Kamm RD. Vascular mechanism for the cardiologist. J Am Coll Cradiol, 1994: 23:1289.

40. Richardson RD, Davies MJ, Born GVR. Influence of plaque configuration and stress distribution on fissuring of coronary atherosclerotic plaques. Lancet, 1989: 2:941.

41. Aoki T, Ku DN. Collapse of diseased arteries with eccentric cross section. J Biomech, 1993:26:133.

42. Alfonso F, et al. Determinats of coronary compliance in patients with coronary artery disease: an intravascular ultrasound study. J Am Coll Cardiol, 1994: 23:879.

43. Fuster V, et al. The pathogenesis of coronary artery disease and the acute coronary syndromes (part I and II). N Eng J Med, 1992: 326:242 and 310.

44. Wilcox JN. Thrombotic mechanisms in atherosclerosis. Cor Art Dis, 1994: 5:223.

45. Taubman MB. Tissue factor regulation in vascualr smooth muscle: a summary of studies performed using in vivo and in vitro models. Am J Cardiol, 1993: 72:55C.

46. Mailhac A, et al. Effect of an eccentric severe stenosis on fibri(ogen) deposition on severily damaged vessel wall in arterial thrombosis. Relative contribution of fibri(ogen) and platelets. Circulation, 1994: 90:988.

47. Meade TW, et al. Haemostatic function and cardiovascular death: early results of a prospective study. Lancet, 1980: 1:1050.

48. Rosengren A, et al. Social influences and cardiovascular risk factor as determinat of plasma fibrinogen concentration in a general population sample of middle age men. BMJ, 1990: 330:634.

49. Stary HC. Composition and classification of human atherosclerotic lesions. Virchows Archiv A Pathol Anat, 1992: 421:277.

50. Glagov S. Compensatory enlargement of human atherosclerotic coronary arteries. N Eng J Med, 1987: 316:1371.

51. Davies MJ, et al. Factors influencing the presence or absence of acute coronary artery thrombi in sudden ischaemic death. Eur Heart J, 1989: 10:203.

52. Merickel MB, et al. Noninvasive quantitative evaluation of atherosclerotic using MRI and image analysis. Arterioscler Thromb, 1993: 13:1180.

53. Toussaint JF, et al. 13C-NMR spectroscopy of human atherosclerotic lesions: relation between fatty acid saturation, cholesteryl ester content, and luminal obstruction. Arterioscler Thromb, 1994: 14:1951.

54. Brown BG, et al. Lipid lowering and plaque regression: new insights into prevention of plaque disruption and clinical events in coronary disease. Circulation, 1993: 87:1781.

55. Scandinavian Simvastatin Survival Study Group. Randomized trial of cholesterol lowering in 4444 patients with coronary artery disease: the Scandinavian Simvastatin Survival Study (4S). Lancet, 1994: 344:1383.

56. Pfeffer MA, et al. Effect of captopril on mortality and morbidity in patients with left ventricular dysfunction after myocardial infarction: results of the Survival and Ventricular Enlargment Trial. N Eng J Med, 1992: 327:669.

57. The SOLVD investigators. Effect of enalapril on survival in patients with reduced left ventricular ejection fractios and congestive heart failure. N Eng J Med, 1991: 325:293.

58. The SOLVD investigators. Effects of enalapril on mortality and the development of heart failure in asymptomatic patients with reduced left ventricular ejection fractions. N Eng J Med, 1992: 327:685.

59. Wright RA, et al. Effects of captopril therapy on endogenous fibrinolysis in men with recent uncomplicated myocartdial infarction. J Am Coll Cardiol, 1994: 24:67.

60. Reddy KG, et al. Evidence that selective endothelial dysfunction may occur in the absence of angiographic or ultrasound atherosclerosis in patients with risk factors for atherosclerosis. J Am Coll Cardiol, 1994: 23:833.

61. Yusuf S, et al. Beta blockade during and after myocardial infarction: an overview of the randomized trials. Prog Cardiovasc Dis, 1985: 27:335.

62. Fuster V, et al. Aspirin as a therapeutic agent in cardiovascular disease. Circulation, 1993: 87:659.

63. Simmons ML, et al. Randomized trial of a GPIIb/IIIa platelet receptor blocker in refractory unstable angina. Circulation, 1994: 89:596.

64. Kleiman NS, et al. Profound inhibition of platelet aggregation with monoclonal antibody 7E3Fab after thrombolytic therapy: results of the thrombolysis and angioplasty in myocardial infarction (TAMI) 8 pilot study. J Am Coll Cardiol, 1993: 22:381.

65. Antman EM, for the TIMI 9A Investigators: Hirudin in acute myocardial infarction. Safety report from the thrombolysis and thrombin inhibition in myocardial infarction (TIMI) 9A trial. Circulation, 1994: 90:1624.

2 SYNDROMES OF ACCELERATED ATHEROSCLEROSIS

Beat J. Meyer, Lina Badimon, James H. Chesebro

The development and progression of coronary artery disease depend on both incorporation of lipid and deposition of fibrin and platelets into the arterial wall, with subsequent growth of fibroblasts and smooth muscle cells, as recently reviewed.[1, 2] Lipid incorporation contributes to luminal narrowing and appears to predispose the vascular wall to vasoconstriction and injury and subsequent thrombus formation. Variable degrees of vascular injury and mural thrombosis lead to repeated subclinical and periodic acute events in the progression of atherosclerosis (*Figure 2.1*). Most of the arterial changes are subclinical without symptoms, but others are clinical and include the acute coronary syndromes of unstable angina, myocardial infarction, and sudden death.

Vascular injury

In a recent review[2] , a pathophysiologic classification of vascular injury of three different degrees has been proposed. Type I consists of functional alterations of endothelial cells without substantial morphologic changes; Type II injury is characterized by endothelial denudation; and Type III is characterized by endothelial denudation with damage to both the intima and the media.

In spontaneous atherosclerosis, the tenet is that chronic minimal injury to the arterial endothelium is caused mainly by a disturbance in the pattern of blood flow in certain parts of the arterial tree, such as bending points and areas near branching vessels.[3, 4] In experiments in animals, chronic mild endothelial injury may also be potentiated by hypercholesterolemia, circulating vasoactive amines, immunocomplexes, infection, and chemical irritants in tobacco smoke.[5] Local variability in endothelial susceptibility to these factors may be as important as flow disturbances in the localization of minimal endothelial injury and atherosclerosis. Such Type I

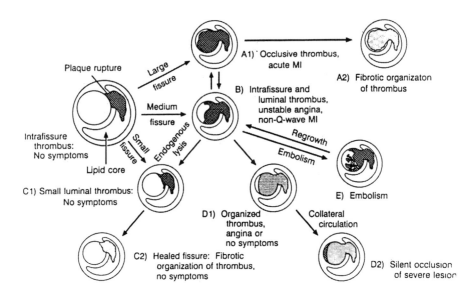

Figure 2.1 **Major pathogenic modes of progression of coronary disease.** *Plaque disruption leads to formation of a fissure with flowing blood contacting intra-arterial structures and forming an intrafissure thrombus. This may not progress or lead to symptoms (except for possible sudden onset of coronary spasm or vasoconstriction associated with arterial injury). The fissure may be small, medium, or large and may progress immediately to various degrees of luminal obstruction (A1,B, or C1). Sudden progression with a large fissure may be due to occlusive thrombus and acute myocardial infarction (MI), A1.*

Fibrotic organization of thrombus may occur (A2) or thrombolysis (exogenous or endogenous) may occur and reopen the lumen to partial obstruction (B). A medium-sized fissure may lead to immediate partial obstruction associated with unstable angina or non-Q-wave (MI) (B); this may progress to total occlusion (A1), partial embolization of thrombus (E), fibrotic organization of thrombus (D1), endogenous lysis to a small thrombus (C1), or no intraluminal thrombus. Residual thrombus may undergo fibrotic or fibromuscular organization (A2, C2, and D1). A severe residual stenosis (D1) may be associated with good collateral circulation and no symptoms. Because of very low antegrade flow and type II injury (endothelial denudation only) but no deep injury, this may silently occlude with a fresh thrombus (D2). A small fissure may lead to a small thrombus without symptoms (C1) and undergo fibrotic organization with progression of disease in the absence of symptoms (C2). With permission from reference 6.

injury enhances the accumulation of lipids and macrophages, which is the initial predominant feature at these sites.[1, 6]

Progressive lipid incorporation into the arterial wall and the release of toxic products by macrophages[7] presumably leads to Type II damage, characterized by the adhesion of platelets.[1, 2, 4, 8] Macrophages and platelets, together with the endothelium, may release various growth factors that lead to the simultaneous migration and proliferation of smooth muscle cells, a process that may contribute to the formation of a fibrotic layer (fibrous capsule) over the luminal side of the lipid core, and ultimately leading to the macroscopic appearance of a fibroatheromatous lesion (Stary, V).[6, 8]

Plaque disruption and thrombosis in rapid coronary disease progression

The processes of lipid accumulation, cell proliferation and extracellular matrix synthesis leading to the progression of coronary artery disease in humans is neither linear nor predictable.[9,10] Angiographic studies show that new high-grade lesions often appear in segments of artery that were normal at previous angiographic examination.[11] Two thirds of the lesions presumably responsible for acute ischemic events (unstable angina or myocardial infarction) have been previously only mildly to moderately stenotic.[10, 11] This rapid and episodic progression can be explained by the occurrence of plaque disruption with subsequent thrombosis and changes in plaque geometry and local rheology leading to intermittent plaque growth.[12]

A lipid lesion surrounded by a thin capsule can be easily disrupted, leading to Type III damage with thrombus formation.[2] Plaque disruption occurs when the strain within the fibrous cap exceeds the deformability of its component material.[13] However, plaque disruption may not always occur at the regions of highest stress, suggesting that local variations in plaque material properties such as thinning of the fibrous capsule with dissolution of collagen to a delicate latticework also contribute to plaque disruption.[14] The plaque disrupts into the arterial lumen (Type III injury), allowing flowing blood to contact deeper arterial structures. The thrombogenic substrates within the intimal plaque and the arterial media are similar and include collagen types I and III, release of tissue thromboplastin, loss of endothelium, decreased prostacyclin, and increased tissue factor, phospholipid from cell membranes of smooth muscle cells and platelets for formation of activator complexes within the coagulation cascade.[2, 15] However, we have recently demonstrated that exposure of the "lipid-rich" core of an atherosclerotic plaque is the most thrombogenic stimulus compared to fibromuscular or other types of plaques.[16]

Macroscopic, platelet-rich mural thrombus occurs with deep or type III arterial injury and covers the region of deep injury.[8, 17]

Platelet and fibrinogen deposition are thrombin dependent and occur within minutes of deep arterial injury.[18, 19] Thrombin is adsorbed to fibrin within thrombus by a binding site that is separate from its catalytic site. Thrombin bound to fibrin becomes internalized in the lesion as the plaque grows; this may also contribute to the thrombogenicity and proliferative activity of some ruptured atherosclerotic plaques.[15]

When thrombi are small they can become organized and contribute to the growth of the atherosclerotic plaque. When thrombi are large and occlusive, they can contribute to acute coronary syndromes such as unstable angina, myocardial infarction, and sudden ischemic death.[20] Ultimately, they become partly lysed or become organized to contribute to chronic fibrotic occlusion, *Figure 2.1.*[15]

Further evidence supporting the role of thrombus incorporation in plaque progression is provided by old and recent studies that used antibodies specifically directed to platelets, fibrin, fibrinogen, and their degradation products.[21-26] Thus, advanced and fibrous plaques, products related to platelets and fibrin were detected in the intima, the neointima, and even in the deeper medial layer, especially in areas of loose connective tissue.

In addition to arterial substrate, the rheology of blood flow is the other major contributor to mural thrombosis. Higher shear forces cause red cells to force platelets to the periphery of the artery. High shear and type III injury that anchors thrombus to the arterial wall increase platelet deposition. Platelet and fibrinogen deposition is maximal within the minimal luminal diameter of the stenosis.[27, 28] These factors increase the risk of occlusion and restenosis in inadequately dilated arteries after percutaneous transluminal coronary angioplasty and after thrombolysis when a high-grade residual stenosis remains.[15]

Systemic factors such as lipids, catecholamines, and lipoproteina also modulate thrombosis but appear to be less potent than thrombogenic substrates and rheology.[2]

An accelerated version of this atherogenic process appears to account for premature coronary disease in patients undergoing heart transplantation, saphenous-vein bypass grafting, or percutaneous transluminal coronary angioplasty. In contrast to the spontaneous atherosclerosis, an acute or subacute Type II or III vascular injury appears to the critical initiating event, followed by intense platelet adherence and thrombus formation, leading to the proliferation of smooth muscle cells and matrix formation. Thus, Type II injury may occur in a saphenous-vein graft in the first postoperative years as a result of the surgical manipulation and the change in intravascular pressure; it may also occur after heart transplantation as a result of immune and other types of injuries of the coronary arteries.[5] Type III injury may also follow coronary angioplasty, with mural thrombosis and subsequent proliferation of smooth muscle cells and fibrotic organization contributing to restenosis.

Restenosis following angioplasty

Percutaneous transluminal coronary angioplasty (PTCA) has become a successful and widely used treatment for patients with coronary disease, since its first clinical application by Gruentzig in 1978.[29] However, late angiographic restenosis, which constitutes the most serious problem after successful angioplasty, occurs in 30-50% of patients within 3 to 6 months after the procedure depending of the clinical concept of restenosis.[30] Advances in technique, equipment and technology have improved the safety and acute success of endovascular therapeutic interventions but regrettably there has been little if any impact on restenosis to date.

The limited human data on the pathology of restenosis obtained at autopsy and atherectomy has revealed that the restenotic tissue is composed predominantly of smooth muscle cells and extracellular matrix with a high proportion of lesions containing thrombus (if examined early after the procedure) [31], and variable and generally limited components of lipid and cellular elements such as macrophages.[32] These findings are similar to the neointimal proliferation and matrix deposition observed in experimental models in response to arterial injury and mural thrombosis.[2]

The role of platelets in the vascular myofibrotic response has been studied with the use of balloon injury-induced thrombosis in the carotid arteries of pigs and rats (rats do not develop acute thrombi with balloon injury). Three phases in the process of myofibrosis have been distinguished *(Figure 2.2)*.[17, 33]

Phase 1 is the deposition of platelet thrombi and fibrin formation, which occurs within minutes of vascular injury and is complete within 24 hours. After approximately 24 hours, smooth muscle cells in the media begin to undergo hypertrophy and proliferate, as detected by increased DNA synthesis and reach peak proliferation at 48 hours. From day 1 on there is a progressive decrease of the mural thrombotic component as the myointimal proliferation increases. The early replication of medial smooth muscle cells has been observed to result from direct mechanical trauma, probably by the release of intracellular non-platelet-dependent basic fibroblast growth factor (b-FGF) more than by the induction of a pathway of autocrine and self-stimulating non-platelet-dependent platelet-derived growth factor(PDGF).[34, 35]

Phase 2 begins on day 2 - 4 and is marked by the migration of smooth muscle cells from the media into the intima. About half of migrating smooth muscle cells proliferate. Cells continue to migrate and proliferate through day 14, when the population approaches its maximum. Platelets may induce the migration of smooth muscle cells by secreting PDGF which is known to have chemotactic as well as mitogenic activity.[36] As in the early proliferation of medial smooth muscle cells, intimal smooth muscle cells may participate in a non-platelet-dependent autocrine pathway of a PDGF-like substance and intimal proliferation.

During phase 3 (day 14 to 3 months), there appears to be an interaction between circulating humoral (i.e. thrombin) and cellular i.e. platelets, monocytes) components, and the deendothelialized surface; such interaction or the lack of regenerated endothelium may contribute to the progression of intimal thickening.[2, 17, 33] This may be due in part to the proliferation and hypertrophy of smooth muscle cells, the attraction of macrophages into organizing thrombus, and the initial platelet secretion of large amounts of transforming growth factor beta, all of which contribute to the accumulation of extracellular matrix, the fibrotic organization of the thrombi, and the composition of growing atherosclerotic plaques.[2]

The role of thrombin in restenosis

The role of thrombin in this three-phase fibrotic organization of the mural thrombus is also emerging. After vascular damage, the enzymatically active thrombin is produced during phase 1 of thrombosis and is absorbed and incorporated into the thrombus and the extracellular matrix.[15, 37-39] Subsequently it may be released gradually in active form during spontaneous fibrinolysis or thrombus organization, or may be active locally when bound to fibrin or arterial matrix. Surface-bound fibrin in particular may act as a reservoir for enzymatically active thrombin.[2, 37, 38, 40] Thus, the existence of a reservoir of slowly released thrombin and possibly new generation of thrombin may explain how, after substantial vascular damage (Type II or III), platelets and ongoing thrombosis are involved in the relatively delayed process of smooth-muscle-cell proliferation and migration (phase 2) and extracellular matrix production (phase 3).[40-42]

In addition recent studies have shown that thrombin may be an important mediator of restenosis not only by promoting and sustaining ongoing mural thrombosis [43] , but also by direct mitogenic effects, or by stimulation the release of growth factors at all stages of the lesion development. Thrombin has very potent effects on both cultured fibroblasts and smooth muscle cells in vitro.[42, 44] Thrombin may also

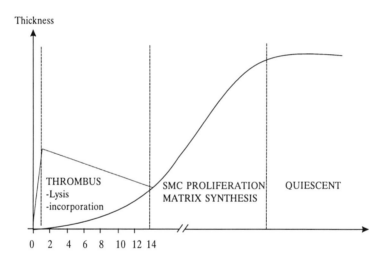

*Figure 2.2 Curves of the hypothetical relation of mural and intramural processes leading to restenosis following angioplasty in a pig model. **Phase 1** (within hours): Vascular injury induces mural thrombosis and direct trauma to the media and the release is mitogens for medial smooth muscle cell proliferation. **Phase 2** (within 2 days to 2 weeks): As a result of mural thrombosis, thrombin generation, and release of PDGF, a myofibrotic response (thrombus organization) may play a role in the restenotic process, and extracellular matrix formation plays a role in the early phase of restenosis. **Phase 3** (2 weeks to 3 months): Until re-endothelialization is complete, interaction between circulating elements (humoral and cellular) and the de-endothelialized surface may play a critical role in the continued progression of the myofibrotic response. Earlier release of growth factors from platelets may promote synthesis of extracellular matrix.*

promote autocrine growth responses since it stimulates the synthesis of fibroblast growth factor (FGF) [45], and PDGF from smooth muscle cells and endothelial cells. These actions of thrombin on smooth muscle cells are most likely mediated by the cellular thrombin receptor. The role of thrombin as a mitogen for vascular cells is supported by the detection of m-RNA for this receptor in human atherosclerotic plaques.[46] When thrombin is neutralized by complex formation with antithrombin III thrombin-induced DNA synthesis and cell proliferation in human arterial smooth muscle cells is completely inhibited.[47] This hypothesis is further supported by studies with specific thrombin and anti-factor Xa inhibitors showing inhibition of arterial thrombosis[18, 19] and restenosis[41, 48] after balloon angioplasty in animals. This suggests a critical role for thrombin in this complex biologic process. Further studies are needed to determine delayed antithrombin effects on cell proliferation and the progression of atherosclerotic lesions.

The development and progression of coronary artery disease depend on both incorporation of lipid and deposition of fibrin and platelets into the arterial wall leading to atherosclerotic plaque formation over decades. Variable degrees of vascular injury induce the formation of thrombin with subsequent platelet activation and mural thrombosis, which may lead to rapid progression of atherosclerosis with periodic acute clinical events. Vascular injury may stimulate smooth muscle cell proliferation via multiple factors relating to thrombus. Thrombin may be an important mediator of rapid progression of atherosclerosis and restenosis not only by promoting and sustaining ongoing mural thrombosis but also by direct or indirect mitogenic effects at all stages of lesion development.

REFERENCES

1. Ross R. The pathogenesis of atherosclerosis: A perspective for the 1990's. Nature 1993: 362: 801.

2. Fuster V, et al. The pathogenesis of Coronary Artery Disease and the Acute Coroanry Syndromes. N Engl J Med 1992: 326; 310.

3. Karino T, et al. Flow patterns in vessels of simple and complex geometries. Ann N Y Acad Sci 1987: 422.

4. Badimon L, et al. Thrombus formation on ruptures atherosclerosis plaques and rethrombosis on evolving thrombi. Circulation 1992: 86 (suppl III):III-74.

5. Ip J, et al. Syndromes of accelerated atherosclerosis. Role of vascular injury and smooth muscle cell proliferation. J Am Coll Cardiol 1990: 15:1667.

6. Stary HC. Composition and classification of human atherosclerosis lesions. Virchows Achiv (Pathol. Anat.) 421: 277.

7. Steinberg D, et al. Beyond cholesterol: modifications of low-density lipoprotein that increase its atherogenicity. N Engl J Med 1989: 320: 915.

8. Davies MJ. A macro and micro view of coronary vascular insults in ischemic heart disease. Circulation 1990: 82 (suppl II): II-38.

9. Bruschke A, et al. The anatomic evaluation of coronary disease demonstrated by coronary angiography in non operated patients. Circulation 1981: 63: 527.

10. Little WC, et al. Can coronary angiography predict the site of a subsequent myocardial infarction in patients with mild, to moderate coronary artery disease. Circulation 1988: 78: 1157.

11. Ambrose J, et al. Angiographic progression of coronary artery disease and the development of myocardial infarction. J Am Coll Cardiol 1988: 12:56.

12. Chesebro JH, Fuster V. Thrombosis in unstable angina. N Engl J Med 1992: 327: 192.

13. Richardson PD, et al. Influence of plaque configuration and stress distribution on fissuring of coronary atherosclerosis plaques. Lancet 1989: 2: 941.

14. Cheng GC, et al. Distribution of circumferential stress in ruptured and stable atherosclerotic lesions. A structural analysis with histopathological correlation. Circulation 1993: 87: 1179.

15. Chesebro JH, et al. Antithrombotic therapy and progression of coronary artery disease. Circulation 86(suppl III):III 100.

16. Fernandez-Ortiz A, et al. Characterization of the relative thrombogenicity of atherosclerotic plaque components: Implications for consequences of plaque rupture. J Am Coll Cardiol 1994: 23:1562.

17. Steele PM, et al. Balloon angioplasty: Natural history of the pathophysiologic response to injury in a pig model. Circ Res 1985: 57:105.

18. Heras M, et al. Effects of thrombin inhibition on the development of acute platelet-thrombus deposition during angioplasty in pigs: heparin versus recombinant hirudin, s specific thrombin inhibitor. Circulation 1989: 79:657.

19. Heras M, et al. Hirudin, heparin and placebo during deep arterial injury in the pig. The in vivo role of thrombin in platelet-mediated thrombosis. Circulation 82: 1476.

20. Fuster V, et al. Atherosclerosis plaque rupture and thrombosis: evolving concepts. Circulation 1990: 82(suppl II):II 47.

21. Woolf N. Interaction between mural thrombi and underlying artery wall. Haemostasis 1979: 8:127.

22. Woolf N, Carstairs KC. Infiltration and thrombosis in atherogenesis: A study using immunofluorescent techniques. Am J Path 1967: 51:373.

23. Woolf N, Carstairs KC. The survival time of platelets in experimental mural thrombi. J Path 1969: 97:595.

24. Woolf N, et al. Experimentalmural thrombi in the pig aorta. the early natural history. B J Exp Path 1968: 49:257.

25. Bini A, et al. Identification and distribution of fibrinogen, fibrin, and fibrin(ogen) degradation products in atherosclerosis: use of monoclonal antibody. Artheriosclerosis 1989: 9: 109.

26. Smith EB, et al. Fate of fibrogen in human arterial intima. Arteriosclerosis 1990: 10:263.

27. Badimon L, Badimon JJ. Mechanisms of arterial thrombosis in non-parallel stramlines. Platelet thrombi grow on the apex of stenotic severely injured vessel wall. J Clin Invest 1989: 84:1134.

28. Mailhac A, et al. Effect on an eccentric severe stenosis on Fibrin(ogen) deposition on severely damaged vessel wall in arterial thrombosis. Circulation, in press.

29. Gruentzig AR. Transluminal dilatation of coronary-artery stenosis. Lancet 1978:1:263.

30. Kuntz RE, Baim DS. Defining coronary restenosis. Newer clinical and angiographic paradigms. Circulation 1993:88 1310.

31. Johnson DE, et al. Primary peripheral arterial stenosis and restenosis excised by transluminal atherectomy: A histopathologic study. J Am Coll Cardiol 15:419.

32. Casscells W. Migration of smooth muscle and endothelial cells: Critical events in restenosis. Circulation 1992:86:723.

33. Clowes AW, et al. Regulation of smooth muscle cell growth in injured arteries. J Cardiovasc Pharmacol 14(suppl 6):S12.

34. Fingerle J, et al. Role of platelets in smooth muscle cell proliferation and migration after vascular injury in rat carotid artery. Proc Natl Acad USA 1989:86:8412.

35. Lindner V, et al. Role of basic fibroblast growth factor in vascular ledion formation. Circ Res 1991:68:106.

36. Ferns GAA, et al. Inhibition of neointimal smooth muscle accumulation after angioplasty by an antibody to PDGF. Science 1991:253:1129.

37. Bar-Shavit R, et al. Binding of thrombin to subendothelial extracellular matrix: Protection and expression of functional properties. J Clin Invest 1989:84:1096.

38. Weitz JI, et al. Clot-bound thrombin is protected from inhibition by heparin-antithrombin III but is susceptible to inactivation by antithrombin III-independent inhibitors. J Clin Invest 1990:86:385.

39. Weitz JI, Hudoba M. Mechanism by which clot-bound thrombin is protected from inactivation by fluid-phase inhibitors. Circulation 1992:86:I-413.

40. Hatton MW, et al. Deendothelialization in vivo initiates a thrombogenic reaction at the rabbit aorta surface. Correlation of uptake of fibrinogen and antithrombin II with thrombin generation by the exposed subendothelium. J Clin Invest 1989:86:452.

41. Ragosta M, et al. Specific factor Xa inhibition reduces restenosis after balloon angioplasty of atherosclerosis femoral arteries in rabbits. Circulation 1994:89:1262.

42. Bar-Shavit R, et al. Thrombin as a multifactorial protein induction of cell adhesion and proliferation. Am J Clin Mol Biol 1992: 6:123.

43. Meyer BJ, et al. Inhibition of the progression of thrombus growth on pre-existing mural thrombus: targeting optimal therapy. J Am Coll Cardiol 1994:23:64A.

44. Graham DJ, Alexander JJ. The effects of thrombin on bovine aortic endothelial and smooth muscle cells. J Vasc Surg 1990: 11:307-13.

45. Weiss RH, Maduri M. The mitogenic effect of thrombin in vascular smooth muscle cells is largely duw to basic fibroblast growth factor. J Biol Chem 1993: 268:5724.

46. Nelken NA, et al. Thrombin receptor expression in normal and atherosclerotic human arteries. J Clin Invest 1992:90:1614.

47. Hedin U, et al. Antithrombin III inhibits thrombin-induced proliferation in human arterial smooth muscle cells. Arterioscler Thromb 1994:14:254.

48. Sarembock IJ, et al. Effectiveness of recombinant desulphatohirudin in reducing restenosis after balloon angioplasty of atherosclerotic femoral arteries in rabbits. Circulation 1991:84:232.

3 LIPOPROTEINS AND APOPROTEINS

Elena Citkowitz, Peter N. Herbert

This chapter describes interrelationship between lipids and vascular disease and is not an extensive review of the literature. Instead, the reader will become familiar with recent research that has led to changing views of the lipid-atherosclerosis association. While a definitive understanding of the way in which dyslipidemias cause atherosclerotic disease is still evolving, the latest research provides new perspectives on lipid pathophysiology and its importance in atherogenesis.

Lipoprotein metabolism

An understanding of lipoproteins is fundamental to any discussion of lipids and atherosclerosis. Cholesterol and triglycerides, the two major constituents of lipoproteins, have been widely emphasized but their absolute levels are less important than the properties of the lipoproteins in which they are carried. For example, a total cholesterol may be elevated because the cholesterol content is abnormally high in one of several lipoproteins, each of which has different prognostic implications for risk of cardiovascular disease. Moreover, many lipoprotein disorders can now be explained by genetic factors that make risk assessment more accurate.[1]

Lipoproteins can be classified by physical methods that separate them by size and charge (electrophoretic mobility) or by density (ultracentrifugation) *(Table 3.1)*. Centrifugation is the traditional method for separating lipoproteins and three of the four major lipoprotein classes derive their names from this method of separation: chylomicrons, very low density lipoproteins (VLDL), low density lipoproteins (LDL), and high density lipoproteins (HDL).

In electrophoresis chylomicrons remain at the origin. LDL migrate slowly with beta globulins and VLDL migrate just ahead with pre-beta globulins. HDL

Table 3.1   *LIPOPROTEIN WEIGHT, DENSITY,*
AND ELECTROPHORETIC MOBILITY

	Molecular Weight $\times 10^6$	Density g/ml	Electrophoretic Mobility
Chylomicrons	0.93	Remains at origin	50-1000
VLDL	0.93-1.006	Pre-b-lipoproteins	10-80
IDL	1.006-1.019	Pre-b-lipoproteins	5-10
LDL	1.019-1.063	b-lipoproteins	2.30
HDL2	1.063-1.125	"a"-lipoproteins	0.360
HDL3	1.125-1.210	"a"-lipoproteins	0.175
Lp(a)	1.040-1.125	Pre-b-lipoproteins	2.6-3.1

Adapted from RJ Havel and JP Kane, Table 56-2 (Ref 4).

migrate significantly ahead of all the other lipoproteins with the alpha globulins. Two minor lipoproteins, intermediate density lipoproteins (IDL) and lipoprotein (a) (Lp(a)), migrate with major lipoproteins: IDL with LDL (beta) and Lp(a) with VLDL (pre-beta). Because of these overlapping regions of electrophoretic migration, quantitation of the cholesterol carried in VLDL, IDL, LDL or Lp(a) can be achieved only by a combination of ultracentrifugation followed by electrophoresis. Because electrophoresis alone is inaccurate as well as expensive, it cannot be recommended except in specialized laboratories that also perform ultracentrifugation.

Lipoproteins are also distinguished by their unique blend of lipids and specific proteins. The lipoprotein core is made up of cholesteryl ester and triglycerides. The surface of lipoproteins contains cholesterol, phospholipids and proteins, called apolipoproteins *(Figure 3.1, Table 3.1)*. Although quantification of apolipoproteins is no more useful than the standard lipid profiles[2], familiarity with the apolipoproteins aids in understanding the physiology and metabolism of the lipoproteins and their constituents. Apolipoproteins act as ligands between lipoproteins and cell receptors; they are cofactors for enzymes in lipid metabolism; and they are structural components of the lipoproteins *(Table 3.2)*. Some apolipoproteins remain bound to the lipoprotein throughout metabolism: apo B-48 with chylomicrons, apo B-100 with LDL, and apo (a) with Lp(a). The non-B apolipoproteins, apolipoproteins A-I, A-II, A-IV, C-I, C-II, C-III, D and E, shuttle between lipoproteins.

Triglyceride-rich lipoproteins (TRL)

The triglyceride-rich lipoproteins (TRL) include chylomicrons and their remnants, very low density lipoproteins (VLDL) and their remnants, and intermediate density lipoproteins (IDL). Chylomicrons and VLDL carry dietary lipids and hepatic lipids, respectively, into the blood stream. During catabolism of chylomicrons and

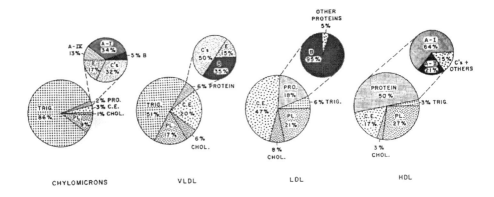

Figure 3.1 Major lipoproteins: composition and primary apolipoproteins.
HDL = high density lipoproteins; LDL = low density lipoproteins;
VLDL = very low density lipoproteins.
CE = cholesteryl ester; CHOL = cholesterol;
PL = phospholipid; PRO = protein; TRIG = triglycerides.

VLDL, triglycerides are broken down to free fatty acids for tissue uptake, particularly by muscle and fat. Cholesterol is delivered to tissues and may be important to the function of steroid-synthesizing organs, particularly the adrenal glands and liver.[3,4]

Chylomicrons and chylomicron remnants

Chylomicrons are the largest lipoproteins and in the nonfasting state are the major triglyceride-carrying lipoproteins *(Figure 3.1)*. After a meal, triglycerides and cholesterol are packaged into chylomicrons by the intestinal mucosal cell and carried via the mesenteric lymphatics and thoracic duct into the blood stream. Chylomicrons possess a unique and defining apolipoprotein, apo B-48, that is present only on chylomicrons and their remnants, and remains with the chylomicron throughout its metabolism. Apo B-48 is identical to the amino-terminal half of apo B-100, the apolipoprotein of low density lipoprotein (LDL) but ends at amino acid 2,152.[5] Apo B-48 is about one half the size of apo B-100 and, lacking the carboxy-terminal portion of apo B-100, has no LDL receptor-binding site.

After mixing with plasma, chylomicrons interact extensively with high density lipoprotein (HDL) and exchange their apo A's for the C and E apolipoproteins in HDL. When chylomicrons acquire apo C-II, which is a necessary cofactor for the enzyme lipoprotein lipase (LPL)[6], the triglycerides are rapidly hydrolyzed to free fatty acids. As chylomicrons are progressively degraded, C apolipoproteins are transferred back to HDL and no further hydrolysis of triglycerides occurs. Chylomicron remnants, which may be atherogenic[7], are removed from the circulation by

Table 3.2   *MOLECULAR WEIGHT, ORIGIN, AND FUNCTION*
OF APOLIPOPROTEINS

Apolipoprotein	Mol. Weight	Sites of Synthesis	Postulated Functions
Apo A-I	28,000	intestine, liver	LCAT cofactor, structural, ligand?
Apo A-II	17,000	intestine, liver	hepatic lipase cofactor, structural, ligand?
Apo A-IV	44,000	intestine, liver	LPL cofactor, LCAT cofactor, ligand?
Apo B-48	250,000	intestine	structural
Apo B-100	550,000	liver	LDL receptor, stuctural
Apo C-I	6,500	liver	LCAT cofactor
Apo C-II	9,000	liver	LPL cofactor
Apo C-III	9,000	liver	inhibitor of LPL ?
Apo D	22,000	?	?
Apo E	34,000	liver	ligand to LDL and LRP receptors
Apo(a)	400,000-800,000	liver	structural (inhibits plasminogen?)

LCAT = lecithin cholesterol acyl transferase, LPL = lipoprotein lipase, LRP = LDL receptor-related protein

cellular receptors specific for apo E. These receptors include the remnant receptor, identified as LDL receptor-related protein [8], and possibly the classical LDL receptor (also known as the B/E or B-100:E receptor) which binds apo E even more avidly than apo B *(Figure 3.2)*. Because chylomicron remnants do not accumulate in patients with homozygous familial hypercholesterolemia who lack LDL-receptors, the role of this receptor in chylomicron remnant clearance is unclear. The development of the genetically engineered mouse in the 1990's, which became a model system for investigating human lipoprotein disorders and atherosclerosis[9], has clarified our uncertainty regarding chylomicron clearance. Mice deficient in apo E have been the focus of several important papers[10], and a "knockout" mouse model with homozygous disruptions of both the apo E and LDL-receptor genes has been particularly helpful in elucidating the clearance mechanisms of chylomicron remnants. Goldstein, Brown and coworkers compared mice lacking apo E, mice lacking the LDL receptor (LDL-R) and mice lacking both proteins.[11] LDL-R-deficient mice had elevations of LDL-C and a marked increase in apo B-100 with a modest increase in apo B-48. Apo E-deficient mice had marked increases in the larger lipoproteins (corresponding to VLDL, chylomicrons and remnants) and increases in apo B-48 but not in apo B-100. Adding the LDL receptor deficiency to the apo E deficiency markedly increased both B-48 and B-100 but had no impact on the degree of hypercholesterolemia of the apo E-deficient mouse.[11] The authors suggested that the dramatic increase of apo B-48 in apo E deficiency compared to LDL-R deficiency and the lack of further boosting of the cholesterol level when the LDL-R deficiency was added to the apo E deficiency, supports the conclusion that the chylomicron remnant is cleared by a receptor other than the LDL-R (probably the LDL-receptor related protein) and that the remnant is removed via the ligand activity of apo E.

Occasionally severe elevations of chylomicrons and their remnants are caused by rare inherited disorders in which lipoprotein lipase (LPL) or its cofactor, apolipoprotein C-II, is absent.[6] But most patients with chylomicronemia have more common abnormalities of lipid metabolism such as uncontrolled diabetes mellitus, alcoholism or oral estrogens which may cause overproduction of VLDL. Decreased clearance of remnants may coexist with overproduction thereby contributing to saturation of lipoprotein lipase which, in turn, causes massive accumulation of chylomicrons.[12] Overexpression or overactivity of apo C-III, a putative inhibitor of lipoprotein lipase, is another potential mechanism causing accumulation of triglyceride-rich lipoproteins *(Table 3.2)*.[13]

VLDL and VLDL Remnants

In the fasting state, VLDL is usually the major triglyceride-carrying lipoprotein *(Figure 3.1)*. VLDL is synthesized in the liver; and newly secreted VLDL, containing apo B-100, take on apo E and apo C's transferred from high density lipopro-

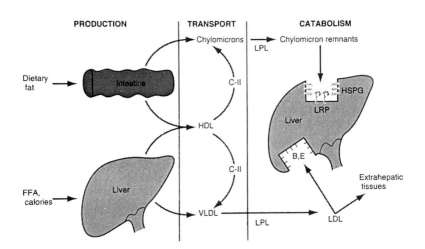

*Figure 3.2 **Normal metabolism of plasma lipoproteins.***

Normal metabolism of plasma lipoproteins. See text for details.

B,E = Membrane receptor for lipoproteins containing apo B and apo E (synonymous with LDL receptor); FFA = free fatty acids;
HDL = high density lipoproteins;

HSPG = heparan sulfate proteoglycan; LDL = low-density lipoproteins;
LRP = LDL-receptor-related protein; VLDL = very low density lipoproteins.

teins. In a pathway analogous to chylomicron processing, lipoprotein lipase hydro-lyzes much of the VLDL triglyceride, generating free fatty acids and VLDL rem-nants. The rapidity of hydrolysis of VLDL triglycerides is significantly less than that for chylomicrons, a consequence perhaps of the smaller size of VLDL which cannot accommodate as many lipoprotein lipase molecules. Compared with LDL clearance, however, VLDL clearance is quite rapid. Larger VLDL generate larger remnants which, because they can accommodate more of the ligand apo E, are cleared more rapidly by cell surface receptors.[4]

Normally approximately half of VLDL remnants are cleared from the circula-tion by apo E-specific cell receptors on hepatic cells, primarily the LDL receptor-related protein. The uptake of remnants is facilitated by removal of the C apolipo-proteins which exposes the receptor-binding domain of apo E. VLDL remnants that are not removed by receptors are further metabolized by a second enzyme, hepatic lipase, yielding LDL. As metabolism of VLDL proceeds, the E apolipoproteins are also lost *(Figure 3.2)*.

Apo E plays a critical role in the regulation of plasma lipoprotein metabolism. Apo E is present on all lipoproteins except LDL and serves as a ligand, binding both chylomicron and VLDL remnants to their receptors. Moreover, unlike B apolipo-proteins, a variable number of apo E's are present on each lipoprotein; and, typical-ly, the greater the number of active apo E, the greater the uptake of the lipoprotein involved. Apo E is synthesized in several tissues including liver, brain, adrenals, ovaries and kidney and may play a role in repair of tissue injury.[14] Like most apo-lipoproteins, a single gene locus codes for the apo E protein; but unlike the other apolipoproteins, the apo E gene is polymorphic and codes for three major isoforms: apo E-2, E-3 and E-4. As a consequence six phenotypes are possible. Of the three isoforms, apo E-3 is usually the most common and apo E-2 the least common.[15] Each isoform has a different impact on serum lipid levels; for example, E-2/E-2 is correlated with lower cholesterol levels and E-4/E-4 with the highest. No correla-tion has been found between the apo E phenotypes and HDL levels (reviewed in 15). It is postulated that E-3 and E-4 have particular affinity for both the LDL receptor-related protein and for hepatic lipase. VLDL remnants containing E-3 or E-4 are either efficiently cleared from the circulation or converted to LDL. VLDL with E-2, however, either accumulate as remnants or are cleared by other mecha-nisms but are not efficiently converted to LDL. Hence, the low cholesterol levels seen in some E-2 homozygotes.

As discussed above, "knockout" mice lacking apo E have elevated serum cho-lesterols (five to eight times that of controls) when fed a normal, low-fat diet; and although LDL cholesterol is somewhat elevated, most of the cholesterol is located in the IDL and VLDL. HDL and triglycerides are minimally affected. Within three months of age, the apo E-deficient mice develop significant atherosclerotic lesions of the coronary (and other) arteries.[16,17] With time, the lesions progress from fatty streaks to mature atherosclerotic plaques made up of smooth muscle cells, foam cells, necrotic debris and fibrous caps, progression that is remarkably similar to that of human atherosclerosis.[18,19] When human apo A-I is transferred to "knockout" mice lacking apo E, HDL increase two- to threefold and atherosclerosis is reduced sixfold in spite of cholesterol levels that are similar to the control mice.[20]

Intermediate density lipoproteins (IDL, β-VLDL)

Patients with type 3 hyperlipoproteinemia (familial dysbetalipoproteinemia) are at increased risk for peripheral vascular disease as well as CAD.[21] Plasma levels of both total cholesterol and triglycerides are increased (often with a low LDL-C), and patients may have palmar xanthomas. The disorder is most confidently diagnosed by demonstrating increased levels of intermediate density lipoprotein (IDL), also known as beta VLDL (β-VLDL). IDL are VLDL remnants and consequently are cholesterol-enriched compared to VLDL. Ultracentrifuge diagnosis of type 3 hyperlipoproteinemia is based on finding a plasma triglyceride:VLDL-cholesterol ratio of 3:1 or less (or a ratio of 1.3:1 if SI units are used).

With very rare exception, the prerequisite for type 3 hyperlipoproteinemia is two copies of apo E-2.[21] But although approximately one percent of Caucasians have E-2/E-2, few of them develop type 3 hyperlipoproteinemia. Typically patients with type 3 hyperlipoproteinemia also have a second condition that causes overproduction or impaired clearance of VLDL such as diabetes, hypothyroidism or obesity. A rare, dominant form of type 3 hyperlipoproteinemia has been identified in which only a single allele of E-2 is necessary for expression of the lipid abnormality and the presence of a secondary condition is not required (See 21 for further discussion).

As already described, apo E-2 binds poorly to lipoprotein receptors, and perhaps to hepatic lipase, thus reducing both direct removal of remants and the conversion of VLDL and IDL to LDL. The accumulated remnants of both chylomicrons and VLDL are cleared by an alternative pathway, probably macrophages, leading to the formation of foam cells and atherosclerotic lesions.[22]

Although not directly relevant to cardiology, brief mention should be made of the recently identified association of apo E and Alzheimer's disease. Apo E-4 appears in greater frequency in patients with Alzheimer's disease and a dose-effect has been documented.[23] Apo E-2, in contrast, is found in lower frequency.[24] Consensus statements have been issued, however, discouraging apo E evaluation to predict risk of future Alzheimer's disease.[25,26]

Low Density Lipoproteins (LDL)

LDL typically carry about 65% of the plasma cholesterol (Figure 3.1). In the catabolism of VLDL remnants to LDL, much of the triglyceride and essentially all apolipoproteins except apo B-100 are removed (Figure 3.2). Apo B-100 is LDL's ligand to the LDL receptor (LDL-R) which is found on both hepatic and extrahepatic cells. Hepatic receptors account for clearance of about two-thirds of plasma LDL. If apo B-100 cannot bind to the LDL-R, plasma LDL cholesterol accumulates. The role of the LDL-R in this process is illustrated by the inherited disorder of familial (monogenic) hypercholesterolemia. Brown and Goldstein received the Nobel Prize for showing that a single, autosomal dominant gene abnormality causes reduced (heterozygote) or absent (homozygote) LDL-R function.[27,28] More than 150 different mutations of the LDL receptor have been identified, and they cause a variety of receptor defects [28]. Heterozygous expression, occurring in approximately 1 in 500 Caucasians and Japanese (and higher frequencies in certain other populations), causes a markedly elevated total cholesterol (TC) (350 to 550 mg/dl) and LDL-cholesterol (LDL-C), a variety of physical findings such as tendon xanthomas, and high risk of premature CAD. In patients homozygous for familial hypercholesterolemia, LDL-C is even higher (600 to 1000 mg/dl) and coronary disease is manifested in childhood.

The mechanism by which many interventions lower LDL-C (low cholesterol diet, low saturated fat diet, resins) is the up-regulation of the LDL-R. The hydroxymethylglutaryl coenzyme A (HMG CoA) reductase inhibitors or statins, which inhibit hepatic cholesterol synthesis, also cause induction of LDL-R transcription. Predictably then, statins are ineffective in patients with homozygous familial hypercholesterolemia in whom inhibition of cellular cholesterol production cannot induce LDL-receptor formation.

Another dominant gene abnormality also impairs binding of LDL to its receptor; but in this condition, familial defective apo B-100 (FDB), the LDL-R is normal and it is a defective apo B-100 that curbs LDL binding activity.[29] FDB is a mutation affecting the binding region of apo B-100 [30]; it causes elevated LDL-C and increased risk of CAD.[31-34] Although other extremely rare mutations have been described[34,35], the most common defect causing FDB results from a single amino acid substitution of glutamine for the 3500th amino acid, arginine.[36,37] In populations of European descent the frequency of FDB may be as high as that for FH, about 1 in 500; but elsewhere FDB appears to be rare. Although one patient with homozygous FDB had only mild hypercholesterolemia[38], many patients with the heterozygous disorder are indistinguishable by physical examination and serum lipids from patients with heterozygous FH[39] and may also have the same risk for CAD.[32,33] Clearly, the full clinical consequences of the defect, including coronary risk, have yet to be determined.

Although the LDL receptor is of primary importance in the genesis of hypercholesterolemia and development of atherosclerosis, a different receptor, the scavenger (or scavenger cell) receptor, also binds LDL and causes cellular uptake of cholesterol. The scavenger receptor is present on monocyte/macrophages and the accumulation of cholesterol transforms them into foam cells [27]. At least 3 classes of scavenger receptor have been identified, and their primary roles may actually be protective rather than damaging; that is, the scavenger receptor may facilitate macrophage ingestion of abnormal or oxidized proteins [40]. Two of the scavenger receptors, type I and type II, were recently isolated [41,42].

High density lipoproteins (HDL)

HDL are unique in several ways. a) They are the only lipoproteins considered to be protective against atherosclerosis. b) They do not carry any form of apo B. c) They are the most dense lipoproteins due to their high protein content *(Figure 3.1)*. HDL appear to be secreted from the liver as discoidal or nascent HDL carrying A apolipoproteins. Immature HDL avidly pick up free cholesterol from tissue or other lipoproteins and may also acquire additional surface apo A-I and phospholipid during chylomicron metabolism by lipoprotein lipase. The enzyme lecithin:cholesterol acyltransferase (LCAT), activated by apo A-I, converts free cholesterol to esterified cholesterol which, being more hydrophobic, moves to the HDL core creating the more spherical HDL3. As HDL3 acquire more free cholesterol, phospholipid and apo A-I, they are gradually transformed into HDL2. HDL2 are acted upon by two different processes. In one, cholesteryl ester transfer protein (CETP) exchanges the cholesterol from HDL2 for triglyceride from VLDL and IDL. In the other pathway, hepatic lipase hydrolyzes HDL core triglycerides and surface phospholipids while apolipoproteins are removed and HDL2 converted back to HDL3 (see review 43).

HDL has been classified not only by its density (HDL2, HDL3), but has also been characterized by whether it contains only A-I or both A-I and A-II.[44] The transgenic mouse model has been used to study the impact of these apolipoproteins on HDL metabolism and atherogenesis[43]; and some[45-47], though not all[48], suggest that HDL containing high levels of apo A-I protect against atherogenesis.

A series of papers suggests that HDL containing high levels of apo A-I are protective against the development of atherosclerosis: a) Overexpression of human apo A-I increased HDL levels and protected against the development of fatty streaks in mice fed an atherogenic diet.[45] b) Overexpresion of both human apo A-I and A-II resulted in a 15-fold increase in atherosclerotic lesions compared to A-I animals despite similar HDL-C levels.[46] c) Overexpression of mouse apo A-II caused increased HDL-C levels but also increased atherosclerotic lesions.[47] On the other hand, in a strain of mice homozygous for an inactive apo A-I gene, total and HDL cholesterol levels were both reduced 25% but the animals did not show increased susceptibility to atherosclerosis.[48] Nonetheless, the significance of this negative finding may be confounded by the abnormal levels of plasma apolipoproteins and, more specifically, by the high apo E content of the HDL which normally contain only trace amounts. Other transgenic mouse models are described by Breslow.[43]

The putative role of HDL in reverse cholesterol transport from peripheral cells to the liver should be apparent from the metabolic pathways described above *(Figure 3.2)*. An HDL receptor may play a part in this process, but this is still a matter of controversy. A protein originally thought to be a scavenger receptor, identified in Chinese hamster ovarian cells, may be an HDL receptor.[49] This protein, SR-BI, displays several characteristics that would be expected of an HDL receptor: 1) It binds HDL. 2) Unlike the LDL receptor, it is not degraded in the process of transferring lipid from the lipoprotein (HDL) into cells. 3) It is most abundant in hepatic and steroid-synthesizing organs (adrenal gland and ovary), tissues that can either dispose or make use of incoming cholesterol. There is unpublished evidence that in the A-I knockout mouse with intact apo A-II and Apo E, cholesteryl ester stores in adrenals are strikingly depleted and steroidogenic responses are decreased.[50] Steinberg suggests that the SR-BI protein, if it is an HDL receptor, does not appear to remove excess cholesterol from peripheral cells because it is not expressed in these cells.[50] But because of its location in hepatocytes, SR-BI could well play a role in the reverse cholesterol transport pathway by facilitating HDL delivery of excess cholesterol to hepatocytes.

HDL may also antagonize the atherosclerotic process by preventing oxidation and aggregation of LDL [51,52], conditions that are thought to promote uptake of LDL by macrophages.[53] This and other mechanisms, such as impact on vasomotor tone and endothelial proliferation, by which HDL may play a cardioprotective were recently discussed.[54]

Lipids and cardiovascular disease

LDL cholesterol and coronary artery disease

The lipid-heart hypothesis holds that an elevated blood cholesterol level *causes* coronary artery disease (CAD) and that lowering cholesterol levels will *decrease* the risk of CAD. Confirmation has come from diverse sources. Animal models, from rodent to primate, have shown that induced hypercholesterolemia can cause atherosclerosis and that lowering the cholesterol level can induce atherosclerotic plaque regression (e.g. 55). The human disorder familial (monogenic) hypercholesterolemia, caused by reduced receptor-mediated clearance of LDL, clarified the critical importance of LDL levels in atherosclerotic plaque formation. In this disorder, cholesterol accumulates and is deposited in macrophages and smooth muscle cells[56]; and the incidence of premature CAD is extremely high. International studies of human populations have shown a strong correlation between cholesterol levels and the incidence and prevalence of CAD.[57-59] Studies of populations migrating from countries with low to countries with high rates of CAD show that the increased prevalence of disease in those who emigrate is related to an increase in their blood cholesterol concentration.[60] Such studies exclude different genetic pools as an explanation of international differences in CAD prevalence.

Cohort studies have provided additional convincing evidence of the link between total and LDL cholesterol and risk for CAD. The Framingham Heart Study, for example, showed that both a high total cholesterol and a low HDL cholesterol are independent risk factors for CAD in men and women.[61-64] Many other studies using multivariate analysis have confirmed this observation.[65] In the Multiple Risk Factor Intervention Trial (MRFIT), more than 300,000 subjects were followed for six years. There was a continuous, graded and strong relationship between serum cholesterol and CHD death rate that was independent of smoking or blood pressure status.[66] This association was further confirmed in a follow-up through 12 years.[67]

Interventional studies have provided the most conclusive evidence of all.[68,69] At least eight such trials, using diet or lipid-lowering medication, have shown significant reductions in nonfatal, fatal, and total myocardial infarction in treated groups compared to controls. Overall, it has been estimated that reducing serum cholesterol levels by 1% will decrease CHD rates by 2-3%.[70-72] Earlier studies, however, were faulted because they generally failed to show an effect on all-cause mortality or in some did not even show a mortality trend in favor of the treated groups. [73,74]

Three recent trials have resolved much of the uncertainty about the efficacy of aggressive treatment of lipid abnormalities and have provided the best support of the lipid-heart hypothesis available to date. The first of these, the Scandinavian Simvastatin Survival Study (4S) [75], involved more than 4,000 men and women (19% of subjects) with CHD treated with either simvastatin or placebo for 5.4 years. Simvastatin lowered the LDL cholesterol 35% (from 188 to 122 mg/dl). At study termination there were 256 deaths in the placebo group (11.5 % of the total) compared to 182 deaths in the treatment arm (8.2 %). Cardiac endpoints, including acute myocardial infarction and revascularization, showed a similar 30 to 40% relative risk reduction. Most importantly, for total mortality the absolute risk reduction was 3.3%; and no increase in morbidity or mortality from cancer or other causes was noted. The number needed to treat (NNT) to save one life was only 30; and at study termination, the difference between the treated and control groups was continuing to increase.

In 1995 the West of Scotland Coronary Prevention Study (WOSCOPS) was published.[76] This was a primary intervention trial of more than 6,500 men, 45-64 years of age, randomized to receive either placebo or pravastatin (40 mg). The average follow-up period was 4.9 years. Pravastatin reduced the LDL cholesterol 26% (from 192 to 142 mg/dl), with a relative risk reduction for definite coronary events of 31%, 248 in the placebo group and 174 in the pravastatin group. The absolute risk reduction was 2.4% and the NNT to prevent one coronary event was 42. Total mortality was 135 vs. 106, absolute risk reduction was 0.9%, and the calculated NNT to save one life was 111. Importantly, no excess of deaths from non-cardiovascular causes in the pravastatin group were noted.

Most recently, the results of another randomized, double-blind, prospective study, the Cholesterol and Recurrent Events (CARE) trial, were published [77]. Patients with a previous myocardial infarction and moderate cholesterol elevations (mean LDL-C 139 mg/dl, range 115 to 174) and fasting triglycerides less than 350 (mean 155 mg/dl) were randomized to pravastatin or placebo. In a five year follow-up of 3583 men and 576 women, LDL-C was reduced 28% compared to controls and was accompanied by a 24% reduction in the primary end point, fatal coronary event or nonfatal myocardial infarction. The number needed to treat (NNT) to prevent one major coronary event was 33. The need for CABG was reduced by 26% and PTCA by 23% in those on active treatment. This was the first trial to show the dramatic efficacy of LDL-C lowering in men and women with only mild hypercholesterolemia, although in subsequent subgroup analysis of the 4S trial relative risk reduction in patients in the lowest quartile of baseline LDL cholesterol (< 170 mg/dl) was the same as that in the highest quartile (> 207 mg/dl).[78] There were two potentially important additional observations in CARE [77]: event rates were reduced only in those with a baseline LDL-C > 125 mg/dl, and the reduction in coronary events was greater among women than among men.

Outstanding questions remain on two important points. First, should the entire adult population be screened for possible cholesterol abnormalities as recommended by the National Cholesterol Education Program Guidelines[79] or should screening be performed only in subjects with multiple risk factors or established coronary disease as recently recommended by the American College of Physicians?[80,81] This question will be easier to answer when we know more about the long-term toxicity of agents such as the statins which are so effective in LDL reduction. The second major question involves who should receive primary intervention and at what age. The NCEP currently recommends that drug treatment be considered for young men (<35 years) and premenopausal women without other risk factors only for an LDL cholesterol in excess of 220 mg/dl. Aggressive drug treatment at lower LDL cholesterol levels is reserved for those with established coronary heart disease (target LDL-C of 100 mg/dl) or middle-aged and older patients with two or more well-defined risk factors (target LDL-C of 130 mg/dl). Are we missing meaningful intervention opportunities? This debate is likely to continue.

LDL cholesterol and angiographic trials

The results of angiographic (regression) trials present a second powerful argument in support of the lipid hypothesis. Regression trials are randomized arteriographic trials of the effect of lipid-lowering intervention on the progression, stabilization and regression of coronary atherosclerotic disease. Lipid-lowering medications have been used in the majority of studies, but lifestyle[82-84] and surgical intervention [85] have also been undertaken. Because these studies require a minimum of two angiographic interventions per patient, the number of patients randomized has usually been less than 400, although two [85,86] enrolled more than 800.

Of 14 randomized, angiographic trials, 11 showed statistically significant arteriographic and clinical benefit.[87] Meta-analysis of the outcomes of all 14 (on a per patient, not per lesion, basis) demonstrated that of control patients, 50% showed disease progression, 41% no change, and 9% regression; compared with treated patients 34% of whom showed disease progression, 48% no change, and 18% regression. All differences were statistically significant and represent an absolute decrease in rate of progression of 16% and an increase in rate of regression of 9% in the treatment arm.[87] Such large differences in absolute risk can be translated into an exceptionally low value for the number needed to treat (NNT). To prevent progression of CAD in one patient, fewer than seven patients would have to be treated; and to achieve regression in one patient, the NNT would be about 11 patients.

As for clinical outcome, among the total of almost 4,000 patients enrolled in the 14 studies, there were 24% cardiovascular events in the control groups compared to 15% in the treatment groups. In a meta-analysis, Rossouw found a highly significant (relative risk) reduction of 47% (odds ratio 0.53; CI 0.45-0.63).[87] The absolute risk reduction was 9% which translates, once again, to a NNT of 11.

The regression trials tell us, unequivocally, that aggressive lipid-lowering is beneficial. The Interdisciplinary Council on Lipids and Cardiovascular Risk Intervention recently reviewed many angiographic studies, as well as the older intervention trials, and concluded that the regression that has been reported probably does represent actual improvement in atherosclerotic disease; but, as the author of the report suggests [88], the trials have not yet answered the question of "whether there is an absolute level of LDL cholesterol below which predictable changes occur or whether the magnitude of the change in LDL cholesterol level is important." This issue was addressed in a subgroup analysis [89] of the Familial Atherosclerosis Treatment Study (FATS), one of the few earlier angiographic trials to show a statistically significant impact on clinical events in addition to arteriographic improvement.[90] Significant benefits from intensive lipid-lowering therapy were seen in patients with LDL cholesterol levels < 152 mg/dl.[89] Reduction of progression was also documented in the subgroup with LDL-C levels between 85 and 147 in the Regression Growth Evaluation Statin Study (REGRESS).[86] A different conclusion was reached in the Harvard Atherosclerosis Reversibility Project (HARP)[91]. Patients with baseline LDL-C of 135 to 140 mg/dl showed no angiographic benefit. Brown et al compared HARP with FATS to find an explanation for the difference in outcome [92]. They found that, first, there was a marginally statistically significant trend in decreased progression in the treated HARP patients. Second, they suggested that FATS, by using the inclusion criterion of an elevated apo B ($\pm$ 25 mg/dl), selected for a dyslipidemic population of patients with a lower HDL-C and higher lipoprotein (a) level than patients in the HARP study. On the other hand, Sachs et al, analyzing 8 angiographic trials that used only cholesterol-lowering as the single intervention, compared baseline LDL to angiographic improvement [93]. Their results suggest that the higher the baseline LDL, the greater the angiographic improvement in treated compared to control groups (r = 0.83). Until angiographic studies are completed that enroll patients with normal to low cholesterol levels and documented CAD, this question will not be resolved.

One compelling issue that has not yet been addressed is the small increase in lumen diameter, less than 0.3 mm or 10%, in the angiograms of treated patients compared to controls. If lesion progression and regression is small, with a minimal, though significant, difference following lipid-lowering intervention, concern is raised that angiographic trials may not, after all, provide much detailed information regarding the process of atherosclerosis.[94]

This point raises one of the most fascinating issues to evolve from the angiographic trials. What is the meaning of the regression documented by quantitative angiography?[95,96] While it is understood that lipid content is an important aspect of plaque composition and behavior[97], the measurable differences in lumen dimension are not enough to explain the rapid decrease in rates of cardiovascular events. In addition, improvement in perfusion abnormalities, determined by rest-dipyridimole positron emission tomography, has been documented after only 90 days of cholesterol-lowering treatment.[98] In another study, significantly fewer cardiovascular events were documented in the initial 26 weeks in primary prevention patients treated with pravastatin compared to controls.[99] Several mechanisms have been proposed to explain how cholesterol lowering can so rapidly influence clinical events with so little regression of stenotic lesions.[100,101] Plaque instability and disruption have received much attention [102,103], especially in the elegant work by Fuster and his colleagues.[104,105] Other productive avenues of investigation are platelet reactivity [106] and, particularly, endothelial dysfunction.[107-114]

Some examples of studies on cholesterol-endothelium interaction are illustrative. Hypercholesterolemia impaired exercise-induced coronary vasodilation in a graded fashion in the normal vessels of patients with and without CAD but did not affect vasomotor response in stenotic vessels.[109] In subjects with and without CAD, cholesterol reduction significantly improved coronary artery vasomotor response to acetylcholine, while the response to nitrates was unchanged.[108,110,112] The difference in response to acetylcholine and nitrates is significant because the former is endothelium-dependent and the latter is endothelium-independent. Similar results were obtained in an important double-blind study of cholesterol lowering with lovastatin in patients with CAD.[111]

The most important mechanism by which hypercholesterolemia impairs endothelium-dependent vascular relaxation is probably a defect in the bioactivity of nitric oxide (endothelium-derived relaxing factor).[115] In addition the statins, in particular, may have cardioprotective effects independent of changes in plasma LDL concentrations [116]. Other evidence suggests that antioxidants provide additional benefit [112,101]. Thus, these and many other studies provide strong evidence that hypercholesterolemia can influence coronary vessel function and that lipid-lowering therapy can modulate that influence; so much so that some have suggested that the definition of regression should include the concept of improvement in abnormal vasomotor function.[117]

A list of key references on reversal of CAD by lipid-lowering intervention was published in 1994.[118]

Femoral and Cerebrovascular Atherosclerosis. The topic of non-coronary atherosclerosis is somewhat removed from the subject of this text but will be briefly examined because of its importance in understanding the patient at risk for atherosclerosis. In spite of the earlier inconclusive data on the correlation of cholesterol levels with stroke incidence [119], more recent regression trials support the conclusion that lipid-lowering reduces peripheral and cerebrovascular disease. Cholesterol lowering has proven effective in decreasing progression of disease in both carotid [120-124] and femoral arteries [125] (although one study found no treatment effect on progression of femoral atherosclerosis)[123]. A recent overview of randomized clinical trials found no benefit of cholesterol lowering on risk of stroke;[126] but a recent meta-analysis of the effect of tIMG-CoA reductase inhibitors demonstrated a statistically significant reduction in stroke risk compared to placebo.[126a] Large-scale randomized trials will be required to delineate the effects of lowering cholesterol levels on risk of stroke; but already the 4S [75] and CARE [77] trials, because of their large study populations and efficient cholesterol reductions, have demonstrated decreases in cerebrovascular events.

HDL cholesterol and coronary artery disease

Information from the Framingham Study provides some of the best evidence regarding the strong inverse relationship between HDL-C and CHD incidence.[127,128] In Framingham, HDL-C had approximately twice the impact on the incidence of CAD as did LDL-C.[129] A ten-year study of cardiovascular disease mortality in men with and without preexisting disease also showed significant correlations between decreasing HDL-C levels and increasing CHD mortality.[65] A similar effect was seen in the Helsinki Heart Trial, a randomized, controlled clinical trial using gemfibrozil.[130] The seeming exception of societies with low HDL-C levels (25 to 35 mg/dl) but low rates of CAD, is explained by the compensating low total and LDL cholesterol levels of approximately 150 and 100, respectively.

Apo A-I levels are highly correlated to HDL cholesterol levels and apo A-II levels are not. While strong associations between CAD and HDL subfractions or apo A levels have also been documented [131,132], these measurements are no more informative than HDL-C. In fact no apolipoprotein measurement or ratio appears to be more accurate in multivariate analysis for prediction of a myocardial infarction than the total cholesterol/HDL cholesterol ratio.[133,134]

A variety of known or possible risk factors for CAD cause low levels of HDL-C: cigarette smoking, type II diabetes mellitus, obesity, physical inactivity and increased androgen levels. Most of these conditions also raise triglyceride levels. Two interventions that may be cardioprotective and for which there is considerable, positive epidemiological data are moderate alcohol intake[135] and estrogen replacement therapy in postmenopausal women.[136-141] Each intervention raises both HDL-C and triglycerides.

The original[142] and revised[79] NCEP guidelines both recognized that a low HDL-C (< 35 mg/dl) is an independent risk factor for CAD, but only the revised guidelines recommend screening for HDL-C along with TC. Evidence from both angiographic and clinical trials suggests that raising a low HDL-C contributes to an improvement in atherosclerosis that is independent of the impact on total or LDL-C[143]; and one of the most recent angiographic trials provided important new evidence that raising the HDL-C and lowering triglycerides had as great an impact on progression of coronary lesions as treatment with statins to lower LDL-C.[144] The American College of Physicians[80,81] and the National Cholesterol Education Program[79] both agree that intervention to raise HDL cholesterol is likely to lower CHD events, and trials are in progress to address this issue. Incontrovertible proof may be hard to come by, however, because most interventions affecting HDL also affect other lipoproteins or CHD risk factors.

Triglycerides and coronary artery disease

The importance of hypertriglyceridemia in the development of coronary artery disease continues to be debated. For most large prospective studies, univariate analysis has shown a strong and statistically significant association between elevated triglycerides and coronary mortality. But multivariate analysis including HDL-C diminishes or eliminates the cardiovascular risk attributable to increased levels of triglyceride [145-152]. Some studies have shown that triglycerides continue to predict cardiovascular events after multivariate analysis that includes HDL-C.[153,154] One analysis of data from a study of men after an eight-year follow-up showed that triglycerides were an independent risk factor for a major coronary event[155], although the previous evaluation after six years could not demonstrate an effect.[150]

A recent report may provoke further controversy in suggesting that familial chylomicronemia caused by mutations in the lipoprotein lipase gene causes premature atherosclerosis.[156] Because each of the four patients reported had one or more other risk factors such as smoking, diabetes and family history of atherosclerosis and because so few patients were identified, the conclusion remains in some doubt.

Although triglycerides are not an independent risk in most multivariate models, recent analyses of data from large interventional and observational studies have shown that for high-risk groups, defined as those individuals with an elevated total cholesterol or LDL-C to HDL-C ratio, hypertriglyceridemia was a powerful additional risk factor.[150,157,158] The Helsinki Heart Study [158], an interventional study, showed that the single most sensitive predictor of cardiac events was an LDL-C/HDL-C >5. Subjects with a combination of this ratio and triglycerides >204 mg/dl (2.3 mmol/l) profited most from gemfibrozil therapy with a 71% lower incidence of coronary heart disease events. However, caution is recommended in the interpretation and generalizability of these analyses, most of which involved post hoc, subgroup analysis.[159] Studies are needed to prospectively assess the impact of elevated triglycerides on incidence of atherosclerosis and, most importantly, to determine if possible whether lowering triglycerides without altering accompanying risk factors, including HDL-C, will diminish risk. As Gerald Reaven reminds us[160], patients with hypertriglyceridemia have a variety of abnormalities that may increase the risk of CHD: hyperinsulinemia, glucose intolerance, decreased fibrinolytic activity and small LDL particles. Also, most conditions that increase the risk of CAD and cause elevated triglycerides also cause a low HDL-C level: type II diabetes mellitis, obesity, sedentary lifestyle, smoking.

Other lipoprotein abnormalities

Oxidized LDL

Although oxidized LDL is widely considered to be a critical factor in atherogene-sis[161-164], its causative role has not yet been conclusively proven. Steinberg and Wit-ztum have been prominent in investigating and describing the properties of oxidized LDL and have proposed a hypothesis for fatty streak formation and atherogenesis that stresses the role of oxidized LDL.[162,165] This model distinguishes oxidized LDL from native LDL by such features as its increased rate of uptake by macrophages via a non-LDL "scavenger" receptor, cytoxicity, chemotactic activity for circulating monocytes, inhibition of macrophage motility, and detrimental effects on coagula-tion pathways and vasomotion - all mechanisms that can potentiate atherogenesis [166]. Oxidation of LDL is presumed to occur in a sequestered environment, primarily in the arterial intima [167,168] and LDL-like particles with the properties of oxidized LDL have been isolated from atherosclerotic lesions but not from normal intima.[169] Oxidized LDL in the subendothelial then attracts monocytes. Upregulation of mono-cyte chemotactic protein 1 is found when modified LDL is added to tissue cultures of smooth muscle cells and endothelial cells.[170] Monocytes differentiate into mac-rophages promoting further LDL oxidation and increased uptake of LDL, with trans-formation of macrophages into foam cells, the precursor for the fatty streak. Smooth muscle cells may also be transformed into foam cells by uptake of oxidized LDL.

Can antioxidants prevent the oxidation of LDL and thereby inhibit or slow atherogenesis?[171] Probucol, an LDL cholesterol-lowering agent that also lowers HDL-C, has been shown to inhibit LDL oxidation[172] and has been employed in many studies. In human cell cocultures, the induction of monocyte chemotactic protein 1 and the stimulation of monocyte transmigration was inhibited by pretreatment of LDL with probucol, β-carotene, α-tocopherol (vitamin E), or HDL[170]. Treating LDL receptor-deficient rabbits (Watanabe heritable hyperlipidemic rabbits) with probu-col significantly reduced atherosclerotic lesions of aorta compared with control an-imals with the same plasma cholesterol levels;[173] and in two uncontrolled trials of patients with homozygous or heterozygous familial hypercholesterolemia, probucol appeared to reduced Achilles tendon xanthomas.[174,175] Probucol was ineffective, however, in slowing the progression of femoral atherosclerosis in a recent large, well-controlled study.[176] On the other hand in another study that looked at vascular function using lovastatin to lower cholesterol in conjunction with either a resin or probucol compared to diet only, the cholesterol-antioxidant (probucol) group showed the greatest improvement in endothelium-dependent vasomotion.[112]

The effects of three major dietary antioxidants, vitamins E, C and beta caro-tene have also been studied. Of these vitamins, the data from trials investigating vitamin E's impact on CAD are the strongest. In vitro oxidation of LDL is prevent-ed by dietary supplementation with vitamin E, but not beta carotene [177-179]; and two large observational studies published in 1993 added important support for the hy-pothesis that oxidation of lipoproteins plays a role in atherosclerosis and that antioxidants may have a therapeutic effect.[180] These studies, with a combined enroll-ment of more than 120,000, showed that use of vitamin E supplements correlated with reductions in the relative risk of coronary disease in both women[181] and men. [182] Statistical significance was maintained after controlling for coronary risk factors and use of other vitamin supplements, including other antioxidants. In both studies [181,182], the benefit of vitamin E was demonstrated only after supplementation with at least 100 international units/day for two or more years, findings that enhance the credibility that a biological effect was the cause of the reduced events. In another large, prospective study of more than 34,000 postmenopausal women, vitamin E consumption was inversely associated with risk of fatal coronary heart disease, par-ticularly in those subjects who did *not* take dietary supplements.[183] A nonrandom-ized angiographic trial of patients taking at least 100 IU of vitamin E showed signif-icantly less progression of coronary atherosclerotic lesions.[184] Appropriate criticism has been raised regarding the strength of these and other epidemiologic observa-tions, even those carried out prospectively.[185]

A few randomized trials have been performed with conflicting results.[186] One negative study, the Alpha-Tocopherol, Beta Carotene (ATBC) trial, received much attention. This was a large, double-blind study that looked at the effect of low dose vitamin E (50 mg/day), beta carotene (20 mg/day) or both on the incidence of cancer in 29,000 Finnish middle-aged male smokers.[187] The vitamin E arm was cor-related with a slight reduction in CAD. The dose of vitamin E was low, and the preselected end points of the study did not include any cardiovascular events, only cancer.[188] Two subsequent randomized trials published in 1996 have shown positive results. In a placebo-controlled study, vitamin E intake was associated with a reduc-tion in the incidence of angina pectoris.[189] The dose of vitamin E in this study was also small (50 mg/d). Although of short duration, the most convincing study to date is the prospective, placebo-controlled Cambridge Heart Antioxidant Study (CHA-OS) that demonstrated a clinically significant reduction in cardiovascular events in men with coronary disease treated with either 400 or 800 IU/d of vitamin E for a median of 510 days, with benefit apparent after one year of treatment.[190]

The data for vitamin C and for beta carotene are considerably weaker. Caro-tenoid intake or serum level has been inversely correlated with risk of coronary events in prospective, cohort trials.[182,191] And in the placebo-controlled Physicians' Health Study of aspirin and beta carotene, preliminary subgroup analysis of men with CAD before randomization appeared to show reduced coronary events in those taking beta carotene [192]; but at study termination, the effect of beta carotene was no longer evident.[193] Other randomized, double-blind trials of beta carotene supple-mentation have also shown no cardiovascular benefit.[194,195] In the beta carotene arm of the ATBC trial discussed above, not only was no benefit detected but total mortality actually increased slightly due to lung cancer and ischemic heart disease.[187] These findings have been questioned on both statistical and biomedical grounds.[188,196] As for vitamin C, most studies show no impact on coronary heart disease.[181-184] In a study of antioxidants in Linxian, China, combined vitamin E, selenium and beta carotene were associated with reduced total mortality due mostly to lower cancer rates; three other arms of the study, one including vitamin C, showed no significant effects.[197] Other classes of antioxidants such as flavonoids (polyphenols), particularly prevalent in tea, onions, apples and red wine, are also being studied.[198]

Finally, several factors that are thought to be important in the promotion or prevention of atherosclerosis have the expected effect of enhancing or inhibiting LDL oxidation. Enhanced LDL oxidation is caused by elevated glucose[199], smoking[200], and replacement of cholesteryl esters with triglyceride in the LDL core (small, dense LDL).[201,202] Inhibition of LDL oxidation is seen with high HDL levels[51,52,170] and estrogen replacement therapy.[203]

The interrelationships of LDL, antioxidants, vasomotion and atherosclerosis are complex. In vitro studies have shown that oxidized LDL inhibits endothelium-dependent vasomotor function[204], probably by inhibiting the release of nitric oxide (endothelium-derived relaxing factor), which plays a key role in vasodilatation.[107] But one cannot assume that all effects of antioxidants on coronary heart disease relate to oxidation of LDL. In normocholesterolemic chronic smokers [205] and patients with CAD [206], *acute* administration of vitamin C improved endothelium-dependent vasomotor function, suggesting an effect on endothelium rather than the oxidative state of lipids. On the other hand, after prolonged exposure to antioxidants that did reduce LDL oxidation in hypercholesterolemic patients, no impact on endothelial dysfunction could be demonstrated.[207] Adding to the complexity of these investigations are the possibly adverse consequences of too much antioxidant. A study using vessels harvested from hypercholesterolemic rabbits showed that high dose alpha-tocopherol worsened endothelial-dependent vasodilation while a lower dose improved it.[208]

Although the topic of antioxidant modulation of vasomotor dysfunction is of considerable interest, further exploration is beyond the scope of this chapter.

Lipoprotein (a)

Lipoprotein (a) [Lp(a)], is a lipoprotein that was not fully characterized until the 1980's (also see reviews 209-214,148). Lp(a) is an LDL particle with a singular difference: its apolipoprotein is composed of apo B-100 (LDL's sole apolipoprotein) covalently linked by a disulfide bond to a high molecular weight glycoprotein, apolipoprotein (a). Lp(a) is between VLDL and LDL in size, and its density ranges from 1.04 to 1.125 g/ml, a range that includes both LDL and HDL. At this density, Lp(a) sinks and was initially labeled "sinking pre-beta lipoprotein" *(Table 3.1)*. In standard lipid analysis, the cholesterol of Lp(a) is included in the calculated LDL-C. Because Lp(a) is such a complex and heterogeneous lipoprotein and because there are no generally accepted reference standards, quantification can be highly inaccurate. ELISA techniques appear to hold the most promise.[209] Also, long-term storage of blood specimens before measurement of Lp(a) may confound results of such studies; stability of the stored lipoprotein and accuracy in its subsequent measurement reportedly require temperatures below -70° C.

The large range in density of Lp(a) is due to the multiple isoforms of apo(a). The mass ranges from 300 to 800 kDa (compared to apo B-100 with 512 kDa), and there appears to be an inverse relationship between the mass of apo(a) isoforms and plasma concentrations of Lp(a).[210] Apo(a) has extensive homology to plasminogen [216]; and, like plasminogen, has domains of structures called kringles, ring-like regions made up of three polypeptide chains linked by disulfide bridges. Plasminogen contains five different kringles (KI to KV); apo(a) contains one copy of kringle KV but, unlike plasminogen, has multiple copies of KIV. It is the number of KIV units that gives Lp(a) its tremendous heterogeneity. Human apo(a) also contains the protease region of plasminogen but with a single amino acid substitution that causes loss of fibrinolytic activity. In vitro studies show that Lp(a) or apo(a) blocks plasminogen activation by interference with both nonphysiologic (streptokinase) and physiologic (urokinase, tissue-type plasminogen activator) enzymes (reviewed in 209). Moreover, Lp(a) binds to fibrin, t-PA, endothelial and mononuclear cells, and platelets; all are actions that could contribute to the attenuation of plasminogen binding and activation.[217] While these characteristics suggest that Lp(a) can augment atherogenic processes by disrupting clot dissolution, there has also been speculation regarding a possible protective role for Lp(a). Brown and Goldstein have suggested that Lp(a), by binding to fibrin, may assist in delivery of cholesterol to sites requiring tissue repair.[218] In addition, in vitro studies have demonstrated that Lp(a) has proteolytic and autocatalytic activity toward fibronectin and apo B, respectively, which could further promote this process.[209]

Like apo B to which it is eventually attached, apo(a) appears to be synthesized in the liver although the site of assembly of Lp(a) is not known with certainty. However, in transgenic mice expressing human apo(a), Lp(a) is formed in the plasma after infusion of human LDL.[219] The metabolic fate of Lp(a) is unknown but does not appear to depend on the LDL receptor. When labeled Lp(a) is injected into patients with homozygous familial hypercholesterolemia, the fractional catabolic rate appears to be normal.[220] Moreover, Lp(a) levels are not reduced by either statins or resins, both of which up-regulate LDL receptors. Niacin, which works by different mechanisms, appears to be the only lipid-lowering medication that is effective in reducing the levels of Lp(a) [221-223]; although postmenopausal estrogen replacement may also be of benefit. Lp(a) levels have been shown to be negatively correlated with estrogen replacement therapy in nonrandomized studies [224-227]; and two randomized, double-blind, crossover trials showed small but statistically significant decreases in Lp(a) [228,229] leading some investigators to suggest that the decreases in Lp(a) levels caused by estrogen may be one of the hormone's cardioprotective mechanisms.

An individual's Lp(a) level is a highly heritable trait that is remarkably resistant to lifestyle intervention with diet, weight loss and smoking cessation. Diabetes mellitus, on the other hand, may be important in determining levels of Lp(a). Some [230-232], but not all [233], studies have shown that elevated Lp(a) levels in diabetic patients correlate with glycemic control. Likewise, higher Lp(a) levels are associated with microalbuminuria in diabetics in several [234,235], but not all studies.[232] Interestingly, patients with nephrotic syndrome, regardless of etiology, have substantial Lp(a) elevations. With remission of the syndrome, Lp(a) decreases dramatically.[236]

Apo(a) has been localized in atherosclerotic plaque and elevations of Lp(a) have been associated with increased risk of coronary, cerebrovascular and peripheral vascular disease - again, in most[209-215, 237-239], but not all [240,241] investigations. In one study, persistent elevations of Lp(a) were no longer a clinical risk after LDL-C reduction with lovastatin.[242] In transgenic mice, expression of human apo(a) causes an almost 20-fold increase in lipid-containing lesions of the aorta.[243] The causative role of Lp(a) in atherogenesis is by no means settled, however, and recommendations for assessment and management of Lp(a) levels await prospective trials demonstrating the efficacy of intervention.

Small, dense LDL

High plasma triglycerides are often accompanied by increases in small, dense LDL, a potentially atherogenic lipoprotein. In the past LDL particles were thought to be uniform in size and composition, but they are now understood to be heterogeneous and are categorized into subpopulations based on size, density and composition. Small, dense LDL are relatively depleted of cholesteryl ester and, hence, more dense than larger LDL.

Austin et al, using gradient gel electrophoresis, have grouped the LDL subpopulations into two major subclasses.[244] Pattern A is defined as LDL with particle diameters predominantly greater than 25.5 nm and pattern B (small, dense LDL), as LDL with diameters primarily less than 25.5 nm. A third subclass, phenotype I (intermediate), was subsequently added.

Of the general population examined to date, the majority are phenotype A and approximately 30% are phenotype B. Austin et al [244] described a case-control analysis in which small, dense LDL (pattern B) was significantly associated with a three-fold increased risk of myocardial infarction (95% CI, 1.7-5.3). Multivariate logistic regression analysis showed that the risk was independent of some cardiac risk factors: age, sex and body mass index, LDL-C and IDL. However, the addition of HDL to the model reduced the risk to 2.2 (95% CI, 1.2-4.1) and addition of triglycerides further reduced the risk to a non-significant 1.6. Angiographic studies assessing significant stenoses of major coronary arteries, as well as further case-control studies of patients with CHD, continue to show an association between pattern B and CAD, although not an independent one.[148]

Interestingly, a 3.5-year prospective, nested case-control study by Austin et al[245] demonstrated that subjects with a predominance of phenotype B LDL had a more than two-fold risk for developing non-insulin dependent, type II, diabetes mellitus. The authors suggested that some of the excess risk of atherosclerosis in type II diabetes that is not accounted for by conventional risk factors, may be explained by the association with small, dense LDL. Reaven and colleagues examined the relationship between LDL pattern and insulin resistance in 100 healthy, nondiabetic adults.[246] When matched for age, BMI and gender, pattern B subjects were shown to have higher glucose and insulin response to an oral glucose challenge and to be more insulin resistant compared with pattern A or intermediate subjects. They also had higher blood pressures and triglycerides and lower HDL-C. The authors concluded that small, dense LDL particles should be added to the cluster of risk factors for CAD that Reaven originally designated syndrome X.[247]

Two recent prospective studies of small, dense LDL found an association with incidence of CAD.[248,154] In one, a nested case-control cohort from the Physicians' Health Study, small, dense LDL was no longer an independent predictor for risk of a myocardial infarction after adjustment for other lipids and coronary risk factors.[154] The other study, which included women as well as men, concluded that small, dense LDL was a strong, graded and independent predictor of CAD risk after controlling for physiological risk factors.[248] But LDL size was no longer statistically significant after adjusting for the total cholesterol:HDL-C ratio which was the strongest independent predictor. As the accompanying editorial elucidates [249], "independence" can signify either etiologic independence (physiologic autonomy) or statistical independence (predictive autonomy). What is the best independent predictor of disease may not be physiologically independent of other biological risk factors. Given the many metabolic interactions that affect LDL size, the task of teasing out a possible causal role for small, dense LDL will be a difficult one.

Lipids and restenosis after angioplasty

Although restenosis following coronary angioplasty may, to some degree, represent elastic recoil of the dilated vessel, the primary mechanisms involved are believed to be an endothelial response to injury causing thrombogenesis, release of growth factors, and smooth muscle proliferation.[250] Whether lipids influence restenosis is an unresolved issue.[251] Simvastatin and fluvastatin inhibit cell migration and smooth muscle proliferation in vitro and intimal hyperplasia in vivo.[252] In humans, although some studies have suggested that cholesterol lowering is beneficial[253], more recent studies have shown no association between cholesterol levels and restenosis. For example, a large, prospective observational study of 2753 patients and 3336 lesions showed no association between coronary restenosis and hypercholesterolemia, LDL, HDL or their ratio[254]; nor did a much smaller study.[255] More importantly, a randomized, placebo-controlled trial of lovastatin failed to decrease restenosis at six months.[256] Whether there is a correlation with other lipoproteins such as Lp(a) or HDL remains unsettled. [257-263]

Fish oils, which lower triglycerides and modulate other factors believed important in atherogenesis, were thought to prevent restenosis following angioplasty; but one of the largest placebo-controlled trials of moderate doses of omega-3 (N-3) fatty acids failed to decrease angiographically determined restenosis.[264] Coronary restenosis and antioxidants has been another focus of investigation.[265] Treatment with probucol, an antioxidant that also lowers both LDL and HDL cholesterol, has produced conflicting results. In a trial of probucol in 118 patients with average LDL cholesterol levels (mean 130 mg/dl), three month restenosis rates were close to 20% and 40% in the treated group and control groups, respectively.[266] A somewhat larger (239 patients), double-blind trial of combined lovastatin and probucol in patients with LDL cholesterol levels of approximately 140 mg/dl failed to prevent restenosis at six months.[267] The impact of antioxidants on restenosis awaits further study, but any documented benefit may occur via lipid-independent mechanisms, just as lipid-lowering may improve cardiovascular outcome through direct endovascular effect rather than simply decreasing cholesterol deposition.

Lipids and cardiac transplantation

There are several reasons to consider dyslipidemias in cardiac transplantation: 1) Many patients have an underlying lipid disorder that contributed to the coronary disease which necessitated cardiac transplantation and that may once again cause severe disease. 2) Dyslipidemias are a common consequence of immunotherapy and present difficult management decisions in this setting. 3) Lipid disorders may play a role in the accelerated form of coronary vascular disease that affects the majority of post-transplant patients.

Cardiac transplant vasculopathy

Although early mortality in cardiac transplant patients has dramatically improved, coronary artery disease remains the major complication and leading cause of death after the first year.[268] The pathophysiology of the vascular disease encountered in cardiac (and also liver, renal, and heart-lung) transplant patients is different from that of classic CAD.[269] The disease in these patients is rapidly progressive, severe, and diffuse. It involves coronary venules as well as arteries and is referred to variously as *accelerated* atherosclerosis or transplant or allograft vasculopathy to distinguish it from non-transplant atherosclerosis. The major, distinguishing angiographic features of allograft vasculopathy are lesions that are diffuse, concentric, distal and obliterative; branch vessels are affected more than epicardial vessels.[270] It is rarely reported before the first year after transplantation; but its incidence and severity increase inexorably at a rate of approximately 10% per year.[271] Long-term survivors also show focal, asymmetric lesions that are indistinguishable from naturally occurring coronary atherosclerosis.[272]

The pathogenesis of allograft vasculopathy continues to be actively explored. The fundamental mechanism is considered to be a response to endothelial injury[273], the same mechanism believed to cause other forms of atherosclerosis, including the "accelerated atherosclerosis" of restenosis secondary to coronary angioplasty or saphenous vein bypass grafting.[274] In allograft vasculopathy, the primary injury is probably immune-mediated because of the selective involvement of vessels in the transplanted organ with sparing of the host vasculature. Advances in immunosuppressive therapy, however, have not had a major impact on the course of post-transplant vascular disease; and a host of other factors have been advanced to explain the development of accelerated atherosclerosis such as donor and recipient age, donor ischemic time, infection, hyperlipidemia and other classic risk factors for CAD. Most authors conclude that the cause is multifactorial and recommend multi-risk factor intervention. To date, however, the only definitive treatment remains retransplantation.[274]

Causes of dyslipidemia

Hyperlipidemia has been reported in 60% to 80% of patients treated with triple-drug immunosuppression.[274] Immunotherapy is the principal offender, although preexisting lipid abnormalities, particularly in patients whose pre-transplantation diagnosis was ischemic cardiomyopathy, contribute to the frequency of post-transplant dyslipidemias. Studies of patients before and after cardiac transplantation on standard, triple-drug immunosuppression have documented an increase in lipids, primarily plasma total cholesterol and triglyceride levels[275-279], but also LDL and HDL cholesterol levels.[276,277] Lipoprotein (a) levels are decreased.[276]

Both steroids and cyclosporine cause lipid abnormalities in transplant patients (reviewed in 268,280). In nontransplant patients, corticosteroids commonly increase serum triglycerides and cyclosporine increases LDL cholesterol and apo B levels.[281] But hypertriglyceridemia is also common in transplant patients treated with cyclosporine.[268] Reduced hepatic clearance of LDL[282,283], and/or cyclosporine-mediated changes in lipoprotein lipase and hepatic lipase[284] are mechanisms that have been postulated to explain these lipid abnormalities. In spite of continued reports, we have not yet advanced very far beyond stating the obvious: elevations in LDL cholesterol and, to a lesser degree, triglycerides are to be expected in these patients. Some of the reasons for the discrepancies between studies are discussed by Miller and include the lack of control for common variables such as diet and weight gain.[268] Also the usual side effects of corticosteroids, weight gain, insulin resistance and glucose intolerance, invoke a dizzying number of mechanisms that alter lipids.

Is hyperlipidemia an important determinant of atherosclerosis only in long-term survivors of cardiac transplantation or does hyperlipidemia also influence accelerated atherosclerosis? Most pertinent studies and reviews do show a relation between hyperlipidemia and post-transplant atherosclerosis[285-289]; and allograft vasculopathy undoubtedly accounts for much of the disease documented. But to prove that hyperlipidemia causes accelerated atherosclerosis requires *surveillance* angiography or intravascular ultrasonography[290,291] to distinguish transplant vasculopathy from classic atherosclerosis. The investigations that have included such definitive descriptions have identified total and LDL cholesterol levels[270,290,292] and triglycerides[270,290] as significant risk factors for transplant vasculopathy. Moreover, as further advances in immune therapy are made and as additional studies of lipid-lowering therapy document reduced morbidity and mortality (see below), hyperlipidemia in the transplant patient may prove to have an even more powerful impact on vasculopathy than previously thought.

Treatment of hyperlipidemia

Treatment of hyperlipidemia appears to improve the clinical outcome of cardiac transplant patients and to reduce allograft vasculopathy. An important paper recently described serial angiography (or autopsy findings) in an open-label trial of 97 patients randomly and consecutively assigned to receive treatment with pravastatin or not following cardiac transplantation.[293] After one year the cholesterol was 193 ± 36 mg/dl in the treated group and 248 ± 49 in the controls. This intervention significantly lowered the incidence of vasculopathy (6% vs 20%), hemodynamically compromised cardiac rejection (6% vs 28%) and mortality, (6% vs 22%). Intimal thickening, measured by intracoronary ultrasound was also reduced, as was natural-killer-cell cytotoxicity. The difference in mortality was so great that the number needed to treat for one year to save one life was only 17.

Treatment of LDL cholesterol elevation

The safety of bile acid sequestrants (resins) makes them an appealing choice, but resins are problematic in patients on a multidose regimens because they interfere with absorption of many other medications, including cyclosporine.[277] On the other hand, if other medications are given at least one hour before or four hours after the resin, no interaction should be anticipated. However, such a schedule would require almost superhuman patient compliance; and, because LDL elevations are so often severe, most clinicians turn to statins. Their use deserves special attention given that concomitant treatment with cyclosporine significantly increases the incidence of myositis and rhabdomyolysis leading to renal failure.[294-296] These reports of severe side effects were published soon after the first statin (lovastatin) was approved and very high doses were used. Most patients were also taking medications that compound the risk of myositis when given with lovastatin (gemfibrozil, niacin and erythromycin). Since that time, studies of cardiac transplant patients on double- or triple-drug immunosuppressive therapy, including cyclosporine, have documented the safety and efficacy of lovastatin and other statins.[277,297-299] Cyclosporine is now understood to increase serum concentrations of the statins, and most authorities advocate a maximal statin dose of 20 mg/day [300], with close monitoring of transaminase and creatine kinase levels; acceptable elevations are 3 times and 10 times the upper limit of normal, respectively.

Treatment of elevated triglycerides

Although cholesterol elevations are more common, hypertriglyceridemia is not rare, particularly if high steroid doses are used. Therapy with gemfibrozil is safe and efficacious in the cardiac transplant patient[277], as is bezafibrate.[299,301] Both fibrates lower triglycerides and raise HDL cholesterol, but bezafibrate also has LDL- and apo B-lowering effects.[299,301] The major precaution for gemfibrozil (and possibly bezafibrate) is its administration with a statin as discussed above.

Niacin is a useful drug in patients with high triglycerides and has the advantage of lowering LDL and raising HDL; but its side effects of hepatotoxicity, exacerbation of peptic ulcer disease, glucose intolerance and uric acid elevations overlap with the side effects of cyclosporine and glucocorticoids, making niacin a poor choice for transplant patients. If statins are also prescribed caution is again necessary because of the increased incidence of myositis.

Treatment with omega-3 polyunsaturated fatty acids (fish oils) is a safe alternative and has no significant harmful side effects or medication interactions. In cardiac transplant recipients they lower triglycerides as well as bezafibrate [301] at a relatively modest dose of 10 g/day and one study showed inhibition of allograft vasculopathy.[302] Fish oils may also have immunosuppressive, antiinflammatory, antihypertensive, antithrombotic and other antiatherosclerotic effects.[303-308] Most recently, n-3 fatty acids were documented to have antiarrhythmic effects.[309,310]

Lipids and cardiovascular disease in women and the elderly

Questions often arise regarding the risks attending hyperlipidemia in two large groups of subjects: women and the elderly. While this subject deserves extensive review (see 311), brief mention will be made of some recent findings.

Women lag approximately ten years behind men in their incidence of CAD, unless they have diabetes which abolishes women's gender advantage.[312-314] The Framingham data provide strong evidence that a woman's risk of CAD rises both with increasing age and hypercholesterolemia. In regression trials that have included women in sufficient numbers[85,315,316] cardiovascular events were significantly reduced in women as well as men. Moreover, recent clinical trials with statins such as 4S and CARE have now shown that statistically and clinically significant reductions in coronary events can be achieved in women when cholesterol levels are reduced.[75,77] Finally, results from the CARE trial suggest that in patients with mildly elevated LDL cholesterol levels, cholesterol lowering benefited women more than men.[77]

Oral estrogens may be considered for treatment of hypercholesterolemia in post menopausal women.[79] Estrogens lower LDL cholesterol, raise HDL cholesterol and triglycerides and, as discussed earlier, reduce Lp(a) and LDL oxidation. Estrogen replacement in women at risk for CAD is particularly attractive given the overwhelming number of epidemiological studies showing that women who use estrogens are less likely to develop CAD than those who do not.[137-141] The addition of a progestin substantially reduces the lipid effects of estrogens[136] but does not appear to attenuate cardioprotective effects.[139,317] Much of the vascular benefit of estrogen is independent of the lipid effects.[318-322]

There is less agreement as to whether elderly subjects with elevated cholesterol levels are at increased risk for CAD.[323-329] In some studies, though by no means all, the advancing age of a population appears to weaken the impact of total and LDL cholesterol levels on the risk of coronary events. One possible explanation is confounding due to comorbid disease which lowers cholesterol levels at a late age. A low HDL-C in a healthy older adult may prove to be the best marker of assessing increased risk for CHD.[330,331] Although the controversy will be more firmly settled with the results of ongoing randomized clinical trials, it is already apparent from the 4S[75] and CARE[77] trials and the pooled analysis[316] that the benefit for those over 60 to 65 is comparable to that for younger subjects.

REFERENCES

1. Dammerman M, Breslow JL. Genetic basis for lipoprotein disorders. Circulation 1995;91:505-12.

2. Rader DJ, Hoeg JM, Brewer Jr HB. Quantitation of plasma apolipoproteins in the primary and secondary prevention of coronary artery disease. Ann Intern Med 1994;120:1012-25.

3. Ginsberg HN. Lipoprotein metabolism and its relationship to atherosclerosis. In Lipid Disorders. Medical Clinics of North America, WB Saunders Co Philadelphia 1994;78:1.

4. Havel RJ and Kane JP. Structure and metabolism of plasma lipoproteins in Scriver CR, Beaudet AL, Sly WS, Valle D, Stanbury JB, Wyngaarden JB, Fredrickson DS, eds. The Metabolic and Molecular Bases of Inherited Disease. McGraw-Hill, New York, 1995.

5. Young SG. Recent progress in understanding apolipoprotein B. Circulation 1990;82:1574.

6. Brunzell JD. Familial lipoprotein lipase deficiency and other causes of the chylomicron syndrome. In: Scriver CR, Beaudet, AL, Sly WS, Valle D, Stanbury JB, Wyngaarden JB, Fredrickson DS, eds. The Metabolic and Molecular Bases of Inherited Disease. McGraw-Hill, New York, 1995;p 1913.

7. Weintraub MS, et al. Clearance of chylomicron remnants in normolipidaemic patients with coronary artery disease: case control study over three years. BMJ 1996;312:935.

8. Kowal RC, et al. Low density lipoprotein receptor-related protein mediates uptake of cholesterol esters derived from apolipoprotein E-enriched lipoproteins. Proc Natl Acad Sci USA 1989;86:5810.

9. Breslow JL. Transgenic mouse models of lipoprotein metabolism and atherosclerosis. Proc Natl Acad Sci 1993;90:8314.

10. Brown MS, Goldstein JL. Koch's postulates for cholesterol. Cell 1992;71:187.

11. Ishibashi S, et al. The two-receptor model of lipoprotein clearance: tests of the hypothesis in "knockout" mice lacking the low density lipoprotein receptor, apolipoprotein E, or both proteins. Proc Natl Acad Sci 1994;91:4431.

12. Chait A, Brunzell JD. Chylomicronemia syndrome. In Advances in Internal Medicine 1991;37:249.

13. Ginsberg HN, et al. Apolipoprotein B metabolism in subjects with deficiency of apolipoprotein CIII and AI. Evidence that apolipoprotein CIII inhibits catabolism of triglyceride-rich lipoproteins by lipoprotein lipase in vivo. J Clin Invest 1986;78:1287.

14. Mahley RW. Apolipoprotein E: cholesterol transport protein with expanding role in cell biology. Science 1988;240:622.

15. Davignon J, Gregg RE, Sing CF. Apolipoprotein E polymorphism and atherosclerosis. Arteriosclerosis 1988;8:1.

16. Plumb AS, et al. Severe hypercholesterolemia and atherosclerosis in apolipoprotein E-deficient mice created by homologous recombination in ES cells. Cell 1992;71:343.

17. Zhang SH, et al. Spotaneous hypercholesterolemia and arterial lesions in mice lacking apo-lipoprotein E. Science 1992;258:468.

18. Nakashima Y, et al. ApoE-deficient mice develop lesions of all phases of atherosclerosis throughout the arterial tree. Arterioscler Thromb 1994;14:133.

19. Reddick RL, Zhang SH, Maeda N. Atherosclerosis in mice lacking apo E. Evaluation of lesional development and progression. Arterioscler Thromb 1994;14:141.

20. Paszty C, et al. Apolipoprotein A1 transgene corrects apolipoprotein E deficiency-induced atherosclerosis in mice. J Clin Invest 1994;94:899.

21. Mahley RW and Rall SC Jr. Type III hyperlipoproteinemia (dysbetalipoproteinemia): the role of apolipoprotein E in normal and abnormal metabolism. In Scriver CR, Beaudet AL, Sly WS, Valle D, Stanbury JB, Wyngaarden JB, Fredrickson DS, eds. The Metabolic and Molecular Bases of Inherited Disease. McGraw-Hill, New York, 1995.

22. Mahley RW, et al. Genetic defects in lipoprotein metabolism. Elevation of atherogenic lipo-proteins caused by impaired catabolism. JAMA 1991;265:78.

23. Roses AD. Apolipoprotein E alleles as risk factors in Alzheimer's disease. Annu Rev Med 1996;47:387.

24. Hardy J. Apolipoprotein E in the genetics and epidemiology of Alzheimer's disease. Am J Med Genet 1995;60:456.

25. American College of Medical Genetics/American Society of Human Genetics Working Group on Apo E and Alzheimer Disease. Statement on use of apolipoprotein E testing for Alzhe-imer disease. JAMA 1995;274:1627.

26. National Institute on Aging/Alzheimer's Association Working Group. Apolipoprotein E geno-typing in Alheimer's disese. Lancet 1996;347:1091.

27. Goldstein JL, et al. Binding site on macrophages that mediate uptake and degradation of acetylated low density lipoprotein, producing massive cholesterol deposition. Proc Nat Acad Sci 1979;76:333.

28. Goldstein JL, Hobbs HH, Brown MS. Familial hypercholesterolemia. In Scriver CR, Beaudet AL, Sly WS, Valle D, Stanbury JB, Wyngaarden JB, Fredrickson DS, eds. The Metabolic and Molecular Bases of Inherited Disease. McGraw-Hill, New York, 1995.

29. Vega GL and Grundy SM. In vivo evidence for reduced binding of low density lipoproteins to receptors as a cause of primary moderate hypercholesterolemia. J Clin Invest 1986;78:1410.

30. Innerarity TL, et al. Familial defective apolipoprotein B-100: low density lipoproteins with abnormal receptor binding. Proc Natl Acad Sci 1987;84:6919.

31. Rauh G, et al. Familial defective apolipoprotein B100: clinical characteristics of 54 cases. Atherosclerosis 1992;92:233.

32. Tybaerg-Hansen A, Humphries SE. Familial defective apolipoprotein B-100: a single muta-tion that causes hypercholesterolemia and premature coronary artery disease. Atherosclero-sis 1992;96:91.

33. Myant NB. Familial defective apolipoprotein B-100: a review, including some comparisons with familial hypercholesterolemia. Atherosclerosis 1993;104:1.

34. Kane JP and Havel RJ. Disorders of the biogenesis and secretion of lipoproteins containing the B apolipoproteins. In Scriver CR, Beaudet, AL, Sly WS, Valle D, Stanbury JB, Wyn-gaarden JB, Fredrickson DS, eds. The Metabolic and Molecular Bases of Inherited Disease. McGraw-Hill, New York, 1995.

35. Bersot TP, et al. A unique haplotype of the apolipoprotein B-100 allele associated with famil-ial defective apolipoprotein B-100 in a Chinese man discovered during a study of the preva-lence of this disorder. J Lipid Res 1993;34:1149.

36. Soria LF, et al. Association between a specific apolipoprotein B mutation and familial defec-tive apolipoprotein B-100. Proc Natl Acad Sci 1989;86:587.

37. McCarthy BJ, et al. An arginine^{3500}–glutamine mutation in familial defective apo-B100 sub-jects with LDL defective in binding to the apo-B,E(LDL) receptor. Circulation 1988;78,II-166 (abstract).

38. März W, et al. Familial defective apolipoprotein B-100: mild hypercholesterolemia without atherosclerosis in a homozygous patient. Lancet 1992;340:1362.

39. Defesche JC, et al. Familial defective apolipoprotein B-100 is clinically indistinguishable from familial hypercholesterolemia. Arch Intern Med 1993;153:2349.

40. Brown MS and Goldstein JL. Scavenging for receptors. Nature 1990;343:508.

41. Kodama T, Freeman M, et al. Type I macrophage scavenger contains α-helical and collagen-like coiled coils. Nature 1990;343:531.

42. Rohrer L, et al. Coiled-coil fibrous domains mediate ligand binding by macrophage scavenger receptor type II. Nature 1990;343:570.

43. Breslow JL. Familial Disorders of High-Density Lipoprotein Metabolism. In Scriver CR, Beaudet AL, Sly WS, Valle D, Stanbury JB, Wyngaarden JB, Fredrickson DS, eds. The Metabolic and Molecular Bases of Inherited Disease. McGraw-Hill, New York, 1995.

44. Silverman DI and Pasternak RC. High-density lipoprotein subfractions. Am J Med 1993;94:636.

45. Rubin EM, et al. Inhibition of early atherogenesis in transgenic mice by human apolipoprotein AI. Nature 1991;353:265.

46. Schultz JR, et al. Protein composition determines th anti-atherogenic properties of HDL in transgenic mice. Nature 1993;265:762.

47. Warden CH, et al. Atherosclerosis in transgenic mice overexpressing apolipoprotein A-II. Science 1993;261:469.

48. Li H, Reddick RL, Maeda N. Lack of apoA-I is not associated with increased susceptibility to atherosclerosis in mice. Arterioscler Thromb 1993;13:1814.

49. Acton S, et al. Identification of scavenger receptor SR-BI as a high density lipoprotein receptor. Science 1996;271:518.

50. Steinberg D. A docking receptor for HDL cholesterol esters. Science 1996;271:460.

51. Parthasarathy S, Barnett J, Fong LG. High-density lipoprotein inhibits the oxidative modification of low-density lipoprotein. Biochim Biophys Acta 1990;1044:275.

52. Khoo JC, et al. Prevention of low density lipoprotein aggregation by high density lipoprotein or apolipoprotein A-1. J Lipid Res 1990;31:645.

53. Steinberg D, et al. Beyond cholesterol. Modifications of low-density lipoprotein that increase its atherogenicity. N Engl J Med 1989;320:915.

54. Hoeg JM. Can genes prevent atherosclerosis? JAMA 1996;276:989.

55. Armstrong ML, Megan MB. Lipid depletion in atheromatous coronary arteries in rhesus monkeys after regression diets. Circ Res 1972;30:675.

56. Ross R. The pathogenesis of atherosclerosis: an update. N Engl J Med 1986;314:488.

57. Keys A. Coronary heart disease in seven countries. Circulation 1970; 41(suppl I):I-199.

58. Wilson PWF. The epidemiology of hypercholesterolemia. A global perspective. Am J Med 1989;87(suppl 4A):5S.

59. Verschuren WMM, et al. Serum total cholesterol and long-term coronary heart disease mortality in different cultures. Twenty-five-year follow-up of the Seven Countries Study. JAMA 1995;274:131.

60. Robertson TL, et al. Epidemiologic studies of coronary heart disease and stroke in Japanese men living in Japan, Hawaii and California. Am J Cardiol 1977;39:244.

61. Kannel WB, et al. Serum cholesterol, lipoproteins and risk of coronary heart disease. Ann Intern Med 1971;74:1.

62. Anderson KM, Castelli WP, Levy D. Cholesterol and mortality: 30 years of follow-up from the Framingham Study. JAMA 1989;257:2176.

63. Kannel WB. Contribution of the Framingham Study to preventive cardiology. J Am Coll Cardiol 1990;15:206.

64. Castelli WP. Epidemiology of triglycerides: A view from Framingham. Am J Cardiol 1992;70:3H.

65. Pekkanen J, et al. Ten-year mortality from cardiovascular disease in relation to cholesterol level among men with and without preexisting cardiovascular disease. N Engl J Med 1990;322:1700.

66. Stamler J, Wentworth D, Neaton JD. Is relationship between serum cholesterol and risk of premature death from coronary heart disease continuous and graded? JAMA 1986;256:2823.

67. Multiple Risk Factor Intervention Trial Research Group. Mortality rates after 10.5 years for participants Multiple Risk Factor Intervention Trial. JAMA 1990;263:1795.

68. The Lipid Research Clinics Program. The Lipid Research Clinics Coronary Primary Prevention Trial results. I. Reduction in incidence of coronary heart disease. JAMA 1984;251:351.

69. Frick MH, et al. Helsinki Heart Study: Primary-prevention trial with gemfibrozil in middle-aged men with dyslipidemia. Safety of treatment, changes in risk factors, and incidence of coronary heart disease. N Engl J Med 1987;317:1237.

70. Davis CE, et al. A single cholesterol measurement underestimates the risk of coronary heart disease: an empirical example from the Lipid Research Clinics mortality follow-up study. JAMA 1990;264:3044.

71. National Cholesterol Education Program. Report of the Expert Panel on Population Strategies for Blood Cholesterol Reduction. Circulation 1991;83:2154.

72. Law MR, Wald NJ, Thompson SG. By how much and how quickly does reduction in serum cholesterol concentration lower risk of ischaemic heart disease? BMJ 1994;308:367.

73. Davey Smith G, Pekkanen J. Should there be a moratorium on the use of cholesterol lowering drugs? BMJ 1992;304:431.

74. Oliver MF. Doubts about preventing coronary heart disease. Multiple interventions in middle aged men may do more harm than good. BMJ 1992;304:393.

75. Randomized trial of cholesterol lowering in 4444 patients with coronary heart disease: the Scandinavian Simvastatin Survival Study (4S). Lancet 1994;344;1383.

76. Shepherd J, et al. for the West of Scotland Coronary Prevention Study Group. Prevention of coronary heart disease with pravastatin in men with hypercholesterolemia. N Engl J Med 1995;333:1301.

77. Sacks FM, et al. for the Cholesterol and Recurrent Events Trial Investigators. The effect of pravastatin on coronary events after myocardial infarction in patients with average cholesterol levels. N Engl J Med 1996;335:1001.

78. Scandinavian Simvastatin Survival Study Group. Baseline serum cholesterol and treatment effect in the Scandinavian Simvastatin Survival Study (4S). Lancet 1995;345:1274.

79. Summary of the second report of the National Cholesterol Education Program (NCEP) Expert Panel on Detection, Evaluation, and Treatment of High Blood Cholesterol in Adults (Adult Treatment Panel II). JAMA 1993;269:3015.

80. Guidelines for using serum cholesterol, high-density lipoprotein cholesterol, and triglyceride levels as screening tests for preventing coronary heart disease in adults. Ann Intern Med 1996;124:515.

81. Garber AM, Browner WS, Hulley SB. Cholesterol screening in asymptomatic adults, revisited. Ann Intern Med 1996;124:518.

82. Ornish D, et al. Can lifestyle changes reverse coronary heart disease? The Lifestyle Heart Trial. Lancet 1990;336:129.

83. Schuler G, et al. Regular physical exercise and low-fat diet. Effect on progression of coronary artery disease. Circulation 1992;86:1.

84. Watts GF, Lewis B, Brunt JNH. Effects on coronary artery disease of lipid-lowering diet, or diet plus cholestyramine, in the St. Thomas' Atherosclerosis Regression Study (STARS). Lancet 1992;339:563.

85. Buchwald H, et al and the POSCH Group. Effect of partial ileal bypass surgery on mortality and morbidity from coronary heart disease in patients with hypercholesterolemia. N Engl J Med 1990;323:946.

86. Jukema JW, et al on behalf of the REGRESS Study Group. Effects of lipid lowering by pravastatin on progression and regression of coronary artery disease in symptomatic men with normal to moderately elevated cholesterol levels. The Regression Growth Evaluation Statin Study (REGRESS). Circulation 1995;91:2528.

87. Rossouw JE. Lipid-lowering interventions in angiographic trials. Am J Cardiol 1995;76:86C.

88. Gotto AM Jr. Lipid lowering, regression, and coronary events. A review of the interdisciplinary council on lipids and cardiovascular risk intervention, seventh council meeting. Circulation 1995;92:646.

89. Stewart BF, et al. Benefits of lipid-lowering therapy in men with elevated apolipoprotein B are not confined to those with very high low density lipoprotein cholesterol. J Am Coll Cardiol 1994;23:899.

90. Brown BG, et al. Regression of coronary artery disease as a result of intensive lipid-lowering therapy in men with high levels of apolipoprotein B. N Engl J Med 1990;323:1289.

91. Sacks FM, et al. for the Harvard Atherosclerosis Reversibility Project (HARP). Effect on coronary atherosclerosis of decrease in plasma cholesterol concentrations in normocholesterolemic patients. Lancet 1994;344:1182.

92. Brown BG, et al. What benefit can be derived from treating normocholesterolemic patients with coronary artery disease? Am J Cardiol 1995;76:93C.

93. Sacks FM, et al. The Project Research Group. Am J Cardiol 1995;76:78C.

94. Hong MK, et al. Limitations of angiography for analyzing coronary atherosclerosis progression and regression. Ann Intern Med 1994;121:348.

95. Brown BG, et al. Regression of atherosclerosis. Does it occur and does it have clinical meaning? Eur Heart J 1995;16:E2.

96. Fuster V, Badimon JJ. Regression or stabilization of atherosclerosis means regression or stabilization of what we don't see in the arteriogram. Eur Heart J 1995;16:E6.

97. Small DM. Progression and regression of atherosclerotic lesions. Insights from lipid physical biochemistry. Arteriosclerosis 1988;8:103.

98. Gould KL, et al. Short-term cholesterol lowering decreases size and severity of perfusion abnormalities by positron emission tomography after dipyridamole in patients with coronary artery disease. A potential noninvasive marker of healing coronary endothelium. Circulation 1994;89:1530.

99. The Pravastatin Multinational Study Group for Cardiac Risk Patients. Effects of pravastatin in patients with serum cholesterol levels from 5.2 to 7.8 mmol/liter (200 to 300) plus two additional atherosclerotic risk factors. Am J Cardiol 1993;72:1031.

100. Waters D. Plaque stabilization: a mechanism for the beneficial effect of lipid-lowering therapies in angiography studies. Prog Cardiovasc Dis 1994;37:107.

101. Levine GN, Keaney JF, Jr, Vita JA. Cholesterol reduction in cardiovascular disease. N Engl J Med 1995;332:512.

102. Brown BG, et al. Lipid lowering and plaque regression. New insights into prevention of plaque disruption and clinical events in coronary disease. Circulation 1993;87:1781.

103. MacIsaac AI, Thomas JD, Topol EJ. Toward the quiescent coronary plaque. J Am Coll Cardiol 1993;22:1228.

104. Falk E, Shah PK, Fuster V. Coronary plaque disruption. Circulation 1995:92:657.

105. Fuster V. Elucidation of the role of plaque instability and rupture in acute coronary events. Am J Cardiol 1995;76:24C.

106. Lacoste L, et al. Hyperlipidemia and coronary disease. Correction of the increased thrombogenic potential with cholesterol reduction. Circulation 1995;92:3172.

107. Flavahan NA. Atherosclerosis or lipid-induced endothelial dysfunction. Potential mechanisms underlying reduction in EDRF/nitric oxide activity. Circulation 1992;85:1927.

108. Leung WH, Lau CP, Wong CK. Beneficial effect of cholesterol-lowering therapy on coronary endothelium-dependent relaxation in hypercholesterolaemic patients. Lancet 1993;341:1496.

109. Seiler C, et al. Influence of serum cholesterol and other coronary risk factors on vasomotion of angiographically normal coronary arteries. Circulation 1993;88:2139.

110. Egashira K, et al. Reduction of serum cholesterol with pravastatin improves endothelium-dependent coronary vasomotion in patients with hypercholesterolemia. Circulation 1994;89:2519.

111. Treasure CB, et al. Beneficial effects of cholesterol-lowering therapy on the coronary endothelium in patients with coronary artery disease. N Engl J Med 1995;332:481.

112. Anderson TJ, et al. The effect of cholesterol-lowering and antioxidant therapy on endothelium-dependent coronary vasomotion. N Engl J Med 1995;332:488.

113. Vogel RA, Corretti MC, Plotnick GD. Changes in flow-mediated brachial artery vasoactivity with lowering of desirable cholesterol levels in healthy middle-aged men. Am J Cardiol 1996;77:37.

114. Henry PD. Hyperlipidemic arterial dysfunction. Circulation 1990;81:697.

115. Casino PR, Kilcoyne CM, et al. The role of nitric oxide in endothelium-dependent vasodilation of hypercholesterolemic patients. Circulation 1993;88:2541.

116. Vaughan CJ, Murphy MB, Buckley BM. Statins do more than just lower cholesterol. Lancet 1996;348:1079.

117. Heistad DD, Armstrong ML. Sick vessel syndrome. Can atherosclerotic arteries recover. Circulaton 1994;89:2447.

118. Brown BG, Maher VMG. Reversal of coronary heart disease by lipid-lowering therapy. Observations and pathological mechanisms. Circulation 1994;89:2928.

119. Bronner LL, Kanter DS, Manson JE. Primary prevention of stroke. N Engl J Med 1995;333:1392.

120. Blankenhorn DH, et al. Beneficial effects of colestipol-niacin therapy on the common carotid artery. Two- and four-year reduction of intima-media thickness measured by ultrasound. Circulation 1993;88:20.

121. Furberg CD, et al. for the Asymptomatic Carotid Artery Progression Study (ACAPS) Research Group. Effect of lovastatin on early carotid atherosclerosis and cardiovascular events. Circulation 1994;90:1679.

122. Crouse JR, et al. Pravastatin, lipids, and atherosclerosis in carotid arteries (PLAC-II). Am J Cardiol 1995;75:455.

123. Salonen R, et al. Kuopio Atherosclerosis Prevention Study (KAPS). A population-based primary prevention trial of the effect of LDL lowering on atherosclerotic progression in carotid and femoral arteries. Circulation 1995;92:1758.

124. Hodis HN, et al. Reduction in carotid arterial wall thickness using lovastatin and dietary therapy. A randomized, controlled clinical trial. Ann Intern Med 1996;124:548.

125. Blankenhorn DH, et al. Effects of colestipol-niacin therapy on human femoral atherosclerosis. Circulation 1991;83:438-47. See also editorial comment: Olsson AG. Regression of femoral atherosclerosis. Circulation 1991;83:698.

126. Hebert PR, Gaziano JM, Hennekens CH. An overview of trials of cholesterol lowering and risk of stroke. Arch Intern Med 1995;155:50.

126a. Bucher HC, Griffith LE, Gyatt GH. Effect of HMGcoA reductase inhibitors on stroke. A meta-analysis of randomized-controlled trials. Ann Intern Med 1998;128:89.

127. Gordon T, et al. High density lipoprotein as a protective factor against coronary heart disease. Am J Med 1977;62:707.

128. Castelli WP, et al. Incidence of coronary heart disease and lipoprotein cholesterol levels. The Framingham Study. JAMA 1986;256:2835.

129. Kannel WB, Castelli WP, Gordon T. Cholesterol in the prediction of atherosclerotic disease. New perspectives in the Framingham Study. Ann Intern Med 1979;90:85.

130. Manninen V, et al. Lipoprotein alterations and decline in the incidence of coronary heart disease in the Helsinki Heart Study. JAMA 1988;260:641.

131. Buring JE, et al. Decreased HDL_2 and HDL_3 cholesterol, apo A-I and apo A-II, and increased risk of myocardial infarction. Circulation 1992;85:22.

132. Reinhart RA, et al. Apolipoprotein A-I and B as predictors of angiographically defined coronary artery disease. Arch Intern Med 1990;150:1629.

133. Stampfer MJ, et al. A prospective study of cholesterol, apolipoproteins, and the risk of mycardial infarction. N Engl J Med 1991;325:373.

134. Kannel WB. Low high-density lipoprotein cholesterol and what to do about it. Am J Cardiol 1992;70:810.

135. Gaziano JM, et al. Moderate alcohol intake, increased levels of high-density lipoprotein and its subfractions, and decreased risk of myocardial infarction. N Engl J Med 1993;329:1829.

136. The Writing Group for the PEPI Trial. Effects of estrogen or estrogen/progestin regimens on heart disease risk factors in postmenopausal women: the Postmenopausal Estrogen/Progestin Interventions (PEPI) trial. JAMA 1995;273:199.

137. Psaty BM, et al. A review of the association of estrogens and progestins with cardiovascular disease in postmenopausal women. Arch Intern Med 1993;153:1421.

138. Manson JE. Postmenopausal hormone therapy and atherosclerotic disease. Am Heart J 1994;128:1337.

139. Grodstein F, Stampfer MJ. The epidemiology of coronary heart disease and estrogen replacement in postmenopausal women. Prog Cardiovasc Dis 1995;38:199.

140. Ettinger B, et al. Reduced mortality associated with long-term postmenopausal estrogen therapy. Obstet Gynecol 1996;87:6.

141. Moerman CJ, et al. for the Working Group on Women and Cardiovascular Disease of the Netherlands Heart Foundation. Eur Heart J 1996;17:658.

142. The Expert Panel. Report of the National Cholesterol Education Program Panel on Detection, Evaluation and Treatment of High Blood Cholesterol in Adults. Arch Intern Med 1988;148:36.

143. Sacks FM. Desirable serum total cholesterol with low HDL cholesterol level. An undesirable situation in coronary heart disease. Circulation 1992;86:1341.

144. Ericsson C-G, et al. Angiographic assessment of effects of bezafibrate on progression of coronary artery disease in young male postinfarction patients. Lancet 1996;347:849.

145. Hulley SB, et al. Epidemiology as a guide to clinical decisions. The association between triglycerides and coronary heart disease. N Engl J Med 1980;302:1383.

146. Austin MA. Plasma triglyceride and coronary heart disease. Arterioscler Thromb 1991;11:2.

147. Austin MA, et al. The hypertriglyceridemias: risk and management. 5. Epidemiology. Am J Cardiol 1991;68:1A.

148. Austin MA, Hokanson JE. Epidemiology of triglycerides, small dense low-density lipoprotein, and lipoprotein (a) as risk factors for coronary heart disease. In Lipid Disorders. The Medical Clinics of North America 1994;78:99.

149. Wilson PWF, et al. Twelve-year incidence of coronary heart disease in middle-aged adults during the era of hypertensive therapy: The Framingham Offspring Study. Am J Med 1991;90:11.

150. Assmann G, Schulte H. Relation of high-density lipoprotein cholesterol and triglycerides to incidence of atherosclerotic coronary artery disease (the PROCAM experience). Am J Cardiol 1992;70:733.

151. Criqui MH, et al. Plasma triglycerides level and mortality from coronary heart disease. N Engl J Med 1993;328:1220.

152. Menotti A, Scanga M, Morisi G. Serum triglycerides in the prediction of coronary artery disease (an Italian experience). Am J Cardiol 1994;73:29.

153. Bainton D, et al. Plasma triglyceride and high density lipoprotein cholesterol as predictors of ischaemic heart disease in British men. The Caerphilly and Speedwell Collaborative Disease Studies. Br Heart J 1992;68:60.

154. Stampfer MJ, et al. A prospective study of triglyceride level, low-density lipoprotein particle diameter, and risk of myocardial infarction. JAMA 1996;276:882.

155. Assmann G, Schulte H, von Eckardstein A. Hypertriglyceridemia and elevated lipoprotein(a) are risk factors for major coronary events in middle-aged men. Am J Cardiol 1996;77:1179.

156. Benlian P, et al. Premature atherosclerosis in patients with familial chylomicronemia caused by mutations in the lipoprotein lipase gene. N Engl J Med 1996;335:848.

157. Castelli WP. The triglyceride issue: a view from Framingham. Am Heart J 1986;112:432.

158. Manninen V, et al. Joint effects of serum triglyceride and LDL cholesterol and HDL cholesterol concentrations on coronary heart disease risk in the Helsinki Heart Study. Circulation 1992;85:37.

159. Austin MA. Joint lipid risk factors and coronary heart disease. Circulation 1992;85:365.

160. Reaven GM. Are triglycerides important as a risk factor for coronary disease? Heart Disease Stroke 1993;2:44.

161. Steinberg D, Witztum JL. Lipoproteins and atherogenesis. Current concepts. JAMA 1990;264:3047.

162. Parthasarathy S, Steinberg D, Witztum JL. The role of oxidized low-density lipoproteins in the pathogenesis of atherosclerosis. Annu Rev Med 1992;43:219.

163. Leake DS. Oxidised low density lipoproteins and atherogenesis. Br Heart J 1993;69:476.

164. Witztum JL. Role of oxidised low density lipoprotein in atherogenesis. Br Heart J 1993;69:S12.

165. Steinberg D, et al. Beyond cholesterol. Modifications of low-density lipoprotein that increase its atherogenicity. N Engl J Med 1989;320:915.

166. Witztum JL, Steinberg D. Role of oxidized low density lipoprotein in atherogenesis. J Clin Invest 1991;88:1785.

167. Witztum JL. The oxidation hypothesis of atherosclerosis. Lancet 1994;344:793.

168. Navab M, et al. The yin and yang of oxidation in the development of the fatty streak. A review based on the 1994 George Lyman Duff Memorial Lecture. Arterioscler Thromb Vasc Biol 1996;16:831.

169. Yla-Herttuala S, et al. Lipoproteins in normal and atherosclerotic aorta. Eur Heart J 1990;11:E88.

170. Navab M, et al. Monocyte transmigration induced by modification of low density lipoprotein in cocultures of human aortic wall cells is due to induction of monocyte chemotactic protein 1 synthesis and is abolished by high density lipoprotein. J Clin Invest 1991;88:2039.

171. Steinberg D and Workshop Participants. Antioxidants in the prevention of human atherosclerosis. Summary of the Proceedings of a National Heart, Lung, and Blood Institute Workshop: September 5-6, 1991, Bethesda, Maryland. Circulation 1992;85:2338.

172. Parthasarathy S, et al. Probucol inhibits oxidative modification of low density lipoprotein. J Clin Invest 1986;77:641.

173. Carew TE, Schwenke DC, Steinberg D. Antiathergenic effect of probucol unrelated to its hypocholesterolemic effect: evidence that antioxidants *in vivo* can selectively inhibit low density lipoprotein degradation in macrophage-rich fatty streaks and slow progression of atherosclerosis in the Watanabe heritable hyperlipidemic rabbit. Proc Nat Acad Sci 1987;84:7725.

174. Yamamoto A, et al. Effects of probucol on homozygous cases of familial hypercholesterolemia. Atherosclerosis 1983;48:157.

175. Yamamoto A, et al. Effects of probucol on xanthoma regression in familial hypercholesterolemia. Am J Cardiol 1986;57:29H.

176. Walldius G, et al. The effect of probucol on femoral atherosclerosis: the Probucol Quantitative Regression Swedish Trial (PQRST). Am J Cardiol 1994;74:875.

177. Reaven PD, et al. Effect of dietary antioxidant combinations in humans. Protection of LDL by vitamin E but not by β-carotene. Arteriosclerosis and Thrombosis 1993;13:590.

178. Jialal I, Grundy SM. Effect of combined supplementation with a-tocopherol, ascorbate, and beta carotene on low-density lipoprotein oxidation. Circulation 1993;88:2780.

179. Gaziano JM, et al. Supplementation with beta-carotene in vivo and in vitro does not inhibit low density lipoprotein oxidation. Atherosclerosis 1995;112:187.

180. Steinberg D. Antioxidant vitamins and coronary heart disease. N Engl J Med 1993;328:1487.

181. Stampfer MJ, et al. Vitamin E consumption and the risk of coronary disease in women. N Engl J Med 1993;328:1444.

182. Rimm EB, et al. Vitamin E consumption and the risk of coronary heart disease in men. N Engl J Med 1993:328:1450.

183. Kushi LH, et al. Dietary antioxidant vitamins and death from coronary heart disease in postmenopausal women. N Engl J Med 1996;334:1156.

184. Hodis HN, et al. Serial coronary angiographic evidence that antioxidant vitamin intake reduces progression of coronary artery atherosclerosis. JAMA 1995;273:1849.

185. Jha P, et al. The antioxidant vitamins and cardiovascular disease. Ann Intern Med 1995;123:860.

186. Hoffman RM, Garewall HS. Antioxidants and the prevention of coronary heart disease. Arch Intern Med 1995;155:241.

187. The Alpha-Tocopheral, Beta Carotene Cancer Prevention Study Group. The effect of vitamin E and beta carotene on the incidence of lung cancer and other cancers in male smokers. N Engl J Med 1994;330:1029.

188. Hennekens CH, Buring JE, Peto R. Antioxidant vitamins - benefits not yet proven. N Engl J Med 1994;330:1080.

189. Rapola JM, et al. Effect of vitamin E and beta carotene on the incidence of angina pectoris. A randomized, double-blind, controlled trial. JAMA 1996;275:693.

190. Stephens NG, et al. Randomised controlled trial of vitamin E in patients with coronary disease: Cambridge Heart Antioxidant Study (CHAOS). Lancet 1996;347:781.

191. Morris DL, Kritchevsky SB, Davis CE. Serum carotenoids and coronary heart disease. The Lipid Research Clinics Primary Prevention Trial and Follow-up Study. JAMA 1994;272:1439.

192. Gaziano JM, et al. Beta carotene therapy for chronic stable angina (abstract). Circulation 1990;82(suppl):III-201.

193. Hennekens CH, et al. Lack of effect of long-term supplementation with beta carotene on the incidence of malignant neoplasms and cardiovascular disease. N Engl J Med 1996;334:1145.

194. Greenberg ER, et al. Mortality associated with low plasma concentration of beta carotene and the effect of oral supplementation. JAMA 1996;275:699.

195. Omenn GS, et al. Effects of a combination of beta carotene and vitamin A on lung cancer and cardiovascular disease. N Engl J Med 1996;334:1150.

196. Correspondence. N Engl J Med 1994;331:611.

197. Blot WJ, et al. Nutrition intervention trials in Linxian, China: supplementation with specific vitamin/mineral combinations, cancer incidence, and disease-specific mortality in the general population. J Natl Cancer Inst 1993;85:1483.

198. Hertog MGL, et al. Dietary antioxidant flavanoids and risk of coronary heart disease: the Zutphen Elderly Study. Lancet 1993;342:1007.

199. Kawamura M, Heineke JW, Chait A. Pathophysiological concentrations of glucose promote oxidative modification of low density lipoprotein by a superoxide-dependent pathway. J Clin Invest 1994;94:771.

200. Scheffler E, et al. Smoking influences the atherogenic potential of low-density lipoprotein. Clin Investig 1992;70:263.

201. de Graaf J, et al. Enhanced susceptibility to *in vitro* oxidation of the dense low density lipoprotein subfraction in healthy subjects. Arteriosclerosis and Thrombosis 1991;11:298.

202. Chait A, et al. Susceptibility of small, dense, low-density lipoproteins to oxidative modification in subjects with the atherogenic lipoprotein phenotype, pattern B. Am J Med 1993;94:350.

203. Sack MN, Rader DJ, Cannon RO III. Oestrogen and inhibition of oxidation of low-density lipoproteins in postmenopausal women. Lancet 1994;343:269.

204. Kugiyama K, et al. Impairment of endothelium-dependent arterial relaxation by lysolecithin in modified low-density lipoproteins. Nature 1990;344:160.

205. Heitzer T, Just H, Münzel T. Antioxidant vitamin C improves endothelial dysfunction in chronic smokers. Circulation 1996;94:6.

206. Levine GN, et al. Ascorbic acid reverses endothelial vasomotor dysfunction in patients with coronary artery disease. Circulation 1996;93:1107.

207. Gilligan DM, et al. Effect of antioxidant vitamins on low density lipoprotein oxidation and impaired endothelium-dependent vasodilation in patients with hypercholesterolemia. J Am Coll Cardiol 1994;24:1611.

208. Keaney JF Jr, et al. Low-dose α-tocopherol improves and high-dose α-tocopherol worsens endothelial vasodilator function in cholesterol-fed rabbits. J Clin Invest 1994;93:844-51.

209. Utermann G. Lipoprotein (a). In Scriver CR, Beaudet AL, Sly WS, Valle D, Stanbury JB, Wyngaarden JB, Fredrickson DS, eds. The Metabolic and Molecular Bases of Inherited Disease. McGraw-Hill, New York, 1995.

210. Utermann G. The mysteries of lipoprotein(a). Science 1989;246:904.

211. Albers JJ, Marcovina SM, Lodge MS. The unique lipoprotein(a): properties and immunochemical measurement. Clin Chem 1990;36/12:2019.

212. Scanu AM, Lawn RM, Berg K. Lipoprotein(a) and atherosclerosis. Ann Intern Med 1991;115:209.

213. Scanu AM. Lipoprotein(a). A genetic risk factor for premature coronary heart disease. JAMA 1992;267:3326.

214. Rader DJ, Brewer HB. Lipoprotein(a). Clinical approach to a unique atherogenic lipoprotein. JAMA 1992;267:1109.

215. Bostom AG, et al. Elevated plasma lipoprotein (a) and coronary heart disease in men aged 55 years and younger. A prospective study. JAMA 1996;276:544.

216. McLean JW, et al. cDNA sequence of human apolipoprotein(a) is homologous to plasminogen. Nature 1987;330:132.

217. Ezratty A, Simon DI, Loscalzo J. Lipoprotein(a) binds directly to human platelets and attenuates plasminogen binding and activation. Biochemistry 1993;32:4628.

218. Brown MS, Goldstein JL. Plasma lipoproteins. Teaching old dogmas new tricks. Nature 1987;330:113.

219. Chiesa G, et al. Reconstitution of lipoprotein(a) by infusion of human low density lipoprotein into transgenic mice expressing human apolipoprotein(a). J Biol Chem 1992;267:24369.

220. Rader DJ, et al. The low density lipoprotein receptor is not required for normal catabolism of Lp(a) in humans. J Clin Inves 1995;95:1403.

221. Gurakar A, et al. Levels of Lp(a) decline with neomycin and niacin treatment. Atherosclerosis 1985;57:293.

222. Noma A, et al. Reduction of serum lipoprotein(a) levels in hyperlipidemic patients with a-tocopheryl nicotinate. Arteriosclerosis 1990;84:213.

223. Lepre F. Low-dose sustained release nicotinic acids (Tri-B$_3$) and lipoprotein (a). Am J Cardiol 1992;70:33.

224. Soma MR, et al. The lowering of lipoprotein(a) induced by estrogen plus progesterone replacement therapy in postmenopausal women. Arch Intern Med 1993;153:1462.

225. Kim CJ, et al. Effects of hormone replacement therapy on lipoprotein(a) and lipids in postmenopausal women. Arterioscler Thromb 1994;14:275.

226. Kim CJ, et al. Changes in Lp(a) lipoprotein and lipid levels after cessation of female sex hormone production and estrogen replacement therapy. Arch Intern Med 1996;156:500.

227. Kim CJ, et al. Effect of hormone replacement therapy on lipoprotein(a) and lipid levels in postmenopausal women. Arch Intern Med 1996;156:1693.

228. Sacks FM, McPherson R, Walsh BW. Effect of postmenopausal estrogen replacement on plasma Lp(a) lipoprotein concentrations. Arch Intern Med 1994;154:1106.

229. Haines C, et al. Effect of oral estradiol on Lp(a) and other lipoproteins in postmenopausal women. Arch Intern Med 1996;156:866.

230. Bruckert E, et al. Increased serum levels of lipoprotein(a) in diabetes mellitus and their reduction with glycemic control. JAMA 1990;263:35.

231. Ramirez LC, et al. Lipoprotein (a) levels in diabetes mellitus: relationship to metabolic control. Ann Intern Med 1992;117:42.

232. Purnell JQ, et al. Levels of lipoprotein(a), apolipoprotein B, and lipoprotein cholesterol distribution in IDDM. Results from follow-up in the Diabetes Control and Complications Trial. Diabetes 1995;1218.

233. O'Brien T, et al. Lipids and Lp(a) lipoprotein levels and coronary artery disease in subjects with non-insulin-dependent diabetes mellitus. Mayo Clin Proc 1994;69:430.

234. Kapelrud H, et al. Serum Lp(a) lipoprotein concentrations in insulin dependent diabetic patients with microalbuminuria. BMJ 1991;303:675.

235. Jenkins AJ, et al. Increased plasma apolipoprotein(a) levels in IDDM patients with microalbuminuria. Diabetes 1991;40:787.

236. Wanner C, et al. Elevated plasma lipoprotein(a) in patients with the nephrotic syndrome. Ann Intern Med 1993;119:263.

237. Schaefer EJ, et al. Lipoprotein(a) levels and risk of coronary heart disease in men. The Lipid Research Clinics Coronary Primary Prevention Trial. JAMA 1994;271:999.

238. Valentine RJ, et al. Lp(a) lipoprotein is an independent, discriminating risk factor for premature peripheral atherosclerosis among white men. Arch Intern Med 1994;154:801.

239. Bostom AG, et al. A prospective investigation of elevated lipoprotein (a) detected by electrophoresis and cardiovascular disease in women. The Framingham Study. Circulation 1994;1688.

240. Ridker PM, Hennekens CH, Stampfer MJ. A prospective study of lipoprotein(a) and the risk of myocardial infarction. JAMA 1993;270:2195.

241. Marburger C, et al. Association between lipoprotein(a) and progression of coronary artery disease in middle-aged men. Am J Cardiol 1994;73:742.

242. Maher VMG, et al. Effects of lowering elevated LDL cholesterol on the cardiovascular risk of lipoprotein(a). JAMA 1995;274:1771.

243. Lawn RM, et al. Atherogenesis in transgenic mice expressing human apolipoprotein(a). Nature 1992;360:670.

244. Austin MA, et al. Low-density lipoprotein subclass patterns and risk of myocardial infarction. JAMA 1988;260:1917.

245. Austin MA, et al. Prospective study of small LDLs as a risk factor for non-insulin dependent diabetes mellitus in elderly men and women. Circulation 1995;92:1770.

246. Reaven GM, et al. Insulin resistance and hyperinsulinemia in individuals with small, dense, low density lipoprotein particles. J Clin Invest 1993;92:141.

247. Reaven GM. Role of insulin resistance in human disease. Diabetes 1988;37:1595.

248. Gardner CD, Fortmann SP, Krauss RM. Association of small, dense lipoprotein particles with the incidence of coronary artery disease in men and women. JAMA 1996;276:875.

249. Coresh J, Kwiterovich PO Jr. Small, dense low-density lipoprotein particles and coronary heart disease risk. A clear association with uncertain implications. JAMA 1996;276:914.

250. Landau C, Lange RA, Hillis LD. Percutaneous transluminal coronary angioplasty. N Engl J Med 1994;330:981.

251. Austin GE. Lipids and vascular restenosis. Circulation 1992;85:1613.

252. Corsini A, et al. Pathogenesis of atherosclerosis and the role of 3-hydroxy-3-methylglutaryl coenzyme A reductase inhibitors. Am J Cardiol 1995;76:21A.

253. Sahni R, et al. Prevention of restenosis by lovastatin after successful coronary angioplasty. Am Heart J 1991;121:1600.

254. Violaris AG, Melkert R, Serruys PW. Influence of serum cholesterol and cholesterol subfractions on restenosis after successful coronary angioplasty. A quantitative angiographic analysis of 3336 lesions. Circulation 1994;90:2267.

255. Roth A, et al. and the Ichilov Magnesium Study Group. Serum lipids and restenosis after successful percutaneous transluminal coronary angioplasty. Am J Cardiol 1994;73:1154.

256. Weintraub WS, et al. and the Lovastatin Restenosis Trial Study Group. Lack of effect of lovastatin on restenosis after coronary angioplasty. N Engl J Med 1994;331:1331.

257. Hearn JA, et al. Usefulness of serum lipoprotein (a) as a predictor of restenosis after percutaneous transluminal coronary angioplasty. Am J Cardiol 1992;69:736.

258. Yamamoto H, et al. Risk factors for restenosis after percutaneous transluminal coronary angioplasty: role of lipoprotein (a). Am Heart J 1995;130:1168.

259. Cooke T, et al. Lipoprotein(a) in restenosis after percutaneous transluminal coronary angioplasty and coronary artery disease. Circulation 1994;89:1593.

260. Desmarais RL, et al. Elevated serum lipoprotein(a) is a risk factor for clinical recurrence after coronary balloon angioplasty. Circulation 1995;91:1403.

261. Shah P, Amin J. Low high density lipoprotein level is associated with restenosis rate after coronary angioplasty. Circulation 1992;85:1279.

262. Rozenman Y, et al. Plasma lipoproteins are not related to restenosis after successful coronary angioplasty. Am J Cardiol 1993;72:1206.

263. Dzavik V, et al. Effect of serum lipid concentrations on restenosis after successful de novo percutaneous transluminal coronary angioplasty in patients with total cholesterol 160 to 240 mg/dl and triglycerides <350 mg/dl. Am J Cardiol 1995;75:936.

264. Leaf A, et al. Do fish oils prevent restenosis after coronary angioplasty? Circulation 1994;90:2248.

265. Godfried SL, Deckelbaum LI. Natural antioxidants and restenosis after percutaneous transluminal coronary angioplasty. Am Heart J 1995;129:203.

266. Watanabe K, et al. Preventive effects of probucol on restenosis after percutaneous transluminal coronary angioplasty. Am Heart J 1996;132:23.

267. O'Keefe JH, et al. Lovastatin plus probucol for prevention of restenosis after percutaneous transluminal coronary angioplasty. Am J Cardiol 1996;77:649.

268. Miller LW. Long-term complications of cardiac transplantation. Prog Cardiovasc Dis 1991;33:229.

269. Hosenpud JD, Shipley GD, Wagner CR. Cardiac allograft vasculopathy: current concepts, recent developments, and future directions. J Heart Lung Transplant 1992;11:9.

270. Gao S-Z, et al. Accelerated coronary vascular disease in the heart transplant patient: coronary arteriographic findings. J Am Coll Cardiol 1988;12:34.

271. Park J-W, et al. Lipid disorder and transplant coronary artery disease in long-term survivors of heart transplantation. J Heart Lung Transplant 1996;15:572.

272. Billingham ME. Cardiac transplant atherosclerosis. Transplant Proc 1987;19,suppl 5:19.

273. Ross R. The pathogenesis of atherosclerosis - an update. N Engl J Med 1986;314:488.

274. Miller LW, et al. 24th Bethesda Conference: cardiac transplantation - Task Force 5: Complications. J Am Coll Cardiol 1993;22:41.

275. Stamler JS, et al. Frequency of hypercholesterolemia after cardiac transplantation. Am J Cardiol 1988;62:1268.

276. Farmer JA, et al. Lipoprotein(a) and apolipoprotein changes after cardiac transplantation. J Am Coll Cardiol 1991;18:926.

277. Ballantyne CM, et al. Hyperlipidemia after heart transplantation: report of a 6-year experience, with treatment recommendations. J Am Coll Cardiol 1992;19:1315.

278. Kubo SH, et al. Factors influencing the development of hypercholesterolemia after cardiac transplantation. Am J Cardiol 1992;70:520.

279. Rudas L, et al. Serial evaluation of lipid profiles and risk factors for development of hyperlipidemia after cardiac transplantation. Am J Cardiol 1990;66:1135.

280. Stamler JS, Vaughan DE, Loscalzo J. Immunosuppressive therapy and lipoprotein abnormalities after cardiac transplantation. Am J Cardiol 1991;68:389.

281. Ballantyne CM, et al. Effects of cyclosporine therapy on plasma lipoprotein levels. JAMA 1989;262:53.

282. Stamler JS, et al. Frequency of hypercholesterolemia after cardiac transplantation. Am J Cardiol 1988;62:1268.

283. Löpez-Miranda J, et al. Low density lipoprotein metabolism in rats treated with cyclosporine. Metabolism 1993;42:678.

284. Superko HR, Haskell WL, Di Ricco CD. Lipoprotein and hepatic lipase activity and high-density lipoprotein subclasses after cardiac transplantation. Am J Cardiol 1990;66:1131.

285. Bieber CP, et al. Complications in long-term survivors of cardiac transplantation. Transplant Proc 1981;13:207.

286. Keogh A, et al. Hyperlipidemia after heart transplantation. J Heart Transplant 1988;7:171.

287. Eich D, et al. Hypercholesterolemia in long-term survivors of heart transplantation: an early marker of accelerated coronary artery disease. J Heart Lung Transplant 1991;10:45.

288. Johnson MR. Transplant coronary disease: nonimmunologic risk factors. J Heart Lung Transplant 1992;11:S24.

289. de Lorgeril M, et al. Platelet aggregation and HDL cholesterol are predictive of acute coronary events in heart transplant recipients. Circulation 1994;89:2590.

290. Escobar A, et al. Cardiac allograft vasculopathy assessed by intravascular ultrasonography and nonimmunologic risk factors. Am J Cardiol 1994;74:1042.

291. Rickenbacher PR, et al. Prognostic importance of intimal thickness as measured by intracoronary ultrasound after cardiac transplantation. Circulation 1995;92:3445.

292. Gao SZ, et al. Retransplantation for severe accelerated coronary artery disease in heart transplant recipients. Am J Cardiol 1988;62:876.

293. Kobashigawa JA, et al. Effect of pravastatin on outcomes after cardiac transplantation. N Engl J Med 1995;333:621.

294. Norman DJ, et al. Myolysis and acute renal failure in a heart-transplant recipient receiving lovastatin. N Engl J Med 1988;318:46.

295. East C, et al. Rhabdomyolysis in patients receiving lovastatin after cardiac transplantation. N Engl J Med 1988:318:47.

296. Corpier CL, et al. Rhabdomyolysis and renal injury with lovastatin use. Report of two cases in cardiac transplantation recipients. JAMA 1988;260:239.

297. Kuo PC, et al. Lovastatin therapy for hypercholesterolemia in cardiac transplant recipients. Am J Cardiol 1989;64:631.

298. Pflugfelder PW, et al. Cholesterol-lowering therapy after heart transplantation: a 12-month randomized trial. J Heart Lung Transplant 1995;14:613.

299. Hidalgo L, et al. Lovastatin versus bezafibrate for hyperlipidemia treatment after heart transplantation. J Heart Lung Transplant 1995;14:461.

300. Valantine HA. Correspondence. N Engl J Med 1996;334:402.

301. Barbir M, et al. *Maxepa* versus *bezafibrate* in hyperlipidemic cardiac transplant recipients. Am J Cardiol 1992;70:1596.

302. Sarris GE, et al. Inhibition of accelerated coronary disease in heart transplant recipients. J Thorac Cardiovasc Surg 1989;97:841.

303. Lee TH, et al. Effects of dietary enrichment with eicosapentaenoic acid and docosahexaenoic acid on in vitro neutrophil and monocyte leukotriene generation and neutrophil function. N Engl J Med 1985;312:1217.

304. Endres S, et al. The effect of dietary supplementation with n-3 polyunsaturated fatty acids on the synthesis of interleukin-1 and tumor necrosis factor by mononuclear cells. N Engl J Med 1989;320:265.

305. Morris MC, Sacks FM, Rosner B. Does fish oil lower blood pressure? A meta-analysis of controlled trials. Circulation 1993;88:523.

306. DeCaterina R, et al. Vascular prostacyclin is increaseed in patients ingesting w-3 polyunsaturated fatty acids before coronary artery bypass graft surgery. Circulation 1990;82:428.

307. Leaf A, Weber PC. Cardiovascular effects of n-3 fatty acids. N Engl J Med 1988;318:549.

308. Leaf A. Cardiovascular effects of fish oils. Beyond the platelet. Circulation 1990;82:624.

309. Billman GE, Hallaq H, Leaf A. Prevention of ischemia-induced ventricular fibrillation by w3 fatty acids. Proc Natl Acad Sci 1994;91:4427.

310. Kang JX, Leaf A. Antiarrhythmic effects of polyunsaturated fatty acids. Circulation 1996;94:1774.

311. LaRosa JC. Dyslipoproteinemia in women and the elderly. Lipid Disorders. Medical Clinics of North America. WB Saunders, Philadelphia, 1994;78:163.

312. Kannel WB. Metabolic risk factors for coronary heart disease in women: Perspective from the Framingham Study. Am J Cardiol 1987;114:413.

313. Krowleski AS, et al. Evolving natural history of coronary artery disease in diabete mellitus. Am J Med 1991;1991(suppl 2A):56S.

314. Kannel WB, Wilson PWF. Risk factors that attenuate the female coronary disease advantage. Arch Intern Med 1995;155:57.

315. Kane JP, et al. Regression of coronary atherosclerosis during treatment of familial hypercholesterolemia with combined drug regimens. JAMA 1990;264:3007.

316. Byington RP, et al. Reduction in cardiovascular events during pravastatin therapy. Pooled analysis of clinical events of the pravastatin atherosclerosis intervention program. Circulation 1995;92:2419.

317. Grodstein F, et al. Postmenopausal esterogen and progestin use and the risk of cardiovascular disease. N Engl J Med 1996;335:453.

318. Sarrel PM, et al. Angina and normal coronary arteries in women: Gynecologic findings. Am J Obstet Gynecol 1992;167:467.

319. Rosano GMC, et al. Beneficial effect of oestrogen on exercise-induced myocardial ischaemia in women with coronary artery disease. Lancet 1993;342:133.

320. Gilligan DM, et al. Acute vascular effects of estrogen in postmenopausal women. Circulation 1994;90:786.

321. Samaan SA, Crawford MH. Estrogen and cardiovascular function after menopause. J Am Coll Cardiol 1995;26:1403.

322. Anderson HV. Estrogen therapy, atherosclerosis, and clinical cardiovascular events. Circulation 1996;94:1809.

323. Benfante R, Reed D. Is elevated serum cholesterol level a risk factor for coronary heart disease in the elderly? JAMA 1990;262:393.

324. Kronmal RA, et al. Total serum cholesterol levels and mortality risk as a function of age. A report based on the Framingham data. Arch Intern Med 1993;153:1065.

325. Aronow WS and Ahn C. Correlation of serum lipids with the presence or absence of coronary artery disease in 1,793 men and women aged ≥ 62 years. Am J Cardiol 1994;73:702.

326. Grover SA, Palmer CS, Coupal L. Serum lipid screening to identify high-risk individuals for coronary death. The results of the Lipid Research Clinics Prevalence Cohort. Arch Intern Med 1994;154:679.

327. Krumholz HM, et al. Lack of association between cholesterol and coronary heart disease mortality and morbidity and all-cause mortality in persons older than 70 years. JAMA 1994;272:1335.

328. Tervahauta M, Pekkanen J, Nissinen A. Risk factors of coronary heart disease and total mortality among elderly men with and without preexisting coronary heart disease. Finnish cohorts of the Seven Countries study. J Am Coll Cardiol 1995;26:1623.

329. Weijenberg MP, Feskens EJM, Kromhout D. Total and high density lipoprotein cholesterol as risk factors for coronary heart disease in elderly men during 5 years of follow-up. The Zutphen Elderly Study. Am J Epidemiol 1996;143:151.

330. Corti M-C, et al. HDL cholesterol predicts coronary heart disease mortality in older persons. JAMA 1995;274:539.

331. Denke MA, Winker MA. Cholesterol and coronary heart disease in older adults. No easy answers. JAMA 1995;274:575.

4 LIPID LOWERING THERAPY

Donald A. Smith

Prevention of coronary heart disease is not only important from the public health point of view. Efforts to prevent disease test our fundamental concepts of etiology. Atherosclerotic coronary heart disease is a complex process of atherosclerotic plaque accumulation and interaction with a thrombotic and fibrinolytic system, which may or may not ultimately result in a clinical syndrome. Because of the slowness and complexity of this lifelong process, preventive interventions may as well seem too weak or too slow in their power to appreciably alter the course of clinical disease. The societal burden of this disease, however, has become so great and its treatment so technologically complex, that even small gains in its prevention applied to large populations can be appreciable in terms of both reduction in human suffering and reduction in health care expenditures.

The primary purpose of this chapter will be to explore the experimental data that justify lipid lowering in preventing the clinical onset and progression of coronary heart disease, i.e., lipid-lowering as a tool of both primary and secondary prevention. Since the cardiologist will predominantly be seeing patients referred with coronary heart disease already, as opposed to the general internist who will predominantly be seeing patients without coronary heart disease, the major focus of this chapter will be on the newer studies on secondary prevention of coronary heart disease. Since improvement in angiographic outcome seems predictive of improvement in clinical outcome, angiographic studies will also be discussed as potential correlates of clinical studies.

Primary prevention

Although there had been many animal and pathological studies suggesting the importance of cholesterol in the development of coronary atherosclerotic plaques, it was the early international epidemiologic studies of Ansel Keys in the Seven Countries Study that demonstrated marked differences in coronary heart disease mortality among countries and related this to median national serum cholesterol levels and intake of saturated fat as percent of calories that began to suggest that the growing epidemic of coronary heart disease might have an important environmental component.[1] The ten year incidence of fatal myocardial infarctions in men aged 40-59 years in Eastern Finland where the group median plasma cholesterol was 265 mg/dL was 14 times higher than that in four cities in Japan and Yugoslavia where the group median cholesterol was 160 mg/dL.[2] Emigration studies as well have suggested that increasing coronary heart disease incidence is related to environmental factors. The Ni-Hon-San study measured total cholesterol levels in Japanese men in mainland Japan, Honolulu, and San Francisco and found the means to be 180, 218, and 228 mg/dL.[3] Corresponding coronary heart disease death rates were 1.3, 2.2, and 3.7 per thousand per year, a threefold increase as Japanese men emigrated from Japan and acculturated to the United States.

The Framingham Study which was initiated in 1948 in Framingham, Massachusetts, and is still ongoing has been one of the most respected and productive studies of the relationship of lipids to coronary heart disease. 5200 men and women in Framingham were originally examined and then followed every two years to determine risk of baseline variables to the onset of cardiovascular disease. At ten years of follow-up total cholesterol was linearly related to incidence of CHD.[4] At the eighteen year followup, total cholesterol was linearly related to both coronary and peripheral vascular disease, but not significantly to cerebrovascular disease.[5] The relationship was a strong one suggesting that for each 1% rise in total cholesterol, the incidence of coronary heart disease increased 2 - 3%.[6] After the age of fifty, in women total cholesterol was no longer an important predictor of coronary heart disease. Lipid subfractions began to be measured in Framingham in 1968.[5] Low density lipoprotein (LDL) cholesterol was significantly related to coronary heart disease incidence in both men and women and at ages older than 50 years.[5] More importantly high density lipoprotein (HDL) cholesterol was found to be a very significant protective risk factor,[7,8] and low levels of it (36 md/dL or less in men or 46 mg/dL or less in women) even in persons with total cholesterol levels less than 200 was associated with a two fold increase (men) and (seven-fold increase in (women) 12 year incidence rates of myocardial infarction when compared to those with HDL-C levels 20 mg/dL higher.[9]

The Multiple Risk Factor Intervention Trial screened 356,222 men age 35 - 57 years for serum cholesterol and followed for six years for CHD mortality. This study showed that the lowest rates of CHD mortality were in the men in the lowest decile of total cholesterol, (167 mg/dL or less) and that risk increased steadily throughout the remaining nine deciles resulting in a 4.1 fold increase in relative risk for those in the tenth decile (total cholesterol = 264 mg/dL and above) compared with those in the first decile.[10]

The importance of the lipid hypothesis to the clinical prevention of CHD gathered momentum as randomized, placebo controlled studies were able to demonstrate the effectiveness of LDL-cholesterol lowering to the reduction in incidence of CHD. One of the most important in terms of clinical impact was the Lipid Research Clinics Coronary Primary Prevention Trial (CPPT) reported in 1984 in which approximately 3800 men aged 35 to 59 with a total plasma cholesterol of 265 mg/dL or greater and an LDL cholesterol level 190 mg/dL or greater were randomly assigned to receive 24 grams of cholestyramine or placebo in conjunction with a lipid lowering diet.[11,12] Subjects were followed for an average of 7.4 years and monitored for sudden cardiac death and non-fatal MI. LDL cholesterol levels decreased from 216 at baseline to 199 and 198 mg/dL at one and seven years in the placebo group and from 216 at baseline to 159 and 175 mg/dL in the cholestyramine group, The cumulative incidence of CHD death or non-fatal MI dropped from 8.6% in the placebo group to 7.0% in the cholestyramine group, a significant (though not earth-shaking) 19% drop in these events. Greater decreases in total or LDL cholesterol resulted in greater decreases in clinical events rate, such that those subjects who took all six packets of cholestyramine per day with a 35% decrease in LDL cholesterol or a 25% decrease in total cholesterol had a 50% decrease in clinical events rate.

The Helsinki Heart Study reported in 1987 [13] was a second important primary prevention trial that demonstrated reductions in CHD morbidity and mortality with primary treatment of hyperlipidemia, this time with gemfibrozil, a fibric acid derivative. Approximately 4000 men, age 40 to 55, and with a non-HDL cholesterol (LDL plus VLDL cholesterol) of 200 mg/dL or more, were randomized to gemfibrozil 600 mg bid or to placebo bid after dietary intervention. They were followed for five years with the primary end point being incidence of CHD death or non-fatal MI. Gemfibrozil treatment resulted in a 10% decrease in total cholesterol, an 11% decrease in LDL cholesterol, a 35% decrease in triglycerides, and an 11% increase in HDL cholesterol. After two years in the trial, the treated group began having fewer clinical events resulting at five years in a 34% reduction in primary events from 84 (4.1%) in the placebo group to 56 (2.7%) in the gemfibrozil group. There was a decreased incidence of events in each of the three Frederickson lipid phenotype patterns , but the largest effect was in those with a IIB phenotype, i.e., with baseline elevations in both LDL cholesterol and triglyceride levels.[14] Later subgroup analysis,[15] showed that participants with triglyceride levels above 200 mg/dL in the presence of an LDL/HDL cholesterol ratio of greater than 5.0 had a 71% reduction in the primary end points. This was one of the first studies demonstrating those persons for whom triglyceride decreases may lower clinical coronary events.

Total mortality in both the CPPT and the Helsinki trials was not lowered significantly because of increases in mortality in deaths from accidents, suicides, and homicides. These data have inspired a surge in research on the behavior-altering effects of cholesterol reduction. This author feels that the increases in these categories of death , although associated with, were not caused by the drugs used nor the cholesterol reduction itself; the Helsinki authors speak to this issue in a letter to the editor and a recent review article goes into an exploration of the issue in quite some detail.[16,17] These data plus a recent meta -analysis looking at mortality outcome by degree of baseline risk [18] do demonstrate, however, how difficult it is to lower total mortality in persons with a small risk of coronary heart disease, e.g., in men before the age of 45 years and in premenopausal women, and thus lipid-lowering recommendations have tended to become more conservative in the pharmacologic approach to primary prevention in these low risk groups. For example the current recommendation of the Expert Panel of the National Cholesterol Education Program Expert Panel on detection, evaluation, and treatment of high blood cholesterol in adults is not to use drugs for LDL cholesterol lowering even if the LDL cholesterol remains in the 190-220 mg/dL range after dietary therapy for men under 35 and for premenopausal women.[19]

Secondary prevention

On the other hand there have been many studies now of the secondary prevention of CHD which show decreases in non-fatal and fatal events in persons with CHD as well as decreases in total morality. At the arterial level, the major expected benefit from LDL-C lowering has been stability or regression in degree of stenosis within arteries already containing atherosclerotic plaques and a diminution in the rate of new plaque formation and progression. Sequential coronary angiography using visual assessment by a panel of cardiologists or by computerized image analysis has been the tool to evaluate sequential changes in percent stenosis (%S), comparing the narrowest point in a vessel with what would appear to be a normal segment, a measure of relative change between two segments in a coronary artery. More recent studies have used minimal and mean lumen diameter changes in coronary artery segments as a measure of atherosclerotic disease activity. These are absolute changes (in mm) in diameters with time and require the presence of a measuring scale on the tip of the catheter as an absolute point of reference. Such studies also measure coronary heart disease morbidity and mortality so that angiographic and clinical outcomes may be compared. There are now many such studies and these will be be presented in brief narrative form with the details summarized in *Tables 4.1-4.3*.

Dietary angiographic trials (Table 4.1)

At least three dietary trials have shown that angiographic improvement can be obtained without pharmacologic help. The Leiden Intervention Trial [20]was an uncontrolled two-year trial in 39 subjects with at least one coronary vessel with greater than a 50% stenosis who were placed on a vegetarian diet consisting of 6.6% saturated fat, less than 30 mg per day of cholesterol, and with a polyunsaturated/saturated (P/S) fat ratio of 2.5. Ninety percent were male with an average age of 49 years. Total cholesterol fell 10% from 267 to 240 mg/dL (6.9 to 6.2 mE/L). Both visual imaging and computer-assisted imaging was used to assess angiograms. Fifty four percent showed progression by both methods with 46 percent showing regression (18%) or no change (28%). The important finding was that lesion growth was associated with average baseline and two-year TC/HDL-C ratios (r=0.5, p< .001) and that there was no progression in those with on trial TC/HDL-C ratios less than 6.9.

Persistent angina was associated with progression and in 3.5 years of follow-up, 5 deaths occurred all of which were in persons with lesions that had progressed.

The recent Lifestyle Heart Trial conducted by Dr. Dean Ornish and coworkers enrolled 48 subjects with coronary atherosclerosis on diagnostic angiography in at least one coronary vessel and randomly placed half of them on a comprehensive lifestyle-change program consisting of a vegetarian diet (7% fat, 12 mg cholesterol per day), stress management exercises for one hour per day, excercise minimally 3 hours per week, and group support meetings twice weekly.[21,22] Eighty nine percent were male with an average age of 58 years, ninety percent of whom were experiencing angina. LDL-cholesterol levels decreased from 152 to 95 mg/dL (3.92 to 2.46 mE/L) in the treatment group with no change in HDL cholesterol levels. Of the 41 subjects who had two comparable angiograms at one year, average stenosis regressed 2.2% in the experimental group and progressed 3.4% in the usual care control group (p<.001). Eighteen percent of subjects in the treatment group had lesions that on average tended to progress compared with 53% of subjects in the control group. It is unclear which part of the intervention was most important or whether the total program is necessary. Those who were most adherent to all part of the program showed the greatest improvement. Angiographic changes were slightly better in women than in men and in lesions where the percentage stenosis was greater than 50%. Only one death occurred in a man assigned to the intervention group who exceeded exercise recommendations in an unsupervised gym. There was a marked decrease in angina in the experimental group within one month of entering the program.

The St. Thomas Athersclerosis Regression Study (STARS) [23] had one arm with dietary intervention showing that more modest changes in diet than the previous two can result in angiographic improvement. Sixty men evaluated angiographically with CHD, average age 49 years, were randomly assigned to dietary therapy (27% total fat, 8-10% saturated fat, cholesterol = 100 mg/1000 calories per day, high soluble fiber) or to diet plus cholestyramine 16 grams per day. In the dietary arm, the average LDL cholesterol decreased from 194 to 162 mg/dL (5.00 to 4.19 mE/L) with no change in HDL cholesterol while cholestyramine therapy in addition to the diet resulted in a decrease in average LDL cholesterol from 204 to 130 mg/dL (5.26 to 3.37 mE/L). After 39 months, the mean luminal diameter decreased .201 mm in the control group but increased .003 mm in the dietary group and .103 mm in the diet plus cholestyramine group (p = .012). On trial LDL/HDL-C ratio and mean blood pressure best predicted the changes in luminal status. In addition although there were 10 of 28 subjects (36%) in the control group who had either an MI, death, angioplasty, coronary artery bypass grafting, or stroke, there were only 11% in the diet group, and 4% in the diet plus cholestyramine group who had such events (p<.05,<.01) respectively.

These three dietary studies , two using vegetarian diets and one using a more standard type II American Heart Association type diet, demonstrate an ability to improve angiographic results assessed at one to 3.3 years. Two of these studies show that angiographic changes are associated with TC/HDL-C or LDL/HDL-C ratios in

Table 4.1   STUDIES OF DIETARY THERAPY OF HYPERLIPIDEMIA

Study	Participants						Intervention	Length of trial (yrs)	Lipid changes Treatment Group	
	n randomized/ angios compared	% angina % MI	% male	Mean age (yrs)	% ASA	% Smoker			LDL-C mg/dl (mE/L)	[-%]
Leiden Interven Trial[20]	53/39	100/69	90	49	–	–	Vegeterian diet: P/S=2,5 Chol=30 mg/day Sat fat=6,6%	2	TC267 (6.9 →6.2)	[-10] →240
Life style Heart Trial[21,22]	48/41	90/-	89	58	–	0	Vegeterian diet: 7% fat 12 mg/day chol Stress management. 1 hr/d + exercise 3 hr/wk + group supp 4 hrs. biw	1	152→95 (3.92 →2.46)	[-37]
St. Thomas Atherosclerosis Regression Study STARS DIET[23]	60/50	69/46	100	49	–	27	27% total fat 8-10% sat fat chol=100 mg/1000 Cal, hi sol fiber	3.3	194→162 (5.00 →4.19)	[-16]

spite of the fact that LDL-C levels attained were quite different — approximately 160 in the Leiden Trial and STARS and 95 mg/dl in the Lifestyle Heart Trial. STARS showed a significant lowering of event rates during the 3.3 years of the study while in the Leiden Study follow-up of 3.5 years, the five deaths occurred only in those with progression on angiography at two years. Thus the dietary studies suggest findings seen in the following studies using more powerful pharmacologic or surgical interventions.

Pharmacologic, surgical angiographic trials

The National Heart, Lung, and Blood Institute (NHLBI) Type II Coronary Intervention Study [24] recruited subjects in the upper 10th percentile of LDL-cholesterol on dietary therapy who had presumed coronary artery disease; 23% had a previous MI and 33 experienced angina (Table 4.2). One hundred and fourty three subjects were randomized to diet plus 24 grams of cholestyramine daily or to diet and matching placebo. The treatment group achieved a 26% drop in LDL-cholesterol to 178 mg/dL (4.60 mE/L) and an 8% increase in HDL-cholesterol to 41 mg/dL (1.06 mE/L); LDL/HDL-cholesterol ratio decreased from 6.1 to 3.9. Angiography was performed 5 years later and 116 subjects had angiograms which were comparable. Thirty two percent of the treatment group had arteries which had progressed compared with 49 percent of the diet only group , p = .03. Regression rates were the same. Although clinical events tended to be less in the treatment group (8 versus 12), the difference was not statistically significant. Best results were seen in lesions where

Table 4.1   STUDIES OF DIETARY THERAPY OF HYPERLIPIDEMIA

ΔHDL-C mg/dl (mE/L)	Δ [Δ%] L/H	Angiographic Change by Patient												Clinical Events			Comments
		MLD diameter			% Progression			% Regression			Δ% S						
		Rx	con-trol	P	Rx	con-trol	P	Rx	con-trol	P	Rx	con-trol	P	Rx	con-trol	P	
39.1 →37.9 (1.01 →0.98)	[-3] (T/H) 7.1-6.4	-.13	–		54	–		18	–		+4.5	–		–			Lession growth assoc with avg TC/HDL-C at 0 and 2yrs, r=0.5 No progression if trial TC/HDL-C < 6.9. 5 deaths in 3.5 yrs F/U occur in progressors only.
39→38 (1.00	[-3] 4.2-2.9				18	53	–	82	42	–	-2.2	+3.4	.001	1	0	–	Angio changes better in women than men, is better in % S > 50. Those most adherent to program had most benefit.
44.1 →44.1 (1.14 →1.14)	[0] 4.5 3.7	0.003	0.201	0.012	15	46	<.02	38	4	0.2	1.1	+5.8	NS	3	10	<.05	Angio changes assoc. with LDL-C/HDL-C in trial and change in mean BP.

stenosis was greater than 50% and subjects in the highest tertile of HDL/T cholesterol ratio during the study independent of treatment classification had 30 to 50% less progression than those in the lowest tertile. In fact the effect of cholestyramine on progression was eliminated when HDL/TC ratio was added to a multivariate regression model confirming in-study lipid HDL-cholesterol and LDL-cholesterol levels as the most important determinants in predicting angiographic progression.

The Cholesterol Lowering Atherosclerosis Study (CLAS) [25], performed at the University of California at Los Angeles under the direction or David Blankenhorn, randomly assigned 188 non-smoking men who had had coronary artery bypass grafting to dietary therapy as the placebo group or to colestipol 30 grams plus niacin 4 grams per day in the treatment group.. There was a major decrease in LDL cholesterol (171 to 97 mg/dL [4.42 to 2.51 mE/L]) and a major increase in HDL cholesterol (45 to 61 mg/dL [1.16 to 1.58 mE/L]) such that the LDL/HDL cholesterol ratio decreased from 4.0 to 1.7 . The percentage of subjects with progression on angiograms two years apart as measured by a visual global evaluation score was 61% in the control group and only 39% in the treated group (p=.001) . Moreover the percentage of subjects with regression was 2% in the control group but was 16% in the treatment group (p=.002). These differences persisted in a subgroup which continued another two years (75% versus 45% of patients progressing and 6% versus 18 % of patients regressing repectively).[26] This was the first study to clearly document angiographic regression and caused quite a bit of excitement. Another exciting finding was that subjects with baseline cholesterol values 240 mg/dL or less did as well as those with values 241 mg/dL and greater. Finally in the treatment group with low

Table 4.2   STUDIES OF PHARMACOLOGIC OR SURGICAL
THERAPY OF HYPERLIPIDEMIA

Study	Participants						Intervention	Length of trial (yrs)	Lipid changes Treatment Group	
	n randomized/ angios compared	% angina % MI	% male	Mean age (yrs)	% ASA	% Smoker			LDL-C mg/dl (mE/L)	[Δ%]
NHLBI[24] Type II Coronary Intervention Study	143/ 116	23/33	81	46	–	39	D+Csty24 gm	5	242→178 (6.25 →4.60)	[-26]
Cholesterol Lowerin Atherosclerosis Study CLAS I[25]	188/ 162	100% CABG	100	54	0	0	D+Colspol 30 gm+Νιασίνη 4 gm	2	171→97 (4.42 →2.51)	[-43]
CLAS II[26] Familial Atherosclerosis Treatment Study	188/ 103		100	54	75	<25		4	171→101 (4.43→2.62)	[-40]
FATS (N+C)[28,29]	146/120	50/72		47			D+Colspol 30 gm+Niac 4 gm		190→129 (4.91 →3.33)	[-32]
FATS (L+C)[43]	146/ 120	42/63	100	48	56	25	D+Colspol 30 gm+Lova 4 gm	2.5	196→107 (5.06 →2.76)	[-45]

LDL cholesterol levels, levels of triglyceride rich particles as measured by seemed to predict angiographic progression whereas in the diet only group, non-HDL cholesterol (that found in LDL and VLDL particles in general) predicted progression. In spite of these impressive angiographic differences, there was no significant difference in event rates.

The same group performed a further angiographic study , the first to test monotherapy with an HMG CoA reductase inhibitor , using a larger subject population called the Monitored Atherosclerosis Regression Study (MARS) which has been recently reported.[27] A total of 270 subjects with two stenotic lesions on coronary angiograms, one being greater than 50%, were randomly assigned to either dietary therapy or to lovastatin 80 mg daily. LDL-cholesterol fell in the treated group from 151 to 93 mg/dL (3.91 to 2.41 mE/L) and HDL cholesterol increased from 42.6 to 45.7 mg/dL (1.10 to 1.18 mE/L) resulting in a decrease in LDL/HDL cholesterol ratio of approximately 3.5 to 2.0. After 2.2 years, there was no significant difference in percent stenosis nor in average mean luminal diameter. In lesions with greater than 50% stenosis, however, both of these parameters were significantly better in the treated group. Using a visual global score, the treated group showed less progression and more regression than the dietary group over the 2.2 years. Clinical coronary events were not different in the two groups although the lovastatin group tended to have fewer.

Table 4.2   STUDIES OF PHARMACOLOGIC OR SURGICAL
            THERAPY OF HYPERLIPIDEMIA

ΔHDL -C mg/dl (mE/L)	Δ [Δ%] L/H	MLD Rx	MLD con-trol	MLD P	% Progression Rx	% Progression con-trol	% Progression P	% Regression Rx	% Regression con-trol	% Regression P	Δ% S Rx	Δ% S con-trol	Δ% S P	Clinical Events Rx	Clinical Events con-trol	Clinical Events P	Comments
38→41 (0.98-1.06)	[+8] 6.1→3.9	32	49	.03	7	7	NS				8	12	NS				High HDL-C/TC best predictor of less progression (30-50% less in top tertile of increase). Best results where % S > 50.
45→61 (1.16-1.58)	[+37] 40→1.7	39	61	.001	16	2	.002				14	18	NS				New lesion formation less in Rx group. Same benefit if baseline TC=185-240 or 241-350
44→60 (1.14→1.55)	[+37] 3.9→1.7	45	75	.001	18	6	.04				4	7	NS				Non-HDL cholesterol predicts progression in PBO group, TG rich particles in RX group.
39→55 (1.01→1.42)	[+41] 4.9→2.3				25	46		39	11	.005	-0.9	+2.1	.005	2	11	.01	↓ apo B, ↓ LDL, ↑ HDL, ↓ Syst. BP predict angio benefit
35→41 (0.90→1.06)	[+17] 5.6→2.6				22	46		32	11	.005	-0.7	+2.1	.02	3	11	.01	Benefit found in all lesions but best where % S > 50. Best results if baseline LDL-C<160

The Familial Atherosclerosis Treatment Study (FATS) directed by Gregory Brown at the Northwest Lipid Research Clinic in Seattle, Washington, used two different pharmacologic interventions to lower LDL-C and raise HDL-C in men less than 62 years of age with high levels of apolipoprotein B (>125 mg/dL), a family history of coronary heart disease, and at least one coronary stenotic lesion greater than 50 % or three greater than 30%.[28] One hundred and fourty six men were randomly assigned to dietary therapy or to colestipol 30 grams plus niacin 4 grams or to colestipol 30 grams plus lovastatin 40 mg per day for two and one half years. LDL cholesterol levels dropped from 190 to 129 mg/dL(4.91 to 3.33 mE/L) in the colestipol/niacin treatment group and moreso in the colestipol/lovastatin group from 196 to 107 mg/dL (5.06 to 2.76 mE/L). There was a larger increase in the HDL-cholesterol in the niacin group (39 to 55 mg/dL [1.01 to 1.42 mE/L]) than in the lovastatin group (35 to 41 mg/dL [0.90 to 1.06]). In-study LDL/HDL cholesterol ratios were approximately the same 2.3 and 2.6 respectively. The percentage of patients with progression using quantitative computerized angiography was 22 - 25% in the treated groups compared with 46% in the diet only group whereas regression was seen in 32 - 39 % in the treated group versus only 11% in the diet only group. Most importantly from the clinical point of view was a 73% reduction in cardiovascular death, nonfatal MI, and angina necessitating angioplasty or bypass. Decreases in LDL cholesterol and systolic blood pressure, and increases in HDL

Table 4.2 (cont)   STUDIES OF PHARMACOLOGIC OR SURGICAL THERAPY
OF HYPERLIPIDEMIA

Study	Participants						Intervention	Length of trial (yrs)	Lipid changes Treatment Group	
	n randomized/ angios compared	% angina % MI	% male	Mean age (yrs)	% ASA	% Smoker			LDL-C mg/dl (mE/L)	[-%]
Program on the Surgical Control of Hyperlipidemia POSCH[31,32]	838/ 838	-/100	91	51	–	35	D+partial ileal bypass	9.7	179→104 (4.62 →2.68)	[-42]
University of California San Francisco, Arteriosclerosis Specialized Center of Research Intervention Trial SCOR[33]	97/72	3/0	43	42	7	17	D+Colstipol 30 gm+Niac 2 gm +Lova 40	2	283→172 (7.32 →4.45)	[-38]
Monitoring Atherosclerosis Regression Study MARS[27]	270/ 247	41/60	91	58	90	80	D+Lova 40	2.2	151→93 (3.91 →2.41)	[-38]

cholesterol were the best predictors of angiographic benefit. Although benefit was seen in all stenotic lesions, those greater than 50% did better than those less stenotic. Surprisingly, subjects with baseline levels of LDL-C less than 160 improved more than those with higher baseline levels.[29]

Partial distal ileal bypass was introduced as a technique to lower serum cholesterol in l963. This operation could lower serum LDL cholesterol by 40% by increasing fecal neutral steroid excretion threefold and fecal bile acid excretion fivefold.[30] The Program on the Surical Control of Hyperlipidemia (POSCH) [31] randomly assigned eight hundred and thirty eight subjects who had had an MI to dietary therapy or to the surgical procedure. Coronary angiograms were performed every two years as the patients were followed for an average of 9.7 years. LDL cholesterol levels fell in the surgical group from 179 to 104 mg/dL while HDL cholesterol levels stayed essentially the same. LDL/HDL cholesterol ratio decreased froom 4.3 to 2.3. A visual global assessment scale was used to compare angiograms. Over the approximate 10 year period, 85% of the control group progressed, while only 55% of the surgical groups did so. Regression rates were 4 and 6% and did not differ. Most importantly the number of sudden coronary heart disease deaths and non-fatal MI's

Table 4.2 (cont)   STUDIES OF PHARMACOLOGIC OR SURGICAL THERAPY
OF HYPERLIPIDEMIA

ΔHDL -C mg/dl (mE/L)	Δ [Δ%] L/H	Angiographic Change by Patient												Clinical Events			Comments
		MLD			% Progression			% Regression			Δ% S						
		Rx	con-trol	P	Rx	con-trol	P	Rx	con-trol	P	Rx	con-trol	P	Rx	con-trol	P	
39.9 →41.8 (1.03 →1.08)	[+5]	4.3→ 2.3			55	85	<.001	6.4	3.8	–				82	125	<.001	Angio progression from Yr 0 to 3 predict 2x ↑ risk all cause and CHD death and CHD death plus non-fatal MI. Approx 60% decrease in CABG, PTCA Men and women had similar results
47→59 (1.22 →1.53)	[+28]	6.0→ 2.9*			20	41	.06	33	13	.06	-1.53	0.80	.04	0	1	NS	Men and women had same results
42.6 →45.7 (1.10 →1.18)	[+8.5]	3.5→ 2.0*	-.03	-.06	NS	29	41	.07	23	12	.04	1.6	2.2	NS	22	31	NS	%S and Δ min lum diam signif better with Rx where % S > 50. Global score 0.9 in PBO, 0.4 in Rx, p=.002, shows less progression with Rx

decreased by 35% in the surgical group; survival analysis showed that the surgical group demonstrated fewer events starting in the third year post surgery. Total death rate decreased in that subgroup of patients who had an ejection fraction of 50% or greater at baseline, one of the first studies showing an actual decrease in death rate with lipid-lowering. There was an approximate 60% decrease in coronary artery bypass grafting and angioplasties in the surgical group. Men and women had similar results. Using an overall global angiographic assessment of change between baseline and year 3, those subjects showing progression had a doubling of risk for subsequent overall mortality, coronary heart disease mortality, and the latter plus nonfatal MI , suggesting that angiographic results can indeed predict clinical events.[32]

John Kane directed the University of California, San Francisco, Arteriosclerosis Specialized Center of Research (SCOR) Intervention Trial,[33] a major lipid lowering trial using multiple drugs in 72 patients with heterozygous familial hypercholesterolemia. This was a primary prevention angiographic trial and the subjects were randomized to dietary therapy or to colestipol up to 30 grams, niacin up to 7.5 grams, and lovastatin up to 60 grams. LDL cholesterol fell from 283 to 172 mg/dL (7.32 to 4.45 mE/L) and HDL cholesterol increased from 47 to 59 mg/dL (1.03 to 1.08 mE/L) in the

Table 4.2 (cont)   STUDIES OF PHARMACOLOGIC OR SURGICAL THERAPY
                    OF HYPERLIPIDEMIA

Study	Participants						Intervention	Length of trial (yrs)	Lipid changes Treatment Group	
	n randomized/ angios compared	% angina % MI	% male	Mean age (yrs)	% ASA	% Smoker			LDL-C mg/dl (mE/L)	[-%]
St Thomas Atherosclerosis Study	90/74	69/46	100	49	–	27	Diet	3.3	194→162 (5.00 →4.19)	[-16]
STARS D[23]										
STARS D+R	90/74	54/79	100	50	–	21	D+Csty 16 gms	3.3	204→130 (5.26 →3.37	[-36]
Canadian[26] Coronary Atherosclerosis Inter- vention Trial CCAIT	331/ 299	66/54	81	53	100	27	D+Lova 20-80 γιι to attain LDL-C<130	2	173→122 (4.47 →3.15)	[-29]
Stanford[35] Coronary Risk Intervention Project SCRIP	300/ 246	73/47	86	57	76	14	D+Exer.+D/C smok.+13 drugs to attain LDL-C<110, TG<100, HDL-C>55	4	159→120 (4.1→3.1)	[-24]
Multicentre[34] Anti-Atheroma StydyMAAS	404/ 381	68/54	88	55	61	25	D+Simv 20	4	170→117 (4.38 →3.02)	[-31]
Pravastain[36,37] Limitation of Atherosclerosis in Coronary Arteries PLAC I	408	–	76	57	–		D+Prav 40	3	162→117 (4.19 →3.03	[-28]

drug treated group. LDL/HDL cholesterol ratio fell from 6.0 to 2.9. Over the two year study there was a trend to more progression in the control versus the treated group (41% versus 20%, p=.06) and to less regression (13 % versus 33%, p=.06). Mean percentage stenosis increased 0.80% in the control group and decreased 1.53% in the drug treated group. There was no difference in clinical events since only one event occurred in the control group, none in the drug treated group. Fifty seven percent of the subjects were women and they did as well or better than the men angiographically. This study is important for the demonstration of salutory effects in coronary angiograms when absolute values of LDL cholesterol are only reduced on average to 172 mg/dL (4.45 mE/L) and suggest that the goal of and LDL cholesterol of 100 mg/dL or less is not absolutely necessary for angiographic improvement.

Table 4.2 (cont)   STUDIES OF PHARMACOLOGIC OR SURGICAL THERAPY
OF HYPERLIPIDEMIA

ΔHDL -C mg/dl (mE/L)	Δ [Δ%] L/H	Angiographic Change by Patient											Clinical Events						Comments
		MLD			% Progression			% Regression			Δ% S							
		Rx	con-trol	P	Rx	con-trol	P	Rx	con-trol	P	Rx	con-trol	P	Rx	con-trol	P		
44.1→44.1 (1.14 →1.14)	[0] 4.5→ 3.7	.003	-.201	.01	15	46	0.02	38	4	0.02	-1.1	5.8	NS	3	10	<0.5		On trial LDL-C/ HDL-C and Δ mean BP best predict Δ % S. Benefit in all lesions but most striking stenotic lesions
48.0→46.1 (1.24 →1.19)	[-4] 4.4→ 2.9	.103	-.201	.012	12	46	0.02	33	4	0.02	-1.9	5.8	NS	1	10	<0.1		
41.3→3.2 (1.07 →1.12)	[+7] 4.2→ 2.8	-.05	-.09	.01	33	50	.02	10	7	NS	+1.66	+2.89	.04	14	18	NS		HDL-C assoc. with improvement, LDL-C with worsening. Fewer new lesions in Rx vs PBO, (16 vs 32%). Angiogr improve only in those with LDL-C >176 (median), and in % S <50. Men and women had similar results.
46.1→51.5 [+12] (1.19 →1.33	3.4→ 2.3	-.10	-.18	.02	50	50	NS	20	10	.07				25	44	.05		Diff in events signif lower in yrs 3,4 in Rx group.
42.6→45.7 [+9] (1.10→ 1.18)	4.2→ 2.7	-.02	-.08	.006	23	32	.02	19	12	.02	1.0	3.6		40	51	NS		Benefit found in all lesions but best where % S > 50.
41→44 (1.06 →1.14)	[+8]													7	18	.01		Fewer new lesions and tot occlusions in Rx group.

The Canadian Coronary Atherosclerosis Intervention Trial (CCAIT) directed by David Waters [26] randomized 331 subjects to diet or to diet plus lovastatin up to 80 mg daily to achieve an LDL-cholesterol less than 130 mg/dL. Two thirds of subjects had at least one stenosis greater than 50% on angiography and approximately one half had had a MI. LDL cholesterol levels fell from 173 to 122 mg/dL (4.47 to 3.15 mE/L) with a minimal increase in HDL cholesterol from 41.3 to 43.2 mg/dL (1.07 to 1.12 mE/L). LDL/HDL cholesterol ratio decreased from 4.2 to 2.8. Drug treated patients over two years showed less progression (33% versus 50%), less diminution in minimal mean luminal diameter (.05 versus .09 mm) and less of an increase in percent stenosis (1.66% versus 2.89%) than diet treated subjects. There was no difference in angiographic regression nor in clinical event rates. On trial higher LDL cholesterol levels were associated with worsening angiograms and higher HDL cholesterol levels with improvement. Fewer new lesions were seen in the drug treated group and men and women did equally well. Unlike previous trials, angiographic improvements were seen only in those with a baseline LDL cholesterol greater than the median of 176 mg/dL, and only in lesions less than 50% stenotic. Since the goal of therapy was an LDL-C of 130 mg/dL, those with lower baseline cholesterol levels had less drug therapy and less of a percentage fall in LDL cholesterol which may have accounted for a lack of beneficial effect of drug treatment in them.

The Multicenter Anti-Atheroma Study (MAAS) [34]directed by M. S. Oliver was very similar to the previous study but used simvastatin 20 mg to reduce LDL cholesterol levels from 170 to 117 mmg/dL (4.38 to 3.02 mE/L) in a random one half of 404 subjects with coronary artery disease similar to that in the above study CCAIT. HDL cholesterol levels increased from 42.6 to 45.7 mg/dL (1.10 to 1.18 mE/L) and LDL/HDL cholesterol ratio decreased from 4.2 to 2.7. After 4 years, simvastatin treated subjects showed less progression (23 versus 32 % of subjects progressed), more regression (19 versus 12%), and less narrowing of mean luminal diameter (.02 versus .08 mm decrease) than subjects given diet only. Benefit was more marked in lesions where stenosis was greater than 50%. There were fewer new lesions and total occlusions in the drug treated group. Disappointingly clinical event rates were not significantly different over the four year period.

The Stanford Coronary Risk Intervention Project (SCRIP) [35] directed by William L. Haskell was a randomized trial of lifestyle changes (diet with less than 20% fat, less than 6% saturated fat, and less than 75 mg of cholesterol daily, exercise, and smoking cessation) plus lipid lowering medication to reduce LDL cholesterol to less than 110 mg/dL (2.4 mE/L), triglycerides to less than 100 mg/dL (1.13 mE/L), and to increase HDL cholesterol to greater than 55 mg/dL (1.42 mE/L). 300 subjects referred for coronary angiography who had at least one coronary stenosis with narrowing between 5 and 69% were randomized to the life style intervention or to usual care. Sixty percent of intervention subjects took a bile-acid binding resin , one third took niacin , one third took an HMG CoA reductase inhibitor, and 20% took a fibric acid at some point in the four years of the trial to achieve these lipid results. Average LDL cholesterol dropped from 159 to 120 mg/dL (4.1 to 3.1 mE/L), HDL cholesterol increased from 46.1 to 51.5 mg/dL (1.19 to 1.33 mE/L) with average LDL/HDL cholesterol ratio dropping from 3.4 to 2.3. Average triglyceride level decreased from 157 to 126 mg/dl (1.77 to 1.42 mE/L). After the four years, the intervention group was 4 kilograms lighter on average with decreased mean fasting glucose and insulin levels and systolic blood pressure was 4 mm Hg less than the usual care group. Minimum lumen diameter decreased less over the four years in the risk reduction group (-.096 versus -.180 mm) than in the usual care group. When each patient was categorized into an exclusive group of progression, regression, no change, or mixed response, the two groups differed significantly (p=.07) with more in the regression category in the risk reduction group (20 versus 10%) and more in the mixed category in the usual care group (21 versus 12 %) with progression and no change groups being identical. There was a thirty nine percent decrease in cardiac events (sudden unexplained death, non-fatal MI, CABG, PTCA) in the risk reduction group (p = .05), which occurred after two years in the study.

Clinical event rates have been reported recently in the Pravastatin to Limit Atherosclerosis in the Coronary Arteries Study (PLAC I). [36,37] This was an coronary angiographic trial assessing progression in 10 coronary segments in 408 subjects (76% male, mean age 57 years) with a history of angina, MI, or PTCA who as well had at least one coronary stenotic lesion 50% or greater. To qualify, subjects had to have LDL-cholesterol levels of 130 to 189 mg/dL (3.36 to 4.90 mE/L) and triglyceride levels of 350 mg/dL or less (3.95 mE/L or less) on a American Heart Association Phase I diet (total fat less than 30%, daily cholesterol less than 300 mg, saturated fat less than 10%). The treatment group received 40 mg pravastatin at night on a randomized, double-blind basis. Follow up was for three years.

In the treatment group LDL-cholesterol dropped from 162 to 117 mg/dL (4.19 to 3.03 mE/L) and HDL cholesterol increased from 41 to 44 mg/dL (1.06 to 1.14 mE/L). Although coronary angiographic changes have not been published, the secondary endpoints of the study, clinical events, have been. [37] Myocardial infarctions were 5 in the pravastatin group and 17 in the diet-only placebo group, a 71% reduction (p = .005). There were 7 myocardial infarctions or CHD deaths in the pravastatin group and 18 in the placebo group, a 61% reduction (p = .014). The angiographic results of this trial are eagerly awaited. Meanwhile another pharmacologic agent has been added to the list of those producing important cardioprotective effects.

Clinical ultrasonographic studies

Two studies have recently been reported examining intimal medial thickness (IMT)in the internal and common carotid arteries and the carotid bifurcation while on lipid-lowering therapy (Table 4.3). The Asymptomatic Carotid Artery Progression Study (ACAPS)[38], a primary prevention Study, screened thousands of people with no history of cardiovascular disease to find subjects with at least one of 12 measurements of IMT of 1.5 mm or more with all measurements less than 3.5 mm (average IMT in middle-age people = 0.6mm).[39] 919 subjects were found with LDL-cholesterol levels on phase I AHA diet of 160 - 189 mg/dL (4.34 -5.13 mE/L) with zero or one coronary risk factor or 130 - 159 mg/dL (3.53 - 4.33 mE/L) with two or more risk factors. Subjects were randomly assigned to lovastatin 10 mg [5%], lovastatin 20 mg (44%) or lovastatin 40 mg (50%) daily to reduce LDL cholesterol to 90 - 110 mg/dL (2.44 - 2.84 mE/L) and were followed on a double-blinded protocol for three years with ultrasonographic readings taken each 6 months.

Average LDL cholesterol fell from 156 to 117 mg/dL (4.0 to 3.0 mE/L) and HDL cholesterol increased from 52 to 54 mg/dL (1.34 to 1.40 mE/L) in subjects on lovastatin. After 12 months, IMT thickening was decreasing at an average of .009 mm per year in the lovastatin group versus increasing an average of 0.006 mm per year in the placebo group (p = .001). The same effect was seen in men and women and in those less than and over 60 years of age. Clinically there were 5 cardiovascular events (myocardial infarctions, strokes, or CHD deaths) in the lovastatin-treated group versus 14 in the placebo group, a 61% decrease (p = .04). There was one death in the lovastatin group and 8 deaths in the placebo group (p = .02). All six cardiovascular deaths were in the placebo group.

Amazingly similar results were obtained in the smaller Pravastatin, Lipids and Atherosclerosis in the Carotid Arteries (PLAC II) study.[40,41] 151 participants (85% male, mean age 63 years) were found with a history of myocardial infarction (63%) or >50% stenosis in one or more coronary arteries, with one or more carotid plaques with IMT 1.3 mm or greater. Subjects had to have an LDL cholesterol on phase I AHA diet of 160 - 190 mg/dL (4.34 - 5.13 mE/L) with triglycerides 350 mg/dL (3.95 mE/L) or less. Pravachol was randomly assigned in doses of 10mg (4%), 20 mg(24%), or 40mg (72%) to decrease LDL cholesterol to 90 - 110 mg/dL (2.44 - 2.84 mE/L). Follow-up was for 3 years in a double-blinded protocol and ultrasound measurements of the carotid artery segments were done each six months.

Average LDL cholesterol decreased from 167 to 120 mg/dL (4.3 to 3.1 mE/L) with no change in HDL cholesterol in the pravastatin treated group. The annual rate of change in mean maximal intimal-medial thickness was no lower in the pravastatin versus placebo group (0.059 versus 0.0675 mm per year, p = .44) using all carotid artery segments. In the common carotid artery, however, the annual rate of thickening of intimal-medial thickness was less in the pravastatin-treated group (0.029 versus 0.046 mm per year , p = 0.03). The decrease in progression rate was correlated with treatment level of LDL cholesterol and results were slightly better in women than men (p= .08).

There were 4 cardiac events (MI plus CHD deaths) in the pravastatin group versus 10 in the placebo group (p = .09). There were 5 MI's plus all deaths in the pravastatin group versus 13 in the placebo group (p= .04) This 60% reduction in cardiac events was identical to that seen in ACAPS described above.

Summary of clinical trials

These lipid-lowering angiographic and ultrasonographic trials present several important general findings.

1. Lipid alterations - specifically LDL-C lowering and HDL-C increases are associated with coronary angiographic benefits to those treated most aggressively, i.e., less progression, more stability, and in some cases more regression in atherosclerotic lesions.

2. These angiographic benefits can occur in all degrees of stenoses but are generally more detectable in lesions where stenoses are greater than 50%.

3. Men and women react similarly to such lipid alterations.

4. Subjects with lower cholesterol levels (TC ≤ 240 mg/dl) react similarly to those

with greater cholesterol levels (TC > 240 mg/dl).

5. The association of improved angiographic findings and lipid improvements are found in several different interventions for lowering lipid levels, i.e., pure dietary, surgical, and pharmacologic.

6. Although on-trial LDL/HDL or TC/HDL ratios or degree of change in LDL or HDL-cholesterol changes from baseline were associated with angiographic or ultrasound findings, no specific target goal for LDL-cholesterol or percentage lowering can be discerned as being absolutely necessary for stabilization of coronary angiograms (*Table 4.4*).

    Average achieved levels of LDL-cholesterol ranged from 93 mg/dl (2.41 mE/L) (MARS) [27] to 178 mg/dl (4.60 mE/L)(NHLBI II). [24] Percentage lowering in baseline LDL cholesterol ranged from 16% (STARS-diet)[23] to 45% (FATS-colestipol plus lovastatin)[28] and average absolute lowering of mean LDL-cholesterol levels ranged from 32 mg/dl (.82 mE/L) (STARS-diet)[23] to 111 mg/dl (2.86 mE/L) (SCOR).[33] In SCOR, the LDL-cholesterol during the study was plotted against mean change in percent area stenosis with a small r value = 0.282, p=.018. At LDL-C levels as low as 100 mg/dl (2.58 mE/L) and as high as 300 mg/dl (7.75 mE/L), one could find subjects with progression and other subjects with regression. This same scatter of points around the regression line of on trial LDL-C and L/H ratio and change in mean absolute width of coronary segment was seen in STARS with r=.4, suggesting that on trial LDL cholesterol only explains 16% of the variance in change in mean absolute width in segments. Similarly one can not discern a target LDL-cholesterol or L/H cholesterol ratio which would guarantee a decrease in events rate; a similar range of achieved values is seen in those with and those without a decrease in event rates. *(Table 4.4)* The studies are very different in their power, study populations with different levels of risk, and follow-up periods and thus are difficult to compare. Yet it is hard to support the current NCEP guideline that an LDL-C goal of < 100 mg/dl (<2.58 mE/L) is necessary to stabilize angiograms and to prevent further clinical events. One might reasonably say from these studies that minimally one needs a drop in LDL-cholesterol of greater than 30 mg/dl (.78 mE/L) or greater than a 25% drop from baseline after routine dietary therapy. A reasonable target range for LDL-cholesterol from all the trials might be 90-120 mg/dl (2.3-3.1 mE/L). This will not universally guarantee either a prevention of progression of angiographic disease or a decrease in clinical events rates but will do so measurably in a portion of the population.

7. Reductions in clinical events do not occur immediately and simultaneously with lipid reduction. Decreases in total mortality occurred by 18-24 months in ACAPS but decreased in POSCH only in the group with ejection fraction > 50 % after 10 years. Decreases in clinical event rates started appearing after 1 year in SCRIP, ACAPS, PLAC II, and FATS, and 3 years in POSCH. Such data suggests a need for rapid initiation of lipid-lowering efforts in the person with coronary disease in order to secure the clinical benefits within one to two

Table 4.3   ULTRASOUND STUDIES OF ATHEROSCLEROSIS REGRESSION

Study	Inclusion criteria	Participants						Intervetion	Length
		n randomized/ angions compared	% angina %MI	% male	Mean age (yrs)	% ASA	% smo-ker		of trial (yrs)
Asymptomatic[38] Carotid Artery Progression Study (ACAPS)	a. No cardiovascular disease b. 1 of 12 IMT's≥ 1,5 mm all< 3,5 mm c. H LDL-C on diet: 160-189 0-1 RF's (4,34-5,13) 130-159≥2RF's (3,53-4,33)	919	0/0	52	62 (40-79)	100% ASA 81 mg	12	Lova to dicrease LDL-C to 90-110 (2,44-2,84) Lova 10: 5% Lova 20: 44% Lova 40: 50%	3
Prevastatin[40,41], Lipids and Atherosclerosis in the Carotid Arteries (PLAC II)	a. Hx of MI (63%) or ή > 50% stenosis in ≥ 1 coronary b. ≥1 carotid artery plaque with IMT≥1,3 mm c. LDL on diet 160-190 (4,34-5,13) TG<350 (3,95)	151	-/63	85	63	–	13	Prava to decrease LDL-to 90-110 (2,44-2,84) Prava 10: 4% Prava 20: 24% Prava 40: 72%	3

years. Any mechanisms for explaining these decreases in clinical events must take into account this delay in protection from clinical events.

8.   Angiographic progression of coronary stenoses increases the risk of subsequent clinical events two to threefold. POSCH was able to demonstrate a relation-ship between progression rates over 3 years and subsequent clinical events. Any subjects - whether in the surgical or control group - who had a global score suggesting progression over the first three years had a doubling of risk for subsequent cardiovascular death and non fatal MI.[32] Tiny increases in global scores often represent a large increase in one stenosis averaged over nine ar-terial segments, eight of which have remained the same. Usually progression measured by such scores reflects a significant measurable increase in one or two stenoses most probably from changes in the plaque, inducing thrombosis, and then incorporating this thrombosis into a larger stenotic lesion. One might hypothesize then that increasing global scores for progression represent a measure of increased plaque instability, which would predictably increase clin-ical events. This notion that measurable single plaque progression represents plaque instability potentially leading to increased clinical events was confirmed in a previous study performed by CCAIT investigatiors who found a relative risk of 7.3 for cardiac death and of 2.3 for cardiac death or non fatal MI in

Table 4.3   ULTRASOUND STUDIES OF ATHEROSCLEROSIS REGRESSION

Lipid Changes-Treatment Group			Ultrasound Change by Patient			Clinical Events	Comment
ΔLDL mg/dl	[Δ%]	ΔHDL mg/dl	[Δ%]	Mean Maximal Intime-Medial Thickness			
				Rx control	P	Rx control P (%decrease)	
156→117 (4.0-3.0)	[-25]	52→54 (1.34→1.40)	[+5]	-0.009 +0.006	.001	MI&CHD death +Stroke ——————— 5 14 .04 (60%)	Same effect men & women, > 60 vs < 60 yrs. 6-12 mo to slow progression
167→120 (4.3→3.1)	[-28]	42→41 (1.09-1.06)	NS	.059 .0675	0.44	MI&CHD death ——————— 4 10 .09 (60%)	Decrease in progression correlated with treatement LDL-C. Women more effective than men.
				(common carotid only) .029 .046	0.03	MI+all death ——————— 5 13 .04 (61%)	

persons who had ≥15% progression in any coronary lession on subsequent angiogram 2 years after the first.[42]

9. Clinical event rates are most likely determined by what happens to the 95% of lesions which are less than 70% stenotic. Most angiographic studies indicate that the greatest improvement in coronary segmental stenoses are in lesions with stenoses greater than 50%. The decrease in event rates, however, most likely has to do with changes associated with the mild (10-39%) or moderate (40-69%) lesions. Thirteen patients in FATS [43] with baseline and follow-up angiograms, had coronary events, 4 in the 74 subjects on niacin/colestipol or cholestipol/lovastatin and 9 in the 46 patients on non-pharmacologic therapy. (Figure 4.1) The rate of progression to clinical event from the baseline severe lesions (70+ % stenosis) was the same in each group - 83/1000 lesions in the drug treated group and 62/1000 in the non-pharmacologically treated group (N.S.). The drug treated group progressed to a clinical event from a mild to moderate lesion at a rate of 1.5/1000, a major reduction from 19.3/1000 in the non-pharmacologic group (p < 0.004). Thus although lesions (> 50%) seem to improve angiographically more than those of a lesser degree, it would seem that some effect, e.g. "stabilization," of plaques less than 70% produce the greatest decrease in subsequent clinical events. This data also suggests that

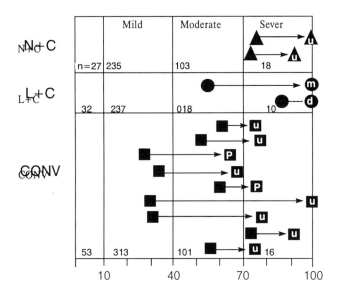

Stenosis Severity

(Baseline→Event) (%S)

Incidence of coronary events per 1000 lesions:

	Mild-moderate	Severe	%severe lesions at baseline
N+C,	1.46	83.3	5.0 (36/719)
L+C	19.3	62.5	3.7 (16/430)
p	<.004	NS	

Figure 4.1 Lesion changes associated with 13 coronary events familiar atherosclerosis Study (FATS)

stenoses > 70% probably have a greater risk of producing a clinical event than a lesion <70%, 62.5 verses 19.3/1000, but that since severe lesions account for only 4-5% of total lesions on angiography, the great bulk of clinical disease is secondary to progression of lesions with less than 70% stenosis.

Clinical nonangiographic secondary prevention trials

The association of angiographic progression with increased clincal events and the association of lipid-lowering with decreased progression suggests that secondary prevention lipid-lowering trials given sufficient time and power should significantly lower clinical events including total mortality.

Table 4.4   *INCIDENCE OF CLINICAL EVENTS IN VARIOUS LIPID-LOWERING TRIALS*

Significant decrease in clinical events LDL-C and L/H ratio achieved

mg/dl	mE/L	% LDL-C lowering	L/H	n	Study
162	4.19	16	3.7	74	STARS-diet[23]
130	3.37	36	2.9	74	STARS-resin[23]
129	3.33	32	2.3	120	FATS (C+N)[28]
120	3.10	24	2.3	246	SCRIP[35]
120	3.10	28	---	151	PLACII[40,41]
117	3.03	28	---	408	PLACI[37]
117	3.00	25	---	919	ACAPS[38]
107	2.76	45	2.6	120	FATS (C+L)[28] (colest+lova)
104	2.68	42	2.3	838	POSCH[31]

No significant decrease in clinical events LDL-C and L/H ratio achieved

Study	n	mg/dl	mE/L	% LDL-C lowering	L/H
NHLBI-II[24]	116	178	4.60	26	3.9
SCOR[33]	72	172	4.45	38	2.9
CCAIT[26]	299	122	3.15	29	2.8
MAAS[34]	381	117	3.02	31	2.7
CLAS[25]	162	97	2.51	43	1.7
Life style[21]	41	95	2.46	37	2.9
MARS[27]	247	93	2.41	38	2.0

n = total subjects with comparable angiograms

The Scandinavian Simvastatin Survival Study has accomplished just that.[44] 4444 subjects (81% male, 19% female), age 35-70 years, with a history of coronary heart disease (80% MI, 20% angina) and with total cholesterols on diet between 220 and 320 mg/dl (5.5 - 8.0 mE/L) were randomized to a daily dose of simvastatin 20mg (63%) or 40mg (37%) that would achieve a total cholesterol less than 200 mg/dl (5.2 mE/L). In the group on simvastatin average LDL-C decreased 35% from 187 to 122 mg/dl (4.86 to 3.15 mE/L) and HDL-C levels increased 8% from 46 to 50 mg/dl (1.2 to 1.3 mE/L). At a median of 5.4 years of follow-up total mortality decreased 30% in the simvastatin group compared with the placebo group (p = .003), all accounted for by decreases in coronary-heart-disease associated deaths with no increase in deaths from any other cause (cancer, trauma, suicide, etc). Definite or probable non-fatal acute MI rates decreased 37%, CABG and angioplasty procedures decreased by 37%, and cerebrovascular events decreased 30%. These differences were evident at one to one and one half years after randomization. No evidence of toxicity for the drug could be found. Decreases in major coronary events (death and non-fatal MI) were significant for women (35%) and for men (34%), for persons $\geq$ 60 yrs (29%) and those < 60 years (39%), and for those in all quartiles of baseline LDL-cholesterol and HDL-cholesterol. This study confirms the previously described decreased clinical events in the angiographic studies and suggests that cholesterol-lowering over a 6 year period not only significantly decreases morbidity and mortality but also is harmless. There were no increases in traumatic, accidental, suicidal deaths or in incidence of any forms of cancer and thus cholesterol-lowering per se seems to be harmless, an important consideration for primary as well as secondary prevention.

The Pravastatin Multinational Study [45] for patients with high risk for coronary heart disease selected 1062 men and women with total cholesterol levels after four weeks on dietary therapy of 5.2 to 7.8 mE/L (200 - 300 mg/dL) plus two additional risk factors for coronary heart disease (including angina, previous myocardial infarction, male gender, hypertension, cigarette smoking, or family history of coronary heart disease.). One-half were randomly assigned to either 20 or 40 milligrams of pravastatin, the larger dose utilized in subjects who on the lower dose had not decreased total cholesterol levels by 15% from baseline or who had not achieved levels less than 5.2mE/L (200 mg/dL). Mean age of the subjects was 55 years, with 76% being male, 48% having hypertension, 29% smoking, 43% having a positive family history of coronary artery disease, 34% having had a previous myocardial infarction and 40% having angina − certainly a high risk group of subjects. Average LDL cholesterol decreased from 4.69 to 3.47 mE/L (181 to 134 mg/dL) in the pravastatin treated group (a 26% decrease) with no change in the placebo group. HDL cholesterol increased from 1.14 to 1.23 mE/L (44 to 48 mg/dL) in the pravastatin group (an 8% increase with only a 3% increase in the placebo group). Over a 26 week period there were 13 serious cardiovascular events (MI, unstable angina, CHF, sudden cardiac death) in the placebo group and only 1 in the treated group (p < .001). The Kaplan-Meier life table analysis of these events diverges within two to three week of the beginning of the randomization suggesting a very statistically improbable event or a major therapeutic effect with onset much earlier than other comparable trials.

All of the primary and secondary prevention studies presented above should be comprehensive enough to convince even the most skeptical of the beneficial effects of lowering LDL cholesterol on clinical and angiographic coronary disease. Future studies will need to focus on some of the details. Although LDL-lowering preventive effects are demonstrable in persons into their mid seventies, do these same effects continue to occur into the mid eighties and nineties? Will they occur at these ages in both those with and without coronary heart disease? Will the benefits of LDL-lowering extend to persons with HDL cholesterol levels below 30 mg/dL whose LDL cholesterol levels are only minimally elevated in the 100 - 130 range but who have experienced coronary heart disease? If so, how low must LDL levels be targeted in these persons with hypoalphalipoproteinemia and coronary heart disease? Will intravascular ultrasound be able to sort coronary lesions and arteries into those that are the most and the least responsive to LDL-lowering?

Hypertriglyceridemia and coronary disease

There is enough evidence at this point that hypertriglyceridemia may be atherogenic that one must be concerned with triglyceride levels for both primary and secondary prevention of CHD. The Framingham Study demonstrated increased risk for coronary heart disease from triglyceride levels greater than 140 mg/dl in the presence of an HDL-C less than 40 mg/dl in both men and women.[46] The Prospective study in Gotenburg, Sweden, has demonstrated over a 20 year follow-up that the highest quartile of triglycerides as a univariate variable are very predictive of subsequent total and coronary heart disease mortality in 1450 females whereas total cholesterol is not such a predictor.[47] The Prospective Atherosclerosis Trial in Muenster, Germany, found an increased incidence of coronary heart disease in persons with triglyceride levels over 200 mg/dl in the presence of an HDL-C less than 35 and a total cholesterol to HDL cholesterol (TC/HDL-C) ratio greater than 5.0.[38] The Helsinki Heart Study placebo group demonstrated a relative risk of 5.0. in those with triglycerides greater than 200 mg/dl in the presence of an LDL-C/HDL-C ratio greater than 5.0.[15] Over the five year study, there was an overall 34% decrease in coronary heart disease in the total gemfibrozil-treated cohort, but a 71% decrease in this subgroup with elevated triglycerides and LDL-C/HDL-C suggesting that intervention with this type of fibric acid drug may be very helpful in primary prevention in persons with this lipid profile.[15]

The positive association of hypertriglyceridemia and risk for coronary heart disease, however is not as clear-cut as the association of high LDL-cholesterol or low HDL-cholesterol. The Lipid Research Clinic Follow-up Study [48] showed a relationship between the natural logarithm of baseline triglyceride level and 12 year coronary heart disease mortality in 4129 men and 3376 women with a relative risk of 1.5 to 1.9 per natural log unit of triglycerides. This relative risk decreased to 1.3

and 1.2 respectively (N.S.) for both sexes when adjusted for HDL and LDL cholesterol, smoking status, systolic blood pressure, BMI, and postmenopausal estrogen use in women. The relative risk further declined to 1.1 and 1.0 (N.S.) when fasting plasma glucose was added to the analysis.

This study points out the predicament of the hypertriglyceridemic phenotype: is it the hypertriglyceridemia or the associated physiologic findings that cause the increased risk. The insulin resistance syndrome is one that combines a variety of risk factors for coronary heart disease, all of which are associated with each other: insulin resistance to glucose disposal with hyperinsulinemia and impaired glucose tolerance or frank hyperglycemia and diabetes, hypertriglyceridemia, low HDL cholesterol, increased waist to hip ratio, hypertension, and hyperuricemia.[49,50] Although hypertriglyceridemia has a univariate relationship with increased risk for coronary heart disease, when its associated physiologic abnormalities are corrected for in multivariate analysis, hypertriglyceridemia often loses its predictive risk.[51,52] In these analyses, the risk factors are correlated and multivariate analysis may significantly underestimate the risk of hypertriglyceridemia. Another type of analysis based on logistic regression analysis, called the projected-slope analysis [53], attempts to control for redundant information in multivariate analysis of correlated risk factors. When applied to the Framingham data on triglycerides, triglycerides become more significant when HDL-cholesterol is considered whereas in the multivariate analysis, triglycerides lose their significance.[46]

Two angiographic trials have implicated triglyceride-rich particles in the progression of coronary atheroslerosis. CLAS pointed toward triglycerides particles in both placebo and drug-treated groups as predictors of progression.[54] Apolipoprotein C-III, an inhibitor of lipoprotein lipase which retards hepatic uptake of triglyceride-rich lipoproteins and their remnants, is transferred from triglyceride-rich apolipoprotein B containing particles (chylomicrons and VLDL) to HDL particles as the former undergo lipolysis. Hence levels of apo C-III associated with HDL my be used as a measure of triglyceride-rich particle catabolism. In CLAS higher levels of apo C-III associated with HDL (and thus presumably better catabolism of triglyceride-rich particles) was shown to decrease the risk of progression in the drug-treated group. In the placebo group, the risk of progression was best associated in multivariate analysis with non-HDL cholesterol which is a measure of cholesterol in both LDL and triglyceride-rich VLDL particles.

MARS [27] was the first to show that LDL/HDL cholesterol ratios best predict progression in stenoses >50% in the treated group with LDL-C < 100 mg/dL, whereas apolipoprotein C-III in the apo-B fraction (LDL plus VLDL) best predicted progression in lesions with <50% stenosis, again implying the potential importance of triglyceride-rich particles in progression, especially when LDL-C levels are low.

It is clinically very clear that some persons with hypertriglyceridemias may have increased risk for coronary heart disease. This happens in Type III dysbetalipoproteinemia in which individuals have an abnormal apoprotein E and hence are unable to clear VLDL particles by the liver.[55] This results in intermediate density lipoproteins with a different electrophoretic mobility which are directly atherogenic.

Goldstein and colleagues described familial combined hyperlipidemia in families of MI survivors in ther early 1970's.[56] Such families have variable lipid phenotypes, varying between Types IIA, IIB, and IV. An individual family member's phenotype may change with time, and different generations in the same family have different lipid phenotypes. Such hypertriglyceridemic families contrast with other families in which only one lipid phenotype, Type IV, is present. These families with what is called familial hypertriglyceridemia, do not characteristically appear to have an increased risk for coronary heart disease. In familial combined hyperlipidemia, several unique features exist which are not present in families with familial hypertriglyceridemia.[57] They have small VLDL particles but increased levels of apoprotein B which suggests an excess of such particles as compared with the large, apparently benign VLDL particles with normal levels of apoprotein B in those with familial hypertriglyceridemia.

Subclasses of LDL particles may be identified by gradient gel electrophoresis which separates particles by size and charge. Pattern B is characterized by small dense LDL particles and this pattern has been associated with increased risk for myocardial infarction.[58] Pattern B is also associated with with decreased levels of plasma HDL-cholesterol and apolipoprotein A1 and increases in triglyceride and apolipoprotein B levels.[59] There is a greatly increased frequency of LDL pattern B in persons with triglyceride levels greater than 141 mg/dL, the level in Framingham above which one sees increasing risk for CHD in the presence of HDL cholesterol levels less than 40 mg/dL.[46] An early community genetic study demonstrated that the frequency of the pattern B allele is .25 in the general population and that the gene segregates in a Mendelian dominant fashion with penetrance mainly seen in males over the age of 20 and females over the age of 50 in the postmenopausal period.[59] More recent data suggest that up to three genes may be involved in expression of LDL subclass patterns.[60]

This LDL pattern B has also been found in families with familial combined hyperlipidemia with a slightly higher gene frequency of 0.3.[61] Family members with this type B pattern have significantly higher levels of triglycerides (184 mg/dL) compared with family members with type A pattern (94 mg/dL) or with spouse controls (90 mg/dL). Hence the gene for LDL pattern may be interactive with another gene for increased apolipoprotein B levels to produce the unique lipid features of persons with combined familial hyperlipidemia which contribute to increased CHD risk. Triglyceride-lowering with gemfibrozil therapy has not been associated with a switch of the type B LDL subclass pattern to type A, but has been associated with some increase in buoyant LDL particles.[62]

Several studies have demonstrated an association of hypertriglyceridemia with a hypercoagulable state. Eighteen patients with a fasting triglyceride level greater than 310 mg/dL (3.5 mM/L) were found to have increased concentrations of factor X and fibrinogen and a lower fibrinolytic activity (100 / clot lysis time in hours).[63]

Triglyceride levels were decreased from 602 to 275 mg/dL (6.8 to 3.l mM/L) over six months with either dietary means or clofibrate therapy. Over the same time course Factor X and factor VII concentrations were significantly reduced and mean fibrin-olytic activity was significantly increased. There was no effect on fibrinogen or fac-tor VIII levels.

High plasma levels of tissue plasminogen activator (t-PA) inhibitor were found in seventy patients three years after a myocardial infarction compared with a healthy control group.[64] Levels of this t-PA inhibitor were associated with triglyceride levels (r= 0.6, p<.001). These two studies suggest that it may be the association of high triglyceride levels with hypercoaguable states rather than the lipoprotein particles themselves that increase CHD risk with hypertriglyceridemia.

Although much epidemiologic evidence points to high triglyceride levels as a CHD risk factor in some persons and some lipid phenotypes, clinical evidence that lowering triglycerides prevents CHD has been scarce. Both niacin and clofibrate were used to lower lipids in the Coronary Drug Project [65], a secondary prevention trial in male survivors of myocardial infarction. Fifty percent of subjects had base-line triglyceride levels greater than 450 mg/dL (5mE/L) and total cholesterol levels greater than 250 mg/dL (6.5 mE/L). Triglyceride levels were lowered 15.6 and 19.4 % by one year in the clofibrate and niacin groups respectively and cholesterol levels by 6.2 and 9.6% respectively. There was no decrease in cardiovascular mortality at 5 years or at 15 years in the clofibrate-treated group. In the niacin group there was a decrease in non-fatal MI at 5 years and a decrease in cardiovascular mortality at 15 years.[66] The group with the greatest protective effects was that with the greatest drop in total cholesterol between baseline and year 1, not in the group showing the greatest drop in triglyceride levels. Such results do not suggest triglyceride-lowering as a major goal of lipid-altering therapy.

On the other hand, there was a great preventive effect of another fibric acid derivative, gemfibozil, in the Helsinki Heart Study primary prevention trial in men with LDL/HDL cholesterol ratio's greater than 5.0 and triglycerides levels greater than 200 mg/dL (2.3 mE/L); MI's and fatal CHD were reduced 70% over a 5 year period.[15] In addition in the Stockholm Ischaemic Heart Disease Secondary Preven-tion Study the combination of clofibrate (one gram BID) and niacin (one gram TID) reduced total mortality 26% and CHD mortality 36% over a five year period in 555 subjects, men (80%) and women (20%), who were discharged having survived an MI. Treatment effects became apparent at two years and reduction in CHD mortality was greatest (>60%) in those with greater than 30% reduction in triglyc-erides. Since HDL cholesterol levels were not measured, one can not sort out the contributions of triglyceride reductions and increases in HDL cholesterol. None-theless the empiric findings of this little-cited study are very clear in persons with elevations of triglycerides greater than 140 mg/dL just after a myocardial infarction, i.e., use of niacin and clofibrate which cause triglyceride reductions (>30%) may have major preventive effects on morbidity and mortality. The authors of this study suggest that the quicker preventive effects in this study compared with the niacin-produced effects in the Coronary Drug Project was that the Stockholm Study included people who enrolled within four months of discharge from an MI whereas the Coronary Drug Project had long term survivors after an MI (69% > 1 year,35% > 3 years). Consequently subjects in the Coronary Drug Project may have been long-term MI survivors with a decreased mortality rate thus requiring a longer time to show further a decrease in mortality.

The Food and Drug Administration has not allowed gemfibozil to be marketed as an effective agent for secondary prevention. For persons excluded from the primary prevention arm of the Helsinki Heart Study because of a history of angina, myocardial infarction, or unexplained ECG changes, there was a request for a secondary prevention trial. 628 middle-aged males, only 15% of whom met the strict original criteria for verifiable CHD, were randomized to gemfibrozil (600 mg BID) or placebo therapy for a period of 5 years which paralleled the primary prevention trial.(Lopid package insert) Using intent to treat analysis, there were 24 cardiac events (fatal or nonfatal MI's or sudden cardiac death) in the placebo group and 35 in the gemfibrozil group (p=.14, NS). 12 of the 35 patients in the gemfibrozil group and 8 of 24 in the placebo group had discontinued the study before the event. If coronary bypass grafting is added to the above cardiac events, and analyzed while in the study or within one year of withdrawal, 28 events occurred in the placebo group and 29 in the gemfibrozil group (N.S.).(Data on file with Parke-Davis) This mixed primary/secondary prevention study thus shows no beneficial effect of gemfibrozil nor does it discount one because of its small size and insufficient power.

In summary, elevated triglyceride levels especially when associated with low HDL cholesterol levels are associated with an increased risk for coronary heart disease. The use of gemfibrozil in primary prevention would seem to provide a major protective effect. Niacin alone and niacin plus clofibrate have shown significant decreases in morbidity and mortality in persons with CHD, the latter but not the former being associated with decreases in triglyceride levels. A small secondary prevention study using gemfibrozil, although showing no beneficial effect, did not have the power to discount one.

This author when seeing a patient with coronary heart disease and lipid patterns IIb or IV does not simply focus on LDL-cholesterol-lowering. Triglycerides are first lowered to less than 200 mg/dl with hopes of a simultaneous increase in HDL-cholesterol. After triglycerides are lowered, the focus shifts to LDL-cholesterol to make sure it is in the 90-120 mg/dl (2.3-3.1 mE/L) range. Niacin has been shown to most consistently reduce further coronary events and improve survival in this situation. There is a suggestion from a primary prevention trial that gemfibrozil may have secondary preventive benefits at least in those with an LDL/HDL cholesterol ratio greater than 5.0, but a large secondary prevention trial will be necessary to document this.

Possible mechanisms of LDL-cholesterol-lowering and prevention of coronary disease

Regression studies in non-human primates such as cynomologous monkeys [67,68]or rhesus monkeys [69] demonstrate that atherosclerotic lesions formed after 18 months on a high cholesterol or high fat diet, have a sequential decrease in lesional cholesterol ester and then in free cholesterol after the animals are placed on regular chow diets depleted of cholesterol and low in fat. In rhesus monkeys this regression process plateaued at approximately 20 months with not much further lesional decrease in either form of cholesterol over the ensuing 20 months. In cynomologous monkeys progression occurs with increasing foam cells filled with cholesterol ester. At 30 months there is much cellular necrosis with the appearance of large amounts of free cholesterol crystals located extracellularly and foam cells located at the periphery of the lesions. With six months of regression, there is a decrease in foam cells and cholesterol esters, but an increase in free cholesterol crystals which themselves are reduced significantly by 12 months.

One might hypothesize that the same thing happens in humans with significant lowering of LDL cholesterol. Both the STARS dietary arm, the Leiden trial, and the Life Style Intervention Trial of Ornish show that with dietary fat restriction, one may obtain angiographic improvements in coronary arteries.

Earlier epidemiologic pathologic studies by Vartiainen and Kanerva in Finland suggested that raised atheromatous aortic plaques found at autopsy between 1940 and 1945 in Finland were 20 to 40 percent diminished from those found in l933 to l938 prior to the war.[70] Simultaneously Strom and Jensen in Norway found a decline from cardiovascular mortality beginning in 1940 with the lowest rates in 1943-45 and increasing in the post-war period.[71] All cardiovascular mortality was decreased 10 to 20 percent but atherosclerotic mortality was decreased 30 to 40 percent. Per capita consumption of fat during l940 to 1945 declined in Oslo by 50%, protein by 20%, and calories by 20%.[71] The similarities in these ecologic epidemiologic findings with those of the experimental nonhuman primate dietary trials are striking.

The unfortunate point of the angiographic trials, however, is that angiographic regression is not seen in most of the studies, rather a lack of progression which correlates well with decreased clinical event rates. Thus a decrease in percent stenosis which might be hypothesized to reduce plaque fragility by reducing turbulent flow may not be the predominant mechanism of event reduction.

It has been demonstrated the the coronary lesions most likely to fissure and thrombose are those with the most extracellular lipid in the central core.[72,73] In an in vitro perfusion chamber it has also been shown that the most thrombogenic substance in arterial plaques is the atheromatous core with abundant cholesterol crystals as compared to foam-cell- rich matrix or collagen-rich matrix.[74] Since the animal experimental data is that cholesterol ester and then cholesterol monohydrate decrease in regression in animals, it is possible that there are significant decreases in lipid plaque core in the most vulnerable plaques which has not been detected by looking at changes in average stenosis of many coronary segments during the angiographic trials. Certainly this issue will be explored as ultrasound and other imaging techniques are used to classify components of plaques within the arterial system.

Lowering serum cholesterol levels has important functional as well as morphologic effects on the vascular wall. It has been shown that hypercholesterolemia and atherosclerosis both impair endothelium-mediated vasodilation in both humans and animals.[75] Recently Treasure et al.[75] have demonstrated that a 26% reduction in LDL cholesterol (mean LDL cholesterol 148 to 110 mg/dL [3.8 to 2.8 mE/L]) using lovastatin 40 mg bid versus placebo in a randomized, double-blind study of 23 patients who had coronary heart disease resulted in significantly improved endothelium-mediated vasodilation within five and one-half months of beginning medication. This improvement did not occur at 12 days after starting medication although LDL reduction had occurred by that time. At five and one-half months improved, but not fully normal, function had been restored, suggesting that more time may be necessary for normalization of function. Gould et al.[76] have shown improved dypiridamole perfusion defects in 12 persons with coronary heart disease after reducing LDL cholesterol levels by 29% (213 to 151 mg/dL [5.5 to 3.9 mE/L] over a three month period. Perfusion defects reverted to the original pattern within 60 days of returning to a baseline LDL cholesterol level.

Although these improvements in endothelial vasodilation measured directly or indirectly with PET scanning occur at 3 to 6 months after LDL lowering, and hence don't have the exact same longer time course for reductions in clinical events (usually occuring after one year), nonetheless it is very possible that such improvement in vascular function may partially explain the beneficial effects of LDL-lowering on clinical events.

Finally it may be that LDL-lowering decreases the thrombogenic potential or increases the fibrinolytic potential involved in the interaction of blood and a fractured plaque which produces the thrombus associated with coronary clinical events. Unfortunately very few studies have examined LDL-lowering and changes in fibrinogen, Factor VII, PAI-I, and other potential thrombogenic or antifibrinolylic factors. It is clear from many studies that Lp(a) is not associated with LDL-lowering.[77] Badimon et al. have shown that feeding rats a high cholesterol diet for 60 days results in increased platelet deposition in an in vitro perfusion chamber under high shear rates.[78] Another report [79] has recently shown that 40 mg of pravastatin for two to three months inducing a drop in LDL cholesterol from 190 to 135 mg/dL (4.9 to 3.5 mE/L) in 18 patients with coronary heart disease decreases platelet deposition in the same in vitro chamber under high and low shear rates, whether taking aspirin or not. These fascinating preliminary studies must be followed by further work to explore the relationship of LDL-cholesterol lowering and thrombogenesis as a mechanism from improved clinical effects.

The data from *Figure 4.1* suggest that lesions less than 70% have less likelihood of rapidly progressing to give an acute syndrome. This might occur if the strength of the fibrous cap were maintained or at least were not undermined. A recent report [80] has shown that in an in vitro system, macrophages grown in tissue culture from peripheral blood monocytes and exposed to fibrous caps dissected from human aortic plaques for 48 hours expressed collagenase type I activity during culture resulting in increased hydroxyproline levels suggesting for the first time that macrophages can induce fibrous plaque breakdown. By lowering plasma LDL cholesterol, one might postulate a decrease LDL penetration into the subendothelial space resulting in less LDL oxidation and thus less stimulus for both endothelium-produced chemoattractants for macrophages such as macrophage chemoattractant protein 1 (MCP 1) and less stimulus for endothelium-produced macrophage colony stimulating factor (MCSF) which activates macrophages. With fewer activated macrophages, one could then postulate less macrophage secretion of metallo-proteases and hence less breakdown of the collagen and elastin within the fibrous cap.

Whatever the mechanism(s) for decreases in LDL-cholesterol-lowering to reduce coronary event rates, the fact that it does so is no longer a matter of speculation. Data are now very suggestive as well that LDL-cholesterol-lowering decreases cerebrovascular events, peripheral vascular disease, and coronary and all-cause mortality. All physicians interested in managing atherosclerotic arterial disease are now under the obligation to aggressively treat lipids and significantly reduce further events.

REFERENCES

1. Keys A, et al. Coronary heart disease in seven countries. Circulation. 1970;41(Suppl I):I-1.

2. Keys Ansel. Seven Countries: A Multivariate Analysis of Death and Coronary Heart Disease. Cambridge,Mass: Harvard University Press, 1980.

3. Robertson TL, et al. Epidemiologic studies of coronary heart disease and stroke in Japanese men living in Japan, Hawaii, and California. Incidence of myocardial infarction and death from coronary heart disease. Amer J Cardiol. 1977;39:239.

4. Kannel WB, et al. Risk factors in coronary heart disease. An evaluation of several serum lipids as predictors of coronary heart disease - The Framingham Study. Ann Int Med. 1964;61:888.

5. Castelli WP. Cardiovascular disease and multifactorial risk:challenge of the 1980's. Am Heart J. 1983;106:1191.

6. Cornfield J. Joint dependence of risk of coronary heart disease on serum cholesterol and systolic pressure: A discriminant function analysis. Fed Proc. 1962;21 (part 2):58.

7. Gordon T, et al. High density lipoprotein as a protective factor againt coronary heart disease. Am J Med. 1977;62:707.

8. Castelli WP, et al. Incidence of coronary heart disease and lipoprotein cholesterol levels, The Framingham Study. JAMA. 1986;256:2835.

9. Abbott RD, et al. High density lipoprotein cholesterol, total cholesterol screening, and myocardial infarction. The Framingham Study. Arteriosclerosis. 1988;8:207.

10. Stamler J, Wentworth D, Neaton JD, MRFIT Research Group. Is the relationship between cholesterol and risk of premature death from coronary heart disease continuous and graded? Findings in the 356,222 primary screenees of the Multiple Risk Factor Intervention Trial (MRFIT). JAMA. 1986;256:2823.

11. Lipid Research Clinics Program. The Lipids Research Clinics Coronary Primary Prevention Trial results I. Reduction in incidence of coronary heart disease. JAMA. 1984;251:351.

12. Lipid Research Clinics Program. The Lipid Research Clinics Coronary Primary Prevention Trial Results II. The relationship of reduction in incidence of coronary heart disease to cholesterol lowering. JAMA. 1984;251:365.

13. Frick MH, et al. Helsinki Heart Study:Primary-prevention trial with gemfibrozil in middLe-aged men with dyslipidemia. N Engl J Med. 1987;317:1237.

14. Manninen V, et al. Lipid alterations and decline in the incidence of coronary heart disease in the Helsinki Heart Study. JAMA. 1988;260:641.

15. Manninen V, et al. Joint effects of serum triglyceride and LDL cholesterol and HDL cholesterol concentrations on coronary heart disease risk in the Helsinki Heart Study. Implications for treatment. Circulation. 1992;85:37.

16. Frick MH, et al. Gemfibrozil and coronary heart disease. N Engl J Med. 1988;318:1275.

17. Law MR, Thompson SG, Wald NJ. Assessing possible hazards of reducing serum cholesterol. BMJ. 1994;308:373.

18. Davey-Smith G, Song F, Sheldon TA. Cholesterol lowering and mortality: the importance of considering initial level of risk. BMJ. 1993;306:1367.

19. Expert Panel. Summary of the second report of the National Cholesterol Education Program (NCEP) Expert Panel on detection, evaluation, and treatment of high blood cholesterol in adults (Adult Treatment Panel II). JAMA. 1993;269:3015.

20. Arntzenius AC, et al. Diet, lipoproteins, and the progression of coronary atherosclerosis. The Leiden Intervention Trial. N Engl J Med. 1985;312:805.

21. Ornish D, et al. Can lifestyle changes reverse coronary heart disease? The Lifestyle Heart Trial. Lancet. 1990;336:129.

22. Ornish D, et al. Can lifestyle changes reverse coronary atherosclerosis? Four year results of the Lifestyle Heart Trial. Circulation. 1993;88 (Suppl 4):I-385.

23. Watts GF, et al. Effects on coronary artery disease of lipid-lowering diet, or diet plus cholestyramine, in the St. Thomas' Atherosclerosis Regression Study STARS. Lancet. 1992;339:563.

24. Levy RI, et al. The influence of changes in lipid values induced by cholestyramine and diet on the progression of coronary artery disease: results of the NHLBI Type II Coronary Intervention Study. Circulation. 1984;69:325.

25. Blankenhorn DH, et al. Beneficial effects of combined colestipol-niacin therapy on coronary atherosclerosis and coronary venous bypass grafts. JAMA. 1987;257:3233.

26. Waters D, et al. Effects of monotherapy with an HMG-CoA reductase inhibitor on the progression of coronary atherosclerosis as assessed by serial quantitative arteriography. The Canadian Coronary Atherosclerosis Intervention Trial. Circulation. 1994;89:959.

27. Blankenhorn DH, et al. Coronary angiographic changes with lovastatin therapy: The Monitored Atherosclerosis Regression Study (MARS). Ann Int Med. 1993;119:969.

28. Brown G, et al. Regression of coronary artery disease as a result of intensive lipid-lowering therapy in men with high levels of apolipoprotein B. N Engl J Med. 1990;323:1289.

29. Stewart BF, et al. Benefits of lipid-lowering therapy in men with elevated apolipoprotein B are not confined to those with very high low density lipoprotein cholesterol. J Am Coll Cardiol. 1994;23:899.

30. Moore RB, Frantz ID, Buchwald H. Changes in cholesterol pool size, turnover rate, and fecal bile acid and sterol excretion after partial ileal bypass in hypercholesterolemic patients. Surgery. 1969;65:98.

31. Buchwald H, et al. Effect of partial ileal bypass surgery on mortality and morbidity from coronary heart disease in patients with hypercholesterolemia. N Engl J Med. 1990;323:946.

32. Buchwald H, et al. Changes in sequential coronary arteriograms and subsequent coronary events. JAMA. 1992;268:1429.

33. Kane JP, et al. Regression of coronary atherosclerosis during treatment of familial hypercholesterolemia with combined drug regimens. JAMA. 1990;264:3007.

34. M.A.A.S.Investigators. Effect of simvastatin on coronary atheroma: the Multicentre Anti-Atheroma Study (MAAS). Lancet. 1994;344:633.

35. Hashell WL, et al. Effects of intensive multiple risk factor reduction on coronary atherosclerosis and clinical cardiac events in men and women with coronary artery disease. The Stanford Coronary Risk Intervention Project (SCRIP). Circulation. 1994;89:975.

36. Pitt B, et al. Design and recruitment in the United States of a multicenter quantitative angiographic trial of pravastatin to limit atherosclerosis in the coronary arteries (PLAC I). Am J Cardiol. 1993;72:31.

37. Pitt B, et al. Pravastatin limitation of atherosclerosis in the coronary arteries (PLAC I). J Amer Coll Cardial. 1994;23 (special issue):131A .

38. Furberg CD, et al. Effect of lovastatin on early carotid atherosclerosis and cardiovascular events. Circulation. 1994;90:1679.

39. Howard G, et al. Carotid artery intimal-medial thickness distribution in general populations as evaluated by B-mode ultrasound. Stroke. 1993;24:1297.

40. Crouse JR, et al. Pravastatin, lipids and atherosclerosis in the carotid arteries (PLAC II). Am J Cardiol. 1995;75:455.

41. Furberg CD, et al. Pravastatin, lipids, and major coronary events. Am J Cardiol. 1994;73:1133.

42. Waters D, Craven TE, Lesperance J. Prognostic significance of progression of coronary atherosclerosis. Circulation. 1993;87:1067.

43. Brown BG, et al. Lipid lowering and plaque regression. New insights into prevention of plaque disruption and clinical events in coronary disease. Circulation. 1993;87:1781.

44. Scandinavian Simvastatin Survival Study Group. Randomized trial of cholesterol lowering in 4444 patients with coronary heart disease: the Scandinavian Simvastatin Survival Study (4S). Lancet. 1994;344:1383.

45. The Pravastatin Multinational Study Group for Cardiac Risk Patients. Effects of pravastatin in patients with serum total cholesterol levels from 5.2 to 7.8 mmol/liter (200-300 mg/dL) plus two additional atherosclerotic risk factors. Am J Cardiol. 1993;72:1031.

46. Castelli WP. The triglyceride issue: A view from Framingham. Am Heart J. 1986;112:432.

47. Bengtsson C, et al. Associations of serum lipid concentrations and obesity with mortality in women: 20 year follow up of participants in prospective population study in Gottenburg, Sweden. BMJ. 1993;307:1385.

48. Criqui M, et al. Plasma triglyceride level and mortality from coronary heart disease. N Engl J Med. 1993;328:1220.

49. Reaven GM. Role of insulin resistance in human disease, Banting Lecture 1988. Diabetes. 1988;37:1595.

50. Haffner SM, et al. Cardiovascular risk factors in confirmed prediabetic individuals. Does the clock for coronary heart disease start ticking before the onset of clinical diabetes. JAMA. 1990;263:2893.

51. Austin MA. Plasma triglyceride and coronary heart disease. Arterioscler Thromb. 1991;11:2.

52. NIH Consensus Development Panel. NIH Consensus conference: triglyceride, high-density lipoprotein, and coronary heart disease. JAMA. 1993;269:505.

53. Abbott RD, Carroll FR. Interpreting multiple logistic regression coefficients. Am J Epidemiol. 1984;119:830.

54. Blankenhorn DH, et al. Prediction of angiographic change in native human coronary arteries and aortocoronary bypass grafts: Lipid and nonlipid factors. Circulation. 1990;81:470.

55. Mahley RW, Rall SC, Jr. Type III Hyperlipoproteinemia (Dysbeta lipoproteinemia): The role of apolipoprotein E in normal and abnormal lipoprotein metabolism. New York: McGraw Hill, 1995.1953.

56. Goldstein JL, et al. Hyperlipidemia in coronary heart disease: II. Genetic analysis in 176 families and delineation of a new inherited disorder, combined hyperlipidemia. J Clin Invest. 1973;52:1544.

57. Brunzell JD, et al. Plasma lipoproteins in familial combined hyperlipidemia and monogenic familial hypertriglyceridemia. J Lipid Res. 1983;24:147.

58. Austin MA, et al. Low density lipoprotein subclass patterns and risk of myocardial infarction. JAMA. 1988;260:1917.

59. Austin MA, et al. Atherogenic lipoprotein phenotype: a proposed genetic marker for coronary heart disease risk. Circulation. 1990;82:495.

60. Austin MA. Genetics of low-density lipoprotein subclasses. Curr Opin Lipidol. 1993;4:125.

61. Austin MA, et al. Inheritance of low density lipoprotein subclass patterns in familial combined hyperlipidemia. Arteriosclerosis. 1990;10:520.

62. Hokanson JE, et al. Plasma triglyceride and LDLheterogenety in familial combined hyperlipidemia. Arterioscler Thromb. 1993;13:427.

63. Simpson HCR, et al. Hypertriglyceridemia and hypercoagulability. Lancet. 1983;1:786.

64. Hamsten A, et al. Increased levels of a rapid inhibitor of tissue plasminogen activator in young survivors of myocardial infarction. N Engl J Med. 1985;313:1557.

65. The Coronary Drug Project Research Group. Clofibrate and niacin in coronary heart disease. JAMA. 1975;231:360.

66. Canner PL, et al. Fifteen year mortality in Coronary Drug Project patients: long-term benefit with niacin. JACC. 1986;8:1245.

67. Small DM, et al. Physicochemical and histological changes in the arterial wall of non-human primates during progression and regression of atherosclerosis. J Clin Invest. 1984;73:1590.

68. Armstrong ML, Megan MB. Arterial fibrous proteins in cynomologous monkeys after atherogenic and regression diets. Circ Res. 1975;36:256.

69. Armstrong ML, Megan MB. Lipid depletion in atheromatous coronary arteries in rhesus monkeys after regression diets. Circ Res. 1972;30:675.

70. Vartiainen I, Kanerva K. Arteriosclerosis and war-time. Ann Med Intern Fenn. 1947;36:748.

71. Strom A, Jensen RA. Mortality from circulatory diseases in Norway 1940-1945. Lancet. 1951;126.

72. Richardson PD, Davies MJ, Born GVR. Influence of plaque configuration and stress distribution on fissuring of coronary atherosclerotic plaques. Lancet. 1989;ii:941.

73. Davies MJ. A macro and micro view of coronary vascular insult in isechemic heart disease. Circulation. 1990;82 (Supp II):II -38.

74. Fernandez-Ortiz A, et al. Characterization of the relative thrombogenicity of atherosclerotic plaque components: implications for consequences of plaque rupture. JACC. 1994;23:1562.

75. Treasure CB, et al. Beneficial effects of cholesterol-lowering therapy on the coronary endothelium in patients with coronary artery disease. N Engl J Med. 1995;332:481.

76. Gould KL, et al. Short-term cholesterol lowering decreases size and severity of perfusion abnormalities by position emission tomography after dipyridamole in patients with coronary disease. Circulation. 1994;89:1530.

77. Scanu AM. Lipoprotein (a) - A genetic risk factor for premature coronary heart disease. JAMA. 1992;267:3326.

78. Badimon JJ, et al. Platelet deposition at high shear rates is enhanced by high plasma cholesterol levels. In vivo study in the rabbit model. Arterioscler Thromb. 1991;11:395.

79. L-Lacoste L, et al. Pravachol decreases thrombus formation in hypercholesterolemic coronary patients in conjunction with improvements in serum lipids. JACC. 1994;23(special Issue):131A.

80. Shah PK, et al. Human monocyte-derived macrophages express collagenase and induce collagen breakdown in atherosclerotic fibrous caps: implications for plaque rupture. Circulation. 1993;88:I-254.

5 SILENT MYOCARDIAL ISCHEMIA

Brian P. Schafer, Thomas C. Andrews, Peter H. Stone

Until recently, our understanding of coronary artery disease has been dominated by the misconception that myocardial ischemia is an inherently painful phenomenon. In 1772, William Heberden described angina pectoris as a "strangling ... most disagreeable sensation in the breast,"[1] and later in the 18th century C.H. Parry associated angina with narrowing of the coronary arteries.[2] It was not until 1950 that silent ischemia was first described when Paul Wood reported 25% of patients with exertional angina who developed asymptomatic repolarization abnormalities of ischemia during exercise electrocardiography.[3] Subsequently, data from the Framingham study has demonstrated that 25 % of myocardial infarctions are clinically silent.[4] Stem and Tzivoni in 1974 were the first to demonstrate silent ischemia using ambulatory monitoring in coronary patients during normal daily activities.[5] Over the past decade silent ischemia has emerged as an important manifestation of ischemic heart disease, and in this chapter we review the current understanding of the pathophysiology, detection, prognostic significance and treatment of this disorder.

Factors affecting the perception of angina

When myocardium becomes ischemic, a cascade of changes take place including metabolic abnormalities, diastolic and systolic ventricular dysfunction, and electrocardiographic abnormalities.[6] The temporal position of angina in this cascade is highly variable and often absent. Some coronary disease patients demonstrate both symptomatic and asymptomatic episodes of ischemia, and others silent ischemia alone. What determines which episodes of ischemia result in angina is incompletely understood.

The perception of ischemia is believed to originate from intramyocardial receptors responding to local chemical mediators released during ischemia. These messages are transmitted via afferent pathways to synapses with dorsal horn neurons which act as gating stations, receiving input both from other visceral and somatic receptors as well as inhibitory messages from brainstem, thalamic and cortical centers. From the dorsal horn the processed stimuli ascend the spino-thalamic tract for processing in higher cortical centers.[7] Several explanations for variability in the perception of ischemic pain arise from this model. First, neuropathic processes may decrease the amount of noxious stimuli arriving at the dorsal horn by damaging the receptors or afferent pathways. The association between silent ischemia and neurologic dysfunction has been well established.[7-11] For example, although an increased incidence of silent ischemia in diabetics has been an inconsistent finding,[8-14] those studies that have focused on patients with diabetic peripheral neuropathy have found a consistent association.[8, 9] Second, afferent input from other visceral or somatic sites into the dorsal horn may lead to filtering out of the pain of myocardial ischemia. Third, higher cortical or thalamic centers may minimize or obscure the perception of ischemia via serotonin, endorphins or other neurotransmitters. Some investigators have suggested that endogenous opioids are elevated in patients with silent ischemia,[15, 16] although this has been an inconsistent finding.[9, 17] In addition, certain patients with silent ischemia have generalized high pain thresholds and other personality traits which may indicate an exaggerated influence of cortically mediated pain inhibition pathways.[18-20] Finally, some studies have suggested that compared with symptomatic ischemia, silent ischemia may simply represent less severe ischemia as measured by the degree of ST depression or hemodynamic changes, the duration of ischemia, or the extent of perfusion defect on thallium.[21-24]

Detection of silent ischemia

Silent myocardial ischemia is defined as objective evidence of ischemia in the absence of clinical symptoms, and such ischemia can be documented by a variety of methods. An occasional patient will demonstrate reversible ST segment depression on serial resting electrocardiograms, but exercise electrocardiography much more frequently documents asymptomatic ST segment depression in patients with coronary artery disease. For example, in the Coronary Artery Surgery Study registry 30% of patients displayed silent ischemia on standard exercise tests.[25] The addition of thallium scintigraphy may increase the sensitivity of exercise testing in diagnosing ischemia, both symptomatic and silent.[26] Mental stress can be used to provoke silent ischemia as shown by Selwyn, Deanfield and colleagues using PET scanning[27] and Rozanski and co-workers using radioventriculography.[28] Ambulatory monitoring of the ECG is the modality most frequently used in the detection and quantification of silent ischemia, and many investigators have shown that approximately 80 to 90% of episodes of ischemia during daily life are asymptomatic.[5, 22, 27, 29, 30]

Ambulatory monitoring is performed by utilizing a two or three channel ECG recorder, usually with a lateral and inferior lead configuration. Continuous

ECG recording is performed for at least 24 hours while the patient is performing routine daily activities with the information stored either on a magnetic tape or digitally and transferred at a later date to a computer workstation for analysis of ST-segment changes. Ischemia is usually reported as number of episodes of ischemia and total duration of ischemia per 24 hours of recording. Twenty-five to 45 percent of patients with coronary artery disease demonstrate ST-segment abnormalities of ischemia on ambulatory ECG monitoring, and the majority of episodes are clinically silent.[5, 22, 27, 29, 30] Hence, the terms "ambulatory ischemia," "daily life ischemia," and "silent ischemia" are often used interchangeably, although it is recognized that not all ambulatory or daily life ischemia is clinically silent. For ease of communication, we will discuss two types of silent ischemia in this review — asymptomatic ST segment depression on exercise testing (by definition 100% of which is silent) and ischemia on ambulatory ECG monitoring (approximately 90% of episodes silent).

Pathophysiology of silent ischemia

In the past decade, much attention has been given to understanding the relative contributions of changes in myocardial oxygen supply and demand in the pathogenesis of silent ischemia. Investigators frequently utilize changes in heart rate prior to onset of ischemia on ambulatory ECG monitoring as a surrogate for changes in myocardial oxygen demand. Many have shown that myocardial ischemia occurs at lower heart rates on ambulatory monitoring compared with ischemia induced by exercise testing, implicating transient coronary vasoconstriction as a significant pathophysiologic contributor to ambulatory ischemia.[31-33] Significant controversy persists regarding the relative contribution of vasoconstriction, with some investigators claiming that the majority of episodes of ischemia are due to vasoconstriction,[31, 32, 34] others claiming most episodes are due to increases in myocardial oxygen demand.[35-37]

Our group analyzed 933 episodes of ambulatory ischemia from 50 patients treated with propranolol, diltiazem, nifedipine or placebo in a randomized, double-blind, cross-over trial to determine the heart rate patterns preceding the onset of ischemia.[38, 39] Examining the mean heart rate activity during the hour preceding each episode of ischemia, 81% of episodes were preceded by a heart rate increase of at least 5 beats per minute, while 19 % were unassociated with preceding heart rate increases and presumably were caused primarily by coronary vasoconstriction. Underscoring the importance of increases in myocardial oxygen demand in the pathogenesis of ambulatory ischemia, we found that the likelihood of developing an episode of ischemia was directly related to the baseline heart rate, the magnitude of the increase in heart rate, and the duration of time the heart rate remained elevated. For example, there was a 4 % likelihood of developing ischemia after a heart rate increase of less than 10 beats per minute lasting less than 10 minutes, compared with a 60% likelihood of developing ischemia after a heart rate increase of greater than 20 beats per minute lasting more than 40 minutes. The heart rate-related episodes were most effectively suppressed by propranolol, while non-heart rate-related episodes (presumably caused by coronary vasoconstriction) were more effectively suppressed by nifedipine. We concluded that most episodes of ischemia occurring in patients with chronic stable angina during daily life are associated with increases in a number of heart rate variables, explaining why therapies that reduce the magnitude and duration of heart rate increases and reduce baseline heart rate (such as beta-adrenergic blocldng agents) effectively reduce ischemia.

Ambulatory ischemia displays a circadian pattern of occurrence, with a primary peak in morning hours as well as a secondary peak in the evening.[40-42] Similar patterns have been observed in myocardial infarction,[43] stroke,[44] sudden cardiac death,[45] platelet aggregability,[46] cortisol levels,[47] catecholamine levels,[47] and heart rate.[39] There is controversy whether the morning peak in ambulatory ischemia is due to heightened coronary tone, increased physical activity, or both. The observation of circadian changes in ischemic thresholds on exercise testing in patients with stable coronary artery disease provides additional indirect evidence for circadian changes in coronary artery tone.[48] Panza and colleagues described the circadian rhythm of forearm vascular tone mediated by changes in alpha-sympathetic activity and postulated that this phenomenon may explain the increased morning incidence of cardiovascular events.[49] Fujita and Franklin described similar circadian changes in coronary tone in conscious dogs.[50] As yet, there have been no direct measurements of circadian changes in human coronary artery tone.

Parker and coworkers studied the effects of physical activity pattems on the morning increase in ambulatory ischemia in 20 patients with stable coronary disease.[51] Ambulatory monitoring was performed on two consecutive days. On day 1 patients adhered to a "regular activity" pattern (awake and assume normal activities at 8:OOAM). On day 2, patients assumed a "delayed activity" pattern (awake at 8:OOAM, arise at 10:OOAM, begin normal activity at noon). During the regular activity day, the usual morning increase in heart rate an ischemic episodes was observed, and this circadian pattem was "phase-shifted" four hours later on the delayed activity day. The majority of episodes of ischemia were associated with preceding increases in heart rate. The investigators concluded that the morning increase in ambulatory ischemia is due to physical activity patterns, not to changes in coronary tone.

Prognosis

In most subgroups of coronary disease patients, the finding of silent ischemia on ambulatory monitoring or exercise testing has been shown to portend a worse prognosis when compared with similar patients who do not demonstrate such ischemia. In this section, we discuss the relationship between silent ischemia and prognosis in four subgroups of coronary disease patients: asymptomatic patients, patients with stable coronary disease, patients recovering from an episode of unstable angina or myocardial infarction, and patients undergoing surgery for peripheral vascular disease.

Asymptomatic Patients

The presence of ischemia on exercise testing in asymptomatic patients has been shown to predict adverse cardiovascular events. In a prospective case-control study, Giagnoni and colleagues performed bicycle ergometry on 10,723 subjects without symptoms of coronary artery disease to find 135 patients with 1mm or greater ST-segment depression. These patients were then matched with control subjects with a negative ergometry test, but with similar cardiovascular risk factors. After a mean follow-up of 6 years, the event rate for the cases was 10. 4 % compared with 0. 8 % in the controls.[52] Similar data from asymptomatic patients enrolled in the Lipid Coronary Primary Prevention Trial demonstrated a cardiovascular mortality rate of 6.7% in patients with a positive treadmill test after 7.4 year mean follow-up compared with 1.3 % in those with a negative test.[53] Other trials have corroborated these results and further demonstrate the prognostic significance of silent ischemia in the asymptomatic population. Limited data is available for the use of ambulatory monitoring and screening of asymptomatic populations.[54-57] Hedblad et al. performed ambulatory monitoring of 394 men born in 1914. There were 341 subjects without known coronary artery disease and of those 79 demonstrated ST segment changes on ambulatory monitoring. Although event rates and predictive values were low, those with silent ischemia on ambulatory monitoring had a significantly increased risk of cardiac events (relative risk= 4.4, p =.005).[58] However, ambulatory monitoring is not recommended as a screening test for silent ischemia due to concerns about false positive tests in a population with low prevalence of true disease.

Stable coronary artery disease

The presence of ischemia on exercise treadmill testing in stable patients with known coronary artery disease has well established prognostic implications.[59-61] Data from the Coronary Artery Surgery Study registry demonstrate that patients with silent ischemia during treadmill testing have a similar prognosis as those with symptomatic ischemia.[25, 59] The presence of ischemia on ambulatory monitoring also provides prognostic information in this patient population. Rocco and coworkers performed ambulatory monitoring on 86 patients with coronary artery disease and ischemia on exercise treadmill testing. Fifty-seven percent experienced ambulatory ischemia, the vast majority of episodes being silent. On mean follow-up of 12.5 months, death, non-fatal myocardial infarction, and/or unstable angina occurred in 41% of patients with ischemia on ambulatory monitoring compared with 3% in the group without ischemia.[62] Late follow-up of this cohort demonstrated an adverse prognosis of ambulatory ischemia at five years as well.[63] In a similar study, Deedwania and Carbajal described 107 veterans, 43 % demonstrating ischemia on ambulatory monitoring (87 % silent). After 23 month mean follow-up, cardiac death occurred in 24 % of the group with ischemia versus 8% of those without ischemia.[64] Similar results have been reported by Tzivoni's group.[65] In contrast, two studies in low risk patients failed to demonstrate a negative prognosis for patients with ischemia on ambulatory monitoring: Quyyumi and colleagues studied 116 patients at low risk for cardiac events based on angiographic markers, 39% of whom demonstrated ischemia on ambulatory monitoring, [66] and Gandhi and coworkers studied a low risk group of patients presenting with new-onset exertional angina.[67] In conclusion, in patients with stable coronary disease, ischemia on exercise testing provides prognostic information independent of symptoms, and ischemia on ambulatory monitoring portends a relatively poor prognosis, except perhaps in low risk subgroups.

Unstable angina and myocardial infarction

Similar to the prognostic signficance of silent ischemia in stable patients, the presence of ischemia on exercise testing in patients recovering from an episode of unstable angina or from myocardial infarction identifies a group of patients at high risk for cardiac events, regardless of the occurrence of symptoms.[68] Ischemia on ambulatory monitoring provides prognostic information for this group of patients as well. Gottlieb and coworkers performed ambulatory monitoring in 70 patients during the initial 48 hours after presentation for unstable angina. Despite similar angiographic severity of coronary disease, the group demonstrating ischemia displayed a 16% rate of myocardial infarction during the subsequent month, compared with a 3% infarction rate in those without ischemia. After two year follow-up, 57% of the patients with ischemia on initial presentation suffered a major cardiac event including death, myocardial infarction, or coronary revascularization.[69, 70] Langer and colleagues demonstrated that the presence of ischemia on ambulatory monitoring in the first 24 hours of presentation for unstable angina predicted higher rate of in-hospital death, myocardial infarction or coronary revascularization.[71] Other investigators have confirmed the findings of these two groups, i.e., that the presence of ischemia, regardless of the presence or absence of associated symptoms, portends a poor prognosis in patients recovering from an episode of unstable angina.[72, 73]

In post-myocardial infarction patients, Gottlieb's group recorded ambulatory monitoring on 103 high risk patients with left ventricular ejection fraction less than 40% and frequent ectopy. At one year follow-up 30% of patients with ambulatory ischemia experienced cardiac death compared with 11% in those without ischemia.[74] Tzivoni and colleagues studied 224 patients after myocardial infarction a mean of 24 months after the index event and 74 patients demonstrated ambulatory ischemia. On mean follow-up of 28 months, those with ischemia had a significantly higher cardiac event rate than those without ischemia.[75] In a small trial Solimene and coworkers also demonstrated the prognostic value of ambulatory ischemia two years after uncomplicated myocardial infarction.[76] In contrast to these previous studies, Goldberg evaluated 103 patients with ambulatory monitoring within the first week of the MI and was unable to find a relationship between silent ischemia and subsequent cardiac events over a 10 month period.[77] Moss and colleagues performed ambulatory monitoring on stable low-risk post-infarction patients 1 to 6 months after the index event and was unable to predict coronary events based on the presence or absence of ambulatory ischemia.[78]

Peripheral vascular disease

Several groups have reported the prognostic value of ambulatory monitoring in patients undergoing surgery for peripheral vascular disease. Raby and colleagues first reported 176 such patients and found that the presence of ischemia on preoperative monitoring was highly predictive of postoperative cardiac events,[79] and these findings have been confirmed by other investigators.[80, 81] In longer term follow-up, Raby's group found that preoperative ischemia remains a negative prognostic marker up to two years postoperatively (risk ratio 5.4),[82] and Mangano's group has confirmed these findings as well.[83] Raby also showed that adverse cardiac events in the postoperative period are invariably preceded by silent ischemia, and he has hypothesized that identification and treatment of silent postoperative ischemia may prevent subsequent events.[84]

Treatment of silent ischemia

While much evidence exists that the presence of silent ischemia portends a poor prognosis in a variety of clinical settings, it is unclear whether silent ischemia should be specifically treated. Every class of medication used to treat symptomatic ischemia has been proven to be effective in the suppression of silent ischemia as well.[38, 85-87] Coronary revascularization has also been shown to be an effective therapy for silent ischemia.[88] A consistent finding in trials of silent ischemia treatment is that medications that lower heart rate, such as β-adrenergic blocking agents, are most effective. For example, in the Angina and Silent Ischemia Study (ASIS), Stone and colleagues showed that propranolol was more effective than either diltiazem or nifedipine in the suppression of silent ischemia when these agents were used at maximum dosages as single agents.[38] As discussed previously, subsequent analyses showed that propranolol was particularly effective in suppressing the 81 % of episodes of ischemia preceded by increases in heart rate (demand related episodes), while nifedipine was more effective in suppressing the 19% of episodes caused by coronary vasoconstriction.[39] Many have postulated that the most effective regimen for suppression of all ischemia would be a combination of a beta-adrenergic blocking agent and a vasodilator.[39]

Three major trials have recently been completed which were designed to determine the effect of treatment of silent ischemia on the occurrence of adverse cardiac events in patients with stable coronary disease. The final results of the Total Ischaemic Burden European Trial (TIBET) have not yet been published. The Atenolol Silent Ischemia Study (ASIST) enrolled 306 patients with mild or no angina, ischemia on exercise stress testing and on ambulatory monitoring.[89] Patients were randomized to atenolol (100 mg daily) or placebo. Atenolol therapy effectively reduced the number and average duration of ischemic episodes compared with placebo, and there was a nonsignificant trend for fewer serious events (death, resuscitation from ventricular tachycardia or fibrillation, myocardial infarction or hospitalization for unstable angina) at one year. Only when the endpoints "aggravation of angina" or "need for revascularization" were added to the composite endpoint was statistical signficance reached for a positive treatment effect of atenolol.

The Asymptomatic Cardiac Ischemia Pilot (ACIP) study enrolled 618 patients from 11 clinical sites in the United States and Canada.[90, 91] The primary endpoint was the suppression of ischemia by three different treatment strategies including: 1) medical therapy titrated to suppress symptomatic ischemia only (angina-guided strategy), 2) medical therapy titrated to suppress both symptomatic ischemia and ischemia on serial ambulatory monitoring (ischemia-guided strategy), and 3) revascularization with angioplasty or bypass surgery. The medical regimens included either diltiazem plus isosorbide dinitrate or atenolol plus nifedipine. After twelve weeks of therapy, ambulatory ischemia was abolished in 39% of patients assigned to the angina-guided strategy, 41 % of patients assigned to the ischemia-guided strategy, and 55 % of patients assigned to revascularization strategy. For most patients in the two medical strategies, angina was controlled with relatively small doses of medication. At one year follow-up, 14 patients (7%) in the angina-guided strategy had died or suffered a myocardial infarction, compared with 12 (6%) in the ischemia-guided strategy and 4 (2%) in the revascularization group (p=0.04). Although the number of events were small and the duration of follow-up short, these results suggest a benefit for revascularization.[88]

There is some evidence that treatment of silent ischemia in patients undergoing surgery for peripheral vascular disease may improve short term prognosis. Using ambulatory monitoring, Andrews and co-workers studied 145 patients undergoing peripheral vascular surgery at a single institution and identified 36 patients with preoperative ischemia. These patients were treated with aggressive medical therapy for ischemia in the postoperative period and suffered significantly fewer postoperative cardiac events compared with similar historical controls.[92] As yet, there have been no randomized trials to examine the role of medical therapy or revascularization in reducing postoperative ischemia and/or cardiac events in this patient population.

Future directions

Most investigators agree that the presence of ischemia on exercise testing or ambulatory monitoring identifies a group of patients at high risk for cardiac events regardless of whether symptoms are also present. Ambulatory ischemia during daily life (most of which is silent) is usually caused by changes in myocardial oxygen demand, although some degree of transient coronary vasoconstriction may also contribute to the pathogenesis. Beta-adrenergic blocking agents are the mainstay of medical therapy, although revascularization is also highly effective. Additional study is necessary to determine whether medical therapy or revascularization to specifically treat the asymptomatic manifestations of ischemia provides benefits on cardiac morbidity or mortality beyond those benefits associated with treatment of more conventional symptomatic ischemia.

REFERENCES

1. Heberden W. Some account of a disorder of the breast. Med Trans Coll Physicians (Lond.) 1772:2:59.

2. Parry C. An inquiry into the symptoms and causes of the syncope anginosa, commonly called angina pectoris. Bath, England: K. Cuttwell, 1799: vol 3 and 4).

3. Wood P, et al. The effort test in angina pectoris. Br Heart J 1950:12:363.

4. Kannel W, Abbott R. Incidence and prognosis of unrecognized myocardial infraction: an update on the Framingham study. N Engl J Med 1984:311:1144.

5. Stern S, Tzivoni D. Early detection of silent ischaemic heart disease by 24-hour electrocardiographic monitoring of active subjects. Br Heart J 1974:36:481.

6. Nesto R, Kowalchuk G. The ischemic cascade: Temporal sequence of hemodynamic, electrocardiographic and symptomatic expressions of aschemia. Am J Cardiol 1987:59:23C-30C.

7. Maseri A, et al. Mechanisms and significance of cardiac ischemic pain. Prog cardiovasc Dis 1992::1.

8. Hartmann A, et al. Stomatic pain threshold and reactive hyperemia in autonomic diabetic neuropathy and silent myocardial ischemia. Int J Cardiol 1993:42:121.

9. Marchant B, et al. Silent myocardial ischemia: Role of subclinical neuropathy in patients with and without diabetes. J Am Coll Cardiol 1993:22:1433.

10. Hikita H, et al. Usefulness of plasma beta-endorphin level, pain threshold and autonomic function in assessing silent myocardial ischemia in patients with and without diabetes mellitus. Am J Cardiol 1993:15:140.

11. Shakespeare C, et al. Differences in autonomic nerve function in patients with silent and symptomatic myocardial ischaemia. Br Heart J 1994:71:22.

12. Chipkin S, et al. Frequency of painless myocardial ischemia during exercise tolerance testing in patients with and without diabetes mellitus. Am J Cardiol 1987:59:61.

13. Callahan P, et al. Exrcise-induced silent ischemia: Age, diabetes mellitus, previous myocardial ifarction and prognosis. J Am Coll Cardiol 1989:14:1175.

14. Nesto R, et al. Silent myocardial ischemia and infarction in diabetics with peripheral vascular disease: assessment by dipyridamole thallium-201 scintigraphy. Am Heart J 1990:120:1073.

15. Miller P, et al. Beta-endorphin response to exercise and mental stress in patients with ischemic heart disease. J Psychosom Res 1993:37:455.

16. Falcone C, et al. Beta-endorphins during coronary angioplasty in patients with silent or symptomatic myocardial ischemia. J Am Coll Cardiol 1993:22:1614.

17. Marchant B, et al. Rexamination of the role of endogenous opiates in silent myocardial ischemia. J Am Coll Cardiol 1994:23:645.

18. Davies R, et al. Relative importance of psychological traits and severity of ischemia in causing angina during treadmill exercise. J Am Coll Cardiol 1993:21:331.

19. Glazier J, et al. Importance of generalized defective perception of painful stimuli as a cause of silent myocardial ischemia in chronic stable angina pectoris. Am J Cardiol 1986:58:667.

20. Droste C, Roskamm H. Experimental pain measurement in patients with asymptomatic myocardial ischemia. J Am Coll Cardiol 1983:1:940.

21. Chierchia S, et al. Impairment of myocardial perfusion and function during painless myocardial ischemia. J Am Coll Cardiol 1983:1:924.

22. Deedwania P, Carbajal E. Prevalence and patterns of silent myocardial ischemia during daily life in stable angina patients receiving conventional antianginal drug therapy. J Am Cardiol 1990:65:1090.

23. Kurata C, et al. Exercise-induced silent myocardial ischemia: Evaluation by thallium-201 emission computed tomography. Am Heart J 1990:119:557.

24. Cecchi A, et al. Silent myocardial ischemia during ambulatory electrocardiographic monitoring in patients with effort angina. J Am Coll Cardiol 1983:1:934.

25. Weiner D, et al. The role of exercise-induced silent myocardial ischemia in patients with abnormal left ventricular function. A report from the Coronary Artery Surgery Study (CASS) registry. Am Herat J 1989:118:649.

26. Fleg J, et al. Prevalence and prognostic significance of exercise-induced myocardial ischemia detected by thallium scintigraphy and electrocadriography in asymptomatic volunteers. Circulation 1990:81:428.

27. Deanfield J, et al. Transient ST-segment depression as a marker of myocardial ischemia during daily life. Am J Cardiol 1984:54:1195.

28. Rozanski A, et al. Mental stress and the induction of silent myocfardial ischemia in patients with coronary artery disease. N Engl J Med 1988:318:1005.

29. Deanfield J, et al. Silent myocardial ischemia due to mental stress. Lancet 1984:2:1001.

30. Schang CJ, Pepine C. Transient asymptomatic ST segment depression during daily activity. Am J Cardiol 1977:39:396.

31. Deanfield J, et al. Myocardial Ischemia during daily life in patients with stable angina: Its relation to symptoms and heart rate changes. Lancet 1983:2:753.

32. Chierchia S, et al. Role of heart rate in pathophysiology of chronic stable angina. Lancet 1984:2:1353.

33. Banai S, et al. Changes in myocardial ischemic threshold during daily activities. Am J Cardiol 1990:66:1403.

34. Chierchia S, et al. Role of the sympathetic nervous system in the pathogenesis of chronic stable angina. Implications for the mechanism of action of Beta-blockers. Circulation 1990:82(suppl II):II71.

35. Quyyumi A, et al. Mechanisms of nocturnal angina pectoris: Importance of increased myocardial oxygen demand in patients with severe coronary artery disease. Lancet 1985:1:1207.

36. Quyyumi A, et al. Nocturnal angina: Precipitating factors in patients with coronary artery disease and those with variant angina. Br Heart J 1986:56:346.

37. Deedwania P. Nelson J. Pathophysiology of silent myocardial ischemia during daily life. Circulation 1990:82:1296.

38. Stone PH, et al. Comparison of propanolol, diltiazem, and nifedipine in the treatment of ambulatory ischemia in patients with stable angina. Circulation 1990:82:1962.

39. Andrews TC, et al. Subsets of ambulatory myocardial ischemia based on heart rate activity: Circadian distribution and response to anti-ischemic medication. Circulation 1993:88:92.

39. Rocco M, et al. Circadian variation of transient myocardial ischemia in patients with coronary artery disease. Circulation 1987:75:395.

40. Mulcahy D, et al. Circadian variation of total ischemic burden and its alteration with anti-anginal agents. Lancet 1988:1:755.

41. Nademanee K, et al. Circadian variation in occurence of transient overt amd silent myocardial ischemia in chronic stable angina and comparison with Prinzmetal angina in men. Am J Cardiol 1987:60:494.

42. Muller JE, et al. Circardian variation in the frequency of onset of acute myocardial infarction. N Engl J Med 1985:313:1315.

43. Marler J, et al. Morning increase in onset of ischemic stroke. Stroke 1989:20:473.

44. Muller JE, et al. Circedian variation in the frequency of sudden cardiac death. Circulation 1987:75:131.

45. Tofler G, et al. Concurrent morning increase in pletelet aggregability and the risk of myocardial infarction and sudden cardiac death. N Engl J MeD 1987:316:1514.

46. Turton M, Deegan T. Circadian variations of plasma catecholamines, cortisol and immunoreactive isnulin concentrations in supine subjects. Clin Chem Acta 1974:55:389.

47. Quyyumi A, et al. Circadian variation in ischemic events: Causeal role of variation in vascular resistance. Circulation 1988:78(Suppl II):II-.

48. Panza J, Epstein S, Quyyumi A. Circadian variation in vascular tone and its relation to alpha-sympathetic vasoconstrictor activity. N Engl J Med 1991:325:986.

49. Fujita M, Franklin D. Diurnal changes in coronary blood flow in conscious dogs. Circulation 1987:76:488.

50. Parker J, et al. Morning increase in ambulatory ischemia in patients with stable coronary artery disease. Circulation 1994:89:604.

51. Giagnoni E, et al. Prognostic value of exercise ECG testing in asymptomatic normotensive subjects: A prospective matched study. N Engl J Med 1983:309:1085.

52. Ekelund L, et al. Coronary heart disease morbidity and mortality in hypercholesterolemic men predicted from an exercise test: The Lipid Research Clinics Coronary Primary Prevention Trial. J Am Coll Cardiol 1989:14:556.

53. McHenry P, et al. The abnormal exercise electocardiogram in apparently healthy men: a predictor of angina pectoris as an initial coronary event during long-term follow-up. Circulation 1984:62:522.

54. Froelicher V, Maron D. Exercise testing and ancillary techniques to screen for coronary heart disease. Prog Cardiovasc Dis 1981:24:261.

55. Bruce R, et al. Enhanced risk assessment of primary coronary heart disease events by maximal exercise testing: 10 years experience of Seattle Heart Watch. J Am Coll Cardiol 1983:2:565.

56. Multiple Risk Factor Intervention Trial Research Group. Exercise electrocardiogram and coronary heart disease mortality in the Multiple Risk Factor Intervention Trial. Am J Cardiol 1985:55:16.

57. Hedblad B, et al. Increased mortality in men with ST segment depression during 24 hour ambulatory long-term ECG recording. Eur Heart J 1989:10:149.

58. Weiner D, et al. Significance of silent myocardial ischemia during exercise testing in coronary artery disease. Am J Cardiol 1987:59:725.

59. Weiner D, et al. Prognostic importance of a clinical profile and exercise test in medically treated patients with coronary artery disease. J Am Coll Cardiol 1984:3:722.

60. Dagenais G, et al. Survival of patients with a strongly positive exercise electrocardiogram. Circulation 1982:65:452.

61. Rocco M, et al. Prognostic importance of myocardial ischemia detected by ambulatory monitoring in patients with stable coronary artery disease. Circulation 1988:78:877.

62. Yeung A, et al. Effects of asymptomatic ischemia on long-term prognosis in chronic stable coronary disease. Circulation 1991:83:1598.

63. Deedwania P, Carbajal E. Silent ischemia during daily life is an independent predictor of mortality in stable angina. Circulation 1990:81:748.

64. Tzivoni D, et al. Comparison of mortality and myocardial infarction rates in stable angina pectoris with and without ischemic episodes during daily activities. Am J Cardiol 1989:63:273.

65. Quyyumi A, et al. Prognostic implications of myocardial ischemia during daily life in low risk patients with coronary artery disease. J Am Coll Cardiol 1993:21:700.

66. Gandhi M, Wood D, Lampe F. Characteristic and clinical significance of ambulatory myocardial ischemia in men and women in the general population presenting with angina pectoris. J Am Coll Cardiol 1994:23:74.

67. Theroux P, et al. Prognostic value of exercise testing soon after myocardial infarction. N Engl J Med 1979:301:341.

68. Gottlieb S, et al. Silent ischemia predicts infarction and death during 2 year follow-up of unstable angina. J Am Coll Cardiol 1987:10:756

69. Gottleib S, et al. Silent ischemia as a marker for early unfavorable outcomes in patients with unstable angina. N Engl J Med 1986:314:1214.

70. Langer A, Freeman M, Armostrong P. ST segment shift in unstable angina: Pathophysiology and association with coronary anatomy and hospital outcome. J Am Cardiol 1989:13:1495.

71. Nadamanee K, et al. Prognostic significance of silent myocardial ischemia in patients with unstable angina. J Am Coll Cardiol 1989:13:1495.

72. Johnson S, et al. Continuous electrocardiographic monitoring in patients with unstable angina: Identification of high-risk subgroups with severe coronary disease, variant angina, and/or impaired early prognosis. Am Heart J 1982:103:4.

73. Gottlieb S, et al. Silent ischemia on holter monitoring predicts mortality in high-risk post-infraction patients. JAMA 1988:259:1030.

74. Tzivoni D, et al. Prognostic significance of ischemic episodes in patients with previous myocardial infarction. Am J Cardiol 1988:62:661.

75. Solimene M, et al. Prognostic significance of silent myocardial ischemia after a first uncomplicated myocardial infarction. Int J Cardiol 1993:38:41.

76. Goldberg A, et al. ST depression of Holter monitor during hospitalization for acute myocardial infarction does not predict subsequent cardiac events. J Am Coll Cardiol 1991:17:66.

77. Moss A, et al. Detection and significance of myocardial ischemia in stable patients after recovery from an acute coronary event. JAMA 199:269:2379.

78. Raby K, et al. Correlation between preoperative ischemia and major cardiac events after peripheral vescular surgery. N Engl J Med 1989:321:1296.

79. Mangano D, et al. Association pf perioperative myocardial ischemia with cardiac morbidity and mortality in men undergoing noncardiac surgery. N Engl J Med 1990:323:1781.

80. Landesberg G, et al. Importance of long-duration postoperative ST-segment depression in cardiac morbidity after vascular surgery. Lancet 1993:341:715.

81. Raby K, et al. Long-term prognosis of myocardial ischemia detectedby holter monitoring in peripheral vascular disease. Am J Cardiol 1990:66:1309.

82. Mangano D, et al. Long term cardiac prognosis following noncardiac surgery. JAMA 1992:268:233.

83. Raby K, et al. Detection and significance of intraoperative and postoperative ischemia in peripheral vascular surgery. JAMA 1992:268:222.

84. Nabel E, et al. Effects of dosing intervals on the development of tolerance to hogh-dose transdermal nitroglycerine. Am J Cardiol 1989:63:663.

85. Nesto R, et al. Effect of nifedipine on total ischemic activity and circadian distribution of myocardial ischemic episodes in angina pectoris. Am J Cardiol 1991:67:128.

86. Imperi G, et al. Effects of titrated beta blockade (metoprolol) on silent myocardial ischemia in ambulatory patients with coronary artery disease. Am J Cardiol 1987:60:519.

87. Rogers W, et al. Asymptomatic Cardiac Ischemia Pilot (ACIP) Study: 1 year follow-up. Circulation 1994:90:i-17.

88. Pepine C, et al. Effecfts of treatment on outcome in mildly symptomatic patients with ischemia during daily life. The Atenolol Silent Ischemia Study (ASIST). Circulation 1994:90:762.

89. Pepine C, et al. The Asymptomatic Cardiac Ischemia Pilot (ACIP) study: Design of a randomized clinical trial, baseline data and implications for a long-term trial. J Am Coll Cardiol 1994:24:1.

90. Knatterud G, et al. Effects of treatment strategies to suppress ischemia in patients with coronary artery disease: 12-week results of the Asymptomatic Cardiac Ischemia Pilot (ACIP) study. J Am Coll Cardiol 1994:24:11.

91. Andrews T, et al. Identification of treatment of myocardial ischemia in patients undergoing peripheral vascular surgery. J Vasc Med Biol 1994:5:8.

6 VASOSPASTIC ANGINA

Attilio Maseri, Gaetano A. Lanza

In 1959 Prinzmetal et al[1] described a variant form of angina, which, in contrast with the more common effort angina, occurs exclusively or predominantly at rest, often without apparent cause, and is characterized by elevation, rather than depression, of the ST-segment on the electrocardiogram (ECG). The authors hypothesized that this form of angina was caused by an increase in "tonus" at the site of a subcritical coronary stenosis.[1] Indeed, no increase in the hemodynamic determinants of myocardial oxygen consumption can be detected by continuous hemodynamic monitoring before the appearance of ischemia.[2,3]

In the mid-1970s coronary angiography, performed during spontaneous or provoked anginal episodes, demonstrated convincingly that variant angina is due to a transmural reduction in myocardial blood flow caused by an occlusive or subocclusive vasospasm of an epicardial coronary artery.[3,4] Angiography also showed that occlusive coronary artery epicardial spasm may occur not only at the site of subcritical stenoses, but also in angiographically normal coronary arteries[5] and at the site of severe stenoses.[6]

Pathogenetic mechanisms of coronary artery spasm

In 1976 we proposed that coronary artery spasm results from the interaction of two components: 1) an abnormality in a localized segment of an epicardial coronary artery, which makes it hyperreactive to vasoconstrictor stimuli, and 2) various vasoconstrictor stimuli, acting on different receptors, which are able to trigger the spasm in the same segment.[7] This hypothesis was subsequently confirmed by several studies.

Enhanced segmental vasoconstrictor reactivity

The segmental nature of the vascular alteration was suggested because ST-segment elevation always occurs in the same ECG leads in any given patient, and was clearly confirmed by the angiographic demonstration that spasm usually occurs in a localized and well indentifiable segment of an epicardial coronary artery. However, spasm can sometimes involve two segments of the same branch or different arterial vessels, or it may involve diffusely multiple branches. Multifocal spasm,[8] as an increased basal tone,[9] appears to be more common in Japanese than in Caucasian patients.[10]

The most fundamental advance in our understanding of the pathophysiology of epicardial coronary artery spasm was the demonstration that it can be induced by a variety of pharmacologic agents,[11] acting by different mechanisms and involving different receptorial systems.[12-17] This indicates that multiple triggers of spasm can exist, but that they can only cause spasm at the site of hyperreactive segments. Therefore, the therapeutic failure of specific receptor blocking agents[18-20] in patients with variant angina is not surprising, as the blockade of a single receptor/agonist interaction leaves other receptors unopposed and capable of eliciting spasm.

Endothelial damage has been proposed as a possible cause of susceptibility to spasm, as it could preclude the vasodilatory response to endothelium-dependent coronary dilator stimuli, thus favouring spasm in response to vasoconstrictor stimuli.[21] However, endothelial damage or dysfunction is common, while coronary spasm is very rare, in patients with coronary stenoses.

It has also been suggested that passive mechanical forces may have a role in the pathogenesis of coronary artery spasm. The concept was that in the presence of eccentric stenoses, lesion geometry, smooth muscle tone and perfusion pressure could interact in such a way to be conducive to spasm.[22] Coronary spasm, however, does not develop in most eccentric stenoses, whereas it occurs often in patients with normal coronary arteries.

Based on the presence of local vascular fibromuscular hyperplasia reported in some cases,[23] an abnormal production of growth factors (by smooth muscle, platelets, etc.) has also been proposed, but coronary angiography in these patients may remain unchanged for several years.

A post-receptorial alteration in vascular smooth muscle cells, for example at the level of the G-protein transduction system, therefore, appears a more likely cause of the local vascular hyperreactivity.[24]

The various triggering stimuli

There are several stimuli capable of inducing occlusive coronary artery spasm, but only when they act at the site of hyperreactive coronary vascular segments.

A heightened nervous adrenergic activity has received a great deal of attention as a possible major trigger of spasm. Indeed, coronary artery spasm may be induced by alpha-agonist drugs[11,12] and by stimuli (e.g., exercise and cold pressor test)[25,26] which increase the sympathetic outflow to coronary arteries, and it can be prevented by alpha-blockers.[27,28] Furthermore, the duration of ischemic episodes was found to increase following therapy with beta-blockers, and this was attributed to facilitation of vasoconstriction by alpha stimulation.[29] Nevertheless, alpha-blockade has been unsuccessful in other studies[18] and levels of coronary catecholamines have been found to increase late during spontaneous ischemic episodes,[30] suggesting an increase that is secondary to ischemia, and questioning the importance of sympathetic activation as a major trigger of spasm.

Conversely, it has also been suggested that an increase in vagal activity can induce spasm,[14] and this hypothesis is supported by the higher incidence of anginal attacks during sleep in most patients,[31] and by the possibility that coronary spasm can be induced with cholinergic drugs.[14] However, the intracoronary administration of vagomimetic substances in order to provoke spasm may lead to high nonphysiologic concentrations at the cellular level, thus determining a condition which may not occur in the clinical setting. Furthermore, the frequent occurrence of ischemic episodes during the night does not mean necessarily that an increase in vagal activation is the trigger. Finally, recent data, analyzing autonomic changes associated with spontaneous ST-segment elevation using heart rate variability, suggest that a vagal withdrawal, rather than activation, may precede the appearance of ischemia.[32]

It has also been hypothesized that an abnormal platelet aggregation, secondary to endothelial damage, with release of vasoconstrictor substances such as $TXA2$[33] and serotonin, may be a major trigger of coronary spasm. However, in one study levels of coronary sinus $TXA2$ metabolites increased late in the course of spontaneous anginal episodes, thus suggesting that they were secondary to the spasm.[34] Furthermore, the administration of $PGI2$[35] and the inhibition of $TXA2$[19] synthesis failed to achieve consistent clinical benefits. Similarly, anti-serotoninergic drugs have also failed to show consistent results in the control of angina.[20] However, platelet activation can perpetuate spasm and also facilitate plug formation, as suggested by the increased levels of fibrinopeptide A during ischemic episodes in patients with variant angina.[36]

Finally, an increased production of endothelin-1 by endothelial cells has recently been proposed as possibly implicated in the mechanisms of spasm,[37] but this substance has a profound vasoconstrictor effect on distal, but not on proximal, coronary vessels.[38]

Clinical features

The incidence of vasospastic angina is low compared with that of chronic stable angina, but it can vary considerably, depending on the frequency provocative tests are performed in patients with an unclear diagnosis.[39]

Patients with variant angina commonly present with recurrent episodes of angina, typically occurring exclusively or predominantly at rest. These episodes are usually of short duration, occur usually in the early morning hours or in the night, and respond promptly to sublingual nitrates.

In most cases variant angina is characterized by 'hot' and 'cold' symptomatic phases, with waxing and waning of symptoms over a period of weeks or months. Symptoms may, however, occasionally persist for years whenever therapy is withdrawn. During 'hot phases', anginal attacks may recur in clusters of two to four episodes within 20-30 minutes and may show a typical circadian distribution, with a peak during the night or early morning hours,[31] although in some cases they may be prevalent in the late evening.

Although exercise capacity is usually preserved, exercise may sometimes provoke anginal episodes.[25] Emotional distress, exposure to cold,[26] eating, alcohol[40] and some medications,[41,42] may all induce spasm, but in most cases there is no apparent triggering cause of angina.

In patients with variant angina risk factors for coronary artery disease include smoking and hypercholesterolemia,[43,44] but, in many patients, no known risk factors can be recognized. In rare cases, variant angina has been associated with systemic vasomotor disorders such as migraine and Raynaud's phenomenon.[45]

Although variant angina usually occurs in the absence of other symptoms, some patients may present with lipothymia or syncope. In such cases variant angina is likely to be associated with severe bradyarrhythmias or ventricular tachyarrhythmias, which can lead to sudden death.[46,47]

Diagnostic assessment

Variant angina should be suspected on the basis of a history of recurrent episodes of spontaneous angina at rest, particularly in patients with preserved effort tolerance, and is confirmed by documentation of transient ST-segment elevation on the ECG during a spontaneous anginal episode. ST-segment elevation can range from 1-2 mm to 20-30 mm and may be associated with QRS widening, and ST-segment and/or T-wave alternance.[48] Transient Q-waves may also develop occasionally disappearing at the end of the episode.[49] After an ischemic episode T-waves may be persistently negative for periods of several minutes or hours. In these cases a sudden transient return to normal (pseudonormalization) during pain is also indicative of acute myocardial ischemia.

When it is either difficult or impossible to perform an ECG during an attack of chest pain, the diagnosis of variant angina can be reached by performing Holter monitoring for 24 or 48 h in patients with relatively frequent attacks.[31] The observation of transient ST-segment elevation or pseudonormalization of inverted T-waves, coincident with symptoms, confirms the diagnosis. The detection of asymptomatic episodes of transient ischemic ST-segment elevation are clearly diagnostic and also confirm the diagnosis of variant angina.

Provocative tests of spasm

When anginal attacks are rare Holter monitoring is likely to be negative. In such cases, provocative tests may be required in order to confirm the clinical diagnosis. They are also necessary when the clinical presentation and ECG findings are non-diagnostic. Provocative tests of spasm are contraindicated in patients with frequent and prolonged ischemic episodes, particularly those not responding promptly to nitrates, because induced spasm may be difficult to resolve.[50]

Although spasm may be induced by exercise stress testing[25] and by the cold pressor test[26] in some patients, the most widely used provocative tests are ergonovine[13] and hyperventilation.[51]

Both these tests can be performed either noninvasively in the coronary care unit or in the exercise stress testing laboratory, or invasively in the catheterization laboratory during coronary angiography. During coronary angiography spasm and its location and extension can be visualized and intracoronary nitrates and calcium antagonists can be administered when it is not relieved promptly by intravenous drugs. However, in patients with a negative exercise stress test, performing the tests noninvasively under careful ECG monitoring is more practical and has no adjunctive risks when high-risk patients are excluded and when the correct procedures are followed.

The sensitivity of the ergonovine test is influenced by the phase of the disease at the time the test is performed, and the dose that induces spasm shows some inverse correlation with the number of anginal episodes. Thus, in patients with a typical history of variant angina, but no symptoms during the last few weeks, ergonovine testing is often negative. The test is usually performed by injecting intravenously incremental doses of ergonovine maleate (25, 50, 100 and 300 µg) at 5 minute intervals. The test should be interrupted as soon as diagnostic ischemic changes appear on the ECG or when the patient complains of pain or other important symptoms such as malaise, nausea or headache, or when other undesirable side effects such as hypertension or arrhythmias are observed.

Hyperventilation is another valid spasmogenic stimulus and, in theory, it is safer than the ergonovine test because the stimulus wanes as soon as the intracellular pH returns to normal. Compared to ergonovine testing, however, hyperventilation requires the full co-operation of the patients and has a lower sensitivity. The test is performed with the patient breathing as deeply as possible 30 times a minute for 5 min so that the arterial pH increases to about 7.60-7.70. The efficacy of hyperventilation can be increased by infusing alkaline solutions.[52]

The negativity of the results of provocative testing does not exclude definitively the diagnosis of variant angina, as occasionally the vasoconstrictor stimuli may not induce spasm, particularly during 'cold' phases of the disease.

Coronary spasm and small vessel disease

In about 20% of patients, with episodes of chest pain typical and severe enough to warrant cardiac catheterization, no significant coronary stenoses can be found.[53]

Some patients report exclusively or prevalently effort-induced angina and develop ischemic ST-segment depression during exercise testing, a clinical condition that has been termed "syndrome X".[54] In most patients, however, chest pain often occurs at rest, with no apparent triggering cause and ECG exercise stress testing may be negative, also during pain.

Although these patients, whose chest pain can be due to different causes, are likely to constitute a heterogeneous population, several studies have shown that a dysfunction of the small coronary arteries not visible at coronary angiography, demonstrated by a reduced coronary blood flow response to a variety of vasodilator stimuli,[55-57] is present in at least some of them. Therefore, myocardial ischemia due to a dysfunction of small coronary vessels (a condition appropriately defined as "microvascular angina")[56] has been proposed as a major cause of angina. In particular, it has been suggested that a primary prearteriolar vasoconstriction constitutes the most likely microvascular abnormality responsible for susceptibility to myocardial ischemia.[54,58] This abnormality may limit the increase in subendocardial blood supply necessary to match the increase in oxygen demand during exercise, but it may also cause myocardial ischemia at rest, because of a critical primary reduction in coronary flow following an exaggerated microvascular constriction.

This exaggerated microvascular constriction is suggested, 1) by the possibility of inducing anginal pain, in association with an impairment in coronary blood flow, by means of vasoconstrictor stimuli;[56,59] 2) by the occurrence of spontaneous ischemic ECG changes in the absence of a significant increase in heart rate in at least some episodes of ST-segment depression during Holter monitoring;[60,61] 3) by the presence, in some patients, of an increased reactivity to vasoconstrictor stimuli, expressed by an increased noncritical reduction in lumen diameter, also in epicardial coronary vessels.[62,63] It is not clear, however, whether a true spontaneous spasm (i.e. a localized, intense and paroxysmal vasoconstriction), may occur at the coronary microvascular level in man.

Clinically, patients with syndrome X must be distinguished from those with variant angina, as they pose very different diagnostic and therapeutic problems. Usually there are no major difficulties in the differential diagnosis. Indeed, in syndrome X, anginal attacks are often effort- or emotion-related, are long-lasting (10-30 min), are never associated with arrhythmias, occur predominantly during the daytime and often do not respond promptly to sublingual nitrates.[64] The absence of ST-segment elevation during pain allows the correct diagnosis to be made.

Prognostic assessment

A high incidence of severe complications, i.e. myocardial infarction (20-30%) and sudden death (about 10%), was reported in the first studies on vasospastic angina.[65,66] The majority of these events occurred during the acute phase of the disease or during the first months after hospitalization, while the complete remission of symptoms was frequent in the follow-up period.[65,66] However, since the use of high doses of calcium antagonists and nitrates has become widespread as a means of relieving and preventing coronary artery spasm[67,68] both the short- and long-term prognosis of variant angina have improved considerably. A number of patients, however, remain at risk of developing myocardial infarction or sudden death.

Two main findings influence the prognosis of variant angina: the presence of coronary artery stenoses and the development of serious brady- or tachyarrhythmias associated with ischemic episodes. Patients with severe and extensive coronary artery disease have a greater chance of developing myocardial infarction and sudden death and have higher mortality rates. Both myocardial infarction and sudden death can, however, also occur in patients with angiographically normal coronary arteries.[69,70] Indeed, thrombosis, as mentioned above, can be initiated by occlusive spasm due to activation of the hemostatic system.[36] Similarly, life-threatening tachy- or brady-arrhythmias may also occur in patients with normal coronary arteries.[46,47]

The reasons why some patients tend to develop arrhythmias are not known, but they are related strictly neither to the frequency, severity and duration of ischemic episodes, nor to the presence or absence of pain, both in different patients and even in the same patient[46,47,65,66] Ventricular tachyarrhythmias may occur either during ST-segment elevation or after its resolution during the reperfusion phase. Complete atrioventricular block and/or sinus arrest are observed less frequently, usually during inferior ischemia. Patients with severe arrhythmias associated with ischemic episodes have a significantly higher risk of sudden death than those not developing such arrhythmias.[65,66]

Therapeutic approach

Attacks of variant angina usually respond promptly to the sublingual administration of short-acting nitrates. In rare cases resistant to this therapy, intravenous nitrates or calcium antagonists are usually effective.

Since the actual causes of coronary artery hyperreactivity to constrictor stimuli remain unknown, treatment of vasospastic angina is based on the use of nonspecific vasodilator drugs (i.e. calcium-antagonists and nitrates).[67,68] Treatment should be aimed not only at the control of anginal episodes, but also at the suppression of all episodes of silent ischemic episodes detected by Holter monitoring and the prevention of ergonovine-induced spasm. This is crucial, particularly in patients with obstructive coronary artery disease at angiography and/or those who develop potentially fatal arrhythmias during ischemia. However, while positive tests indicate clearly that treatment is inadequate, negative tests do not offer absolute guarantees that treatment will be completely effective in preventing completely ischemic attacks.

Chronic therapy of variant angina is based on the administration of calcium-antagonists. Indeed, several controlled studies have demonstrated that they significantly improve prognosis.[69] Commercially available calcium-antagonists are likely to be equally as effective, although experience is wider with the more traditional drugs verapamil, nifedipine and diltiazem.[70-72] The choice among these depends on their efficacy and side-effects, as assessed by follow-up in individual patients. A complete or substantial suppression of ischemic episodes can be obtained in more than 80% of patients with the administration of the appropriate dosage (i.e., diltiazem and verapamil 360-480 mg/day and nifedipine 60-80 mg/day).

In some patients who continue to develop ischemic episodes in spite of the usual maximal doses of calcium-antagonists, the addition of long-acting nitrates (i.e. isosorbide dinitrate or mononitrate) may improve the efficacy of treatment.[73] Chronic administration of nitrates should be scheduled to cover the period with the highest number of ischemic episodes, leaving a drug-free interval of 10-14 hours in order to prevent tolerance.

While the use of nonspecific vasodilator drugs has been consistenly effective, all attempts to block specific individual stimuli have been therapeutically unsatisfactory. This may be either because the blockers used were inappropriate or insufficient or, more likely, because other constrictor stimuli were left unopposed. Thus, alpha-adrenergic and serotoninergic blockers failed to reduce substantially the number of anginal attacks, although they may be effective in some patients.[27,28] Conceptually, β-blockers are not indicated and are usually avoided in patients with vasospastic angina, based on the assumption that β-blockade may facilitate α-adrenergic stimulation and favour coronary artery spasm,[29] although data on this point are controversial.[46] Other types of treatment which have had inconsistent results include aspirin[18] and intravenous infusion of prostacycline.[35]

In rare cases, coronary artery spasm may be refractory to the usual medical treatment. In the past, some of these patients have been treated with cardiac denervation, but uncertain results have been obtained.[74,75] However, in our experience, very high doses of calcium-antagonists (i.e. diltiazem 960 mg/day, or verapamil 800 mg/day, each associated with nifedipine 100 mg and ISDN 80 mg) may be effective in most patients.[76] In the very rare cases in which these doses are insufficient, the addition of appropriate doses of either guanethidine or clonidine may improve symptoms.[77]

Finally, revascularization procedures (i.e. coronary angioplasty or by-pass surgery)[78,79] should be considered for patients with spasm at the site of a flow-limiting coronary stenosis in patients with a positive exercise test at a low workload or with the persistence of inducible spasm despite full medical therapy.

REFERENCES

1. Prinzmetal M, et al. Angina pectoris. I. The variant form of angina pectoris. Am J Med 1959: 27: 375.

2. Guazzi M, et al. Left ventricular performance and related haemodynamic changes in Prinzmental's variant angina pectoris. Br Heart J 1971: 33: 84.

3. Maseri A, et al. Coronary spasm as a cause of acute myocardial ischemia in man. Chest 1975: 68: 625-33.

4. Oliva, PB, et al. Coronary arterial spasm in Prinzmetal angina : documentation by coronary arteriography. N Engl J Med 1973: 288: 745-50.

5. Cheng TO, et al. Variant angina of Prinzmetal with normal coroanry arteriograms. A variant of the variant. Circulation 1973: 47: 476.

6. Maseri A, et al. "Variant" angina : one aspect of a continuous spectrum of vasospastic myocardial ischemia. Am J Cardiol 1978: 42: 1019.

7. Maseri A, et al. Transient transmural reduction of myocardial blood flow, demonstrated by thallium-201 scintigraphy., a cause of variant angina. Circulation 54: 280.

8. Fujii H, et al. Hyperventilation-induced simultaneous multivessel coronary spasm in patients with variant angina : an echocardiographic and arteriographic study. J Am Coll Cardiol 1988: 12: 1184.

9. Hoshio A, et al. Significance of coronary artery tone in patients with vasospastic angina. J Am Coll Cardiol 1989: 14: 604.

10. Kaski JC, et al. Comparison of epicardial coronary artery tone and reactivity in Prinzmetal's variant angina and chronic stable angina pectoris. J Am Coll Cardiol 1991: 17: 1058.

12. Kaski JC, et al. Spontaneous coronary artery spasm in variant angina results from a local hyperreactivity to a generalized constrictor stimulus. J Am Coll cardiol 1989: 14: 1456.

13. Yasue H, et al. Prinzmetal's variant form of angina as a manifestation of alpha-adrenergic receptor mediated coroanry artery spasm : documentation by coronary arteriography. Am Heart J 1976: 91: 148.

14. Crea, F, et al. Dopamine-induced coronary spasm. Circulation 1985: 72:III-415.

15. Yasue H, et al. Induction of coronary artery spasm by acetylcholine in patients with variant angina : possible role of the parasympathetic nervous system in the pathogenesis of coronary artery spasm. Circulation 74: 955-63.

16. Heupler F, et al. Ergonovine maleate provocative test for coronary arterial spasm. Am J Cardiol 1978: 41: 631.

17. McFadden EP, et al. Effect of intracoronary serotonin on coronary vessels in patients with stable angina and patients with variant angina. N Engl J Med 1992: 324:648.

18. Ginsburg R, et al. Histamine provocation of clinical coronary artery spasm: implications concerning the pathogenesis of variant angina pectoris. Am Heart J 102: 819.

19. Chierchia S, et al. Alpha-adrenergic receptors and coronary spasm : an elusive link. Circulation 1984: 8.

20. Chierchia S, et al. failure of thromboxane A2 blockade to prevent attacks of vasospastic angina. Circulation 1982: 66:702.

21. De caterina R, et al. A double-blind, placebo-controlled study of ketanserin in patients with Prinzmetal's angina. Evidence against a role for serotonin in the genesis of coronary vasospasm. Circulation 1984: 69: 889.

22. Vanhoutte PM, Shimokawa H. Endothelium-derived relaxing factor and coronary vasospasm. Circulation 1989: 80:1.

23. Mc Alpin RN. Contribution of dynamic vascular wall thickening to luminal narrowing during coronary arterial constriction. Circulation 1980: 71: 296.

24. Roberts WC, et al. Sudden death in Prinzmetal's angina with coronary spasm documented by angiography. nalysis of three necropsy patients. Am J Cardiol 1982:50:203.

25. Maseri A, et al. Coronary artery spasm and vasoconstriction. The case for a distinction. Circulation 1990: 81: 1983.

26. Specchia G, et al. Coronary arterial spasm as a cause of exercise-induced ST-segment elevation in patients with variant angina. Circulation 1979: 59: 948.

27. Raizner AE, et al. Provocation of coronary artery spasm by the cold pressor test. Hemodynamic arteriographic and quantitative angiographic observations. circulation 1980, 62: 925.

28. Winniford MD, et al. Alpha-adrenergic blockade for variant angina : a long-term double-blind, randomized trial. Circulation 1983: 67: 1185.

29. Tzivoni D, et al. Prazosin therapy for refractory variant angina. Am Heart J 1983: 105: 262-6.

30. Robertson RM, et al. Exacerbation of ischemia in vasotonic angina pectoris by propranolol. Am J Cardiol 47: 463.

31. Robertson RM, et al. Arterial and coronary sinus catecholamines in the course of spontaneous coronary artery spasm. Am Heart J 1983: 105: 901.

32. Waters D, Miller D. Circadian variation in variant angina. Am J Cardiol 1984: 54: 61.

33. Lanza GA, et al. Role of Autonomic Tone in the Induction of Coronary Spasm in Patients With Variant Angina With or Without Obstructive Coronary Stenoses. J Am Coll Cardiol 1995: 25 (Abstr Suppl.): 195A.

34. Tada M, et al. Elevation of thromboxane B2 levels in patients with classic and variant angina pectoris. Circulation 1981: 64: 1107.

35. Robertson RM, et al. Thromboxane A2 in vasotonic angina. N Engl J Med 1981: 304: 998.

36. Chierchia S, et al. Increased fibrinopeptide A during anginal attacks in patients with variant angina. J Am Coll Cardiol 1989: 14: 589.

37. Irie T, et al. Increased fibrinopeptide A during anginal attacks in patients with variant angina. J Am Coll Cardiol 1989: 14: 589.

38. Toyo-Oka T, et al. Increased plasma level of endothelin-1 and coronary spasm induction in patients with vasospastic angina pectoris. Circulation 1991: 83: 476.

39. Larkin SW, et al. Intracoronary endothelium induces myocardial ischemia by small vessel constriction in the dog. Am J Cardiol 1989: 64: 956.

40. Bertrand M, et al. Frequency of provoked coronary arterial spasm in 1089 consecutive patients undergoing coronary angiography. Circulation 1982: 65: 1299.

41. Fernandez D, et al. Alcohol-induced Prinzmetal variant angina. Am J Cardiol 1973: 32: 238.

42. Shimokawa H, et al. Cimetidine induces coronary artery spasm in patients with vasospastic angina. Canad J Cardiol 1987: 3:177.

43. Miwa K, et al. Exercise-induced angina provoked by aspirin administration in patients with variant angina. Am J Cardiol 1981: 47: 1210.

44. Scholl JM, et al. Comparison of risk factors in vasospastic angina without significant fixed coronary narrowing to signigicant fixed coronary narrowing and no vasospastic angina. Am J Cardiol 1986: 57: 199.

45. Caralis DG, et al. Smoking is a risk factor for coronary spasm in young women. Circulation 1992: 85: 905.

46. Miller D, et al. Is variant angina the coronary manifestation of a generalized vasospastic disorder ? N Engl J Med 1981: 304: 763.

47. Kerin NZ, et al. Arrhythmias in variant angina pectoris. Relationships of arrhythmias to ST segment elevation and R wave changes. Circulation 1979: 60: 1343.

48. Maseri A, et al. Role of coronary arterial spasm in sudden coronary ischemic death. Ann NY Acad Sci 1982: 382: 204.

49. Rozanski J, et al. Non-mechanical ST segment alternance in Prinzmetal·s angina. Am Int Med 1978: 89: 76.

50. Meller J, et al. Transient Q waves in Prinzmetal·s angina. Am J Cardiol 1975: 35: 691.

51. Buxton AE, et al. Refractory ergovine induced coronary vasospasm : importance of intracoronary nitroglycerin. Am J Cardiol 1980: 46:329.

52. Magarian GJ, Mazur DJ. The Hyperventilation challenge test. Chest 1991: 99:199.

53. Yasue H, et al. Coronary arterial spasm and Prinzmetal·s variant angina induced by hyperventilation and Tris-buffer infusion. Circulation 1978: 58:56.

54. Phibbs B, et al. Frequency of normal coronary arteriograms in three academic mediacal centers and one community hospital. Am J Cardiol 1988: 62: 472-74.

55. Maseri A, et al. Mechanisms of angina pectoris in syndrome X. J Am Coll Cardiol 1991: 17: 499.

56. Opherk D, et al. Reduced coronary dilatory capacity and ultrastructural changes of the

myocardium in patients with angina pectoris but normal coronary arteriograms. Circulation 1981 : 63: 817.

57. Cannon RO, Epstein SE. "Microvascular angina" as a cause of chest pain with angiographically normal coronary arteries. Am J Cardiol 1988: 61: 1338.

58. Egashira K, et al. Evidence of impaired endothelium-dependent coronary vasolidation in patients with angina pectoris and normal coronary angiograms. N Engl J Med 1993: 328: 1659.

59. Epstein SE, Cannon RO. Site of increased resistance to coronary flow in patients with angina pectoris and normal epicardial coronary arteries. J Am Coll Cardiol 1986: 8:459.

60. Chauhan A, et al. Effect of hyperventilation and mental stress on coronary blood flow in syndrome X. Br Heart J 1993: 69: 516.

61. Kaski JC, et al. Transient myocardial ischemia during daily life in patients with syndrome X. Am J Cardiol 1986: 58:1242.

62. Lanza GA, Stazi F. Circadian variation of ischemic threshold in syndrome X. Am J Cardiol 1995: 683.

63. Vrints CJM, et al. Impaired endothelium-dependent cholinergic coronary vasolidation in patients with angina and normal coronary arteries. J Am Coll Cardiol 1992: 19:21.

64. Bugiardini R, Pozzati A. Vasotonic angina : a spectrum of ischemic syndromes involving functional abnormalities of the epicardial and microvascular coronary circulation. J Am Coll Cardiol 1993: 22: 417.

65. Kaski JC, Rosano GMC. Cardiac syndrome X : clinical characteristics and left ventricular function. Long-term follow-up study. J Am Coll Cardiol 1995: 25: 807.

66. Severi S, et al. Long-term prognosis of "variant" angina with medical treatment. Am J Cardiol 1980: 46:226.

67. Waters DD, et al. Factors influencing the long-term prognosis of treated patients with variant angina. Circulation 1983: 68: 258.

68. MacAlpin R. Treatment of vasospastic angina. In : Golgberg S (ed). Coronary Artery Spasm and Thrombosis. Philadelphia, F A Davis, 1983, p.129.

69. Maseri A, et al. Rational approach to the medical therapy of angina pectoris : the role of calcium antagonists. Prog Cardiovasc Dis 1983: 15: 269.

70. Yasue H, et al. Long-term prognosis for patients with variant angina and influential factors. Circulation 1988: 78: 1.

71. Previtali M, et al. Treatment of angina at rest with nifedipine : a short-term controlled study. Am J Cardiol 1980 : 45: 875.

72. Johnson SM, et al. A controlled trial of verapamil for Prinzmetal's variant angina. N Engl J Med 1981: 304: 862-66.

73. Feldman RL, et al. Short- and long-term responses to diltiazem in patients with variant angina. Am J cardiol 1982: 49: 554.

74. Hill JA, et al. Randomized double-blind comparison of nifedipine and isosorbide dinitrate in patients with coronary arterial spasm. Am J Cardiol 1982: 49: 431.

75. Bertrand ME, et al. Complete denervation of the heart (autotransplantation) for treatment of severe, refractory coronary spasm. Am J Cardiol 1981: 47: 1375.

76. Clark DA, et al. Coronary artery spasm : medical management, surgical denervation, and autotransplantation. J Thorac Cardiovasc Surg 1977: 73: 332.

77. Lefroy DC, et al. Medical treatment of refractory coronary artery spasm. Cor Art Dis 1992: 3: 745.

78. Frenneaux M, et al. Refractory variant amgina relieved by guanethidine and clonidine. Am J Cardiol 1988: 62: 832.

79. Bertrand ME, et al. Percutaneous transluminal coronary angioplasty in patients with spasm superimposed on atherosclerotic narrowing. Br Heart J 1987: 58: 469.

80. Bertrand ME, et al. Surgical treatment of variant angina : use of plexectomy with aortocoronary bypass. Circulation 1980: 61: 877.

7 THE ROLE OF NITRIC OXIDE IN CORONARY DISEASE

Todd J. Anderson, Ian T. Meredith, François Charbonneau,
Peter Ganz, Andrew P. Selwyn

The vascular endothelium is capable of modulating many biological responses through the release of locally derived vasoactive factors.' One of the most important is nitric oxide, the endothelium-derived relaxing factor (EDRF).[2] Nitric oxide is synthesized by endothelial cells from the essential amino acid I-arginine by nitric oxide synthase (NOS). Three forms of nitric oxide synthase have been sequenced: a constitutive form from vascular endothelium; a constitutive form from the central nervous system; and an inducible enzyme derived from macrophages in response to cytokines.[5] Together, these enzymes, through the release of nitric oxide, control a great variety of processes, in both health and disease. Nitric oxide is important as an inhibitor of platelet aggregation, smooth muscle cell proliferation and endothelial-leukocyte interaction.[6,7,8] However, one of the most important actions of nitric oxide is in the regulation of both basal and stimulated arterial tone.[9,10] In response to a number of pharmacological and physiological stimuli, the activation of constitutive nitric oxide synthase releases nitric oxide, leading to vasodilation. However, in patients with atherosclerosis or cardiac risk factors, vasodilation is attenuated and this may be important in the pathogenesis disturbances in regional and coronary blood flow leading to coronary ischemia.[11] Although many other locally produced vasoactive substances including prostacyclin, endothelium-derived hyperpolarizing factor, endothelin, and thromboxane, are important in controlling vascular tone, nitric oxide plays a key role *(Figure 7.1)*. This chapter will thus focus, on the role of endothelium-derived nitric oxide in the control of coronary conduit vessel vasomotion and coronary blood flow and the abnormalities in this system which are seen with atherosclerosis and related conditions.

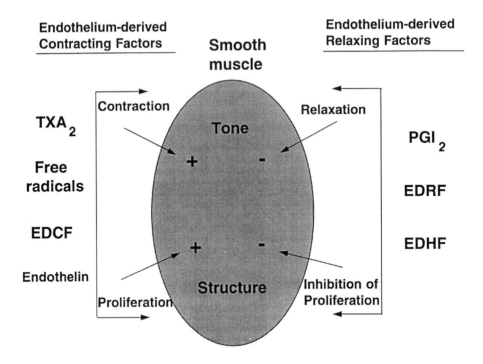

Figure 7.1 Factors acting on vascular smooth muscle cells causing contraction or relaxation. TxA₂=thromboxane A₂, EDCF=endothelium derived contraction factor, EDRF=endothelium-derived relaxing factor, EDHF=endothelium-derived hyperpolarization factor.

Nature of endothelium-derived relaxing factor

In 1980, Furchgott and Zawadski, discovered that acetylcholine-induced relaxation of rabbit aortic strips required an intact endothelium.[2] They concluded that acetylcholine stimulated muscarinic receptors on the endothelium, leading to the release of a non-prostanoid relaxing factor, which they named endothelium-derived relaxing factor.

A diffusible substance with a half-life of several seconds,[12] endothelium-derived relaxing factor can be inhibited by heme-containing proteins[13] and destroyed by oxygen free radicals.[14] It activates soluble guanylate cyclase and increases the concentration of cyclic guanosine monophosphate.[15] Collectively, these characteristics led to the simultaneous observation by Ignarro and Furchgott that endothelium-derived relaxing factor was strikingly similar to nitric oxide.[16,17]

The first proof that nitric oxide was at least one of the relaxing factors resulted from studies by Palmer and colleagues.[4] Using a chemiluminescence assay, they demonstrated that cultured endothelial cells release nitric oxide when exposed to bradykinin. In this assay, nitric oxide is specifically detected by its reaction with ozone. Results of these studies provided strong evidence that endothelium-derived relaxing factor is nitric oxide or a chemically related compound. Recent findings suggest that endothelium-derived relaxing factor may also be similar to a labile nitroso compound (S-nitroso-L-cysteine).[18]

Mechanism of action of endothelium-derived relaxing factor

Palmer et al. have demonstrated that nitric oxide is synthesized from the guanidino nitrogen of the amino acid, L-arginine.[4] In response to shear stress or receptor activation of the endothelium there is a resulting influx of calcium. Receptor activation often occurs in conjunction with signal transduction proteins (the G protein family).[19] Serotonin receptors, for example, interact with the pertussis-sensitive Gi (inhibitory) protein to modulate an increase in intracellular calcium. The increase in calcium results in stimulation of constitutive nitric oxide synthase and the production of nitric oxide. This enzymatic process can be effectively inhibited by an arginine analogue, NG- monomethyl-L-arginine, which is an important tool to investigate the importance of nitric oxide in biological events.[3] Following release from the endothelium, endothelium-derived relaxing factor diffuses across the extracellular space into the smooth muscle cell, and stimulates guanylate cyclase leading to an increase in the intracellular concentration of cyclic guanosine monophosphate.[20] *(Figure 7.2)*.

Cyclic Guanosine 3'-, 5'-Monophosphate System: Intracellular Second Messenger

Cyclic guanosine monophosphate is formed from guanosine 5'-triphosphate by the activation of soluble guanylate cyclase. This process is calcium-independent. Purified soluble guanylate cyclase has been shown to contain heme, which is now thought to be the receptor site for nitric oxide.[21] Local thiol groups are necessary to reduce the heme iron atom to the ferrous state, thus facilitating the nitric oxide-heme interaction.

The net result of the activation of soluble guanylate cyclase is the formation of cyclic guanosine monophosphate, which then activates a serine/threonine protein kinase (cG-Pk).[22] Several proteins may be phosphorylated by cG-Pk, resulting in smooth muscle relaxation. Cyclic guanosine monophosphate also stimulates calcium efflux and calcium uptake by intracellular stores. It may also inhibit calcium influx across the plasma membrane by decreasing production of diacyl glycerol (DAG) and inositol 1,4,5-triphosphate (IP_3) which result in a decrease in protein kinase C activity.[23]

Role of nitric oxide in maintaining vasomotor tone

Experimental evidence

Conduit vessels: Nitric oxide can be released in response to a variety of stimuli *(Table 7.1)*.[24] A substantial body of basic research has established the importance of

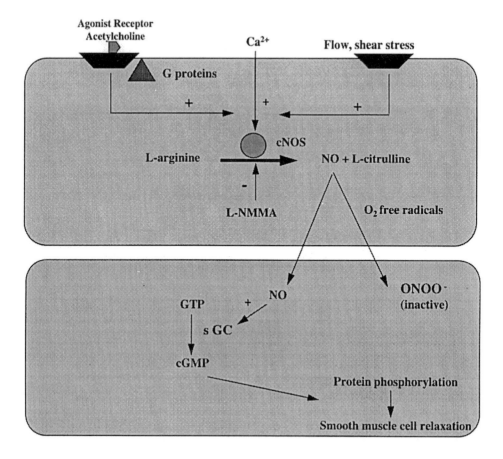

Figure 7.2 The metabolic pathway of aginine; No leads to smooth muscle cell relaxation

nitric oxide release in both basal and stimulated control of vascular tone in large conduit vessels. Studies have demonstrated that basal cyclic GMP levels are higher in aortic strips when the endothelium is intact than when it has been denuded and bioassay techniques have also demonstrated the basal release of NO from large conduit vessels.[13] When the nitric oxide synthase inhibitor, L-NMMA is applied to preconstricted arterial tissue, there is a prompt increase in tension, as a result of inhibition of endothelium-derived nitric oxide.[25] Despite tissue and species differences, endothelium-dependent agonists such as acetylcholine predominantly cause vascular relaxation. The role of nitric oxide as the mediator is supported by experiments that used endothelium-dependent agonists in the presence of inhibitors of nitric oxide. Martin et al. demonstrated in vascular rings from rabbit aortas that hemoglobin and methylene blue abolished the endothelium-dependent relaxation induced by acetylcholine and the calcium ionophore A23187.[13] They believed this

Table 7.1   ENDOTHELIUM-DERIVED VASODILATORS

Acetylcholine	Catecholamines
Histammine	Substance P
Serotonin	Peptide of calcium related gene
ADP, ATP	Platelet activations factor
Bradykinin	Ionophoretic Ca [A23187]
Thrombin	Increased flow, shear stress

was caused by a direct inhibitory effect on guanylate cyclase, as cyclic GMP levels did not rise in the presence of acetylcholine and A23187. The same results have been obtained with L-NMMA as the inhibitor of nitric oxide.[25] Increasing flow and subsequently shear stress are also important mediators of endothelium-dependent vasodilation. It has been shown in the canine femoral and coronary artery, that removal of the endothelium by balloon injury prevents the flow-mediated increase in diameter, demonstrating that the response is endothelium dependent.[26,27]

The vasodilation seen in arterial strips exposed to endothelium-dependent agonists is markedly attenuated in the presence of atherosclerosis.[28] In a study by Heistad et al., an augmented response to vasoconstrictor stimuli was observed in atherosclerotic primates.[29] Similar results have been observed in rabbit models of atherosclerosis.[30] Cholesterol feeding for as little as two weeks resulted in abnormal arterial relaxation to acetylcholine.[31] Recent studies have shown an impairment of endothelium-dependent relaxation with incubation of arterial strips with LDL or particularly oxidized LDL.[32] These studies have shown that abnormalities occur without the need for structural atherosclerosis.

Resistance vessels. In vitro studies have used microscopy, to demonstrate dilation of resistance vessels in an response to acetylcholine from rabbit ear,[33] rat cremaster muscle,[34] and canine coronary resistance vessels.[35] In vivo studies employing rabbit hind limbs, isolated buffer- perfused rabbit heart, and primates employing nitric oxide inhibitors have confirmed that nitric oxide mediates vasodilation in the microcirculation.[36,37] Studies have also shown that resistance vessels are able to dilate in response to increases in flow and shear stress by endothelium-dependent mechanisms.[38] Studies that employed systemic doses of NG-monomethyl-L-arginine have shown an increase in blood pressure and reflex bradycardia in the rabbit 39 the rat,[40] and the guinea pig,[41] suggesting that the basal release of endothelium-derived relaxing factor is important at the resistance vessel level in regulating systemic blood pressure. However, studies in canine coronary arteries have suggested that other mediators besides NO may be important in the control of basal and stimulated coronary blood flow.[42]

As in the conduit vessels, both lipoproteins and cholesterol-induced atherosclerosis impair resistance vessel vasorelaxation compared to controls. This has been demonstrated in both primate and rabbit models.[31,37]

Human studies

Conduit vessels. In vitro studies using human coronary arteries have shown endothelium-dependent relaxation in response to acetylcholine in normal arteries and impaired relaxation in atherosclerotic coronary arteries.[43] In vivo studies of conduit vessel vasomotion have focused on the coronary circulation.[44] Ludmer and colleagues first demonstrated coronary vasodilation in response to acetylcholine in patients with normal coronary arteries and no risk factors for atherosclerosis. It has recently been shown that acetylcholine induced coronary conduit vessel dilation can be inhibited by free reduced hemoglobin and L-NMMA, strongly suggesting that the response is mediated by nitric oxide.[45,46] L-NMMA also causes a small (5%) decrease in coronary diameter suggesting some role of nitric oxide in maintaining basal tone. A number of subsequent studies also showed that other agonists, including substance P, serotonin, and histamine, can increase the coronary artery diameter in normal subjects. Flow mediated vasodilation has also been demonstrated in human coronary arteries.[47] Physiological stimuli that lead to an increase in coronary blood flow, by bicycle exercise, [48] cold pressor testing, [49] atrial pacing,[50] and mental arithmetic, [51] have all been shown to increase coronary artery diameter in patients without atherosclerosis or risk factors. The parallel response of coronary arteries to the physiological stimuli and to acetylcholine led investigators to the conclusion that these stimuli were endothelium-dependent. However, studies employing nitric oxide inhibitors have not been done to confirm the role of nitric oxide in flow-mediated vasodilation, in the coronary circulation.

Important differences in the coronary response to endothelium-dependent stimuli have been observed between patients with smooth arteries and those with atherosclerosis. In the original study by Ludmer et al., it was shown that irregular coronary arteries and those with stenoses constricted in response to acetylcholine.[43] The in vivo vasomotor response to acetylcholine is a balance between the direct vasoconstricting effects on the smooth muscle mediated via muscarinic receptors, and the vasodilating effects of nitric oxide released by the endothelium. In patients with atherosclerosis, there is an impairment of the release or action of nitric oxide, and the observed effect is vasoconstriction. Subsequent to this, Wems et al., showed abnormal vasodilator responses in smooth coronary arteries in patients with atherosclerosis in other vessels.[52] Abnormal endothelium -dependent dilation to acetylcholine in the conduit vessels has also been shown in patients with smooth coronary arteries and documented ischemia (Syndrome X).[53] Attenuation of normal flow-mediated vasodilation has also been demonstrated in response to exercise, pacing, cold pressor testing and mental stress. In fact, in patients provoked with mental stress, constriction at sites of stenoses can be demonstrated.[51]

More recent data has shown, that even in the presence of risk factors for atherosclerosis, endothelial dysfunction may occur. In patients with smooth coronary arteries, there is a good relationship between serum cholesterol, and total number of risk factors, and the endothelium-dependent vasomotor response to acetylcholine.[54] The conduit vessel response to bicycle exercise is also related to serum cholesterol levels in patients with normal coronary arteries.[55] This relationship is more complex in patients with established atherosclerosis, where other parameters of lipid abnormalites such as the size and density of LDL particles and its susceptibility to oxidation may be more important.[56] Recent studies using intravascular ultrasound, also demonstrate that endothelial dysfunction is present before there is any evidence of intimal thickening. This confirms the in vitro findings that the physical presence of atherosclerosis is not a prerequisite for a dysfunctional endothelium. In addition, impairment in endothelium-dependent vasodilator responses to acetylcholine have also been demonstrated in patients with hypertension, and dilated cardiomyopathy.

Resistance vessels. Vasodilatation in resistance vessels is assessed by measuring blood flow. For a constant pressure and cardiac output, changes in flow represent changes in resistance vessel vasomotor tone. Importantly, any stimulus that relaxes resistance vessels and increases flow, will result in a mild increase in conduit vessel diameter as a consequence of flow-mediated vasodilation. Resistance vessel dilation therefore effects changes in conduit vessels through flow-mediated dilation.

In the coronary circulation, Zeiher et al. measured blood flow in response to acetylcholine and papaverine in patients with various degrees of atherosclerosis.[57] Patients with early atherosclerosis showed an impaired blood flow response to acetylcholine, compared with normal controls. A recent study by Ryan et al. also showed that patients with atherosclerosis had impaired blood flow response to substance P and not to adenosine.[58] These studies suggest that endothelium-dependent vasodilator function is impaired in the microvasculature of patients with nonobstructive coronary artery disease. In addition, studies have also demonstrated an impairment of resistance vessel dilation in patients with coronary risk factors such as hypercholesterolemia, hypertension and increasing age.[59,60] Lefroy et al. used coronary sinus oxygen saturation as a measure of coronary blood flow to demonstrate that L-NMMA inhibited the dilation of coronary conduit vessels in response to acetylcholine, but it did not abolish the blood flow (resistance vessel dilation) increase in response to acetylcholine.[46] They suggested that EDRF may not be the only mediator of acetylcholine-induced increase in blood flow in the coronary microvasculature. Other mediators, such as EDHF may be involved, or the contribution of nitric oxide is small, and was not detected. Dysfunction of endothelium-dependent vasomotion in resistance vessels has been demonstrated in patients with hypertension, [61,62] and also in patients with chest pain and normal coronary angiograms (syndrome X).[63]

The role of abnormal vasomotion in coronary heart disease

There is abundant evidence to suggest that proximal coronary lesions play an active role in causing ischemia by intermittently interfering with coronary blood flow.[64,65] Selwyn et al., used rubidium-82 positron emission tomography to study changes in regional myocardial perfusion in patients with stable coronary artery disease.[66] The data from these studies provided evidence that regional coronary blood flow decreased at the onset and during clinical ischemia. More recently and in support of these studies, positron emission tomography also demonstrated absolute decreases in regional myocardial perfusion during exercise, cold pressor stimulation and mental arithmetic in patients with coronary heart disease. The decreases in perfusion occurred in the distribution of stenosed epicardial coronary arteries implying vaso-constriction at the stenotic site.[67]

In the studies of endothelial function in large epicardial coronary arteries, employing physiological stimuli, we have shown that there are important differences in the behavior of angiographically smooth arteries and those containing atherosclerosis. Smooth arteries without angiographic evidence of atherosclerosis generally dilate in response to these provocative tests while irregular and/or stenosed arteries usually constrict.[47-51] Gage et al. demonstrated that stenoses constricted in response to exercise, and Yeung demonstrated similar findings in patients with a mental stress protocol.[51,68] It is very likely that this abnormality in endothelium-dependent vasomotion in the setting of moderate to severe stenoses is an important cause of ischemia.

Endothelial dysfunction: possible mechanisms

Endothelial vasodilator dysfunction has been demonstrated in vitro and in vivo in animal and human studies in a wide range of conditions *(Table 7.2)*. A detailed discussion is beyond the scope of this chapter, but several reviews are available.[9] The mechanism of this vasodilator dysfunction is unclear, and since the actions of endothelium-derived relaxing factor are complex, abnormalities could occur at many sites of actions: i) impairment of endothelial membrane receptors which interact with agonists or physiological stimuli to release nitric oxide; ii) diminished levels or impaired utilization of I-arginine, the substrate for NO synthesis; iii) reductions in nitric oxide synthase, the enzyme responsible for the conversion of I-arginine to nitric oxide iv) impaired release of nitric oxide from the endothelium in its most active form (ie. nitrosothiols); v) enhanced degradation of nitric oxide by oxygen free radicals; vi) impaired transport from endothelium to smooth muscle cell (functional barrier); vii) impaired interaction of nitric oxide with guanylate cyclase and subsequent increase in cyclic guanosine monophosphate and viii) decrease in generalized smooth muscle cell sensitivity to vasodilators.

The best studied conditions associated with endothelial dysfunction are hypercholesterolemia and atherosclerosis. Hypercholesterolemia inhibits endothelium-dependent relaxation evoked by receptor-dependent stimuli, but this generally does not inhibit the direct relaxing effect of nitroglycerin. Studies in hypercholesterolemic porcine coronary arteries have demonstrated that the activity of the pertussis toxin-sensitive Gi protein-dependent receptor pathway is reduced in hypercholesterolemic endothelial cells.[69] This may be one of the mechanisms of endothelial dysfunction in the early stages of the atherosclerotic process.[70] Hypercholesterolemic rabbits have also been demonstrated to produce excessive quantities of superoxide

Table 7.2   *CONDITIONS RELATED TO ENDOTHELIAL DYSFUNCTION*

Atherosclerosis	Syndrome X
Hypercholesterolemia	Variant angina
Hypertension	Dilated cardiomyopathy
Diabetes Mellitus	Cocaine use
Smoking	Chagas disease
Saphenous vein graft atherosclerosis	

anion, by an endothelium-dependent process.[71] As will be discussed below, this is a second mechanism by which hypercholesterolemia could impair endothelium-dependent vasodilation.

The synthesis of nitric oxide involves the oxidation of a guanidino nitrogen on l-arginine by means of specific nitric oxide synthases. Several groups have suggested that a depletion of l-arginine is responsible for this endothelial dysfunction in hypercholesterolemia. It was shown in rabbit hind limbs that L-arginine administration potentiated the acetylcholine-induced increase in hind limb flow in rabbits with dietary hypercholesterolemia.[72] Two studies have addressed this issue in human coronary arteries. Drexler et al. were able to demonstrate an improvement in the flow response (resistance vessel function) to acetylcholine after l-arginine infusion but did not demonstrate any effect on large vessel vasomotion.[73] In contrast, Dubois Rande showed an improvement in the large vessel response to acetylcholine following l-arginine infusion.[74] Therefore, in certain situations, depletion or impaired utilization of l-arginine may contribute to the dysfunction seen in hypercholesterolemia, however, a deficiency of the substrate has not been proven by measurements of intracellular concentrations.

Rubanyi et al. have shown that superoxide anions can inactivate endothelium-derived relaxing factor.[14] In hypercholesterolemic rabbits, an excess amount of superoxide anions are generated from the endothelial cells. In states in which excessive free radicals are generated, an increase in oxidation of low density lipoproteins (LDL) would also result. Oxidized LDL itself has been shown to be a potent inhibitor of endothelium-dependent relaxations through mechanisms that are transduction dependent.[75]

Other potential mechanisms of endothelial dysfunction include intimal thickening, which acts as a barrier to the diffusion of endothelium-derived relaxing factor, and the increased production of vasoconstrictor substances that offset the balance toward vasoconstriction. Endothelin may be one such factor. However, the role of these vasoconstrictors has not been well-defined. Thus, even though the normal physiology of endothelium-derived relaxing factor has been extensively studied, the mechanisms involved in its failure are incompletely understood at this time.

Treatment of endothelial dysfunction

The treatment of endothelial dysfunction would be a desireable end-point. A healthy endothelium, not only maintains vasodilation but has important anti-coagulant and anti-proliferative properties. Before overt atherosclerosis develops, treatment of endothelial dysfunction might prevent or delay its onset. Once atherosclerosis is present, a healthier endothelium could potentially slow atherosclerosis progression, or lessen the risk of unstable coronary syndromes. Based on our understanding of the pathogenesis of endothelial dysfunction, a variety of potential strategies have been advocated for its long-term treatment *(Table 7.3)*.

Cholesterol lowering therapy

Harrison et al. were among the first to demonstrate that reversal of the impairment in endothelium-dependent vasodilation was possible.[76] In primates who were rendered atherosclerotic by cholesterol feeding, the institution of a normal cholesterol diet allowed a return to baseline in the dilator responses of isolated arterial strips to acetylcholine. This occurred despite the continued presence of intimal thickening, suggesting that complete regression was not necessary for improvement in function. Osborne and colleagues also demonstrated after 2 weeks of cholesterol feeding in rabbits, that abnormalities in vasodilator responses were observed. Importantly, this could be prevented by supplementation with lovastatin.[31] Williams et al., were able to demonstrate an improvement in coronary endothelium-dependent vasodilation to acetylcholine in vivo. In atherosclerotic primates who were then fed a low cholesterol diet, a significant attenuation of the initial vasoconstriction to acetylcholine was seen after cholesterol lowering diet therapy.[77]

The first human study to suggest that lipid modification might be useful in improving endothelial dysfunction employed omega-3 fatty acids. In a small group of patients (n=8), treated for 6 months with large doses of fish oils, an improvement in the coronary conduit vessel vasomotor response to acetylcholine was demonstrated.[78] More recently, Leung and colleagues have shown that the coronary vasodilator response to acetycholine could be improved after 6 months of cholesterol lowering therapy in patients with no evidence of atherosclerosis.[79] Patients in this study (n=25) had hypercholesterolemia, but no angiographic evidence of atherosclerosis. At baseline there was a 25% constriction to acetylcholine which improved to 5% dilation after therapy,

*Table 7.3   STRATEGIES FOR POTENTIAL TREATMENT
            OF ENDOTHELIAL DYSFUNCTION*

Cholesterol lowering
Antioxidant therapy
Administration of L-arginine
Omega-3 fatty acids
N-acetylcysteine
Estrogen replacement therapy

with only 6 months of therapy. There was no control group employed, and regression to the mean might explain part of the improvement in vasodilator function.

Preliminary data has been recently presented on the effect of cholesterol lowering on endothelial function in patients with established coronary atherosclerosis. Treasure and his colleagues randomized 19 patients to 6 months of therapy with lovastatin or placebo and measured the coronary conduit vessel vasomotor response to acetylcholine.[80] By measuring up to 5 coronary segments per patients they were able to demonstrate an improvement in response only in the most constricting segment. Although the most constricting segment may contain the most interesting biology and have important implications for the patient, this study suggested that the effect of lovastatin therapy was not that strong in patients with atherosclerosis treated for 6 months. Initial data was also presented from our laboratory from a randomized study employing a control group, an LDL cholesterol lowering group (lovastatin and cholestyramine) and an LDL+ oxidized LDL lowering group (lovastatin and probucol).[81] Patients with atherosclerosis were treated for one year. Preliminary analysis demonstrated that patients treated with drug therapy had a significant attenuation of acetylcholine induced vasoconstriction compared to patients in the diet group. The relative magnitude of improvement in the two treatment groups awaits final analysis. The weight of data suggests that endothelial dysfunction may be improved with strategies aimed at lowering cholesterol.

Recent angiographic regression studies have demonstrated decreased progression and more regression in patients treated with cholesterol lowering regimes. However, the difference in the % diameter stenosis between treatment and control groups is only 3-5%. Despite this, the majority of these studies have shown a marked reduction in clinical events.[82] This has led to the speculation that cholesterol lowering results in a decrease in the cholesterol content of plaques resulting in stabilization and a decreased tendency for plaque rupture. However, the above data, suggests that an improvement in endothelial function might be another mechanism for the clinical benefits observed with cholesterol lowering studies.

Anti-oxidant therapy

The oxidation of LDL cholesterol is now thought to play a primary role in the pathogenesis of atherosclerosis developement.[83] Antioxidants might improve endothelium-dependent dilation by two distinct mechanisms. Oxygen free radicals themselves are potent inactivators of nitric oxide, and oxidized LDL markedly attenuated endothelium-dependent vasodilation. Ohara et al., have shown that rabbits fed high cholesterol diets produce an excessive amount of superoxide anions from the endothelium, and that these arterial strips demonstrate impaired relaxation.[71] Subsequent to this they demonstrated that treating these rabbits with a low cholesterol diet could decrease the production of free radicals and improve dilator responses. A recent study by Keaney and colleagues has nicely demonstrated that cholesterol fed rabbits demonstrated impaired endothelium-dependent relaxation to acetylcholine and A231.[87] However, if the rabbits were supplemented with a-tocopherol, this dysfunction was markedly decreased.[84] Probucol, is a cholesterol lowering agent with a potent antioxidant effect. It has been shown to protect LDL particles against oxidation, and may have important effects at the level of the endothelial cell.[85] A recent study has demonstrated that probucol is able to improve vasodilator responses in arterial strips from cholesterol fed atherosclerotic rabbits.[86]

Little is known about the role of free radical scavengers or anti-oxidants in treating endothelial dysfunction in patients. A study from our laboratory addressed the role of short term infusion of superoxide dismutase, an oxygen free radical scavenger on endothelium-dependent vasomotion in coronary arteries. This study demonstrated that superoxide dismutase could attenuate the vasoconstriction seen with acetylcholine in patients with atherosclerosis.[87] One explanation of these results, is that oxygen free radical inactivation of nitric oxide, is an important mechanism of the impairment of endothelium-dependent vasodilation seen in atherosclerosis. Although there is no current data which addresses the long-term efficacy of anti-oxidant therapy of endothelial function, results will be available soon from our randomized study employing the anti-oxidant probucol.[81]

Estrogen replacement therapy

There is extensive evidence suggesting that estrogen replacement in post-menopausal women reduces cardiac mortality by about 50%.[88] While part of this benefit might simply be related to a favorable change in the cholesterol profile, other factors are likely involved. Favorable in vitro effects on both endothelium-dependent and independent processes have been shown.[89] In cholesterol fed primates, Williams has shown that long-term estrogen replacement improves coronary vasodilator responses to acetylcholine.[90] More recently, they have shown that a short term infusion of estrogen (20 minutes) results in a blunting of acetylcholine induced vasoconstriction, through unknown mechanisms.[91] These studies have been repeated by several groups in post-menopausal women in cardiac catheterization laboratories, including our own laboratory. All have shown that a 10-15 minute infusion of either estradiol or premarin result in an improvement in the conduit and resistance vessel dilator response to acetylcholine.[92] Long-term studies of estrogen replacement have not been done as yet. Keaney and colleagues have presented preliminary data which demonstrates that 17β-estradiol improves dilator responses to acetylcholine in atherosclerotic swine, with an associated decrease in the susceptibility of LDL oxidation in estradiol treated pigs.[93] This provides some evidence that an anti-oxidant effect of estrogen may play a role in endothelium-dependent processes. Other mechanisms such as a calcium-channel blocking effect may also be operating.[94]

Future directions

During the past decade, studies have focused on the development of catheterization techniques to study endothelium-dependent dilation in humans. The range of responses in health and disease have been characterized and we have begun to look at mechanisms of endothelial dysfunction and approaches to the treatment of this problem. The focus has been mainly on epicardial conduit vessels, however more recent technical improvements have allowed a more accurate measurement of coronary blood flow. Future studies will be better able to assess both large and small vessel responses.

Much needs to be learned about the relationship between cardiac risk factors, endothelial dysfunction and atherosclerosis. The evidence to date suggests that endothelial dysfunction precedes and may be important in the pathogenesis of atherosclerosis. However, longitudinal studies are needed to establish this link. Newer methods are also required to identify those patients at risk before atherosclerosis has developed. A new ultrasound technique which assesses flow-mediated brachial artery vasodilation holds promise for studying patients' endothelial function non-invasively.[95] We have shown a good relationship between coronary responses to acetylcholine and brachial artery responses, suggesting that this technique can be used as a surrogate for coronary endothelial function testing.[96] However, the reproducibility of this ultrasound technique must be established, and the long-term significance of endothelial dysfunction in patients with no evidence of atherosclerosis needs to be determined.

With respect to treatment of impaired vasodilator responses, the optimal approach and duration of therapy is not known at this time. And perhaps most importantly it will be necessary to determine if an improvement in coronary endothelial function can result in an attenuation of cardiac ischemic events or a slowing of the progression of atherosclerosis, which will have a lasting benefit for the patient.

Methods of assessing other aspects of nitric oxide's beneficial effects would also be desireable. To date, we cannot properly assess the important anti-platelet effects of nitric oxide in human studies. This is likely an important mechanism for the beneficial effects of preserved endothelial function, and ways to assess this are required.

Conclusion

The l-arginine-nitric oxide pathway plays an important role in mediating vasodilation of both coronary conduit and resistance vessels. Important abnormalities are present in this pathway in patients with cardiac risk factors and established atherosclerosis, and this endothelial dysfunction may play an important role in the ischemic sequelae which are common in these patients. Current research which focuses on the mechanisms responsible for the impairment in vasodilator responses will allow the development of rational treatment strategies, aimed at improving endothelial function and decreasing ischemia in patients with atherosclerosis.

REFERENCES

1. Moncada S, Higgs A. The L-arginine-nitric oxide pathway. N Eng J Med:329: 2002.
2. Furchgott RF, Zawadzki JV. The obligatory role of endothelial cells in the relaxation of arterial smooth muscle by acetylcholine. Nature. 1980:288:373.

3. Palmer RMJ, Ferrige AG, Moncada S. Nitric oxide accounts for the biological activity of endothelium-derived relaxing factor. Nature. 1987:327:524.

4. Palmer RMJ, Ashton D, Moncada S. Vascular endothelial cells synthesize nitric oxide from L-arginine. Nature. 1988:333:666.

5. Moncada S. The L-arginine-nitric oxide pathway. Acta Physiol Scand 1992:145:201.

6. Azuma H, Ishikawa M, Sekizaki S. Endothelium-dependent inhibition of platelet aggregation. Br J Pharmacol. 198:88:411.

7. Garg UC, Hassid A. Nitric oxide generating vasodilarors and 8 bromo-cylic guanosine monophosphate inhibit mitogensis and proliferation of cultured rat vascular smooth muscle cells. J Clin Invest 1989:83:1774.

8. Kubes P, Suzuki M, Granger DN. Nitric oxide: an endogenus modulator of leukocyte adhension. Proc Natl Acad Sci USA 1991:88:451.

9. Rubanyi GM. Cardiovascular Significance of Endothelium-Derived Vasoactive Factors. Mount Kisco, NY:Furura Publishing Co:1991.

10. Ignarro LJ. Biological actions and properties of endothelium-derived nitric oxide formed and released from artery and vein. Circ Res. 1989:5:1.

11. Meredith IT, et al. Role of impaired endothelium-dependent vasodilation in ischemic manifestations of coronary artery disease. Circulation 1993:87[suppl V]: v56.

12. Griffith TM, Edwards DH, et al. The nature of endothelium-derived vascular relaxant factor. Nature. 1984:308:45.

13. Martin W, Villani GM, Jothianandan D, Furchgott RF. Selective blockade of endothelium-dependent and glyceril trinitrate-induced relaxation by hemoglobin and by methylene blue in the rabbit aorta. J Pharmacol Exp Ther. 1985:232:708.

14. Rubanyi GM, Vanhoutte PM. Superoxide anions and hypoxia inactivate endothelium-derived relaxing factor. Am J Physiol. 1986:250:H822.

15. Rapoport RM, Murad F. Agonist-induced endothelium-dependent relaxation in rat theoratic aorta may be mediated through cGMP. Circ Res. 1983: 352-357.

16. Ignarro LJ, Byrns Buga GM, Wood KS. Endothelium-derived relaxing factor from pulmonary artery and vein possess pharmacologic and chemical properties identical to those of nitric oxide radical. Circ Res. 1987:1:879.

17. Furchgott RF, Khan MT, Jothiananadan D. Comparison of endothelium dependent relaxation and nitric oxide induced relaxation in rabbit aorta. Fed Proc. 1987:41:385.

18. Myers PR, et al. Comparative studies on nitrosothiols: similarities between EDRF and S-nitroso-1-cysteine (cysNO). FASEB J. 1989:3:533.

19. Flavahan NA. G-proteins and endothelial responses. Blood Vessels. 1990:27:218.

20. Katsuki S, et al. Stimulation of guanylate cyclase by sodium nitroprusside, nitroglycerin and nitric oxide in various tissue preparations and comparison to the effect of sodium azide and hydroxylamine. L Cyclic Nucleotide Protein Phosphor Res. 1977:3:23-35.

21. Craven PA, DeRubertis FR, Pratt DW. Electron spin resonance study of the role of nitric oxide-catalase in the activation of guanylate cyclase by NaN3 and Nh2OH: modulation of enzyme responses by heme protein and their nitrosyl derivatives. J Biol Chem. 1979:254:8213.

22. Lincoln TM, Corbin JD. Characterization and biological role of the cyclic guanosine monophosphate-dependent protein kinase. Adv Cyclic Nucleotide Res. 1983:15:139-192.

23. Ahlner J, et al. Glyceryltrinitrate inhibits phosphatidylinositol hydrolysis and protein kinase C activity in bovine mesetrenic artery. Life Sci. 1988:43:1241.

24. Luscher TF. Endothelial Vasoactive Substances and Cardiovascular Disease. Basel , Switzerland: Karger Publishers: 1988.

25. Rees DD, et al. A specific of nitric oxide formation from l-arginine attenuates endothelium-dependent relaxation. Br j Pharmacol 1989:9:418.

26. Pohl U, et al. Crurial role of endothelium in the vasodilator response to increased flow in vivo. Hypertension. 198:8:37.

27. Inoue T, et al. Endothelium determines flow-dependent dilation of the epicardial coronary in dogs. J Am Coll Cardiol. 1988:11:187.

28. Freiman PC, et al. Atherosclerosis impairs endothelium-dependent vascular relaxation to acetylcholine and thrombin in primates. Circ Res 1986:58:783.

29. Heistad DD, et al. Augmented responses to vasoconstrictor stumuli in hypercholesterolemic and artherosclerotic monkeys. Circ Res 1984:54:711.

30. Verbeuren TJ, et al. Effect of hypercholesterolemia on vascular reactivity in the rabbit. Circ Res 198:552.

31. Osborne JA, et al. Cardiovascular effects of acute hypercholesterolemia in rabbits. Reversal with lovastatin treatment. J Clin Invest 1989:83:45.

32. Tanner FC, et al. Oxidized low density lipoproteins inhibit relaxations of porcine coronary arteries - Role of scavenger receptor and endothelium-derived nitric oxide. Circulation 1991:83:2012.

33. Owen MP, Bevan JA. Acetylcholine induced endothelial dependent vasodilation increases as the artery diameter decreases in rabbit ear. Experientia. 1985:41:1057.

34. Kaley G, Wolin MS, Messina EJ. Endothelium-derived relaxing factors in the microcirculation. Blood Vessels. 198:23:81.

35. Myers PR, et al. Characteristics of canine coronary resistance arteries: importance of endothelium. Am J Physiol. 1989:257:H03.

36. Forstermann U, Dudel C, Frolich JC. Endothelium-derived relaxing factor is likely to modulate the tone of resistance arteries in the rabbit hindlimb in vivo. J Pharmacol Exp Ther. 1987:243:1055.

37. Sellke FW, Armstrong ML, Harrison DG. Endothelium-dependent vascular relaxation is abnormal in the coronary microcirculation of atheroschlerotic primates. Circulation. 1990:81:158.

38. Kuo L, Davis MJ, Chilian WM. Endothelium-dependent, flow-induced dilation of isolated coronary arterioles. Am J Physiol 1990:259:H103.

39. Ress DD, Palmer RMJ, Moncada S. Role of endothelium-derived nitric oxide in the regulation of blood pressure. Proc Natl Acad Sci USA. 1989:8:3375.

40. Whittle BJR, Lopez-Belmonte J, Rees DD. Modulation of the vasodepressor actions of acetylcholine, bradykinin, substance P and endothelin in the rat by a specific inhibitor of nitric oxide formation. Br J Pharmacol. 1989:98:4.

41. Aisaka K, et al. NG-Methylarginine, an inhibitor of endothelium-derived nitric oxide synthesis, is the potent pressor agent in the guinea pig: does nitric oxide regulate blood pressure in vivo? Biochem Biophys Res Commun. 1989:10:881.

42. Chu A, et al. Nitric oxide modulates epicardial coronary basal vasomotor tone in awake dogs. Am J Physiol 1990:258:H1250.

43. Forstermann U, et al. Selective attenuation of endothelium-mediated vasodilatation in atherosclerotic human coronary arteries. Circ Res. 1988:2:185.

44. Ludmer PL, et al. Paradoxical vasoconstriction induced by acetylcholine in atherosclerotic coronary arteries. N. Engl j Med. 1986:315:104.

45. Collins P, et al. Hemoglobin inhibits endothelium-derived relaxation to acetylcholine in human coronary arteries in vivo. Circulation. 1993:87:80-86.

46. Lefroy DC, et al. Effects on nitric oxide in the human coronary circulation. Circulation. 1993:88:I-43.

47. Nabel EG, Selwyn AP, Ganz P. Large coronary arteries in humanw are responsive to changing blood flow: an endothelium dependent mechanism that fails in patients with atherosclerosis. J Am Coll Cardiol 1990:349:35.

48. Gordon JB, et al. Atherosclerosis and endothelial function influence the coronary response to exercise. J Clin Invest. 1989:83:194.

49. Nabel EG, et al. Dilation of normal and constriction of atherosclerotic coronary arteries caused by the cold pressor test. Circulation. 1988:77:43.

50. Nabel EG, Selwyn AP, Ganz P. Paradoxical narrowing of atherosclerotic arteries induced by increases by heart rate. Circulation 1990:81:850.

51. Yeung AC, et al. The effect of atherosclerosis on the vasomotor response of coronary arteries to mental stress. N Engl J Med. 1991:325:1551.

52. Werns SW, et al. Evidence of endothelial dysfunction in angiographically normal coronary arteries of patients with coronary artery disease. Circulation 1989:79:287.

53. Vrints C, et al. Paradoxical vasoconstriction as the result of acetylcholine and serotonin in diseased human coronary arteries. Eur Heart J 1992:13:824.

54. Vita JA, et al. The coronary vasomotor response to acetylcholine relates to risk factors for coronary artery disease. Circulation 1990:81:491.

55. Seiler C, et al. Influence of serum cholesterol and other coronary risk factors on vasomotion of angiographically normal coronary arteries. Circulation 1993:88:2139.

56. Dyce MC, et al. The relationship between endothelial vasodilator function and LDL particle size, density and number in human coronary atherosclerosis. Circulation in press.

57. Zeiher AM, et al. Endothelial dysfunction of the coronary microvasculate is associated with impaired coronary blood flow regulation in patients with early atherosclerosis. Circulation 1991:84:1984.

58. Ryan TJ Jr, et al. Impaired endothelium-dependent dilation of the coronary microvasculature in patients with atherosclerosis. Circulation 1991:84:II-624.

59. Egashira K, et al Impaired coronary blood flow response to acetylcholine in patients with coronary risk factors and proximal atherosclerotic lesions. J Clin Invest 1993:91:29.

60. Zeiher AM, et al. Endothelium-mediated coronary blood flow modulation in humans: Effects of age, atherosclerosis, hypercholesterolemia, and hypertension. J Clin Invest 1993:92:52.

61. Treasure CB, et al. Hypertension and left venticular hypertrophy are associated with impaired endothelium-mediated relaxation in human coronary resistance vessels. Circulation 1993:87:8.

62. Brush JE, Jr., et al. Abnormal endothelial-dependent coronary vasomotion in hypertensive patients. J Am Coll Cardiol 1992:19:809.

63. Quyyumi AA, et al. Endothelial dysfunction in patients with chest pain and normal coronary arteries. Circulation 1992:8:184.

64. Brown GB, et al. The mechanisms of nitroglycerin actions: Stenosis vasodilatation as a major component of the drug response. Circulation 1981:4:1089.

65. Chierchia S, et al. Impairment of myocardial perfusion and funtion during painless myocardial ischemia. J Am Coll Cardiol 1983:16:1359.

66. Selwyn AP, et al. Patterns of disturbed myocardial perfusion in patients with coronary artery disease. Circulation 1981: 4:83.

67. Deanfield JE, et al. Silent myocardial ischemia due to mental stress. Lancet 1984: 2:1001.

68. Gage JE, et al. Vasoconstriciton of stenotic coronary arteries during dynamic exercises in patients with classic angina pectoris: reversibility by nitroglycerin. Circulation 198: 73:865.

69. Shimokawa H, Flavahan NA, Vanhoutte PM. Loss of endothelial pertussis toxin-sensitive G-protein function in atherosclerotic porcine coronary arteries. Circulation. 1991:83:652.

70. Flavahan NA. Atherosclerosis or lipoprotein-induced endothelial dysfunction: potential mechanisms underlying reduction in endothelium-derived relaxing factor/nitric oxide activity. Circulation 1992:85:1927.

71. Ohara Y, Peterson TE, Harrison DG. Hypercholesterolemia increases endothelial superoxide anion production. J Clin Invest 1993:92:254.

72. Cooke JP, et al. Arginine restores cholinergic relaxation of hypercholesterolemic rabbit aorta. Circulation. 1991:83:1057.

73. Drexler H, et al. Correction of endothelial dysfunction in coronary microcirculation of hypercholesterolaemic patients by L-arginine. Lancet. 1991:338:154.

74. Dubois-Rande J-L, et al. Effects of infusion of L-arginine into the left anterior descending coronary artery on acetylcholine-induced vasoconstriction of human atheromatous coronary arteries. Am J Cardiol. 1992:70:1269.

75. Flavahan NA, Mooney T. Lyseolecithin inhibits a G protein-dependent pathway in porcine endothelial cells. FACEB J. 1991:5:A1729.

76. Harrison DG, et al. Restoration of endothelium-dependent relaxation by dietary treatment of atherosclerosis. J Clin Invest 1987: 80:1808.

77. Williams JK, et al. Psychosocial Factors Impair Vascular Responses of Coronary Arteries. Circulation 1991: 84:214.

78. Vekshtein VI, et al. Fish oil improves endothelium-dependent relaxation in patients with coronary artery disease Circulation 1989:80:II-434A.

79. Leung W-H, Lau C-P, Wong C-K. Beneficial effect of cholesterol-lowering therapy on coronary endothelium-dependent relaxation in hypercholesterolaemic patients. Lancet 1993:341:1496.

80. Treasure CB, et al. Coronary endothelial responses are improved with aggressive lipid lowering therapy in patients with coronary atherosclerosis. Circulation 1993:88:I-38.

81. Anderson TJ, et al. Cholesterol lowering therapy improves endothelial function in patients with coronary atherosclerosis. Circulation 1993:88:I-368.

82. Brown BG, et al. Lipid lowering and plaque regression: New insights into prevention of plaque disruption and clinical events in coronary disease. Circulation 1993:87:1781.

83. Steinberg D. Antioxidants and atherosclerosis: A current assessment. Circulation 1991:84:1420.

84. Keaney JF Jr, et al. Dietary anti-oxidants preserve endothelium-dependent vessel relaxation in cholesterol-fed rabbits. Proc Natl Acad Sci USA 1993:90:11880.

85. Parthasarathy S, et al. Probucol inhibits oxidative modification of low density lipoprotein. J Clin Invest 1986:77:641.

86. Plane F, et al. Probucol and other anti-oxidants prevent the inhibition of endothelium-dependent relaxation by low density lipoproteins. Atherosclerosis 1993:103:73.

87. Meredith IT, et al. Superoxide dismutase restores endothelial vasodilator function in human coronary arteries in vivo. Circulation 1993:88:I-467.

88. Barrett-Connor E, Bush TL. Estrogen and coronary heart disease in women. JAMA 1991:25:181.

89. Jiang C, et al. Endothelium-independent relaxation of rabbit coronary artery by 17-B-oestradiol in vitro. Br J Pharmacol 1991:104:1033.

90. Williams JK, Adams MR, Klopfenstein HS. Estrogen modulates responses of atherosclerotic coronary arteries. Circulation 1990:81:1680.

91. Williams JK, et al. Short-term administration of estrogen and vascular responses of atherosclerotic coronary arteries. J Am Coll Cardiol 1992:20:452-7.

92. Reis SE, et al. Ethinyl estradiol acutely attenuates abnormal coronary vasomotor responses to acetylcholine in postmenopausal women. Circulation 1994:89:52.

93. Keaney JF, et al. 17b-Estradiol preserves endothelial vasodilator function and limits low-density lipoprotein oxidation in hypercholesterolemic swine. Circulation 1994:89:2251.

94. Collins P, et al. Cardiovascular protection by oestrogen-a calcium antagonistic effect? Lancet 1993:341:1264.

95. Celermajer DS, et al. Non-invasive detection of endothelial dysfunction in children and adults at risk of atherosclerosis. Lancet 1992:340:1111.

96. Anderson TJ, et al. Relationship of endothelial function in the coronary and brachial circulation. Circulation in press.

8 THROMBOLYTIC AND ANTITHROMBOTIC THERAPIES FOR ACUTE CORONARY SYNDROMES

Christopher P. Cannon, Joseph Loscalzo

The spectrum of myocardial ischemia

Over the past decade, many advances have been made in the understanding of acute coronary syndromes and in the development of thrombolytic and antithrombotic regimens used to improve clinical outcome. Based on their similar pathophysiology, clinical presentation, and treatment strategies, the acute coronary syndromes can be viewed as part of a spectrum of myocardial ischemia, which ranges from stable angina to acute Q wave myocardial infarction (MI). *(Figure 8.1)* These ischemic syndromes share the same underlying pathophysiology, i.e., the long-term asymptomatic development of atherosclerotic plaques followed by acute plaque activation leading to rupture with superimposed local thrombosis.[1-3] Based on the large number of ruptured and healed plaques with layers of thrombus found at autopsy, it is estimated that the vast majority of ruptured plaques are clinically silent, producing only a mild degrees of coronary stenosis.[4] In some patients, however, the amount of local thrombosis is more extensive and a flow limiting coronary stenosis results; this process leads to myocardial ischemia, with or without some degree of myocardial necrosis, clinically manifest as unstable angina or a non-Q wave MI. If plaque rupture and thrombosis are extensive, complete occlusion of the coronary artery can occur, producing clinically persistent ischemic pain and ST segment elevation, in patients without adequate collateral circulation, which usually evolves into a Q-wave MI.

The clinical course of all acute ischemic syndromes can be complicated by recurrent unstable angina, progression to myocardial infarction or recurrence of myocardial infarction, or death, which can occur in 5-15% of patients depending on the patient's baseline characteristics and the severity of the initial and recurrent event(s).[5-10] *(Figure 8.2)* Following an initial acute event, patients remain at risk for

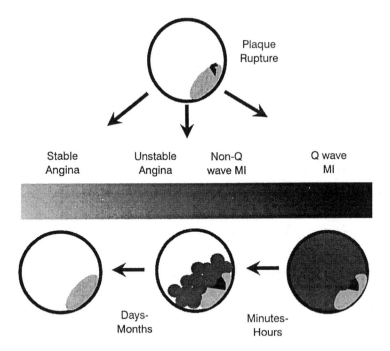

Figure 8.1 **The spectrum of myocardial ischemia.** *The various clinical syndromes of coronary artery disease can be viewed as a spectrum, ranging from patients with stable angina to those with acute Q wave MI. Across the spectrum of the acute coronary syndromes, atherosclerotic plaque rupture leads to coronary artery thrombosis: in acute Q wave MI, which usually presents with ST segment elevation on the electrocardiogram, complete coronary occlusion is present. In those with unstable angina or non-Q wave MI, a flow-limiting thrombus is usually present. In patients with stable angina, thrombus is rarely seen. The overall treatment objective is to move the patients back to a stable lesion. In acute ST elevation MI, the objective over the first minutes to hours is to open the artery and achieve reperfusion. In patients with unstable angina and non-Q wave MI, the goal is to stabilize or "passivate" the active thrombotic lesion over a period of hours to days. Then, over a period of months to years, the goal is to try to heal the lesion with risk factor reduction with treatment of hypercholesterolemia, hypertension, diabetes and smoking cessation, in an attempt to reduce the likelihood of subsequent rupture of the coronary plaques.*

recurrent events: In the TIMI studies, approximately 25% of patients developed recurrent unstable angina by one year following acute Q wave MI,[10] and a similar percentage developed recurrent unstable angina following admission for unstable angina or non-Q wave MI [7,8])

Thus, the treatment objectives for acute coronary syndromes share many similarities, but involve a temporal hierarchy.*(Figure 8.1)* For patients with acute ST segment elevation, indicative of acute coronary occlusion, the objective is to restore coronary perfusion as quickly as possible using thrombolytic therapy (or primary angioplasty). In conjunction with this treatment regimen, antithrombotic therapy (with aspirin, heparin or newer antithrombotic agents) is used to stabilize and "passivate" the acute coronary lesion, thereby preventing reocclusion, and allowing endogenous (or exogenously initiated) fibrinolysis to dissolve the thrombus and reduce the degree of coronary stenosis.[5,11] Antithrombotic therapy is continued long-term so that if future events occur, the agents can limit the degree of thrombosis and/or prevent the progression to a complete occlusion. In addition, after the acute event is stabilized, the many factors that led to the event need to be reversed, i.e., treatment of atherosclerotic risk factors such as hypercholesterolemia, hypertension and cessation of smoking, each of which contributes to healing of the endothelium, improvement in endothelial function and stabilization of the cholesterol-laden plaque.[12,13]

In reviewing the utility of thrombolytic-antithrombotic therapies for acute coronary syndromes, aspirin and heparin (and potentially newer antithrombotic agents)

Clinical Course of
Acute Coronary Syndromes

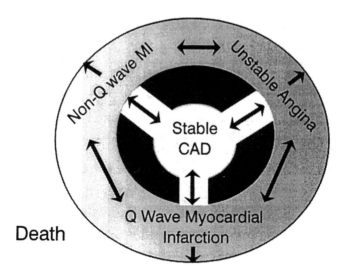

Figure 8.2 **The clinical course of acute coronary syndromes.** *Patients with any of the acute coronary syndromes have a significant risk of developing recurrent ischemic events. For example, a patient who presents with non-Q wave MI could progress to develop post-infarction unstable angina, or progress to develop a Q wave MI. A patient with a Q wave MI could develop a recurrent infarction, and all syndromes carry a significant risk of mortality. The goal of therapy is to treat the ischemia and thrombosis, and thereby return the patient to having stable coronary artery disease.*

have benefits in all patients with atherothrombotic coronary disease. Indeed, oral therapy with aspirin (and/or warfarin as a substitute for heparin) may provide outcome benefits in patients with stable angina[14] and in both primary[15,16] and secondary prevention.[17-20] *(Figure 8.3)* Thrombolytic therapy, however, appears to be beneficial only in patients with acute MI with ST segment elevation, (i.e., in achieving reperfusion of occluded arteries); no benefit was observed in patients with unstable angina or non-Q wave MI.[6] We will now review the data that support these conclusions.

Aspirin

The first and foremost antithrombotic agent in the treatment of acute coronary syndromes is aspirin. Numerous major studies within the past ten years have demonstrated clear beneficial effects of aspirin in these disorders.*(Figure 8.4)* In patients with unstable angina/non-Q wave MI, aspirin administration results in an approximately 50% reduction in the risk of death or MI.[21-25] Following acute MI, aspirin also has been show to reduce reocclusion of patent infarct related arteries,[26], as well as reinfarction,[27] and mortality, both independently and additively with thrombolytic therapy[27].*(Figure 8.4)*

These data, together with the benefits observed in primary prevention,[15,16,18]

Treatment Regimens for Acute Coronary Syndromes

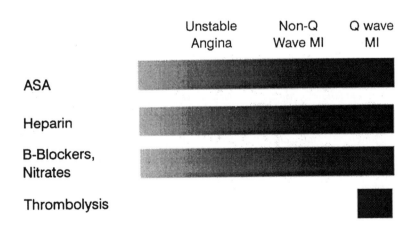

Figure 8.3 **Medical treatments across the spectrum of myocardial ischemia.**
Aspirin, heparin, beta-blockers and nitrates are all uniformly beneficial across the spectrum; thrombolytic therapy is only beneficial in patients presenting with acute MI with ST segment elevation (or new left bundle branch block).

secondary prevention,[17,18,20] and stable angina,[14] support the view that aspirin is now standard therapy for all patients with coronary artery disease. It is therefore important to administer aspirin (150-325 mg) as soon as possible in all patients with acute coronary syndromes, and to continue (or initiate) aspirin therapy (181-325 mg daily) in patients with known or suspected coronary disease. This abundance of supporting data also are consistent with a primary role of platelets in acute coronary syndromes, and suggest that more potent platelet inhibitors may provide additional benefits.

Heparin

Given the importance of fibrin in addition to platelets in forming a thrombus in acute coronary syndromes, the addition of effective anticoagulant therapy to antiplatelet therapy could be of potentially greater benefit than antiplatelet therapy alone. Heparin is a heterogeneous mixture of sulfated polysaccharide chains.[28-30] The majority of heparin's anticoagulant activity is derived from its interaction with antithrombin III.[31] Heparin binds to antithrombin III and induces a conformational change at the arginine center of the serpin, thereby leading to 1000-fold acceleration of the binding of antithrombin III to thrombin.[29,31] Heparin also acts as a catalytic template surface on which thrombin is brought in close proximity to antithrombin III.[28,32] As a result of these interactions, thrombin a reactive-center arginine in antithrombin III reacts with an active site serine in thrombin thereby irreversibly inhibiting the protease.[28] Heparin also catalyzes the antithrombin III-de-

Figure 8.4 Trials showing benefit of aspirin across the spectrum of myocardial →
ischemia. The risk of subsequent MI was reduced by aspirin compared with placebo in healthy subjects and thus was effective primary prevention.[15] Similarly, patients with stable angina had a reduced incidence of MI.[14] In unstable angina, the incidence of death or MI was reduced by over 50% in each of three trials.[22-24] In acute MI, aspirin reduced reocclusion of the infarct-related artery,[26] reinfarction and mortality.[27] Data from the following trials, respectively: Steering Committee of the Physicians' Health Study Research Group. Final report on the aspirin component of the ongoing Physicians' Health Study. N Engl J Med 1989;321:129; Ridker et al. Low-dose aspirin therapy for chronic stable angina. A randomized, placebo-controlled clinical trial. Ann Intern Med 1991;114:835; Cairns JA, et al. Aspirin, sulfinpyrazone, or both in unstable angina. N Engl J Med 1985;313:1369; Theroux P, et al. Aspirin, heparin or both to treat unstable angina. N Engl J Med 1988;319:1105; The RISC Group. Risk of myocardial infarction and death during treatment with low dose aspirin and intravenous heparin in men with unstable coronary artery disease. Lancet 1990;336:827-30; Roux S, Christeller S, Ludin E. Effects of aspirin on coronary reocclusion and recurrent ischemia after thrombolysis: a meta-analysis. J Am Coll Cardiol 1992;19:671-7.; ISIS-2 Collaborative Group. Randomised trial of intravenous streptokinase, oral aspirin, both, or neither among 17,187 cases of suspected acute myocardial infarction: ISIS-2. Lancet 1988;2:349-60.

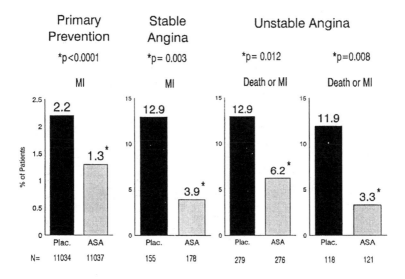

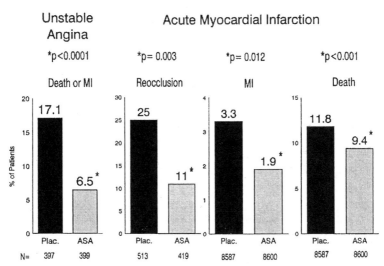

pendent inhibition of factors IXa, Xa, XIa and XIIa, although the next most susceptible to inhibition, factor Xa, is an order of magnitude less sensitive to inhibition
than is thrombin.[29,31,32]

The anticoagulant effects of heparin are known to be variable,[32,33] owing to the
chemical variability of the individual heparin molecules themselves and to the neu-

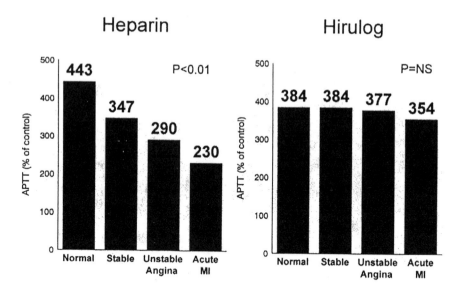

*Figure 8.5 **Heparin resistance**. Among patients with acute coronary syndromes, the APTT prolongation for a fixed dose of heparin is blunted relative to normal or stable patients. In contrast, direct thrombin inhibitors, such as hirulog, have a more stable and predictable level of anticoagulation. (Data from Maraganore, et al.: Heparin variability and resistance: Comparisons with a direct thrombin inhibitor.(abstract) Circulation 1992;86 (Suppl. I):I-386.)*

tralization of heparin by circulating plasma factors and by proteins released by activated platelets, such as platelet factor 4.[32,34-36] This variability in the biochemical activity of commercial heparin underlies the so-called "heparin resistance" syndrome, illustrated by the data in *Figure 8.5*. In blood samples obtained from patients with a variety of coronary syndromes, fixed amounts of heparin or the direct thrombin inhibitor, hirulog, were added to plasma that would prolong the activated partial thromboplastin time (aPTT) to 400% of baseline in normal plasma. In patients with the acute coronary syndromes, the aPTT response with heparin was markedly attenuated, reaching only 290% of control in unstable angina patients and 230% of control in acute myocardial infarction patients (p<0.001 compared with normals and stable angina patients).[37] Of note, the direct thrombin inhibitor provided a stable anticoagulant response in all patients.

Given the problems of variation in bioactivity of different heparin preparations and the attenuation of the anticoagulant response to heparin in acute coronary syndromes, the best strategy at present is to administer a standard initial dose of heparin and utilize very frequent monitoring of the anticoagulant response, usually by the aPTT. We recommend that an aPTT be checked at 6, 12, and 24 hours, and daily thereafter, with titrations made according to a standardized nomogram,

Table 8.1 *NOMOGRAM FOR TITRATION OF INTRAVENOUS HEPARIN*

aPTT (sec)	Repeat Bolus Dose	Stop Infusion (Minutes)	Rate Change (cc/hr)*	Rate Change (U/HR)
< 55	5000 IU	0	+4	+200
55-80	0	0	0	0
81-95	0	0	-2	-100
96-120	0	30	-2	-100
> 120	0	60	-4	-200

* assuming a concentration of 50 units/cc of heparin

APTT should be checked at 6, 12, 24 hours post initiation of heparin, daily thereafter, and 4-6 hours after any adjustment in dose.

such as that provided in *Table 8.1*. The use of a standardized nomogram minimizes the variability in the dosing adjustments given by various physicians, and has been shown to improve the achievement of a target APTT.[32,38,39]

Unstable angina

In the treatment of unstable angina, two initial small studies suggested a reduction in cardiac events by heparin.[40,41] The larger Montreal Heart Institute trial showed that heparin reduced refractory angina and myocardial infarction compared to placebo.[23,25] A follow-up report extending enrollment in that trial found a reduction in the risk of subsequent myocardial infarction by heparin compared to aspirin alone.[42] The RISC trial failed to demonstrate a significant benefit of heparin compared with aspirin alone, but noted that during heparin therapy (i.e., over the first 5 days) patients receiving both aspirin and heparin had the lowest rate of death or MI.[24]

More recently, the Antithrombotic Therapy for Acute Coronary Syndromes (ATACS) Study Group evaluated the role of combination antithrombotic therapy compared to aspirin alone in patients with acute ischemic syndromes who were not prior aspirin users.[43] They observed a trend toward fewer ischemic events (death, MI, recurrent ischemia with electrocardiographic changes) at 12 weeks in patients receiving aspirin and heparin (and subsequently warfarin), 20 (19%) of 105 patients, compared with 31 (28%) of 109 patients receiving aspirin alone (p=0.09).[43] A meta-analysis of the Montreal Heart Institute,[23] RISC,[24] and the ATACS[43] trials found that during the five days of active treatment with aspirin and heparin, the risk of death or MI was lower than for aspirin alone, (odds ratio 0.44, 95% C.I. [0.21-0.93]).[43] These data support the notion that combination of heparin plus aspirin is beneficial in unstable angina/non-Q wave MI. Thus, although not definitively proven, intravenous heparin in addition to aspirin is recommended in accord with the Unstable Angina Guideline.[5]

Heparin and Patency Following t-PA Therapy

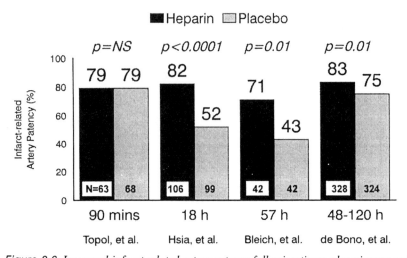

Figure 8.6 *Improved infarct related artery patency following tissue plasminogen activator with heparin compared with placebo (Data from Topol EJ, et al.: A randomized controlled trial of intravenous tissue plasminogen activator and early intravenous heparin in acute myocardial infarction. Circulation 1989;79:281.; Hsia J, et al. A comparison between heparin and low-dose aspirin as adjunctive therapy with tissue plasminogen activator for acute myocardial infarction. N Engl J Med 1990;323:1433; Bleich SD, et al: Effect of heparin on coronary patency after thrombolysis with tissue plasminogen activator in acute myocardial infarction. Am J Cardiol 1990;66:1412; and de Bono DP, et al.: Effect of early intravenous heparin on coronary patency, infarct size, and bleeding complications after alteplase thrombolysis: results of a randomized double blind European Cooperative Study Group trial. Br Heart J 1992;67:122)*

Acute myocardial infarction

In acute MI with ST segment elevation, heparin has not been used extensively as the sole agent, but rather as an adjunct to thrombolytic therapy where it plays an important role in some thrombolytic regimens. In conjunction with tissue plasminogen activator (t-PA), intravenous heparin improves late infarct-related artery patency, as shown in *Figure 8.6* which summarizes the results of four trials.[44-47] At 90 minutes, no difference was observed in patency;[44] however, between 18 hours and 5 days there was higher patency in patients randomized to receive intravenous heparin compared with placebo.[45-47] Of note, the difference in late patency was more pronounced in the two trials that used either no aspirin[46] or a small initial dose (80 mg)[45] in the control arm; however, even when adequate doses of aspirin were administered, as in the European Cooperative Study Group (ECSG)-6 trial, patency was significantly better in patients treated with heparin compared with placebo.[47] Since 90 minute patency was similar, the benefit of heparin is felt to be due largely to decreased reocclusion. Of note, two trials have examined the issue of the required duration of intravenous heparin, and found that infarct-related artery patency at 5-10 days was similar following either a 24-hour or 3-5-day infusion.[48,49] The GISSI-2 and ISIS-3 trials examined the role of subcutaneous heparin, and found no difference in mortality, with an increase in bleeding.[50,51] Thus, subcutaneous heparin does not appear to be beneficial,[52] likely because the heparin is absorbed slowly making the level of anticoagulation inadequate over the first 24 hours,[53-55] a critical time during the early phase of which fibrinolysis leads to thrombin generation and reocclusion.[56-58]

With streptokinase, the role of intravenous heparin is less clear.[52] In the GUSTO-I trial no difference between intravenous heparin or subcutaneous heparin was observed in mortality[59] or infarct-related artery patency[60] in patients receiving streptokinase and aspirin. Interestingly, no increase in bleeding or intracranial hemorrhage was noted with the use of intravenous heparin, compared with subcutaneous heparin, and streptokinase.[59] A potential reason for the difference in the need for heparin between t-PA and streptokinase probably relates to the half-life of the agents: 5-10 minutes for t-PA and 30 minutes for streptokinase.[61,62] In addition, streptokinase generates a greater systemic lytic state with more fibrin degradation products, which, themselves have anticoagulant and antiplatelet properties. Thus, based on the available data, the use of intravenous heparin is optional as initial adjunctive therapy with streptokinase, but is indicated for treatment of recurrent ischemic events.

Heparin dosing

The standard dosing regimen of heparin is a 5000-U bolus followed by a 1000-U /hr infusion, which is then titrated according to the aPTT.[32,63] In the setting of thrombolysis for acute MI, this regimen has been extensively used and appears to be safe.[63] The use of weight-adjusted heparin has suggested as a means of improving safety and been tested in patients with deep venous thrombosis.[64] In one study, weight adjusted heparin, administered as a 80-U/kg bolus and a 18-U/kg/hr infusion, was more successful in achieving an aPTT in the therapeutic range in the early phase of treatment, and in maintaining the aPTT in the target range.[64] Weight adjusted heparin in this dosing scheme was used in two small thrombolytic trials [65,66], one showing promising results [65] and the other not.[66] Furthermore, using a two-step weight-adjustment in heparin dosing, the larger TIMI 9A and GUSTO IIa trials found a higher than expected rate of hemorrhage with heparin.[67,68] Compared with the broad experience with the more standard dosing (5000-U bolus and 1000-U/hr infusion), there has been some reluctance to adopt the weight-adjusted heparin regimen for all patients with acute coronary syndromes, especially those treated with thrombolytic therapy. However, it should be noted that, based largely on the experience in patients with deep venous thrombosis, a weight-adjusted dosing regimen was recommended for patients with unstable angina/non-Q wave MI in the Unstable Angina Guidelines.[5]

Therapeutic range. In addition to the optimal dose of heparin, the exact level of anticoagulation that constitutes the "therapeutic range" is still under evaluation. At present, although the most widely used test to monitor heparin is the activated partial thromboplastin time (aPTT), there are actually only sparse data correlating aPTT and outcome in patients with acute coronary syndromes. With regard to efficacy, analyses from two studies of heparin vs. placebo following t-PA for acute MI[69,70] found that infarct-related artery patency was greatest in patients who had an aPTT >60 seconds[69] or > 2 times control[70]. More recently, a preliminary analysis from GUSTO-I suggested that an aPTT of 50-70 seconds was associated with the lowest mortality.[71] Based on these studies, a lower level of approximately 2 times control or 55-60 seconds appears to be a lower boundary for the therapeutic range. For the upper boundary, an APTT of >90 seconds appears to be associated with an increased risk of hemorrhage, with the majority of data derived from thrombolytic trials. In TIMI 5 in which patients received t-PA, aspirin and heparin, an aPTT of >90 seconds led to a doubling of the risk of hemorrhage.[72] Similar results were observed in the TIMI 4 trial.[73] In the larger TIMI 2 trial, in a time-dependent analysis, patients with an aPTT >90 seconds had an odds ratio for major hemorrhage of 1.7 (p<0.01).[74] Thus, in TIMI 9 and 10 of acute MI, heparin was titrated to maintain an aPTT between 55-80 sec,[67,75] and in ongoing trials between 50-70 sec.

In unstable angina, similar data are not yet available regarding heparin dosing, although a preliminary analysis from TIMI III suggests that the lower range for aPTT may lower than seen in thrombolytic trials.[76] In TIMI IIIB, all patients were treated with aspirin and intravenous heparin titrated to an aPTT 1.5 to 2 times control. When comparing patients who experienced a recurrent ischemic event (death, MI, or recurrent rest pain with ECG changes), there was no difference in the median aPTT.[76] Furthermore, when patients who had all aPTT values _60 seconds were compared with those with one or more aPTT values <60 seconds, there was no difference in the rate of recurrent ischemic events.[76] Thus, these observations suggest that in unstable angina/non Q wave MI, once heparin is administered intravenously with a target of 1.5 - 2 times control, there is no apparent advantage of higher levels of anticoagulation. Thus, for patients with unstable angina, the target range for the aPTT can be approximately 10 seconds lower than for acute MI treated with thrombolytic therapy. In the Unstable Angina Guideline, the target range is an aPTT between 46 and 70 seconds.[5]

Thrombolysis

Thrombolytic therapy is now firmly established as primary therapy for acute MI with ST segment elevation. The pathophysiology of acute MI is well defined: atherothrombotic acute coronary occlusion leads to myocardial necrosis, left ventricular dysfunction, and in some cases death.[77] Thrombolytic therapy is meant to *interrupt* the thrombotic cascade of events and thereby reestablish perfusion. Coronary reperfusion leads to a limitation in infarct size and decreases the extent of left ventricular dysfunction.[77] Most importantly, survival is improved, an effect which correlates strongly with the successful achievement of early reperfusion.[78-81] Over recent years, the more aggressive thrombolytic-antithrombotic regimen of front-loaded t-PA with intravenous heparin and aspirin, has been shown to improve survival further compared with standard thrombolytic regimens, as described below.[59,73]

Open artery hypothesis

Angiographic trials noted that benefit of thrombolytic therapy was related to successful achievement of coronary reperfusion, which became the basis for the so-called "open artery hypothesis".[77,80,81] In the TIMI 1 trial, patients with a patent infarct related artery 90 minutes after the start of thrombolytic therapy, had a lower 1 year mortality compared with those with an occluded artery(8.1% vs. 14.8%).[82] Furthermore, for patients with both early *and sustained* patency through hospital discharge, the subsequent mortality was extremely low, 3.8% at 1 year.[82]

In order to evaluate more carefully the reperfusion achieved by thrombolytic therapy, a grading system of coronary perfusion was developed in the TIMI 1 trial.[83] TIMI grade 0 flow indicates complete occlusion of the coronary artery, while TIMI grade 1 flow denotes some penetration of the obstruction by contrast material, but no perfusion of the distal coronary bed. TIMI grade 2 flow denotes perfusion of the entire coronary artery, but with delayed flow compared to a normal artery, and TIMI grade 3 flow denotes full perfusion with normal flow. TIMI flow grade at 90 minutes following the start of thrombolytic therapy has been shown to correlate well with subsequent mortality: in the TIMI patients with TIMI grade 3 flow had the lowest mortality, 4.7%, compared to 7.0% for patients with TIMI grade 2 flow and 10.6%for patients with occluded arteries (TIMI grade 0 or 1 flow).[84] Rapid reperfusion of the infarct-related artery, especially with TIMI grade 3 flow, has been shown to be associated with smaller infarct size,[85,86], improved left ventricular function,[87,88] a lower rate of reocclusion [89-91] and most importantly, improved survival.[60,73,81,82,84,89,91-95] Thus, these findings have helped establish the achievement of rapid and complete coronary reperfusion (i.e. TIMI grade 3 flow) as the major goal of current and new thrombolytic regimens.

Acute myocardial infarction with ST elevation

At present four thrombolytic agents are approved in the United States for use in acute MI, streptokinase, anistreplase (APSAC [anisoylated plasminogen-streptokinase activator complex]), tissue-type plasminogen activator (t-PA), and r-PA. The first three have been shown to reduce mortality compared with placebo[27,96-98] and the latter has been shown to be equivalent to other thrombolytics.[158-162] Urokinase and single chain urokinase (saruplase) are also available outside the United States. Thrombolytic therapy is clearly indicated in patients with ischemic pain with new or presumably new ST segment elevation or new left bundle branch block, in a time window that extends to 12 hours.[99] Importantly, age is no longer a contraindication to the use of thrombolysis. Several contraindications to thrombolytic therapy remain, however, including active bleeding, a history of recent stroke, or persistently elevated blood pressure at the time of presentation. Of note, patients with remote prior stroke or transient ischemic attack are at increased risk of intracranial hemorrhage.[100] However, many physicians feel that it is beneficial to treat patients with a remote history of stroke. A second risk factor for intracranial hemorrhage is acute hypertension with a blood pressure >180/110.[100-102] One possible guideline for the treatment of patients at increased risk for intracranial hemorrhage is to use a less aggressive thrombolytic regimen, such as streptokinase and aspirin without heparin.

After intravenous thrombolytic therapy was shown to be effective in achieving early coronary reperfusion and improving mortality, comparative trials of the different agents were performed. The GISSI-2/International [50,103] and ISIS-3 trials [51] showed no difference in mortality among t-PA, streptokinase, and anistreplase (anisoylated plasminogen streptokinase activator complex [APSAC]) when these agents were given without intravenous heparin. Thus, any of the three regimens, streptokinase 1.5 MU over 60 minutes, anistreplase 30 U over 2-5 minutes, or t-PA 100 mg over 3 hours, can be considered a "standard" thrombolytic regimen.

Front-loaded t-PA

Given the importance of achieving early reperfusion, (the basis of the so-called "open artery hypothesis"[80]) it was postulated that more aggressive regimens that achieve greater patency would be of additional clinical benefit for patients. After the TIMI 1 trial demonstrated that t-PA provided a higher reperfusion rate than streptokinase,[83] interest grew in developing a "front-loaded" dosing regimen of t-PA, which as currently identified consists of the administration of 100 mg over 90 minutes, using a 15 mg bolus, followed by 50 mg over 30 minutes and 35 mg over 60 minutes (with weight-adjustment for patients <65kg).[59,73,104-106] The GUSTO-I[59] and TIMI 4 trials[73] compared front-loaded t-PA with other standard regimens and demonstrated significantly improved early patency, survival, and overall clinical outcome, thereby establishing this more aggressive regimen as the new "gold standard" in thrombolysis.

The GUSTO-I Trial

The GUSTO-I trial set out to evaluate four regimens of thrombolytic therapy. The reference arms were two regimens of streptokinase, one using subcutaneous heparin (12,500 units subcutaneously every 12 hours beginning at 4 hours) and the other using intravenous heparin. The third arm studied was front-loaded t-PA and intravenous heparin and the fourth used combination thrombolytic therapy, which had shown promise in reducing reocclusion of the infarct-related artery,[107] and consisted of approximately 2/3 the doses of t-PA and of streptokinase with intravenous heparin. All patients received aspirin, 325 mg. daily.

A total of 41,021 patients were enrolled in the GUSTO-I trial, with its primary endpoint being 30-day mortality. Mortality was significantly lower in the front-loaded t-PA arm as compared with each of the three other arms.*(Table 8.2)*[59] Counting the number of lives saved as a clear end point, treatment with front-loaded t-PA, intravenous heparin and aspirin was shown to save an additional 10 lives per 1000 treated, representing a 40% improvement over standard thrombolytic regimens. The improvement in mortality was noted after only 24 hours, with t-PA-treated patients having a significantly lower mortality rate than patients in the other arms of the trial.[108] In addition, other major complications were decreased by t-PA use, including cardiogenic shock, congestive heart failure, and ventricular arrhythmias.*(Table 8.2)*[59]

Intracranial hemorrhage is the most dreaded complication of thrombolytic therapy, although it is fortunately relatively rare. For each of the streptokinase arms in GUSTO-I, 0.5% of patients suffered an intracranial hemorrhage as compared with 0.7% of patients treated with front-loaded t-PA and 0.9% of patients treated with combination thrombolytic therapy.[59] In order to balance the improved efficacy with these adverse effects, the so-called "net clinical benefit" parameter was evaluated, i.e., the occurrence of either death or a disabling stroke. When comparing the net clinical benefit among the four regimens, front-loaded t-PA remained superior to the other three regimens.*(Table 8.2)*[59]

The benefit of t-PA was seen in nearly every subgroup analyzed, including patients with anterior and inferior MIs, in men and in women, and in the young as well as the elderly. Interestingly, in evaluating the effect of time to treatment (with the final "cleaned" data base[109]), t-PA maintained its benefit over streptokinase throughout the first 6 hours.[109]

To understand fully the benefits of the various thrombolytic regimens, an angiographic substudy was carried out in the GUSTO-I trial.[60] Over 2,400 patients were randomized to undergo cardiac catheterization at either 90 minutes, 180 minutes, 24 hours, or 5-7 days. At the important 90-minute time point, the front-loaded t-PA-treated patients had a significantly higher patency rate and a much higher rate of infarct-related artery patency, as well as TIMI grade 3 flow.*(Table 8.2)*[60] At the other three time points there were no significant differences among the four thrombolytic regimens. As such, the principal benefit of front-loaded t-PA was that of achieving an *early* open infarct-related artery.

The TIMI 4 trial

The TIMI 4 trial examined the same front-loaded t-PA regimen[104] and the results were very consistent with those of the GUSTO-I trial. The TIMI 4 trial was a double-blind trial comparing front-loaded t-PA with APSAC and combination thrombolytic therapy (t-PA and APSAC).[73] All patients received aspirin and IV heparin and underwent cardiac catheterization at 90 minutes and 18-36 hours, with clinical follow-up in hospital and at 6 weeks and 1 year. Front-loaded t-PA was found to have a 78% patency rate after only 60 minutes compared to only 59% for APSAC and combination thrombolytic therapy.[73]*(Figure 8.8)* At 90 minutes, patency and

Table 8.2   RESULTS FROM THE GUSTO-I TRIAL.

Outcome	SK and SQ Heparin	SK and IV Heparin	Front-loaded t-PA and IV heparin	t-PA and SK heparin	P value * both SK regimens
n	9796	10,377	10,344	10,328	
30 day mortality (%)	7.2	7.4	6.3*	7.0	*0.005
Net clinical benefit (death or disabling stroke) (%)	7.7	7.9	6.9*	7.6	*0.006
24 hour mortality (%)	2.8	2.9	2.3*	2.8	*0.005
Intracranial hemorrhage	0.5	0.5	0.7*	0.9	*0.03
Congestive heart failure	17.5	16.8	15.2*	16.8	* <0.001
Cardiogenic shock	6.9	6.3	5.1*	6.1	* <0.001
		Angiographic Substudy			
n	293	283	292	299	
Infarct-related artery patency (TIMI grade 2 or 3 flow) at 90 mins (%)	54	60	81*	73	* <0.001
TIMI grade 3 flow) at 90 mins (%)	29	32	54*	38	* <0.001

TIMI grade 3 flow were both significantly better in the front-loaded t-PA arm compared with the other two. Overall clinical outcome using a composite end point,[110] was 41.3% for t-PA compared with 49.0% for APSAC and 53.6% for the combination (p=0.19, t-PA vs. APSAC; p=0.06, t-PA vs. combination). Mortality at one year was lowest in the t-PA-treated patients, 5.3%, compared to 11.0% for APSAC

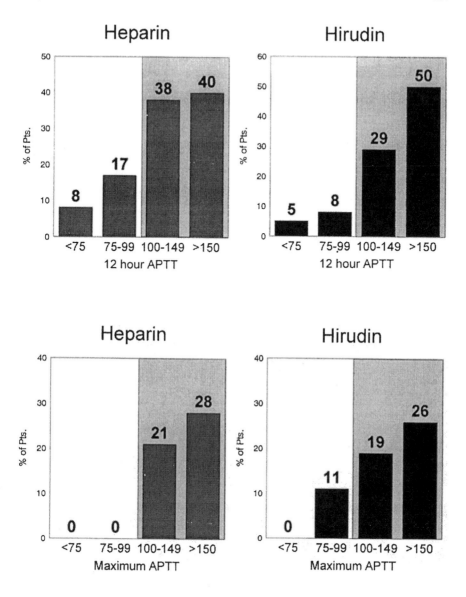

Figure 8.7 Relationship of activated thromboplastin time (aPTT) to major hemorrhage following thrombolytic therapy in the TIMI 5 trial. Major hemorrhage was more common when the 12 hour (Panel A) or the maximum aPTT during the five-day infusion was >100 seconds.(Data from Cannon, et al.: Usefulness of aPTT to predict bleeding for hirudin (and heparin).(abstract) Circulation 1994;90[Pt. 2]:I-563.)

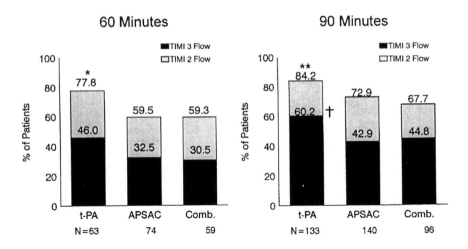

Figure 8.8 Angiographic findings from the TIMI 4 trial.(Reproduced with permission from Cannon, et al.: Comparison of front-loaded recombinant tissue-type plasminogen activator, anistreplase and combination thrombolytic therapy for acute myocardial infarction: results of the Thrombolysis in Myocardial Infarction (TIMI) 4 trial. J Am Coll Cardiol 1994;24:1602-10.)

and 10.5% for combination thrombolytic therapy (p=0.07, t-PA vs. APSAC; p=0.13, t-PA vs. combination).[73]

Thus, GUSTO-I and TIMI 4 demonstrated that front-loaded t-PA achieved significantly higher rates of reperfusion at 60 and 90 min, and was associated with improved overall clinical benefit and survival compared to a standard thrombolytic regimen, or to regimens involving combinations of thrombolytic agents. While further research into other combinations of thrombolytic agents continues,[111] the two regimens tested in GUSTO-I and TIMI 4 appeared to fail in improving outcome because they did not improve early infarct-related artery patency. In addition, these trials add further support to the early open artery hypothesis, and suggest that further improvements in outcome of patients with acute myocardial infarction might be achieved with more effective thrombolytic-antithrombotic regimens.[95]

Time as an adjunctive agent in thrombolysis

Given the importance of rapid reperfusion achieved with different thrombolytic agents, it should be recalled that another way to accelerate reperfusion is to reduce the time to administration of thrombolytic therapy. As such, time can be considered an adjunctive agent to thrombolysis.[112] The quicker the thrombolytic agent is administered, the faster the infarct-related artery will be opened. In the TIMI II trial, time to treatment was an important factor in relation to mortality following acute

MI: For each hour that a patient was treated earlier, there was a decrease in the absolute mortality by 1%.[113] A similar relationship was observed in the GUSTO-1 trial.[109] In addition, the benefit of front-loaded t-PA over streptokinase was additive to that of decreasing the time to treatment.[109,112] As such, time becomes a very important adjunctive agent to thrombolytic therapy, and efforts to speed up the administration of thrombolysis will, thus, improve the efficacy of the overall thrombolytic regimen.[112,114]

Unstable angina

Because thrombolytic therapy is beneficial in the treatment of patients with acute MI presenting with ST elevation, it was hoped that it might play a role in the other acute ischemic syndromes. The TIMI III trials examined the effects of t-PA (0.8 mg/kg over 90 minutes, with 1/3 as a bolus) in patients treated with aspirin and heparin. In TIMI IIIA, 391 patients with acute ischemic chest pain and documented coronary artery disease underwent a baseline coronary arteriogram.[115] Of these, thrombus was clearly visualized in only 35% of patients, a number much lower than previously reported, although an additional 40% of patients had mural opacities or eccentric lesions classified as possible thrombus.[115] Measurable improvement in lesion severity was observed in a similar proportion of patients, 25% following t-PA vs. 19% following heparin alone (p=0.25), suggesting that the overall impact of thrombolysis in patients with acute ischemic syndromes would be minimal.[115]

In TIMI IIIB, 1473 patients with unstable angina and non-Q wave MI were randomized to receive either t-PA or placebo.[6] There was no difference between t-PA and placebo in the primary composite end point: the incidence of death, post-randomization infarction, or recurrent, objectively documented ischemia through six weeks of follow-up (54.2% for t-PA and 55.5% for placebo, p=NS).[6] The incidence of death or MI through 42 days of follow-up was actually higher in patients treated with t-PA compared with placebo (8.8% vs. 6.2%, p=0.05).[6] In addition, t-PA was associated with a 0.55% incidence of intracranial hemorrhage.[6] Thus, in the presence of antiplatelet, anticoagulant, and anti-ischemic therapy, the addition of t-PA does not improve clinical outcome, and is not indicated in unstable angina or non-Q wave MI.

New antithrombotic agents

Platelet IIb/IIIa receptor antagonists

Given the important role of platelets in arterial thrombosis and the dramatic benefits of aspirin in patients with coronary atherthrombotic syndromes, it has been hypothesized that more aggressive antiplatelet regimens will further improve the outcome of patients with acute coronary syndromes. Although thromboxane receptor antagonists have been recently tested,[116] most attention has been focussed on platelet fibrinogen receptor antagonists, the glycoprotein IIb/IIIa inhibitors. These

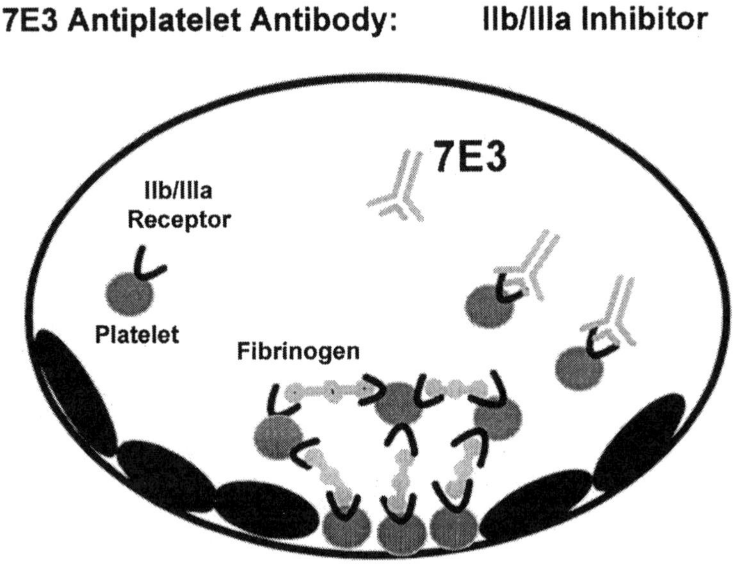

7E3 Antiplatelet Antibody: IIb/IIIa Inhibitor

Figure 8.9 Diagram depicting the action of 7E3, a monoclonal antibody to the platelet glycoprotein IIb/IIIa receptor. Primary hemostasis is achieved by platelets adhering to a damaged vessel wall. Platelets aggregate with fibrinogen binding to the platelet IIb/IIIa receptor. The monoclonal antibody 7E3 (or other peptide inhibitors) bind to the IIb/IIIa receptor and thereby prevent platelets from aggregating and forming a thrombus.

agents block the final common pathway of platelet aggregation, thereby preventing the platelet from participating in thrombus formation/extension.*(Figure 8.9)* The monoclonal antibody to the IIb/IIIa receptor, so-called 7E3 or abciximab,[117-120] is the first agent to be approved for clinical use, but several other tripeptide ihibitors of the IIb/IIIa receptor have been recently developed, including eptifibatide,[121,122] tirofiban,[123] and others.[124]

In a pilot trial of patients receiving t-PA, heparin and aspirin (The Thrombolysis and Angioplasty in Myocardial Infarction [TAMI]-8 trial), 7E3 was administered between 6-24 hours after the start of thrombolytic therapy.[118] Patency of the infarct-related artery at 5 days was higher in patients treated with 7E3 than controls treated with heparin and aspirin.[118] Recurrent ischemic events tended to be lower in patients treated with 7E3. In a larger trial of 7E3 during high risk angioplasty, similar reductions in ischemic events were observed,[119] including among patients with acute MI undergoing primary or rescue PTCA.[125] A recent pilot trial of integrelin as an adjunct to thrombolysis has also been reported, with preliminary findings showing that at higher doses, infarct-related artery patency appeared improved compared to that observed with aspirin and heparin as adjunctive therapy to t-PA.[126]

GP IIb/IIIa Inhibition in Ustable Angina and Non-Q Wave MI

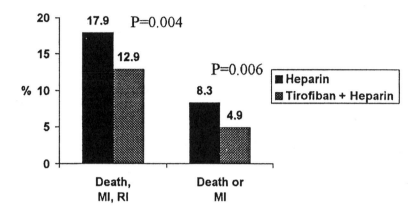

Figure 8.10 Primary results from the PRISM-=PLUS trial at 7 days. Data from: The PRISM-PLUS Investigators. Inhibition of platelet glycoprotein IIb/IIIa with tirofiban in unstable angina and non Q wave myocardial infarction. N Engl J Med (in press);. (MI=myocardial infarction, RI=Recurrent refractory ischemia)

In unstable angina, the IIb//IIIa inhibitors appear to reduce recurrent ischemic events in pilot trials[120,124], and recent Phase III trials. [127-129] In one trial, the combination of heparin and Ib/IIIa antagonist significantly reduced the rate of death, MI or recurrent refractory angina[127] *(Figure 8.10)*. Thus, more potent antiplatelet therapy with the inhibition of the IIb/IIIa receptor function appears to have beneficial effects in reducing recurrent ischemic events among patient within the spectrum of acute coronary syndromes.

However, these improvements in improving efficacy have to be balanced with bleeding risks. In the EPIC trial, the regimen that improved outcome also was associated with a doubling in the rate of major hemorrhage.[119] Additional studies are planned with 7E3 to refine the adjunctive heparin dose in an attempt to reduce the bleeding risk. In addition, further phase III trials are now in progress with the other IIb/IIIa antagonists to determine if the benefits suggested by the pilot trials prove to persist in larger patient populations.

Direct thrombin inhibitors

Following "primary hemostasis" affected by platelets, the second integral component of arterial thrombosis is the coagulation cascade of which thrombin is the final common pathway for generation of the fibrin thrombosis.[54] Given the central role of thrombin in acute thrombosis, the development of more potent and direct thrombin inhibitors like hirudin has led to the so-called "thrombin hypothesis": that more effective inhibition of both soluble and clot-bound thrombin will translate into better clinical outcome for patients with acute coronary syndromes. The prototypical agent in this regard is hirudin, a polypeptide first isolated from the medicinal leech.[130] In contrast to heparin, which acts as a catalyst for antithrombin III (see above), hirudin and the related compound hirulog[131] both bind directly to thrombin in a 1:1 relationship at two sites: 1) the substrate recognition site, the domain of thrombin that recognizes fibrinogen [132] or the platelet [133] and 2) the catalytic site of thrombin.[131,132,134] (Figure 8.11) Hirudin and hirulog have been shown to inhibit all the major thrombotic actions of thrombin, including thrombin-induced generation of fibrin, thrombin-induced platelet activation, as well as thrombin's autocatalytic reaction.[134-138] Potential advantages of these direct thrombin inhibitors over heparin are that they can inhibit clot-bound thrombin,[134,139] they are not inhibited by activated platelets,[134,140] and they do not require a co-factor and, thus, may provide a more stable anticoagulant response.[134,138]

Hirudin

Hirudin is derived from (and named after) the medicinal leech, *Hirudo medicinalis*. Hirudin is now made by recombinant technology and is a 65-amino acid polypeptide that binds with a high affinity directly to thrombin.[95] Inhibition of thrombin, the last step in the coagulation cascade, inhibits both clot formation and thrombin's stimulation of platelets. In addition, hirudin is able to inhibit thrombin that is found within a thrombus (and inaccessible to heparin),[139] making it a very potent antithrombotic agent.

Stability of anticoagulant response

One important advantage of hirudin (and hirulog[134]) have compared with heparin is the ability to achieve a more consistent level of anticoagulation. Unlike heparin, which is frequently associated with wide fluctuations in APTT, hirudin has been found in several trials to maintain a more stable APTT throughout the infusion period.[95,141,142] In the TIMI 5 trial, heparin maintained an APTT within a range of 30 seconds (similar to the target range of 55-85 secs) in only 13% of patients.[95] In contrast, hirudin maintained a stable APTT in nearly 3 times as many patients, 55% (p=0.004). When the range is widened to 40 seconds, still only 19% of heparin-treated patients maintained a stable APTT compared with 55% of hirudin-treated patients (p=0.002).[95] A similar advantage for hirudin was observed in the TIMI 6 trial[141] and in a trial of hirudin vs. heparin in unstable angina.[142] The ability to achieve a more stable APTT may be an important mechanism of benefit, since it will avoid periods of inadequate anticoagulation which have been shown to predispose to reocclusion (with its consequent adverse clinical consequences).[69,70,143]

Acute MI

The effects of hirudin as an adjunct to thrombolysis were first tested in the TIMI 5 trial.[95] In this trial, patients with acute MI received front-loaded t-PA and aspirin and were randomized to intravenous heparin or hirudin at one of four doses. The primary end point of the trial, achievement of TIMI grade 3 flow at both 90 minutes and 18-36 hours without death or reinfarction, was improved by hirudin compared with heparin: 62% of hirudin-treated patients achieved what might be termed "optimal thrombolysis" compared to 49% of heparin-treated patients (p=0.07).[95] Importantly, reocclusion of the infarct-related artery was reduced from 6.7% for heparin-treated patients to 1.6% for hirudin-treated patients (p=0.07). The TIMI 6 pilot trial, which compared hirudin and heparin in conjunction with streptokinase and aspirin.[141]

Unstable Angina. A pilot trial of hirudin was also carried out in unstable angina and non-Q wave MI.[142] One hundred sixty six patients with rest pain and ECG changes, and angiographic evidence of coronary thrombus were randomized to one of two doses of heparin (either a target APTT of 65-90 seconds, or a target of 90-110 seconds) or hirudin at one of four doses (infusion dose ranging from 0.05 to 0.3 mg/kg/hr) for 3-5 days. The primary end point, average cross-sectional area of the coronary lesion improved more in hirudin-treated patients (0.32 mm^2)compared with heparin-treated patients (0.08 mm^2) (p=0.08).[142] Other indices of lesion severity also showed improvement.

Although this angiographic trial was not designed to evaluate clinical endpoints, no deaths occurred in either treatment arm, and a lower incidence of post-randomization myocardial infarction occurred in hirudin-treated patients, 2.6% compared to 8.0% for heparin-treated patients (p=0.11).[142] These data suggest that hirudin is more effective in promoting the resolution of coronary thrombus, as judged by various measures of lesion severity which may in turn be associated with clinical benefits in patients with unstable angina and non-Q wave MI.

Safety. Although hirudin appeared to be quite safe in the initial pilot trials, a bolus dose of 0.6 mg/kg followed by an infusion of 0.2 mg/kg/hr together with a thrombolytic agent and aspirin in the TIMI 9A and GUSTO IIa trials was associated with an excess of bleeding (as was a higher dose of heparin). The incidence of intracranial hemorrhage was 1.7% in hirudin-treated patients and 1.9% in heparin-treated patients (p=NS).[67] Major spontaneous hemorrhage was also higher than expected, 4.9% for heparin and 8.7% for hirudin and (p=0.05).[67] Similar findings were observed in the GUSTO IIa and HIT III trials.[65,68] These findings have led to a reduction of the dose of hirudin in TIMI 9B and GUSTO IIb to a bolus of 0.1 mg/kg followed by an infusion of 0.1 mg/kg/hr, as well as a reduction of the heparin dose to the standard 1000-U/h infusion without weight-adjustment. Further, because the APTT appears to correlate with hemorrhagic events[72], the hirudin and heparin infusions are adjusted to maintain an APTT of 55-85 seconds, using the nomogram in *Table 8.1*. In the Phase III TIMI 9B trial, a trend in lower reinfarction was observed in-hospital, 2.3% vs. 3.4%, p=0.07, but no difference was observed in the primary endpoint, death, MI or severe CHF/shock at 30 days 12.9% for hirudin vs. 11.9% for heparin (p=NS).[141a] Similarly, death or MI was not different between the two anticoagulants, 9.7% vs. 9.5% (p=NS). Hirudin was tested in over 12.000 patients across the full spectrum of acute coronary syndromes in the Gusto IIb trial. There was a reduction in reinfarction (5.4% vs. 6.3% for heparin, p=0,04), but only a trend toward reduction in death or MI at 30 days, 8.9% vs. 9.8% (p=0.06).[141b] Thus, there has not been a dramatic improvement in clinical outcome with direct thrombin inhibitors in acute coronary syndromes. There are several ongoing trials evaluating direct thrombin inhibitors.

Hirulog

Hirulog is a 20 amino acid, synthetic peptide that was designed based on structural studies of hirudin.[131] Hirulog also selectively binds to thrombin and is a direct, specific, and reversible inhibitor of thrombin.*(Figure 8.11)*[144] Hirulog has a shorter half-life than either heparin or hirudin, approximately 35-40 minutes.[144,145]

Acute myocardial infarction. Hirulog has been evaluated as adjunctive therapy to streptokinase for acute MI in an angiographic pilot trial.[146] Forty-five patients were enrolled in this trial, 30 patients received hirulog at 0.5 mg/kg/hr for 12 hours, fol-

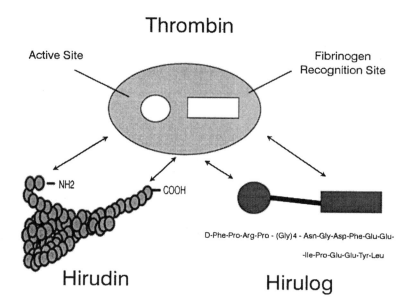

Figure 8.11 Diagram of hirudin and hirulog binding to thrombin. Hirudin and hirulog, unlike heparin, are direct thrombin inhibitors which bind to thrombin at two sites, including the active site where thrombin cleaves fibrinogen to fibrin.

lowed by 0.1 mg/kg/hr for 5 days, and 15 received a heparin infusion (without a bolus) at 1000 U/h titrated to an APTT of 2 to 2.5 times control. Patency of the infarct-related artery at 90 minutes was significantly higher in hirulog-treated patients compared with heparin-treated patients (77% vs. 47%, p<0.05).[146] TIMI grade 3 flow was present in 67% of hirulog-treated patients compared with 40% of heparin-treated patients (p=0.08).[146] Clinical events also tended to be lower in hirulog-treated patients: The incidence of a composite end point (death, recurrent MI, severe congestive heart failure or cardiogenic shock, recurrent ischemia or stroke) occurred in 7% of the hirulog group compared with 27% of the heparin group (p=0.06).[146]

A second dose-ranging trial was conducted by the same investigators, who randomized patients to intravenous heparin or 0.5 mg/kg/hr or 1.0 mg/kg/hr of hirulog. Interestingly they found that patients treated with the higher dose 1.0 mg/kg/hr had a lower patency rate than a dose of 0.5 mg/kg/hr.[147] They hypothesized that *too* effective inhibition of thrombin could prevent thrombin from binding to thrombomodulin and, hence may inhibit the protein C pathway from playing its natural anticoagulant role. These observations are currently being tested further in a larger angiographic trial. Nonetheless, the more effective antithrombotic effects of hirulog with streptokinase appear to improve the rate of early infarct-related artery patency, which could potentially translate into improved clinical outcome for patients with acute MI, which is being tested in the HERO-2 trial.

Unstable Angina. Two pilot trials of hirulog in patients with unstable angina demonstrated overall high rates of clinical success in preventing recurrent ischemic events.[148,149] The TIMI 7 trial was a multicenter, double-blind, dose-ranging trial of hirulog in patients with unstable angina.[150] Patients received a 72 hour intravenous infusion of one of four doses of hirulog: 0.02. 0.25, 0.5 and 1.0 mg/kg/hr. Comparing the patients who received the lowest dose of hirulog (N=160) with patients who collectively received one of the higher doses of hirulog (N=250), the incidence of death or MI through hospital discharge was 11.0% in the low-dose group and 4.0% in the aggregate high-dose group (P<0.004).[150] At 42 days, death or MI occurred in 13.0% of the low dose group compared to 6.0% of the higher dose group (p<0.013).[150] Since those who received the higher doses of hirulog (which achieve aPTT values in the range of 65-90 seconds) appeared to have an improved outcome compared with patients who received the low dose of hirulog (which achieved aPTT values of approximately 40 seconds) aspirin plus a direct thrombin inhibitor at a certain level of anticoagulation (apparently similar to what is considered the therapeutic range for heparin) may be more effective than aspirin and a low level of anticoagulation (or aspirin alone).

Low molecular weight heparin

A major advance in the use of heparin has been in the development of low molecular weight heparins (LMWH), which are combined thrombin inhibitors and Factor Xa inhibitors, thereby inhibiting both thrombin activity and its generation. Low molecular weight heparin has been found to significantly reduce death or MI compared with aspirin alone, 1.8% vs. 4.8% (p=0.001)[150a] and one agent, enoxaparin has been shown to be superior to heparin plus aspirin: In the ESSENCE trial, the primary endpoint, death, MI or recurrent ischemia at 14 days was significantly reduced by enoxaparin compared with heparin (16.6% vs. 19.8%, p=0.019)[150b]. In addition, in ST elevation MI, enoxaparin has recently been shown to reduce the incidence of death, MI or recurrent ischemia following thrombolytic therapy[150c].

Rebound following thrombin inhibition

A phenomenon termed "rebound", whereby a recrudescence of ischemic symptoms was noted soon after stopping a thrombin inhibitor. This clinical syndrome was described following heparin (without aspirin) treatment for unstable angina,[25] and in a pilot trial of the direct thrombin inhibitor argatroban for unstable angina,[151] In the latter trial, 43 patients with unstable angina were treated with a 4 hour infusion of argatroban. After stopping the infusion, they noted recurrent ischemia in 9 of 43 (23%) patients. This was accompanied by increases in direct markers of thrombosis: thrombin-antithrombin complexes rose above their already elevated baseline levels and fibrinopeptide A levels rose back to their elevated levels prior to treatment. Similar observations of increased biochemical markers of thrombosis have been noted with heparin,[152] and hirulog.[148,149]

However, this clinical phenomenon appears to be abolished when aspirin is taken concomitantly.[25] Of note, no *clinical* "rebound" phenomenon has been observed following hirudin[95,142], hirulog,[134,148,149] or low molecular weight heparin[1516]. These and other biochemical observations[153,154] suggest that the clotting system remains in a "prethrombotic state"[54] following the acute ischemic event, with a greater propensity for thrombosis than a patient with stable coronary artery disease. Therefore, following acute stabilization of the patient with aspirin and antithrombin agents, continuation of aspirin is important to prevent recurrent events, and the potential exists that long-term therapy with antithrombotic agents such as low molecular weight heparin might further improve the outcome of patients with acute coronary syndromes.

Novel thrombolytic agents/regimens

Several new thrombolytic agents are recently approved (r-PA[157,158]) or under development, including staphylokinase,[155,156] and other variants of t-PA, TNK-tPA,[159,160] and n-PA (lanoteplase).[163] Reteplase (r-PA). contains the kringle-2 and protease domains, but lacks the finger-, epidermal growth factor, and kringle-1-domains and has a prolonged half-life such that it can be given in a double-bolus regimen.[157,158] The primary goal of all the newer agents is to improve the early establishment of patency, especially TIMI grade 3 flow.

TNK-tPA. A new, modified form of tissue-type plasminogen activator, so called TNK-tPA, has recently been developed which appears to offer several potential advantages over current thrombolytic agents. First, TNK-tPA has a more prolonged half-life compared to standard t-PA, and can thus be administered as a single intravenous bolus.[159] Second, TNK-tPA is more than 10 times more fibrin specific than t-PA.[159-161] Finally, TNK-tPA has an 80-fold higher resistance to inhibition by plasminogen activator inhibitor 1 (PAI-1).[159] In animal testing, TNK-tPA compared favorably to front-loaded t-PA in achieving early reperfusion.[160] Thus, TNK-tPA appears to be a promising new thrombolytic agent for use in treatment of acute MI, and was tested in the TIMI 10 trials.[160,161] In TIMI 10B, the 40 mg signle bolus dose of TNK-tPA was able to achieve similar patency as front-loades t-PA.[161] TNK-tPA is now being tested for equivalence to t-PA in a large mortality trial.

Conclusions. The past several years have witnessed dramatic growth in the field of atherothrombosis. Atherosclerotic plaque rupture and thrombosis has been identified as the major etiology of acute coronary syndromes. Accordingly, major advances in the treatment of unstable angina and acute MI have been made with the use of more effective thrombolytic-antithrombotic regimens. Aspirin is a key component of all antithrombotic therapy, and its benefit across the spectrum of atherthrombotic coronary syndromes suggests that more potent antiplatelet agents may be even more effective. Heparin is important in the treatment of unstable angina/ non-Q wave MI, and as an adjunct to t-PA. It is important to monitor closely the degree of anticoagulation with heparin in an attempt to minimize the bleeding risk. In acute MI with ST elevation, the achievement of early infarct-related artery patency is the key objective, and front-loaded t-PA (with aspirin, intravenous heparin and rapid time to treatment) is the best regimen to achieve this goal at present. If current research efforts are successful in identifying more potent and faster-acting thrombolytic agents, it should be possible to improve further the outcome of patients with acute myocardial infarction. Similarly, all patients with acute coronary syndromes may be significantly improved with the application of newer, safer antiplatelet and antithrombin agents to their treatment regimens.

REFERENCES

1. Fuster V, et al. The pathophysiology of coronary artery disease and the acute coronary syndromes. N Engl J Med 1992;326:242, 310.

2. Falk E. Unstable angina with fatal outcome: dynamic coronary thrombosis leading to infarction and/or sudden death. Circulation 1985;71:699.

3. Davies MJ, Thomas A. Plaque fissuring - the cause of acute myocardial infarction, sudden ischemic death, and crescendo angina. Br Heart J 1985;53:363.

4. Davies MJ. New insights from pathology studies. presented at the George Washington University Symposium on Thrombolysis and Interventional Therapy in Acute Myocardial Infarction. Dallas, Texas: November, 1994: .

5. Braunwald E, et al. Unstable Angina: Diagnosis and Management. Clinical Practice Guideline Number 10.Rockville, MD: Agency for Health Care Policy and Research and the National Heart, Lung, and Blood Institute, Public Health Service, U.S. Department of Health and Human Services, 1994:154.

6. The TIMI IIIB Investigators. Effects of tissue plasminogen activator and a comparison of early invasive and conservative strategies in unstable angina and non-Q-wave myocardial infarction: Results of the TIMI IIIB Trial. Circulation 1994;89:1545.

7. Anderson HV, et al. One-year results of the Thrombolysis in Myocardial Infarction (TIMI) IIIB clinical trial. A randomized comparison of tissue-type plasminogen activator versus placebo and early invasive versus early conservative strategies in unstable angina and non-Q-wave myocardial infarction. J Am Coll Cardiol 1995;26:1643.

8. Stone PH, et al. Influence of race, sex, and age on management of unstable angina and non-Q-wave myocardial infarction: The TIMI III Registry. JAMA 1996;275:1104..

9. TIMI Research Group. Immediate vs delayed catheterization and angioplasty following thrombolytic therapy for acute myocardial infarction. TIMI II A results. JAMA 1988;260:2849.

10. Williams DO, et al. One-year results of the Thrombolysis in Myocardial Infarction Investigation (TIMI) phase II trial. Circulation 1992;85:533.

11. Braunwald E, et al. Diagnosing and Managing Unstable Angina. Circulation 1994;90:613.

12. Vita JA, et al. Coronary vasomotor response to acetylcholine relates to risk factors for coronary artery disease. Circulation 1990;81:491.

13. Anderson TJ, et al. The effect of cholesterol-lowering and antioxidant therapy on endothelium-dependent coronary vasomotion. N Engl J Med 1995;332:488.

14. Ridker PM, et al. Low-dose aspirin therapy for chronic stable angina. A randomized, placebo-controlled clinical trial. Ann Intern Med 1991;114:835.

15. Steering Committee of the Physicians' Health Study Research Group. Final report on the aspirin component of the ongoing Physicians' Health Study. N Engl J Med 1989;321:129.

16. Manson JE, et al. A prospective study of aspirin use and primary prevention of cardiovascular disease. JAMA 1991;266:521.

17. Klimt CR, et al. Persantine-Aspirin Reinfarction Study. Part II. Secondary coronary prevention with persantine and aspirin. J Am Coll Cardiol 1986;7:251.

18. Willard JE, Lange RA, Hillis LD. The use of aspirin in ischemic heart disease. N Engl J Med 1992;327:175.

19. Smith P, Arnesen H, Holme I. The effect of warfarin on mortality and reinfarction after myocardial infarction. N Engl J Med 1990;323:147.

20. Antiplatelet Trialist' Collaboration. Collborative overview of randomised trials of antiplatelet therapy - I: prevention of death myocardial infarction and stroke by prolongued antiplatelet therapy in various categories of patients. BMJ 1994;308:81.

21. Lewis HD, et al. Protective effects of aspirin against acute myocardial infarction and death in men with unstable angina. N Engl J Med 1983;309:396.

22. Cairns JA, et al. Aspirin, sulfinpyrazone, or both in unstable angina. N Engl J Med 1985;313:1369.

23. Theroux P, et al. Aspirin, heparin or both to treat unstable angina. N Engl J Med 1988;319:1105.

24. The RISC Group. Risk of myocardial infarction and death during treatment with low dose aspirin and intravenous heparin in men with unstable coronary artery disease. Lancet 1990;336:827.

25. Theroux P, et al. Reactivation of unstable angina after the discontinuation of heparin. N Engl J Med 1992;327:141.

26. Roux S, Christelier S, Ludin E. Effects of aspirin on coronary reocclusion and recurrent ischemia after thrombolysis: a meta-analysis. J Am Coll Cardiol 1992;19:671.

27. ISIS-2 (Second International Study of Infarct Survival) Collaborative Group. Randomised trial of intravenous streptokinase, oral aspirin, both, or neither among 17,187 cases of suspected acute myocardial infarction: ISIS-2. Lancet 1988;2:349.

28. Tollefsen DM. Heparin: Basic and clinical pharmacology. In: Hoffman R, Benz EJJ, Shattil SJ, Furie B, Cohen HJ, ed. Hematology: Basic principles and practice. New York: Churchill Livingstone, 1991, p1436-45.

29. Verstraete M. Heparin. In: Messerli FH, ed. Cardiovascular drug therapy. Philadelphia: W.B. Saunders Company, 1990, p1457.

30. Majerus PW, et al. Anticoagulant, thrombolytic, and antiplatelet drugs. In: Gilman AG, Rall TW, Nies AS, Taylor P, ed. The pharmacological basis of therapeutics. 8th ed. New York: Pergamon Press, 1990, p 102.

31. Rosenberg RD. The heparin-antithrombin system: a natural anticoagulant mechanism. In: Colman RW, Marder VJ, Salzman EW, Hirsh J, ed. Hemostasis and Thrombosis: Basic Principles and Clinical Practice. 2nd ed. Philadelphia: J.B. Lippincott Company, 1987, p1373.

32. Hirsh J. Heparin. N Engl J Med 1991;324:1565.

33. Ogilby JD, et al. Variability of effective anticoagulation for PTCA is dependent upon heparin potency. Circulation 1991;84:(Suppl II):II-592.

34. Bock PE, et al. The multiple complexes formed by the interaction of platelet factor 4 with heparin. Biochem J 1980;191:769.

35. Lijnen HR, Hoylaerts M, Collens D. Heparin binding properties of human histidine-rich glycoprotein: mechanism and role in the neutralization of heparin in plasma. J Biol Chem 1983;258:3803.

36. Preissner KT, Muller-Berghaus G. Neutralization and binding of heparin by S-protein/vitronectin in the inhibition of factor Xa by antithrombin III. J Biol Chem 1987;262:12247.

37. Maraganore JM, et al. Heparin variability and resistance: Comparisons with a direct thrombin inhibitor.(abstract) Circulation 1992;86 (Suppl. I):I-386.

38. Cruikshank MK, et al. A standard nomogram for the management of heparin therapy. Arch Intern Med 1991;151:333.

39. Flaker GC, et al. Use of a standardized nomogram to achieve therapeutic anticoagulation after thrombolytic therapy in myocardial infarction. Arch Intern Med 1994;154:1492.

40. Williams DO, et al. Anticoagulant treatment in unstable angina. Br J Clin Pract 1986;40:114.

41. Tedford AM, Wilson C. Trial of heparin versus atenolol in prevention of myocardial infarction in intermediate coronary syndrome. Lancet 1981;1:1225.

42. Theroux P, et al. Aspirin versus heparin to prevent myocardial infarction during the acute phase of unstable angina. Circulation 1993;88:2045.

43. Cohen M, et al. Combination antithrombotic therapy in unstable rest angina and non-Q-wave infarction in nonprior aspirin users. Primary end points analysis from the ATACS trial. Circulation 1994;89:81.

44. Topol EJ, et al. A randomized controlled trial of intravenous tissue plasminogen activator and early intravenous heparin in acute myocardial infarction. Circulation 1989;79:281.

45. Hsia J, et al. A comparison between heparin and low-dose aspirin as adjunctive therapy with tissue plasminogen activator for acute myocardial infarction. N Engl J Med 1990;323:1433.

46. Bleich SD, et al. Effect of heparin on coronary patency after thrombolysis with tissue plasminogen activator in acute myocardial infarction. Am J Cardiol 1990;66:1412.

47. de Bono DP, et al. Effect of early intravenous heparin on coronary patency, infarct size, and bleeding complications after alteplase thrombolysis: results of a randomized double blind European Cooperative Study Group trial. Br Heart J 1992;67:122.

48. Thompson PL, et al. A randomized comparison of intravenous heparin with oral aspirin and dipyridamole 24 hours after recombinant tissue-type plasminogen activator for acute myocardial infarction. Circulation 1991;83:1534.

49. Aguirre F, et al. Influence of intravenous heparin duration on clinical outcome of patients receiving accelerated weight-adjusted rt-PA for acute myocardial infarction: preliminary results of the Multicenter Randomized t-PA Heparin Duration Trial.(abstract) Circulation 1993;88[Pt. 2]:I-201.

50. Gruppo Italiano per lo Studio della Sopravvivenza nell'Infarto Miocardico: GISSI-2. A factorial randomised trial of alteplase versus streptokinase and heparin versus no heparin among 12,490 patients with acute myocardial infarction. Lancet 1990;336:65.

51. ISIS-3 (Third International Study of Infarct Survival) Collaborative Group. ISIS-3: a randomised comparison of streptokinase vs tissue plasminogen activator vs anistreplase and of

aspirin plus heparin vs aspirin alone among 41,299 cases of suspected acute myocardial infarction. Lancet 1992;339:753.

52. Ridker PM, et al. Are both aspirin and heparin justified as adjunctions to thrombolytic therapy for acute myocardial infarction? Lancet 1993;341:1574.

53. Kroon C, et al. Highly variable anticoagulant response after subcutaneous administration of high-dose (12,5000 IU) heparin in patients with myocardial infarction and healthy volunteers. Circulation 1992;86:1370.

54. Handin RI, Loscalzo J. Hemostasis, thrombosis, fibrinolysis, and cardiovascular disease. In: Braunwald E, ed. Heart Disease, 4th ed. Philadelphia: W.B. Saunders, 1992, p1767.

55. Goldhaber SZ. Conjunctive heparin therapy. Limitations of sucutaneous administration. Circulation 1992;86:1639.

56. Scharfstein JS, et al. Usefulness of fibinogenolytic and procoagulant markers during thrombolytic therapy in predicting clinical outcomes in acute myocardial infarction. Am J Cardiol 1996;78:503.

57. Ohman EM, et al. Consequences of reocclusion after successful reperfusion therapy in acute myocardial infarction. Circulation 1990;82:781.

58. Gibson CM et al. Angiographic predictors of reocclusion after thrombolysis: results from the Thrombolysis in Myocardial Infarction (TIMI) 4 trial. J Am Coll Cardiol 1995;25:582.

59. The GUSTO Investigators. An international randomized trial comparing four thrombolytic strategies for acute myocardial infarction. N Engl J Med 1993;329:673-82.

60. The GUSTO Angiographic Investigators. The comparative effects of tissue plasminogen activator, streptokinase, or both on coronary artery patency, ventricular function and survival after acute myocardial infarction. N Engl J Med 1993;329:1615-22.

61. Loscalzo J, Braunwald E. Tissue plasminogen activator. N Engl J Med 1988;319:925.

62. Marder VJ, Sherry S. Thrombolytic therapy: current status. N Engl J Med 1988;318:1512, 1585.

63. Hirsh J, Fuster V. Guide to anticoagulation therapy. Part 1: heparin. Circulation 1994;89:1449.

64. Raschke RA, et al. The weight-based heparin dosing nomogram compared with a "standard care" nomogram. Ann intern Med 1993;119:874.

65. Neuhaus K-L, et al. Safety obervations from the pilot phase of a randomized trial: r-Hirudin for Improvement of Thromboysis (HIT-III) Study. A study of the Arbeitsgemeinschaft Leitender, Kardiologischer Koinkenhausarzte (ALKK). Circulation 1994;90:1638.

66. O'Connor CM, et al. A randomized trial of intravenous heparin in conjunction with anistreplase (Anisoylated Plasminogen Streptokinase Activator Complex) in acute myocardial infarction: the Duke University Clinical Cardiology Study (DUCCS). J Am Coll Cardiol 1994;23:11.

67. Antman EM, for the TIMI 9A Investigators. Hirudin in acute myocardial infarction: Safety report from the Thrombolysis and Thrombin Inhibition in Myocardial Infarction (TIMI) 9A trial. Circulation 1994;90:1624.

68. The Global Use of Strategies to Open Occluded Coronary Arteries (GUSTO) IIa Investigators. A randomized trial of intravenous heparin versus recombinant hirudin for acute coronary syndromes. Circulation 1994;90:1631.

69. Hsia J, et al. Heparin-induced prolongation of partial thromboplastin time after thrombolysis: relationship to coronary artery patency. J Am Coll Cardiol 1992;20:31.

70. Arnout J, et al. Correlation between level of heparinization and patency of the infarct-related coronary artery after treatment of acute myocardial infarction with alteplase (rt-PA). J Am Coll Cardiol 1992;20:513.

71. Granger C, et al. Activated partialthromboplastin time and outcome after thrombolytic therapy for acute myocardial infarction: results from the GUSTO-I Trial. Circulation 1996;93:870.

72. Cannon CP, et al. Usefulness of APTT to predict bleeding for hirudin (and heparin).(abstract) Circulation 1994;90[Pt. 2]:I-563.

73. Cannon CP, et al. Comparison of front-loaded recombinant tissue-type plasminogen activator, anistreplase and combination thrombolytic therapy for acute myocardial infarction: results of the Thrombolysis in Myocardial Infarction (TIMI) 4 trial. J Am Coll Cardiol 1994;24:1602.

74. Bovill EG, et al. Hemorrhagic events during therapy with recombinant tissue-type plasminogen activator, heparin, and aspirin for acute myocardial infarction. Results of the Thrombolysis in Myocardial Infarction (TIMI), Phase II trial. Ann Intern Med 1991;115:256.

75. Cannon CP, et al. The Thrombolysis in Myocardial Infarction (TIMI) Trials - the first decade. J Intervent Cardiol 1995;8:117.

76. Becker R, et al. Relationship between systemic anticoagulation as determined by activated partial thromboplastin time and heparin measurements and in-hospital clinical events in unstable angina and non-Q wave myocardial infarction. Am Heart J 1996;1131:421.

77. Braunwald E. Myocardial reperfusion, limitation of infarct size, reduction of left ventricular dysfunction, and improved survival: Should the paradigm be expanded? Circulation 1989;79:441.

78. Braunwald E. Unstable angina: a classification. Circulation 1989;80:410.

79. Califf RM, Topol EJ, Gersh BJ. From myocardial salvage to patient salvage in acute myocardial infarction. The role of reperfusion therapy. J Am Coll Cardiol 1989;14:1382.

80. Braunwald E. The open-artery theory is alive and well - again. N Engl J Med 1993;329:1650.

81. Cannon CP, Braunwald E. GUSTO, TIMI and the case for rapid reperfusion. Acta Cardiol 1994;49:1.

82. Dalen JE, et al. Six- and twelve-month follow-up of the Phase I Thrombolysis in Myocardial Infarction (TIMI) Trial. Am J Cardiol 1988;62:179.

83. TIMI Study Group. The Thrombolysis in Myocardial Infarction (TIMI) Trial; Phase I findings. N Engl J Med 1985;312:932.

84. Flygenring BP, et al. Does arterial patency 90 minutes following thrombolytic therapy predict 42 day survival? J Am Coll Cardiol 1991;17 (Suppl. A):275A.

85. Karagounis L, et al. Does Thrombolysis in Myocardial Infarction (TIMI) perfusion grade 2 represent a mostly patent artery or a mostly occluded artery? Enzymatic and electrocardiographic evidence from the TEAM-2 Study. J Am Coll Cardiol 1992;19:1.

86. Gibson CM, et al. TIMI frame count: a quantitive method of assessing coronary artery flow. Circulation 1996;93:879.

87. Belenkie I, et al. Importance of effective, early and sustained reperfusion during acute myocardial infarction. Am J Cardiol 1989;63:912.

88. Anderson JL, et al. TIMI perfusion grade 3 but not grade 2 results in improved outcome after thrombolysis for myocardial infarction: ventriculographic, enzymatic and electrocardiographic evidence from the TEAM-3 Study. Circulation 1993;87:1829.

89. Badger RS, et al. Usefullness of recanalization to luminal diameter of 0.6 millimeter or more with intracoronary streptokinase during acute myocardial infarction in predicting "normal" perfusion status, continued arterial patency and survival at one year. Am J Cardiol 1987;59:519.

90. Gibson CM, et al. Consequences of TIMI 2 vs 3 flow at 90 minutes following thrombolysis. J Am Coll Cardiol 1993;21 (Suppl. A):348A.

91. Lincoff AM, et al. Significance of a coronary artery with Thrombolysis in Myocardial Infarction grade 2 flow "patency" (Outcome in the Thrombolysis and Angioplasty in Myocardial Infarction (TAMI) Trials). Am J Cardiol 1995;75:81.

92. Kennedy J, Ritchie J, et al. The Western Washington randomized trial of intracoronary streptokinase in acute myocardial infarction: a 12-month follow-up report. NEJM 1985;312:1073.

93. Stadius ML, et al. Risk stratification for 1 year survival based on characteristics identified in the early hours of acute myocardial infarction. Circulation 1986;74:701.

94. Vogt A, et al. Impact of early perfusion status of the infarct-related artery on short-term mortality after thrombolysis for acute myocardial infarction: retrospective analysis of four German multicenter studies. J Am Coll Cardiol 1993;21:1391.

95. Cannon CP, et al. A pilot trial of recombinant desulfatohirudin compared with heparin in conjunction with tissue-type plasminogen activator and aspirin for acute myocardial infarction: Results of the Thrombolysis in Myocardial Infarction (TIMI) 5 Trial. J Am Coll Cardiol 1994;23:993.

96. Gruppo Italiano per lo Studio della Streptochinasi nell'Infarto Miocardico (GISSI). Effectiveness of intravenous thrombolytic treatment in acute myocardial infarction. Lancet 1986;1:397.

97. AIMS Trial Study Group. Effect of intravenous APSAC on mortality after acute myocardial infarction: Preliminary report of a placebo-controlled clinical trial. Lancet 1988;2:545.

98. ASSET Study Group. Trial of tissue plasminogen activator for mortality reduction in acute myocardial infarction. Anglo-Scandinavian Study of Early Thrombolysis (ASSET). Lancet 1988;2:525.

99. Fibrinolytic Therapy Trialists (FTT) Collaborative Group. Indications for fibrinolytic therapy in suspected acute myocardial infarction: collaborative overview of early mortality and major morbidity results from all randomised trials of more than 1000 patients. Lancet 1994;343:311.

100. Gore JM, et al. Intracerebral hemorrhage, cerebral infarction, and subdural hematoma after acute myocardial infarction and thrombolytic therapy in the Thrombolysis in Myocardial Infarction Study. Thrombolysis in Myocardial Infarction, Phase II, pilot and clinical trial. Circulation 1991;83:448.

101. Simoons ML, et al. Individual risk assessment for intracranial hemorrhage during thrombolytic therapy. Lancet 1993;342:1523.

102. Maggioni AP, et al. The risk of stroke in patients with acute myocardial infarction after thrombolytic and antithrombotic treatment. N Engl J Med 1992;327:1.

103. International Study Group. In-hospital mortality and clinical course of 20,891 patients with suspected acute myocardial infarction randomised between alteplase and streptokinase with or without heparin. Lancet 1990;336:71.

104. Neuhaus K-L, et al. Improved thrombolysis with a modified dose regimen of recombinant tissue-type plasminogen activator. J Am Coll Cardiol 1989;14:1566.

105. Neuhaus K-L, et al. Improved thrombolysis in acute myocardial infarction with front-loaded administration of alteplase: results of the rt-PA-APSAC Patency Study (TAPS). J Am Coll Cardiol 1992;19:885.

106. Carney RJ, et al. Randomized angiographic trial of recombinant tissue-type plasminogen activator (alteplase) in myocardial infarction. J Am Coll Cardiol 1992;20:17.

107. Grines CL, et al. A prospective, randomized trial comparing combination half-dose tissue-type plasminogen activator and streptokinase with full-dose tissue-type plasminogen activator. Circulation 1991;84:540.

108. Kleiman NS, et al. Mortality within 24 hours of thrombolysis in myocardial infarction. The importance of early reperfusion. Circulation 1994;90:2658.

109. Topol EJ, et al. More on the GUSTO trial. N Engl J Med 1994;331:277.

110. Braunwald E, Cannon CP, McCabe CH. An approach to evaluating thrombolytic therapy in acute myocardial infarction. The 'Unsatisfactory Outcome' end point. Circulation 1992;86:683.

111. Zarich SW, et al. Sequential low dose conbination thrombolytic therapy: results of the Prourokinase and t-PA Enhancement of Thrombolysis (PATENT) trial.(abstract) Circulation 1994;90[Pt. 2]:I-562.

112. Cannon CP, et al. Time as an adjunctive agent to thrombolytic therapy. J Thromb Thrombolysis 1994;1:27.

113. Timm TC, et al. Left ventricular function and early cardiac events as a function of time to treatment with t-PA: A report from TIMI II. Circulation 1991;84:II-230.

114. National Heart Attack Alert Program Coordinating Committee - 60 Minutes to Treatment Working Group. Emergency department: rapid identification and treatment of patients with acute myocardial infarction. Ann Emerg Med 1994;23:311.

115. The TIMI IIIA Investigators. Early effects of tissue-type plasminogen activator added to conventional therapy on the culprit lesion in patients presenting with ischemic cardiac pain at rest. Results of the Thrombolysis in Myocardial Ischemia (TIMI IIIA) Trial. Circulation 1993;87:38.

116. The RAPT Investigators. Randomized trial of ridogrel, a combined thromboxane A_2 synthase inhibitor and thromboxane A_2/prostaglandin endoperoxide receptor antagonist, versus asprin as adjunction to thrombolysis in patients with acute myocardial infarction. The Ridogrel Aspirin Patency Trial (RAPT). Circulation 1994;89:588.

117. Coller BS, Scudder LR. Inhibition of dog platelet function by in vivo infusion of F(ab')$_2$ fragments of a monoclonal antibody to the platelet glycoprotein IIb/IIIa receptor. Blood 1985;66:1456.

118. Kleiman N, et al. Profound inhibition of platelet aggregation with monoclonal antibody 7E3 Fab after thrombolytic therapy. Results of the Thrombolysis and Angioplasty in Myocardial Infarction (TAMI) 8 pilot study. J Am Coll Cardiol 1993;22:381.

119. The EPIC Investigators. Use of a monoclonal antibody directed against the platelet glycoprotein IIb/IIIa receptor in high risk angioplasty. N Engl J Med 1994;330:956.

120. Simoons ML, et al. Randomized trial of a GPIIb/IIIa platelet receptor blocker in refractory unstable angina. Circulation 1994;89:596.

121. Schulman SP, et al. Effects of Integrelin, a platelet glycoprotein IIb/IIa antagonist, in unstable angina. A randomized multicenter trial. Circulation 1996;94:2083.

122. Nicolini FA, et al. Combination of platelet fibrinogen receptor antagonist and direct thrombin inhibitor at low doses markedly improves thrombolysis. Circulation 1994;89:1802.

123. Kereiakes DJ, et al. Randomized, double-blind, placebo-controlled dose-ranging study of tirofiban (MK-383) platelet IIb/IIIa blockade in high risk patients undergoing coronary angioplasty. J Am Coll Cardiol 1996;27:536.

124. Theroux P, et al. Platelet membrane receptor glycoprotein IIb/IIIa antagonism in unstable angina. The Canadian Lamifiban Study. Circulation 1996;94:899.

125. Lefkovits J, et al. Effects of platelet glycoprotein IIb/IIIa receptor blockade by a chimeric monoclonal antibody (abciximab) on acute and six-month outcomes after percutaneous transluminal coronary angioplasty for acute myocardial infarction. Am J Cardiol 1996;77:1045.

126. Ohman EM, et al. Combined accelerated tissue-plasminogen activator and platelet glycoprotein IIb/IIa integrin receptor blockade with integrilin in acute myocardial infarction. Circulation 1997;95:846.

127. The PRISM-PLUS Investigators. Inhibition of platelet glycoprotein IIb/IIIa with tirofiban in unstable angina and non-Q wave myocardial infarction. N Engl J Med in press.

128. White HD. Platelet Receptor Inhibition for Ischemic Syndrome Management. presented at the American College of Cardiology Scientific Sessions. Anaheim, CA, 1997.

129. Topol EJ. The Platelet Glycoprotein IIb/IIIa in Unstable Angina: Receptor Suppression Using Integrillin Therapy (PURSUIT) trial. presented at the The European Society of Cardiology Congress. Stockholm, Norway, August 1997.

130. Markwardt F. Isolierung uber Hirudin. Naturwissenschafter 1955;42:537.

131. Maraganore JM, et al. Design and characterization of hirulogs: A novel class of bivalent peptide inhibitors of thrombin. Biochemistry 1990;29:7095.

132. Rydel TJ, et al. The structure of a complex of recombinant hirudin and human alpha-thrombin. Science 1990;249:277.

133. Vu T H., et al. Domains specifying thrombin-receptor interaction. Nature 1991;353:674.

134. Cannon CP. Hirulog. In: Messerli FH, ed. Cardiovascular Drug Therapy. 2nd ed. Philadelphia: W.B. Saunders Company, 1996:1498.

135. Talbot M. Biology of recombinant hirudin (CGP 39393): a new prospect in the treatment of thrombosis. Semin Thromb Hemost 1989;15:293.

136. Markwardt F. Past, present and future of hirudin. Haemostasis 1991;21:11.

137. Ofosu FA, et al. Inhibition of the amplification reactions of blood coagulation by site-specific inhibitors of alpha-thrombin. Biochem J 1992;283:893.

138. Cannon CP. Thrombin inhibitors in acute myocardial infarction. In: Kleiman NS, ed. Cardiology Clinics: Acute Myocardial Infarction. Philadelphia: W.B. Saunders Company, in press.

139. Weitz JI, et al. Clot-bound thrombin is protected from inhibition by heparin-antithrombin III but is susceptible to inactivation by antithrombin III-independent inhibitors. J Clin Invest 1990;86:385.

140. Fareed J, et al. Some objective considerations for the neutralization of the anticoagulant effects of recombinant hirudin. Haemostasis 1991;21(Suppl. 1):64.

141. Lee LV, for the TIMI 6 Investigators. Initial experience with hirudin and streptokinase in acute myocardial infarction: results of the Thrombolysis in Myocardial Infarction (TIMI) 6 trial. Am J Cardiol 1995;75:7.

141a. Antman EM, for the TIMI 9B Investigators. Hirudin in acute myocardial infarction: Thrombolysis and Thrombin Inhibition in Myocardial Infarction (TIMI) 9B trial. Circulation 1996;94:911.

141b. The Global Use of Strategies to Open Occluded Coronary Arteries (GUSTO) IIb Investigators. A comparison of recombinant hirudin with heparin for the treatment of acute coronary syndromes. N Engl J Med 1996;335:775.

142. Topol EJ, et al. Recombinant hirudin for unstable angina pectoris. A multicenter, randomized angiographic trial. Circulation 1994;89:1557.

143. Kaplan K, et al. Role of heparin after intravenous thrombolytic therapy for acute myocardial infarction. Am J Cardiol 1987;59:241.

144. Cannon CP, et al. Anticoagulant effects of Hirulog, a novel thrombin inhibitor, in patients with coronary artery disease. Am J Cardiol 1993;71:778.

145. Fox I, et al. Anticoagulant activity of Hirulog™, a direct thrombin inhibitor, in humans. Thromb Haemost 1993;69:157.

146. Lidon R-M, et al. A pilot, early angiographic patency study using a direct thrombin inhibitor as adjunctive therapy to streptokinase in acute myocardial infarction. Circulation 1994;89:1567.

147. Theroux P, et al. Randomized double-blind comparison of two doses of hirulog with heparin as adjunctive therapy to streptokinase to promote early patency of the infarct-related artery in acute myocardial infarction. Circulation 1995;91:2132.

148. Sharma GVRK, et al. Usefulness and tolerability of Hirulog, a direct thrombin-inhibitor, in unstable angina pectoris. Am J Cardiol 1993;72:1357.

149. Lidon R-M, et al. Initial experience with a direct antithrombin, Hirulog, in unstable angina: anticoagulant, antithrombotic and clinical effects. Circulation 1993;88:1495.

150. Fuchs J, Cannon CP, and the TIMI 7 Investigators. Hirulog in the treatment of unstable angina: results of the Thrombin Inhibition in Myocardial Ischemia (TIMI) 7 trial. Circulation 1995;92:727.

151. Gold HK, et al. Evidence of a rebound coagulation phenomenon after cessation of a 4-hour infusion of a specific thrombin inhibitor in patients with unstable angina pectoris. J Am Coll Cardiol 1993;21:1039-47.

151a. FRISC Study Group. Low molecular weight heparin (Fragmin) during istabillity in coronary artery disease (FRISC). Lancet 1996;347:561.

151b. Cohen M, Demers C, Gurfinkel EP, et al. A comparison of low-molecular-weight heparin with unfractionated heparin for unstable coronary artery disease. N Engl J Med 1997;337:447.

151c. Baird SH, McBride SJ, Trouton TG, Wilson C. Low-molecular-weight heparin versus unfractionated heparin following thrombolysis in myocardial infarction. J Am Col Cardiol 1998;31 (Suppl. A):191A.

152. Granger CB, et al. Rebound increase in thrombin generation and activity after cessation of intravenous heparin in patients with acute coronary syndromes. Circulation 1995;91:1929.

153. Merlini PA, et al. Persistent activation of coagulation mechanism in unstable angina and myocardial infarction. Circulation 1994;90:61.

154. Herren T, et al. Fibrin formation and degradation in patients with arteriosclerotic disease. Circulation 1994;90:2679.

155. Collen D, Lijnen HR. Staphylokinase, a fibrin-specific plasminogen activator with therapeutic potential? Blood 1994;84:680.

156. Vanderschueren S, et al. A randomized trial of recombinant staphylokinase versus alteplase for coronary artery patency in acute myocardial infarction. Circulation 1995;92:22044.

157. Bode C, et al. Randomized comparison of coronary thrombolysis achieved with double-bolus reteplase (recombinant plasminogen activator) and front-loaded, accelerated alteplase (recombinant tissue plasminogen activator) in patients with acute myocardial infarction. Circulation 1996;94:891.

158. The Global Use of Strategies to Open Occluded Coronary Arteries (GUSTO III) Investigators. A comparison of reteplase with alteplase for acute myocardial infarction. N Engl J Md 1997;337:1118.

159. Keyt BA, et al. A faster-acting and more potent form of tissue plasminogen activator. Proc Natl Acad Sci USA 1994;91:3670.

160. Cannon CP, et al. TNK-tissue plasminogen activator in acute myocardial infarction: Results of the Thrombolysis in Myocardial Infarction (TIMI) 10A dose-ranging trial. Circulation 1997;95:351.

161. Cannon CP, et al. TNK-tissue plasminogen activator compared with front-loaded tissue plasminogen activator in acute myocardial infarction: Primary results of the TIMI 10B trial. (abstract) Circulation 1997;96(Suppl. I):I-206.

162. International Joint Efficacy Comparison of Thrombolytics. Randomised, double-blind comparison of reteplase double-bolus administration with streptokinase in acute myocardial infarction (INJECT): trial to investigate equivalence. Lancet 1995;346:329.

163. Lopez-Sendon JL, on behalf of the In TIME Investigations. Intravenous nPA for Treatmen of Infarction Myocardium Early: the In TIME study Eur Heart J 1997;18:454.

9 DEVELOPMENT OF COLLATERAL CORONARY CIRCULATION

Olga Hudlicka, Margaret Brown

The collateral circulation of the heart provides blood supply to myocardium, the original arterial supply to which has become restricted either partially or totally. As such, the extent of and capacity to develop collateral circulation will determine the ability of myocardium to survive ischaemia and become revascularized respectively. The existence of collateral circulation varies markedly between species, being greatest in the guinea pig, in which it is almost impossible to produce an infarct, and least in the pig.[1] It also differs in vessel type, existing as larger epicardial arterioles in the dog, 20-60μm in diameter, but as small subendocardial capillary-like vessels in the pig, and in man, the collateral circulation resembles most closely that of the pig, consisting primarily of subendocardial capillaries. [2,3]

In normal adult hearts, growth of vessels is seldom observed. Labelling of endothelial cells by ^{3}H-thymidine, indicating the presence of cells in the synthetic phase prior to mitosis, is below 0.14% in heart capillaries[4], and even less in smooth muscle cells. It can be stimulated in normal hearts by exercise training, mainly in young animals, but is almost absent in heart hypertrophy due to pressure or volume overload[5], and the fact that growth of capillaries under these conditions does not match myocyte growth results in an insufficient oxygen supply and eventually leads to heart failure. The development of collateral vessels in the case of gradual narrowing or ligation of coronary arteries has been described by many authors in several species. However, growth of capillaries in both surviving myocardium, which undergoes hypertrophy, and the border zone is inadequate following infarction.[6]

The mechanisms by which coronary vessels are stimulated to grow are currently being investigated with a view to possible therapeutic interventions. In this chapter, we will review briefly the conditions under which growth of capillaries and larger vessels occurs, both physiological and pathological. We will also discuss the likely factors involved in the triggering of angiogenesis:myocyte-derived metabolic factors as a result of ischaemic/hypoxia, mechanical factors such as shear stress and vessel wall tension resulting from changes in coronary blood flow and/or myocyte contractile function, or mitogenic growth factors, which could be activated by any of the preceding. Much of the data will be drawn from experiments on animals, in which it is possible both to manipulate angiogenic stimuli more specifically and to quantify vascular supply precisely.

Growth of vessels in normal hearts

This has been studied primarily in response to exercise training. Large coronary arteries show enlargement after training in dogs[7] and in human elite athletes[8] The capacity of the coronary arterial bed may be inferred from measurements of blood flow, and it has been shown that maximal coronary conductance is increased by training.[9] However, this could reflect an increased ability to dilate rather than larger vascular capacity. Evidence from animal studies suggests that collateral circulation in the normal heart is not altered by training programs[10], but there have been reports of increases in the number of arteriolar vessels.[9] (Figure 9.1) Although it appears possible to stimulate growth of capillary vessels in young but not adult rat hearts by training[11], other authors have found either unaltered or decreased capillary supply in this species, and also in pigs and dogs after a variety of exercise training regimes.[5] Thus, exercise seems to stimulate growth of larger vessels to a greater extent than that of capillaries.

The increased metabolic demands of physical exercise lead to increased coronary blood flow, which could be a triggering mechanism for the growth of vessels. However, although capillary density was higher when coronary flow was increased on a long-term basis by administration of vasodilating substances such as dipyridamole[12], ethanol[13], adenosine or a xanthine derivative, propentofylline, it is unlikely that there was accompanying growth of larger vessels since maximal coronary blood flow was not increased.[14] (Figure 9.2).

Another possible stimulus to vessel growth in exercise may arise from the bradycardia which is linked with training. It has been shown that so-called 'athletic' animals such as hare or wild rat have lower heart rates and higher capillary densities than similar domesticated species (rabbit, laboratory).[15,16] Bradycardia induced by chronic administration of either a bradycardic drug alinidine[17] or propranolol[18] resulted in increased capillary density, although other authors did not report such a finding with propranolol.[19] A significant increase in capillary supply - capillary density up to 70% greater than normal - was observed in rabbit hearts in which long-term bradycardia was induced by electrical pacing.[20] (Figure 9.3) A similar method has also been used recently in pigs where it increased capillary density by 30%.[21] There are no reports about growth of larger vessels specifically in relation to bradycardia other than that an increased density of arterioles was found in rabbit hearts treated by propranolol.[19] Bradycardial pacing did not increase maximal coronary

Training in pigs

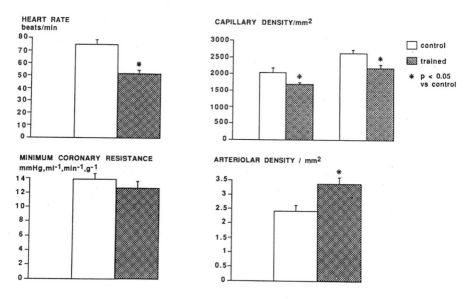

Figure 9.1 *Decreased capillary density and increased arteriolar density, in the absence of changes in minimal coronary resistance, in the hearts of pigs exercise-trained by 3 months on a treadmill. For capillary density, left hand columns are from the left ventricular subendocardium, and right hand columns from the subepicardium (based on data from ref. 9). Training was accompanied by a significant bradycardia. *p<0.05 v. control values. (Breisch et al, J. Appl. Physiol. 60: 1259-1267, 1986)*

blood flow, which, if this can be taken as a reasonable estimate of growth of arterioles or enlargement of larger arteries, suggests that it did not affect growth of either of these vessel categories.[22]

Growth of vessels in heart hypertrophy

Vascular growth in response to cardiac hypertrophy due to volume or pressure overload can occur in young animals and humans, but is much reduced if the hypertrophic stimulus is only present during adult life.[23,24] A review of capillary supply in various types of cardiac hypertrophy demonstrated a decrease in capillarization either on the. basis of estimated capillary density or capillary/fibre ratio.[25] While it may be difficult to ascertain whether this is due to the enlargement of myocytes or whether there is a real loss of capillaries, a transient increase in ^{3}H-thymidine labelling index was found in the hearts of rats with genetic hypertension.[26] Furthermore, some careful morphometric studies on pressure overload heart hypertrophy of various durations in dogs have demonstrated that capillary density declines at first, but

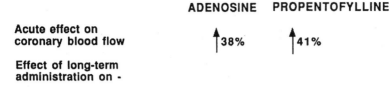

Acute effect on coronary blood flow

Effect of long-term administration on -

CAPILLARY DENSITY

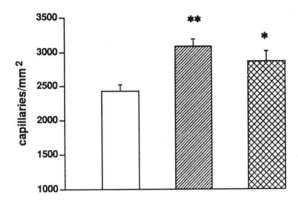

MAXIMAL CORONARY BLOOD FLOW

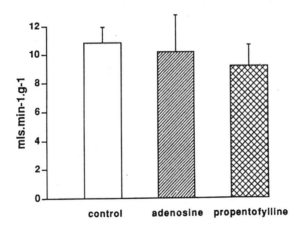

*Figure 9.2 The effects of long-term (3-5 weeks) administration of coronary vasodilators adenosine (hatched columns) and propentofylline (cross-hatched columns) on left ventricular capillary density and maximal coronary blood flow, in comparison with control values (open columns)7 (reference 14) p<0.02, **p<0.001 v. control values.*

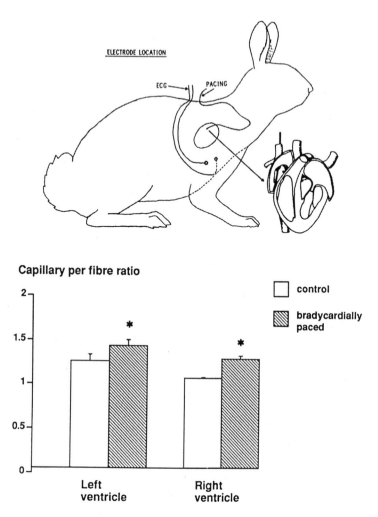

Figure 9.3 Top figure shows right atrial location of electrodes in the rabbit heart for bradycardial pacing. Pacing stimuli were delivered linked to endogenous depolarizations so that every second mechanical beat was eliminated. Subcutaneous ECG electrodes were used to monitor heart rate reduction, which was maintained at ~ 50%[38]. Bottom figure shows left and right ventricular capillary-per-fibre ratios after 2-4 weeks pacing-induced bradycardia. *$p < 0.05$ v. control values.

is normalized after longer (7 months) duration hypertrophy.[23] Kayar & Weiss[27] have confirmed these findings by reporting an increased total capillary length in rabbit hearts with renal hypertension. In a recent review, Hudlicka et al[5] noted that capillary growth does occur in the heart enlargement due to anaemia, which is due to hyperplasia rather than hypertrophy of myocytes.

Even where capillary supply is decreased, the number of arterioles in the hypertrophied heart is either unaffected[28,29] or may be increased if the hypertrophic stimulus is of sufficient duration.[30] The decrease in wall/lumen ratio[31] which is responsible for increased minimal coronary vascular resistance in hypertrophic heart[32] can, to a certain degree, be compensated for by the increased lumen of large epicardial arteries.[30] In humans, volume overload due to aortic valve insufficiency also resulted in increased size of coronary arteries which regressed after valve replacement.[33] *(Figure 9.4)* Gerova et al[34], on the other hand, did not find any change in coronary artery diameter in volume overload hypertrophy in rabbits, but observed changes in the ultrastructure of smooth muscle cells, suggesting remodelling from contractile towards a "synthetic" phase.

Several studies have examined whether exercise can remedy the deficiency in capillary supply of the hypertrophied heart but have found it ineffective.[35] However, capillary supply can be normalized in the hypertrophic heart by treatments which eliminate or block sympathetic nerve influences[36] or by vasodilators such as nifedipine.[37] Furthermore, long-term treatment with a bradycardic drug, alinidine, actually increased capillary per fibre ratio above normal levels in the hypertrophied hearts of rats with renal hypertension[17], and long-term bradycardial pacing of hearts with volume overload hypertrophy in rabbits increased significantly capillary density, although not maximal coronary flow[38], indicating that a capacity for microvascular growth exists even under conditions of pathological hypertrophy.

Growth of vessels in ischemic hearts

Growth of collateral vessels after narrowing of the left circumflex coronary artery, assessed on the basis of retrograde flow, was described in dogs by Eckstein in 1957.[39] More direct evidence was later provided by Rees and Redding[40] using resin perfusion and angiography *(Figure 9.5)*, and by Schaper[2], using either angiography or incorporation of ^{3}H-thymidine in collateral vessels in dogs with the left circumflex coronary artery gradually occluded by an ameroid constrictor. The labelling index increased to 8% in the intima within 2 days of occlusion and gradually decreased to 1-3% after 5 days, while the labelling index in the media increased from 0 to about 2% within the same period.[41] However, in view of the similarity between pig and human coronary vascular anatomy, it may be more appropriate to study the responses of this species. For example, constriction of the cicumflex artery in dogs leads to enlargement of pre-existing epicardial vessels whereas in pigs, as in humans, there is a development of a subendocardial plexus.[3] Growth of collaterals in pigs, assessed by DNA labelling index, was most intensive 2 weeks after ameroid occlusion and declined steadily to levels similar to sham-operated animals (close to zero) 8 weeks after the operation, by which time collateral flow was established.[42] *(Figure 9.6)* In human hearts, Schaper and colleagues[3] have described endothelial cell division at the time of critical stenosis during gradual arterial occlusion with thin-walled vein-like vessels appearing 6-12 weeks after complete occlusion.

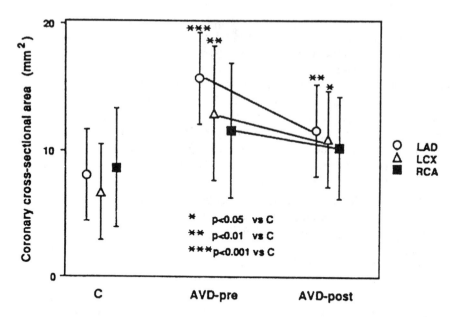

Figure 9.4 *Coronary arteries: area before (AVD-pre) and after (AVD-post) aortic valve
replacement.* *Taken from Villari et al[33], showing enlargment of coronary arteries in
patients with volume-overload cardiac hypertrophy due to aortic valve disease, and
partial regression of enlargment following surgical valve replacement. Reproduced with
permission of Circulation, copyright 1992, the American Heart Association, and the
authors.*

Larger vessels show growth after ischemia, but capillaries show a deficit both
in the infarct border zone and in the non-infarcted myocardium, which undergoes
hypertrophy[6] indicating that their growth response is limited. Physical training for 4
weeks after coronary ligation in rats normalized capillary supply in the border zone[43]
and long-term bradycardial pacing resulted in slightly but not significantly higher
capillary density in rabbit hearts with subendocardial necroses.[44] In pigs, long-term
electrically-induced bradycardia significantly increased capillary density both in the
border zone and in the unaffected part of the left ventricle.[45] In contrast to the
normal heart, it appears that exercise may enhance collateral development in animals.[10] Although Cohen[46] reported an increased collateral blood flow in trained
dog hearts, he considered clinical studies on the effects of exercise on collateral
circulation in humans to be inconclusive.

Many studies have investigated interventions aimed at reducing infarct size
and/or increasing collateral blood flow, but few have examined the long-term effects of these on collateral growth. The development of collaterals in response to
repeated bouts of ischemia was accelerated by heparin treatment in both animals
and patients[47,48], but collateral flow was not improved by removal of constrictor

influences by prior sympathectomy in rabbits.[49] Vasodilators such as glycerol trini-trate enhanced collateral flow[47,48], but nifedipine failed in this respect, possibly because the reactivity of collaterals differs from that of normal vessels.[50] Prior long-term β-blockade was found to reduce infarct size in dogs[51] and from clinical studies, it is clear that β-blockade offers the most effective long-term cardioprotection post-infarct[52] Whether this is due to enhancement of collateral growth is not known, but β-blockade combines positive effects on coronary perfusion with bradycardia, both of which can induce vascular growth.

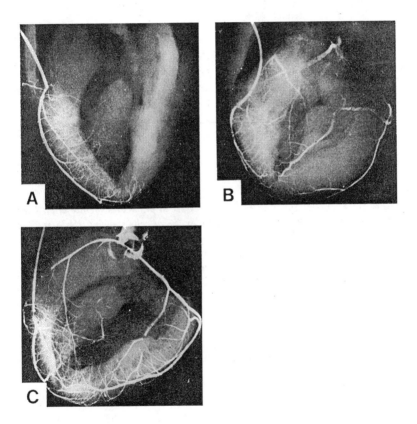

Figure 9.5 Post-modern angiographic evidence of collateral development in dog hearts, taken from Rees and Redding[40], by permission of Cardiovascular Research, copyright 1967. A normal heart after injection through left anterior descending artery (LAD), showing good filling of fine arterioles, no retrograde filling of other coronary vessels. B and C - hearts taken at intervals after ligation of the LAD distal to the large septal branch. C - 10 days post-ligation, showing enlarged anastomoses around the obstruction with retrograde filling of other main coronary arteries. B - 3 months after ligation, showing larger anastomoses at the apex and retrograde filling.

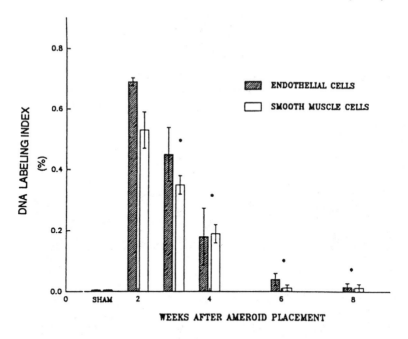

Figure 9.6 DNA labeling index in collateral vessels in pig hearts (White et al, Circ. Res, 71: 1490-1500, 1992). DNA labelling index (% of cells showing 3H-thymidine incorporation in relation to all cells observed) of endothelial and smooth muscle cells in coronary collateral vessels in pig hearts at intervals during gradual occlusion of the left anterior descending coronary artery by an ameroid constrictor. Closure of the ameroid occurs at approximately 3 weeks. Reproduced by permission of Circulation Research, copyright 1992, the American Heart Association, and the authors[42].

Factors involved in growth of vessels

Mechanical factors. The stimulus for growth of coronary collateral vessels has been sought for many years. The comparatively rapid response of collateral circulation to acute coronary artery occlusion - 1-3 days[53] - suggests that ischemia itself may trigger angiogenesis. Indeed, it has been shown subsequently that repetitive brief occlusions of a major coronary artery in dogs lead to progressive augmentation of collateral blood flow [54]. However, ischemia and/or increased metabolic demand such as during exercise also lead to increases in blood flow, which was identified long ago as an important factor in the growth of the vascular bed.[55,56] The contribution of flow to remodelling of large arteries has been recently reviewed[57] and the role of flow-related factors in capillary growth was reviewed by Hudlicka et al.[5]

Increased blood flow could be an important physical stimulus for vessel growth by increasing shear stress across the endothelial surface, or by increasing vessel wall tension, both of which could trigger the angiogenic cascade. In capillaries, this latter involves disturbance of the basement membrane by proteolytic enzymes, followed by endothelial cell migration, mitosis and formation of sprouts[58] while in larger vessels, the internal elastic lamina could be disturbed by leucocyte elastase or plasminogen activators, the matrix between the smooth muscle cells lysed, and some smooth muscle cells possibly undergo necrosis, thereby making space for new growth and arterial enlargement.[59] The initial release/activation of proteolytic enzymes may come either from the luminal side of the vessel in response to shear stress, and possibly increased wall tension as a result of increased blood flow, or alternatively from the abluminal side via stretch and wall tension or tissue damage.

Increased shear stress results from increased vessel diameter and velocity, and could operate as an angiogenic stimulus in situations where blood flow is increased, such as exercise training or administration of vasodilators. For example, capillary growth was induced in both normal and infarcted hearts by long-term administration of dipyridamole, which was shown to increase the velocity of flow through capillaries[60], and significantly elevated shear stress, calculated from the available data on capillary diameters and velocities. There is also direct evidence from tissue culture for the role of shear stress in the inducement of endothelial cell growth[61] and for the link between shear stress and endothelial cell proliferation being plasminogen activator.[62] It is unlikely, however, that shear stress could explain capillary growth induced either by long-term bradycardial pacing or growth of collaterals in ischemic hearts. In the first case, maximal coronary blood flow was not increased, and a relatively small increase in shear stress due to increased blood flow during the prolonged diastole could not offset the much greater shear stress occurring during systole [64]. In the second case, evidence of cell proliferation was located not only in arteries, but also in veins where the shear stress would be low, due to a low velocity of flow.[3]

Increased capillary wall tension as a stimulus to vessel growth can be due to either increased pressure or diameter, and it could lead to disruption of the basement membrane and release of various proteolytic enzymes. This could be operative during capillary growth in response to endurance training, which is linked with bradycardia, and pacing- or drug-induced bradycardia, since capillary diameters, and hence wall tension, are wider during diastole (which is prolonged) than during systole.[63] Again, such a hypothesis is corroborated by the finding, in tissue culture experiments, that endothelial cells are more proliferative when stretched or undergoing cyclic strain, this proliferation being mediated via protein kinase C, which catalyzes protein phosphorylation and can be activated either directly by diacyloglycerol or indirectly by IP_3, both of which are released by endothelial cells in cultures in response to increased shear stress or repeated stretch.[22]

Repeated stretch is quite clearly acting all the time in a beating heart. However, if the force of contraction is increased, which is certainly the case during exercise training or any form of bradycardia which prolongs diastolic filling, capillaries, which are nominally quite tortuous in the heart *(Figure 9.7)*, will be stretch for a prolonged period of time, which could again lead to a disturbance of their basement membrane. Indeed, in experiments where increased force of contraction was induced by chronic administration of a positive inotropic drug dobutamine[65], capillary growth occurred in the absence of bradycardia or increased coronary blood flow.

To what extent mechanical factors are involved in the growth of arterioles or larger coronary vessels remains open to speculation. Schaper[2] originally suggested

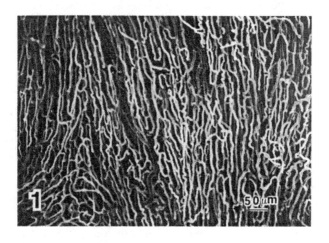

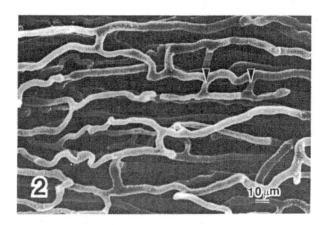

Figure 9.7 Vascular corrosion casts of the capillary bed in the rat left ventricle examined by scanning electron microscopy at low (top) and high (bottom) magnification. Reproduced by permission of Scanning Electron Microscopy 1986/IV, Hossler et al[76].

increased wall tangential stress or differences in pressure gradients as a stimulus for collateral growth, but later discounted this because cellular proliferation was observed in veins which would have low shear stress and pressure.[3] However, high shear stress can cause proliferation of endothelial cells in large vessels, and high pressure is notorious as a stimulus for growth of smooth muscle cells.[5]

Growth factors. A low molecular (about 300 Daltons) factor has been identified in infarcted human hearts at a time when collaterals are presumably growing[66] and also in bradycardially-paced hearts in which capillary growth is intensive.[67] More recently, growth factors studied in connection with the heart include both acidic and basic fibroblast growth factors (aFGF and bFGF), transforming growth factor beta (TGFbeta) and vascular endothelial growth factor (VEGF).[68] It appears that aFGF, TGFbeta, and VEGF are located mainly in myocytes, while bFGF-like activity is found mainly in blood vessels in capillary and venular endotbelium.[69] TGFbeta usually inhibits angiogenesis but contributes to formation of collagen, while a and bFGF and VEGF are all mitogenic for endothelial cells. Elevated expression of aFGF, VEGF and TGFbeta, but not bFGF, has been shown ischemic collateralized porcine myocardium, indicating a role in angiogenesis, but their specific functions have yet to be defined.[68]

Interaction between the mechanical and growth factors. Fibroblast growth factors are supposedly stored in the basement membrane, but since neither aFGF nor bFGF genes have the signal peptide to direct their secretion, it is assumed that they can only stimulate angiogenesis if they are released when the basement membrane is injured - a mechanism suggested by e.g. D'Amore & Orlidge.[70] It has been recently shown that increased hydrostatic pressure can induce release of bFGF from endothelial cells in cultures[71], and thus increased capillary pressure or wall tension could trigger its activation. Similarly, stretch of the capillary basement membrane during increased myocyte lengthening or more forceful contraction may disturb the basement membrane and release some of the stored growth factor. However, since Parker and Schneider[72] did not find expression of FGFs in hearts exposed to increased haemodynamic load, and our preliminary results did not demonstrate any relationship between mRNA for bFGF and capillary supply in bradycardially-paced hearts with increased capillary density[64], it is not clear whether these factors induce angiogenesis in normal hearts.

In contrast, the presence of mRNA for both aFGF and TGFβ in ischemic hearts suggests that they are released from myocytes in the vicinity of necrotic areas. While angiogenic molecules, such as a and bFGF, stimulate production of collagenase and plasminogen activators, which would degrade the basement membrane and thus initiate capillary growth[73] TGFβ accentuates matrix accumulation[74] and possibly prevents endothelial proliferation by mediating the inhibitory effect of pericytes on endothelial cells.[75] A tight balance between these factors would then help to maintain a relatively constant vascularization in the normal heart, which would be disturbed by ischemia. Release of FGFs could then stimulate growth of vessels, while TGFβ would stimulate accumulation of collagen and thus contribute to the healing of the infarcted tissue.

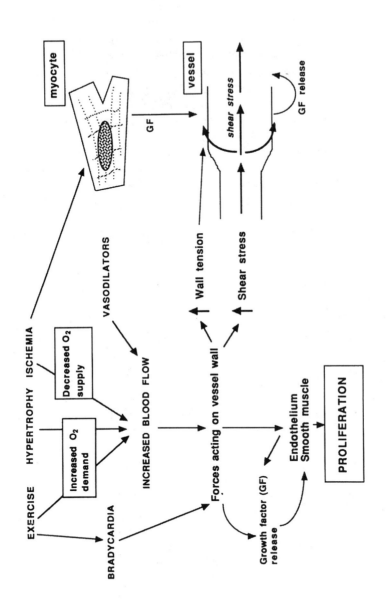

Figure 9.8 Schematic representation of physical factors which act upon blood vessel walls - shear stress and wall tension - in response to increased blood flow and/or bradycardia - and their interaction with growth factors in determining the proliferation of endothelial and smooth muscle cells.

In conclusion, evidence from studies in adult hearts under both normal and pathological conditions shows that both large and small vessels have some capacity to grow in response to either increased metabolic demand on the myocardium (exercise, hypertrophy) or decreased oxygen supply (following coronary vessel occlusion). However, the growth may be selective, involving either enlargment of pre-existent collateral vessels, and/or development of larger vessels and/or capillaries. The duration of stimulus is clearly important in determining the extent to which growth progresses in e.g. hypertrophy. It is becoming increasingly accepted that physical forces such as shear stress and circumferential tension acting on the blood vessel wall, as a result of increased blood flow and/or bradycardia, have a significant impact on both endothelium and vascular smooth muscle and can modulate the proliferative state of these cells *(Figure 9.8)*. The interaction of these forces with growth factors, present either in surrounding myocytes or the blood vessels themselves, requires further investigation to establish the specific nature of their relationship under different conditions of vascular growth. In terms of therapeutic interventions which may promote vessel growth in the vascularly-compromised heart, a combination of vasodilatation with bradycardia should be considered since this would provide the angiogenic stimuli which have already been identified as important for coronary vascular proliferation.

This work was supported by British Heart Foundation and Wellcome Trust.

REFERENCES

1. Maxwell MP, Hearse DJ, Eellon DM. Species variation in the coronary collateral circulation during regional myocardial ischaemia: a critical determinant of the rate of evolution and extent of myocardial infraction. Cardiovasc Res 1987:21:737.

2. Schaper W. "The Collateral Circulation of the Heart". North Holland, Amsterdam, 1971.

3. Schaper W., et al. The collateral circulation of the heart. Progr. Cardiovasc. Dis. 1988:31:57.

4. Engerman RL, Pfaffenbach D, Davis MD. Cell turnover in capillaries. Lab Invest 1967: 17:738.

5. Hudlicka O, Broen M, Egginton S. Angiogenesis in skeletal and cardiac muscle. Physiol. Rev., 1992:72:369-417.

6. Anversa P, et al. Mechanisms of myocyte and capillary growth in the infracted heart. Eur Heart J 1990:11, (Suppl.8) 123.

7. Wyatt HL, Mitchell J. Influences of physical cinditioning and deconditioning on coronary vasculature of dogs. J Appl Physiol 1978:45:619.

8. Pelliccia A, et al. Corornary arteries in physiological hypertrophy: echocardiographic evidence of increased proximal size in elite athletes. Int J Sports Med 1990:11:120.

9. Breisch EA, et al. Exercise-induced cardiac hypertrophy: a correlation of blood flow and microvasculature. J Appl Physiol 1986:60:1259

10. Laughlin MH, McAllister RM. Exercise training-induced coronary vascular adaptation. J Appl Physiol 1992:73:2209.

11. Tomanek RJ. Effects on the extent of the myocardial capillary bed. Anat. Rec., 1970:167:55.

12. Tornling G. Capillary neoformation in the heart of dipyridamole treated rats. Acta Pathol Microbiol Scand 1982:90:269.

13. Mall G, et al. Morphometric analysis of the rabbit myocardium after chronic ethanol feeding - early capillary vhanges. Basci Res Cardiol 1982:77:57.

14. Ziada AMAR, et al. The effect of long-term vasolidation on capillary growth and performance in rabbit heart and skeletal muscle. Cardiovasc Res 1984:18:724.

15. Wachtolva M, Rakusan K, Poupa O. The coronary terminal vascular bed in the heart of the hare (*Lepidus europeus*) and the rabbit (*Oryctolagus domesticus*). Physiol Bohemoslov 1965:14:328.

16. Wachtlova M, et al. The terminal bed of the myocardium in the wild rat (*Rattus norvegicus*) and the laboratory rat (*Rattus norvegicus Lab*). Physiol Bohemoslov 1967:16: 548.

17. Brown MD, Cleasby MJ, Hudlicka O. Capillary supply of hypertrophied rat hearts after chronic treatment with the bradyvardic agent alinidine. J Physiol 1990:427:40P.

18. Tasgal J, Vaughan Williams EM. The effect of prolonged propranolol administration on myocardial transmural capillary density in young rabbits. J Physiol 1981:315:353.

19. Acad BA, et al. Effect of prolonged propranolol administration and withdrawal on perfusion of the myocardial capiallry bed. Cardiovasc Res 1988:22: 793.

20. Wright AJA, Hudlicka O. Capillary growth and changes in heart performance induced by chronic bradycardial pacing in the rabbit. Circ Res 1981:49:469.

21. Brown MD, et al. Long-term bradycardia in the conscious pig produced by electrical pacing: effects on myocardial capillary supply. J Physiol 1994:475:62P.

22. Hudlicka O, Brown MD. Physical forces and angiogenesis. In "Mechanoreception by the Vascular Wall", Ed. GM Rubanyi, Futura Publishing Co Inc Mount Kisco, NY 1993. p.197.

23. Tomanek RJ. Age as a modulator of coronary capillary angiogenesis. Circulation, 1992:86:320.

24. Rakusan K, et al. Morphometry of human coronary capillaries during normal growth and the effect of age in left ventricular pressure-overload hypertrophy. Circulation, 1992:86: 38.

25. Rakusan K. Microcircfulation in the stressed heart. In "The Stressed Heart", Ed. MJ Legato, Boston, MA Nijhoff, 1987, p.107.

26. Tomanek RJ, Searls JC, Lachenbruch PA. Quantitative changes in the capillary bed during developing peak and stabilized hypertrophy in a spontaneously hypertensive rat. Circ Res 1982:51:295.

27. Kayar S. Weiss HR. Diffusion distances, total capillary length and mitochondrial volume in pressure-overload myocardial hypertrophy. J Mol Cell Cardiol 1992:24:1155.

28. Rakusan K, Wicker P. Morphometry of the small arteries and arterioles in the rat heart: effects of chronic hypertnesion and exercise. Cardiovasc Res 1990:24:278.

29. Tomanek RJ. Response of the coronary vasculature to myocardial hypertrophy. J Am Coll Cardiol 1990:15:528.

30. Tomanek RJ, et al. Morphometry of canine coronary arteries, arterioles and capillaries during hypertnesion and left ventricular hypertrophy. Circ Res 1986:58: 38.

31. Strauer BE. The concept of coronary vascular reserve. J. Cardiovasc. Pharmacol 1992:19:S 67.

32. Tomanek RJ, et al. Coronary blood flow in senescent rats with late onset hypertension. Am J Physiol 1993:264: H1854.

33. Villari B, et al. Regression of coronary artery dimensions after successful aortic valve replacement. Circulation, 1992:85:972.

34. Gerova M, et al. Remodelling and functional alterations of the rabbit coronary artery in volume overloaded heart. Cardiovasc Res 1993:27: 2005.

35. Rakusan K, et al. Failure of swimming exercise to improve capillarization in cardiac hypertrophy of renal hypertensive rats. Circ Res 1987:18:641.

36. Torry RJ, et al. Sympathectomy sti,ulates capillary but not precapillary growth in hypertrophic hearts. Am J Physiol 1991:260:H1515.

37. Turek Z, et al. Improved myocardial capillarisation in spontaneously hypertensive rats treated with nifedipine. Cardiovasc Res 1987:21: 725.

38. Wright AJA, Hudlicka O, Brown MD. Beneficial effect of chronic bradycardial pacing on capillary growth and heart performance in volume overload heart hypertrophy. Circ Res 1989:64: 1205.

39. Eckstein RW. Effect of exercise and coronary artery naroowing on coronary collateral circulation. Circ Res 1957:5:230.

40. Rees JR, Redding VJ. Anastomotic blood flow in experimental myocardial infarction. Cardiovasc. Res 1967:1: 169.

41. Rasyk S, et al. DNA synthesis in coronary collaterals after coronary artery occlusion in conscios dog. Am J Pgysiol 1982:242: H1031.

42. White FM, et al. Coronary collateral development in swine after coronary artery occlusion. Circ Res 1992:71: 1490.

43. Przyklenk K, Groom AAC. Effects of exercise frequency, intensity and duration on revascularization in the transition zone of infracted rat hearts. Can J Physiol Pharmacol 1985:63: 273.

44. Brown MD, Hudlicka O. Protective effects opf long-term bradycardial pacing against catecholamine-induced myocardial damage in rabbit hearts. Circ Res 1988:62: 965.

45. Brown MD, et al. A novel method of experimental bradycardia applied to hearts with myocardial infraction: effects on capillary supply. Br Heart J in press.

46. Cohen MV. Exercise and coronary collaterals. Am Heart J 1993:125: 1807.

47. Fujita M, . Improvement of treadmill capacity and collateral circulation as a result of exercise with heparin pretreatment in patients with effort angina. Circulation 1988:77: 1022.

48. Fujita M, et al. Effects of glycerol trinitrate on functionally regressed newly developed collateral vessels in conscious dogs. Cardiovasc Res 1988:22: 639.

49. Matsuki T, et al. Chronic whole body sympathectomy fails to protect ischemic rabbit hearts. Am J Physiol 1989:256: H 1322.

50. White FC, Roth DM, Bloor CM. Coronary collateral reserve during exercise induced isschemia in swine. Basic Res Cardiol 1989:84: 42.

51. Euler DE, Hughes PJ, Scanlon PJ. Comparison of the effects of acute and chronic betablockade on infract size in the fodg after circumflex occlusion. Cardiovasc Drugs Ther 1988:2: 2310.

52. Kendall MJ. Beta blockade and cardioprotection. Science Press Ltd., London, 1991.

53. Schaper W., et al. Molecular biologic concepts of coronary anastomoses. J. Am. Coll. Cardiol 1990:15: 513.

54. Sasayama S, Fujita M. Recent insights into coronary collateral circulation. Circulation 1992:85: 1197.

55. Thoma R. Untersuchungen ber die Histogenese und Histomechanik des Gef systems. Enke Verlag, Stuttgart, 1893.

56. Clark ER. Studies on the growth of blood vessels in the tail of the frog. Am J Anat 1918:23: 37.

57. Langille B. Remodelling of developing and mature arteries - ebdothelium, smooth muscle and matrix. J Cardiovasc Pharmacol 1993:21: 1: S11.

58. Folkman J, Klagsbrun M. Angiogenic factors. Science 1987:235: 442.

59. Schaper W. Angiogenesis in adult heart. In "Endothelial mechanisma of vasomotor control" Eds. H. Drexler, AM Zeiher, E Bassenge & H Just, Steinkopff Verlag, Darmstadt, 1991, p51.

60. Tillmans H, et al. The effect of coronary vasolidators on the microcirculation of the ventricular myocardium. In "Microcirculation of the heart". Eds. H Tillmans, W Kobler, H Zebe, Springer Verlag, Berlin, Heidelberg, 1982, p305.

61. Ando J, Nomura H, Kamiya A. The effect of fluid shear stress on the migration and proliferation of cultured endothelial cells. Microvasc Res 1987:33:62.

62. Diamond SL, et al. Tissue plasminogen activator messenger RNA levels increase in cultured human endothelial cells exposed to laminar shear stress. J Cell Physiol 1987:173: 364.

63. Tillmans TH, et al. Microcirculation in the ventricle of the dog and turtle. Circ Res 1974:34: 561.

64. Hudlicka, O. Mechanical factors involved in the growth of the heart and its blood vessels. Cell Mol Biol Res in press.

65. Brown MD, Hudlicka O. Capillary supply and cardiac performance in the rabbit after chronic dobutaminhe treatment. Cardiovasc Res 1991:25: 909.

66. Kumar S, et al. Angiogenesis factor from human myocardial infracts. Lancet, 1983:2: 354.

67. Hudlicka O, et al. Can growth of capillaries in the heart and skeletal misucle be explained by the presence of an angiogenic factor? Br J Exp Pathol 1989:70: 237.

68. Sharma HS, Zimmerman R. Growth factors and development of coronary collaterals. In "Growth factors and the cardiovascular system". Ed. P. Cummins, Kluwer Academic Publishers, Boston, 1993, p119.

69. Casscels W, et al. Isolation, characterization and localization of heparin-binding growth factors in the heart. J Clin Invest 1990:85: 433.

70. D'Amore PA, Orlidge A. Growth factors and pericytes in microangiography. Diabetes Metab 1988:14: 495.

71. Acevedo AD, et al. Morphological proliferative responses of endothelial cells to hydrostatic pressure - role of fibroblast growth factor. J Cell Physiol 1993:157: 603.

72. Parker TG, Schneider MD. Growth factors, proto-oncogenes and plasticity of the cardiac phenotype. Ann Rev Physiol 1991:53: 179.

73. Folkman J, Shing Y. Angiogenesis. J Biol Chem 1992:267: 10931.

74. Davidson JM, Zoia O, Liu JM. Modulation of transforming growth factor-beta-1-sti,ulatede elastin and collagen production and proliferation in porcine vascular smooth muscle cells and skin fibroblasts by basic fibroblast growth factor alpha and insulin-like growth factor-1. J Cell Physiol 1993:155: 149.

75. Antonelli-Orlidge A, et al. An activated form of TGFbeta is produced by co-cultures of endothelial cells and pericytes. Proc Natl Acad Sci USA, 1989: 86: 4544.

76. Hossler FE, Douglas JE, Douglas CE. Anatomy and morphology of myocardial capillaries studied with vascular corrosion casting and scanning electron microscopy: a method used for rat hearts. Scanning Electron Microscopy 1986, p1469.

Section B
HYPERTENSION

10 INSULIN RESISTANCE, AND HYPERTENSION

Frederick B. Slogoff, Eric J. Wasserman, Robert A. Phillips

The clinical states of non-insulin dependent diabetes mellitus (NIDDM), essential hypertension, and cardiovascular disease are major causes of morbidity and mortality in the United States. The prevalence of NIDDM in the U.S. currently approaches 5 to 7 percent.[1] In 1992 this resulted in a cost to the health care system of approximately \$45 billion.[2] On a similar scale, cardiovascular disease contributes to approximately 900,000 deaths per year in the United States, nearly 40 percent of deaths due to all causes.[3] Furthermore, essential hypertension is perhaps the most prevalent cardiovascular disease affecting an estimated 50 million Americans.[3]

Over the past 25 years each of these conditions has been linked to the presence of either insulin resistance or its resulting hyperinsulinemia, and this may contribute to the clustering of these diseases in certain individuals. Indeed, insulin resistance may be the common etiologic factor which underlies this constellation of diseases. The insulin resistance syndrome (IRS), or Syndrome X, are terms now used to define the association between insulin resistance and NIDDM, essential hypertension, dyslipidemia and cardiovascular disease.

Insulin action and the causes of insulin resistance

Insulin is the central hormone of intermediary metabolism, responsible for directing the utilization of glucose and its conversion to stored glycogen. The predominant target tissues for insulin action, with respect to the storage and breakdown of glucose, are liver, skeletal muscle, and fat. Insulin resistance is traditionally defined as a diminished ability of insulin to stimulate glucose disposal. The insulin receptor is composed of two α-subunits and two β-subunits. Mutations in the insulin receptor leading to insulin resistance are exceedingly rare and are not the cause of insulin resistance in most subjects.[4] After the a-subunits bind insulin, a signal is sent to the b-subunits to initiate autophosphorylation, which leads to phosphorylation of other intracellular.[5] This cascade of post-receptor events activates the enzymes and transport proteins which lead to the intracellular utilization and storage of glucose, amino acids, and fatty acids.[6] At the same time, gluconeogenesis, lipolysis, and protein breakdown are inhibited. Most evidence suggests that insulin resistance is a result of post-receptor abnormalities. It is thought that the most important defect that leads to insulin resistance is a defect in the conversion of glucose to glycogen within the cell.[5,7]

Because plasma glucose is the predominant feedback regulator of insulin secretion, insulin resistance is usually defined as resistance to insulin-stimulated glucose uptake, predominantly in skeletal muscle.[8-10] Of the various IRS conditions, the progression to NIDDM best illustrates the manner in which insulin resistance evolves into clinical disease. Initially, a genetically predisposed individual is exposed to the proper environmental stimuli and acquires a resistance to insulin action. Consequently, the failure of skeletal muscle to utilize glucose leads to enhanced insulin secretion by pancreatic beta cells, in an effort to overcome this target tissue resistance. The result is a compensatory hyperinsulinemia, which can be demonstrated both in the fasting state and in the course of an oral glucose tolerance test (OGTT).[10,11] In this early stage, essential hypertension, dyslipidemia or cardiovascular disease may occur in the absence of NIDDM, representing a manifestation of insulin resistance. After an undetermined length of time, pancreatic insulin output is insufficient to overcome peripheral tissue resistance, leading to the clinical state known as impaired glucose tolerance (World Health Organization (WHO) criteria: fasting plasma glucose < 140 mg/dl and 2-hour plasma glucose between 140 and 200 mg/dl).[12] It is at this stage in the pathogenesis of NIDDM that hyperglycemia can first be detected by an OGTT. Ultimately, beta cells are thought to "burn out" under the constant state of enhanced feedback stimulation. This final step of increasing beta cell failure is characterized by fulfillment of the WHO criteria for diabetes mellitus (i.e., fasting plasma glucose $\geq$140 mg/dl and/or plasma glucose $\geq$200 mg/dl 2 hours after a 75-gram oral glucose load).[12]

Methods of evaluating insulin resistance

A number of methods have been developed to measure insulin action *in vivo*. First, the commonly used oral glucose tolerance test (OGTT), involves the administration of a 75-gram oral glucose load following an overnight fast. Plasma glucose and insulin levels are then measured at 0, 30, 60, 90, and 120 minutes. The presence of impaired glucose tolerance or NIDDM is determined from plasma glucose levels using the WHO criteria. The ratio of insulin to glucose (I/G) at these various intervals as well as a comparison of area under the curve (AUC) of the glucose and insulin levels measured during the test, may also be used to compare glucose tolerance and insulin action among study populations.[13] In a non-diabetic population, AUC of insulin reflects the degree of insulin sensitivity. However, due to variations in glucose absorption, the OGTT is poorly reproducible. Another limitation of the OGTT is the fact that the I/G ratio is dependent upon both the secretion and clearance of insulin, a factor which complicates the assessment of beta cell function.[14] Despite these drawbacks, the OGTT is the simplest test to perform, making it the current test of choice for assessing glucose tolerance in the office setting.

A second test for measuring insulin action is known as the insulin tolerance test (ITT). After determining an individual's plasma glucose level at time zero, an insulin bolus is administered intravenously and the declining plasma glucose is subsequently measured over the next 15 minutes. From these measurements the rate of decline can be calculated, and is known as the k_{ITT} value. A high value indicates a more rapid utilization of glucose. Measurements of plasma glucose are not obtained beyond 15 minutes because they are known to be affected by the counter-regulatory hormonal response that is triggered by insulin-induced hypoglycemia. It is interesting that the k_{ITT} correlates well with estimates of insulin sensitivity obtained from a euglycemic-insulin clamp [15] since it is unlikely that the exogenously administered insulin is acting within 15 minutes; receptor binding and initiation of glucose transport takes at least 30 minutes. The main disadvantages of the ITT, however, are the potential risk of severe insulin-induced hypoglycemia..

A third test, the frequently sampled intravenous glucose tolerance test (FSIGT), utilizes a physiologic "minimal model" as developed by Bergman et al. in 1979.[16,17] This model is used to derive indices of insulin action and secretion. Plasma glucose and insulin are frequently sampled over a 180-minute period, following an intravenous bolus of glucose. The minimal model analyzes these data and calculates an insulin sensitivity (S_I) index, which essentially reflects the rate of glucose disposal per unit of insulin. In a modified version of the FSIGT, tolbutamide, which enhances insulin secretion, is administered at 20 minutes in order to increase insulin concentrations and improve the accuracy of the model. The FSIGT accuracy has been shown to be comparable to the euglycemic-insulin clamp [18-20] (discussed below), and yet it is an easier test to perform. Therefore, this approach lends itself to relatively large population-based assessments of insulin action.

A fourth test, which is considered to be the "gold standard" for measuring insulin action, is the euglycemic-insulin clamp [21]. In this test a constant infusion of insulin is administered for at least 90 minutes, during which time the plasma glucose is held at a constant level by varying the infusion of exogenous glucose. The amount of exogenous glucose required to maintain isoglycemia therefore reflects whole-body glucose disposal, assuming that endogenous glucose production is suppressed. During the insulin infusion, an individual who requires a low amount of exogenous glucose to maintain the steady state has impaired glucose disposal and is insulin resistant. By contrast, an individual who requires a high amount of exogenous glucose to maintain steady state glucose levels during the insulin infusion is insulin sensitive. There are, however, limitations to this approach. First, euglycemic insulin clamp studies are labor intensive, expensive, and require considerable technical skill, curtailing their use in large population-based investigations.[19] Second, a clamp study typically assesses the steady-state response observed two hours after a constant infusion of insulin [21]. It is uncertain whether results obtained under these circumstances can be applied to the normal physiologic state, in which insulin secretion varies according to glucose concentration. Despite these limitations, the euglycemic-insulin clamp is universally accepted as the most accurate measure of insulin sensitivity.

A variation of the euglycemic-insulin clamp, which has been used by some investigators to assess insulin resistance, is known as the insulin suppression test.[22] In this method endogenous insulin secretion is suppressed by an infusion of somatostatin. As in the euglycemic-insulin clamp, a constant infusion of insulin is administered in order to achieve insulinemia in the high physiologic range. This hyperinsulinemia in turn suppresses hepatic glucose output. Exogenous glucose is infused at a constant rate and the steady-state plasma glucose is determined during the last 30 minutes of a 180 minute test period. This value is used to characterize the degree of resistance to insulin stimulated glucose uptake. For instance, a high plasma glucose value reflects impaired glucose disposal due to a greater degree of insulin resistance. Due to the costliness of using somatostatin and the variability in insulin levels achieved, the insulin suppression test is less practical than the euglycemic-insulin clamp.

Evidence for the existence of an insulin resistance syndrome

Cross-sectional studies have provided substantial evidence linking insulin resistance to IRS disorders, [10,11,23] but none can inherently prove that insulin resistance is the cause rather than a consequence. By contrast, the landmark, prospective San Antonio Heart Study conducted by Haffner *et al.*, provides evidence for a causal relationship between insulin resistance and the subsequent development of NIDDM, essential hypertension, and dyslipidemia. In this study 1,288 Mexican Americans and 929 non-Hispanic whites aged 25 to 64 years were evaluated between 1979 and 1982.[12] Baseline examination in this study consisted of plasma lipid, lipoprotein, insulin, and glucose determinations; OGTT; systolic and diastolic blood pressures; and anthropometric measurements (height, weight, subscapular and triceps skinfolds). In 1987 an eight year follow-up study of the 1979-1982 cohort was begun to ascertain the incidence of NIDDM, essential hypertension, and dyslipidemia.

Since there was no statistical evidence for ethnic differences in fasting insulin levels, both Mexican Americans and non-Hispanic whites were pooled and then divided into fasting insulin level quartiles. Fasting insulin was used as a marker of insulin resistance and the subjects with the highest and lowest quartiles of fasting insulin were compared to determine the relative risk of developing various endpoint conditions. Subjects in the highest quartile had a significantly higher incidence of hypertension, hypertriglyceridemia, low HDL-cholesterol, and NIDDM than subjects in the lowest quartile. The odds ratios (OR) were 2.04, 3.46, 1.63, and 5.62, respectively. However, when the two groups were adjusted for age, sex, ethnicity, body mass index (BMI)[1], and centrality index[2], fasting insulin remained associated with the incidence of NIDDM (OR 2.52), hypertriglyceridemia (OR 2.00), and low HDL-cholesterol (OR 1.60) concentrations, but was no longer significantly related to hypertension incidence (OR 1.48, p < 0.140). When the analysis was restricted to lean (BMI < 27 kg/m^2), normoglycemic subjects without a parental history of diabetes, fasting insulin was again found to be independently related to all four endpoints. Therefore, the authors concluded that fasting insulin levels predict the development of all four metabolic abnormalities in this lean, normoglycemic subgroup, and three of the four in the overall study population. It is likely that the results from this study are most likely conservative. That is, the "true" association between insulin resistance and the incidence of metabolic abnormalities could be even stronger if insulin resistance were measured with greater precision, such as with an FSIGT, rather than estimated imperfectly by a single fasting insulin value.

Insulin resistance and essential hypertension

Epidemiological and physiological evidence

One of the first studies to report elevated plasma insulin levels in patients with essential hypertension was performed by Welborn and colleagues in 1966.[24] Since then, many authors have subsequently confirmed these observations.[25,26] In 1987 Reaven and Hoffman proposed that insulin resistance, and more specifically hyperinsulinemia, might be causally related to the development of hypertension.

In that same year, a cross-sectional study by Ferrannini et al. compared 13 young subjects (38 ± 2 years of age) with untreated essential hypertension, but otherwise normal body weight and normal glucose tolerance, with 11 normotensive control subjects, who were matched for age and body weight.[10] To test whether hypertension is associated with insulin resistance independently of obesity, the authors measured insulin sensitivity using the euglycemic-insulin clamp technique, glucose turnover, and whole-body glucose oxidation. While all subjects demonstrated normal tolerance to a 75-gram load of oral glucose, the hypertensive subjects showed significantly higher 2-hour plasma insulin and glucose concentrations than did the normotensive subjects. During the hyperinsulinemic euglycemic clamp, the hypertensive group demonstrated several features of insulin resistance, including: 1) the hypertensive group required significantly lower amounts of exogenous glucose to maintain plasma glucose at 80 mg/dl; 2) whole-body glucose utilization during the second hour of the clamp study was markedly impaired (by 40 percent) in

---

[1] BMI is computed as weight in kilograms/height in meters squared.

[2] Centrality index is computed as the ratio of subscapular to triceps skinfolds.

the patients with hypertension as compared with the control subjects. Total glucose utilization was found to be inversely related to both systolic and mean blood pressure (r = 0.76 for both, p < 0.001). Indirect calorimetry[1] was used to explore the site of insulin resistance in these hypertensive subjects. It was found that both groups displayed similar rates of glucose oxidation and ability to inhibit lipid oxidation. However, only hypertensives showed a significant deficit in nonoxidative glucose disposal (i.e., glycogen synthesis). The authors suggest that this implicates skeletal muscle as the major site of insulin resistance. Other studies have concurred with this viewpoint, [9,10,27] and it may explain the observation that exercise specifically improves insulin sensitivity by enhancing skeletal muscle blood flow and glucose uptake.[16]

Strong prospective evidence for a relation between insulin resistance and hypertension is a study by Salomaa et al.[28] This showed that individuals who later develop hypertension tend to have relatively impaired glucose tolerance up to 18 years before hypertension becomes clinically manifest.[28] This implies that preclinical insulin resistance may precede and contribute to the development of essential hypertension.

Mechanisms of the relation between insulin resistance and hypertension

There are a number of mechanisms that have been proposed to explain the role of insulin resistance in the pathogenesis of essential hypertension (Figure 10.1). Resnick and colleagues proposed the "ionic hypothesis", which suggests that both insulin resistance and essential hypertension share a common abnormality in cellular ion handling.[29] In their analysis it was shown that systolic and diastolic blood pressure correlate directly with intracellular red blood cell calcium and sodium concentrations and inversely with intracellular magnesium and pH. Recent studies have extended these observations to adipose tissue,[30] pancreatic beta cells,[31] skeletal muscle,[7] vascular smooth muscle,[32] and brain.[13] Altogether, these data suggest that an underlying disturbance in the handling of cellular ions appears to have consequences that are specific to the target tissue involved. This hypothesis would explain the various manifestations seen in the insulin resistance syndrome, such as vasoconstriction and increased arterial blood pressure in vascular tissue, resistance to insulin-stimulated glucose uptake in skeletal muscle and fat, augmented insulin secretion in pancreatic beta cells, and enhanced neurotransmitter release and sympathetic nerve activity in neural tissue.[29]

Through a number of hormonally mediated and impaired counterregulatory mechanisms, hyperinsulinemia may elevate blood pressure as a result of increased sodium reabsorption or decreased sodium excretion. During a hyperinsulinemic euglycemic clamp insulin exerts an anti-natriuretic effect on the kidney.[33] This effect may be mediated directly by insulin's action on the proximal or distal tubule.[34] Increased sympathetic nervous system activity associated with insulin resistance may lead to enhanced angiotensin II-mediated aldosterone production and hence volume expansion.[35] Counterregulatory mechanisms to these effects may be impaired. For example, Abouchacra *et al.* compared 10 hypertensive, insulin resistant patients with 12 normotensive, insulin sensitive subjects on the basis of urinary sodium excretion. They found that the former group displayed a blunted natriuretic response to atrial natriuretic peptide (ANP).[36] Furthermore, other investigators have demonstrated that Type 1 (insulin-dependent) diabetics exhibit significantly lower plasma levels of ANP in response to isotonic NaCl.[37]

Vascular abnormalities, particularly at the level of the endothelial cell, might result in increased peripheral vascular resistance (hypertension) and insulin resistance. Phillips et al. *(Figure 10.2)*, have recently shown that in non-obese patients with borderline hypertension, peripheral vascular resistance is inversely related to insulin sensitivity.[38] Although this relationship might not be causal, there are mechanisms which could link these phenomenon. Insulin causes vasodilation by increasing nitric oxide production.[39] Abnormal vascular function in insulin resistant states with abnormal endothelial function, such as obesity, IDDM and NIDDM can manifest as a blunted vasodilatory response to hyperinsulinemia [40-43] or as an exaggerated pressor response to vasoconstrictors.[44] Hence, in these states the vasodilatory action of insulin might be blunted, and this could result in an elevation of peripheral resistance. Hypertensives have lower basal nitric oxide production [45], and this might make them less sensitive to the vasodilatory actions of insulin.

In turn, abnormal vascular structure or endothelial dysfunction associated with hypertension might promote insulin resistance. Defective insulin-mediated skeletal muscle vasodilatation may account for a significant portion of the insulin resistance associated with obesity and NIDDM, as well as for the range of insulin sensitivity in

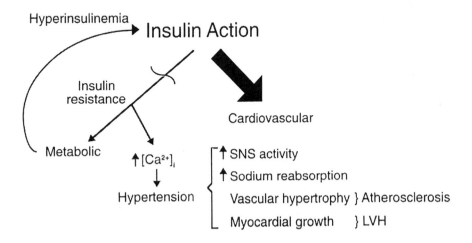

Figure 10.1 Relationship between insulin resistance, hyperinsulinemia and cardiovascular complications. Reprinted with permission from the American Heart Journal [144].

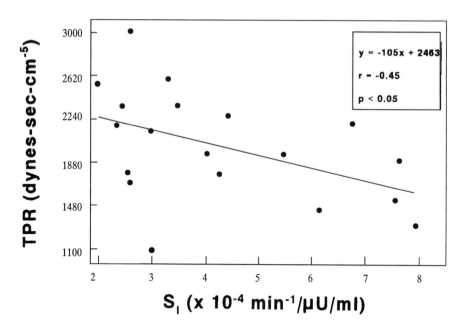

Figure 10.2 Relation between total peripheral resistance (TPR) and insulin sensitivity index (S$_I$). Subjects with lower insulin sensitivity had higher total peripheral resistance. Reprinted with permission from Blood Pressure [38].

normotensives.[40-42] Individuals with low basal nitric oxide production tend to be more insulin resistant.[46] The endothelium is a barrier for insulin transport to the interstitium[47], and blunted transendothelial transport of insulin might result in insulin resistance.[48] The combination in hypertensives of endothelial dysfunction, increased peripheral vascular resistance, and vascular rarefaction might decrease delivery of insulin, leading to impaired glucose uptake and relative insulin resistance.[49,50]

Julius et al. have suggested that elevated sympathetic nervous system tone in hypertension could reduce skeletal blood flow and causes insulin resistance.[49] In support of this concept, Jamerson et al. demonstrated that reflex sympathetically mediated vasoconstriction of the forearm or direct norepinephrine infusion into the forearm causes insulin resistance of that muscle bed.[51,52]

However, the role of the sympathetic nervous system in insulin resistance remains controversial. Insulin infusion significantly raises circulating levels of norepinephrine.[53] Phillips et al. demonstrated that in non-obese patients with borderline hypertension, peripheral vascular resistance, plasma renin activity and circulating levels of catecholamines are related to insulin sensitivity.[38] However, Anderson et al. demonstrated that although insulin infusion in borderline hypertensives causes a marked increase sympathetic nervous system activity, peripheral vascular resistance and blood pressure decreases during the infusion.[54] A study by Supiano et al.[55] found no statistical difference in plasma norepinephrine between normotensive and hypertensive subjects, despite the documented insulin resistance in the latter group. Finally, Baron et al. demonstrated that systematically infused norepinephrine improves insulin sensitivity despite an overall rise in total peripheral vascular resistance.[44] This may be a result of a complex hemodynamic scenario in which splanchnic vascular resistance increases while leg vascular resistance decreases, leading to increased blood flow and improved insulin sensitivity in the leg skeletal muscle bed.

Insulin resistance and coronary artery disease

A noted cross-sectional study completed in 1989 by Zavaroni et al. provided significant evidence linking hyperinsulinemia to risk factors for coronary artery disease (CAD).[56] 247 healthy, normotensive, non-obese subjects with normal glucose tolerance and with no family history of diabetes mellitus were selected from among 732 factory workers and evaluated in order to determine the relationship of plasma insulin to lipid levels and blood pressure. Based on plasma insulin levels, the subjects were divided into hyperinsulinemic and normoinsulinemic subgroups[2] and were matched for age, sex, and BMI, resulting in two final study groups of 32 subjects each. When compared, it was observed that the hyperinsulinemic group had higher concentrations of plasma glucose one hour after an oral glucose challenge, higher plasma triglycerides, lower HDL-cholesterol concentrations, and elevations of systolic and diastolic blood pressure. Other studies had previously shown that the plasma insulin response during an OGTT correlates significantly with resistance to insulin-stimulated glucose uptake.[57,58] Therefore, in this study the authors concluded that hyperinsulinemia directly reflects insulin resistance and is independently associated with a dyslipidemic profile and elevated blood pressures, both of which contribute to CAD risk. Similar findings have been documented in other cross-sectional studies, such as the Bogalusa Heart Study, [59] which evaluated 2,856 children, and the CARDIA Study, [60] which analyzed data from 5,115 participants aged 18-30 years. The main drawback of the above study by Zavaroni and colleagues is its inability to predict which of the subjects will eventually develop the endpoint condition of cardiovascular disease. This is an inherent limitation of its cross-sectional design.

Three prospective studies have examined the relationship between insulin levels and the development of cardiovascular disease. In the Helsinki Policemen Study completed in 1980, Pyorala et al. followed a cohort of 982 men who were 35-64 years of age and free of coronary heart disease (CHD) upon entry into the study.[61] At the baseline examination an OGTT was performed, and fasting, 1-hour, and 2-hour plasma insulin determinations were obtained. Results at follow-up 9 years later revealed that both fatal and non-fatal myocardial infarctions (MI) were more common in those subjects who had the highest fasting, 1-hour, 2-hour, and total plasma insulin responses to a glucose load. Furthermore, multivariate analyses showed that high 1-hour and 2-hour plasma insulin levels were independent predictors of CHD, when blood glucose, plasma cholesterol levels, triglyceride levels, blood pressure, and BMI were taken into account.

A strength of this study by Pyorala *et al.* is its excellent survey response rate of 98.5%, 9 years after the initial examination. Additionally, the endpoints of fatal and non-fatal (MI) were documented in all cases. However, the use of (MI) as the criterion for classifying an individual with CHD ignores the lesser manifestations of CHD (e.g., angina pectoris). This may lead to an underestimation of the true association between insulin levels and cardiovascular disease (i.e., misclassification bias). Another possible drawback of this study is the issue of generalizability; Helsinki policemen may not be representative of other general populations. Despite these limitations, this important study provides convincing evidence that hyperinsulinemia independently contributes to the atherosclerotic process which culminates in cardiovascular disease.

Further prospective evidence for this association is derived from the Paris Prospective Study of 7,534 men aged 43-54 working in the Paris civil service.[62] In this study Fontbonne *et al.* found that the highest incidence of CHD occurred in those subjects with the highest fasting and 2-hour plasma insulin levels. Insulin to glucose (I/G) ratios, both fasting and at 2 hours, were also related to CHD incidence. A limitation of both the Paris Prospective and Helsinki Policemen studies, however, is that neither cohort included women, raising the question of whether gender differences exist in the relationship of hyperinsulinemia to cardiovascular disease. Addressing this concern, a third prospective study by Welborn et al. of 3,390 Western Australians demonstrated that the plasma insulin level was significantly related to the development of CHD in men aged 60-69 years, but not in women of any age.[63]

The mechanism through which insulin contributes to atherogenesis in the evolution of cardiovascular disease is not completely understood, but experimental studies have provided some clues. Early evidence from animal studies demonstrated that insulin, when injected into an artery, causes proliferative and atherosclerotic changes not observed in a saline-injected artery.[64] Subsequently, cell culture studies have shown that insulin stimulates the proliferation of human vascular smooth muscle cells, possibly by interacting with the insulin-like growth factor-1 (IGF-1) receptor.[65] Also, insulin and other growth factors are known to enhance the accumulation of intracellular cholesterol *in vitro* by increasing LDL-receptor activity and decreasing HDL-receptor activity in human fibroblasts.[66] Insulin causes release of endothelin [67], which may lead to coronary vasoconstriction and reduce coronary flow reserve. While the *in vivo* relevance of these findings in humans has yet to be

---

[1]   "Indirect calorimetry" is a technique in which oxygen consumption and carbon dioxide production are measured with an airtight canopy around the subject's neck, in this case during the euglycemic clamp period. Rates of whole-body carbohydrate and lipid oxidation, as well as overall energy consumption can then be calculated from these values.

[2]   Hyperinsulinemia was defined as a fasting or post-glucose load plasma insulin level > 2 S.D. higher than the mean of the 247 index subjects. Normoinsulinemia was within 1 S.D. of this mean.

determined, the existing evidence strongly supports a direct role for insulin in the multifactorial process of atherogenesis that underlies cardiovascular disease.

An important clinical syndrome intimately related to the discussion of insulin resistance and CAD is characterized by the presence of anginal chest pain by history, a positive exercise stress test, and a lack of significant evidence for CAD by angiogram.[9] Due to the absence of large vessel disease, this clinical triad has been referred to as microvascular angina, and is alternatively termed the cardiologist's Syndrome X. In view of the confusion engendered by this latter name, it is important to distinguish this from the metabolic Syndrome X which has been the focus of this current review. The immediate defect responsible for the myocardial ischemia observed in patients with this syndrome appears to be functional in nature, and may involve an impairment in the vasodilatory reserve of the coronary arteries.[68] Important observations in patients with microvascular angina have been that they are both hyperinsulinemic in response to a glucose challenge[69] and insulin resistant when assessed by the euglycemic-insulin clamp.[70] Thus, it appears that some individuals may manifest microvascular coronary disease, rather than developing the large vessel atherosclerosis more commonly associated with the metabolic Syndrome X.

Insulin resistance and left ventricular hypertrophy

Increased blood pressure and other hemodynamic factors are signals for myocardial growth.[71] However, for the same level of blood pressure there is wide variation among individuals both in the degree of left ventricular mass and vascular damage. Careful hemodynamic evaluations indicate that differences in blood pressure, wall stress and wall force account for only about 40% (r=0.66, p <0.001) of the variation in LV mass in hypertensives.[72] This implies that left ventricular mass may be partly determined by nonhemodynamic factors.[73]

There is preliminary evidence that insulin resistance independently contributes to left ventricular mass in non-obese, glucose-tolerant subjects in the early stages of hypertension.[74] In addition, normotensive non-insulin dependent diabetics with insulin resistance are more likely to have left ventricular hypertrophy than insulin-sensitive diabetics.[75] Fasting glucose levels are directly related to the degree of LV hypertrophy in hypertensive non-insulin dependent diabetic subjects.[76] Insulin levels and other less specific indices of insulin resistance have been directly related to left ventricular mass in obese normotensives and in previously treated hypertensives, the majority of whom were obese.[77,78] In the Techumseh Blood Pressure Study of normotensive subjects, higher fasting insulin levels were found in men whose LV mass was in the upper 10th percentile of the population.[79] However, quantitative measures of insulin sensitivity were not performed. Insulin resistance measured by euglycemic clamp has been related to left ventricular wall thickness in a population of mild to moderate hypertensives that included obese subjects.[80] In that study, however, obesity was also directly related to wall thickness and neither LV mass measurement nor its relation to insulin sensitivity was reported. Despite limitations of previous studies, taken together they suggest that hyperglycemia, hyperinsulinemia, or the insulin resistance associated with NIDDM or obesity, may have a significant effect on LV mass.

Insulin resistance and the polycystic ovary syndrome

First identified by Stein and Leventhal in 1935, the polycystic ovary syndrome (PCOS) was described as a clinical triad of hyperandrogenism, chronic anovulation, and obesity in women with enlarged, polycystic ovaries.[81] Dunaif *et al.* demonstrated with the euglycemic-insulin clamp that women with PCOS have marked insulin resistance similar in magnitude to individuals with NIDDM and independent of the degree of obesity.[82] Zimmerman *et al.* showed that women with PCOS, when compared to age- and weight-matched control subjects, did not demonstrate elevated blood pressure despite their profound insulin resistance and hyperinsulinemia.[83] This contrasts with the consistent observation in individuals with Syndrome X that increased blood pressure correlates positively and significantly with hyperinsulinemia and insulin resistance.[84-86] The authors of this study suggested that populations characterized by insulin resistance without hypertension, such as PCOS women and Pima Indians, may possess a more pervasive form of insulin resistance. In other words, whereas the more common form of insulin resistance predominantly affects the skeletal musculature, in these unique individuals their pattern of insulin resistance may also involve sites of blood pressure regulation (e.g., the sympathetic nervous system and the kidney). This would effectively protect these individuals from the insulin-mediated increase in blood pressure which is otherwise observed in essential hypertensive subjects.

Another avenue of investigation raised by the polycystic ovary syndrome is the relationship between insulin resistance and plasma androgen levels. The major determinants of androgen action which have been studied are the plasma free and total testosterone levels, as well as sex hormone binding globulin (SHBG) levels. The latter protein is produced by the liver, primarily under the regulation of insulin, rather than sex steroids.[35] The relationship between these factors and insulin resistance has been found to differ in men and women. For instance, investigators have reported that increased concentrations of plasma testosterone and decreased concentrations of SHBG are associated with hyperinsulinemia in both pre-[87] and postmenopausal women.[88] Furthermore, low levels of SHBG have also been observed to predict the development of NIDDM in women.[89,90] In contrast, a 1994 study by Haffner *et al.* demonstrated in a group of 87 middle-aged men that total testosterone and SHBG were positively associated with insulin sensitivity, measured as wholebody glucose disposal.[91]

Pharmacological treatment of cardiovascular disease in the setting of insulin resistance

Recognizing the existence of an insulin resistance syndrome has had important implications for the treatment of individuals with essential hypertension who either carry a diagnosis of NIDDM or are at high risk for insulin resistance. A number of studies have demonstrated differential effects on glucose tolerance and lipid metabolism by the various beta-adrenergic antagonists, diuretics, ACE inhibitors, calcium channel antagonists, and alpha-1 selective adrenergic antagonists.

In 1993 the Joint National Committee on Detection, Evaluation, and Treatment of High Blood Pressure (JNC V) published their updated recommendations on the choice of initial therapies for essential hypertension.[92] In a controversial decision this committee proposed that in the absence of a contraindication, a diuretic or beta blocker should serve as the first-line agent. This suggestion was based on the fact that these drugs have been the antihypertensive agents in several long-term prospective trials demonstrating their effectiveness at decreasing morbidity and mortality in individuals with hypertension. Therefore, until similar data have been obtained on the newer antihypertensive agents, speculation as to their efficacy must be reserved. Fortunately, a 5 to 7 year trial sponsored by the National Institutes of Health, known as the Antihypertensive and Lipid-Lowering Treatment to Prevent Heart Attack Trial (ALLHAT), is underway and should provide important answers by the beginning of the next decade.

In the absence of results from this important trial, it is debatable if beta-blockers and diuretics are the optimal choices for patients at high risk for coronary artery disease. This notion has arisen from the results of several clinical trials, which have demonstrated that while blood pressure reduction with these agents significantly diminishes the incidence of stroke, congestive heart failure, and renal failure, [93-96] there has been a less than expected effect on the rate of myocardial infarction.[94,97,98] For instance, a meta-analysis by Collins et al., which evaluated the long-term effects of treatment for hypertension, found a 33-50 percent reduction in non-fatal stroke, [99] a figure which matched predictions based on epidemiological data. However, the same study found that clinical trials have demonstrated only a 14 ± 5 percent reduction in CHD events, which is about half of that predicted. A number of factors may have contributed to this discrepancy, including an inadequate duration of follow-up and the possibility that hypertension is a less prominent risk factor for coronary artery disease than it is for cerebrovascular disease. However, some have suggested that the use of beta blockers and diuretics, with their adverse effects on insulin sensitivity and plasma lipids, may have contributed to this finding.

Studies by a number of investigators have documented that diuretics and beta blockers do in fact impair lipid metabolism, as measured by changes in plasma total- and LDL-cholesterol and triglycerides, as well as insulin sensitivity.[100-102] Pollare et al. in 1989 confirmed that patients on hydrochlorothiazide for the treatment of essential hypertension experienced significant increases in plasma total cholesterol,

LDL-cholesterol, and total and VLDL triglyceride levels, along with an impairment in insulin sensitivity, when compared with placebo.[100] The evidence that beta blockers can also impair insulin sensitivity and lipid metabolism in hypertensive patients has been equally as convincing, and according to a follow-up to the 1989 study by Pollare et al., regardless of whether selective or nonselective beta-1 antagonists were utilized, insulin sensitivity was diminished by about 25%.[103] Furthermore, a review by Lithell et al., in which each of the five major classes of antihypertensives were evaluated by IVGTT, found that beta blockers that are selective (metoprolol and atenolol), nonselective (propranolol), or non-selective with intrinsic sympathetic activity (pindolol) each significantly impaired insulin sensitivity.[104] Metoprolol and atenolol decreased the insulin sensitivity index by 27% and 23%, respectively, while propranolol's effect was 30% and pindolol's reduction was about 17%.

The use of diuretics in diabetics is controversial. Concern that diuretics may be deleterious in diabetics was raised by a retrospective analysis by Warram et al. In a 1991 publication from the Joslin Diabetes Center they found that diabetics treated with diuretics for control of hypertension had a 3.8 times higher risk of cardiovascular mortality than patients with untreated hypertension.[105]

While this finding raises concern, due to the retrospective nature of the study it is important to consider the possibility that diuretic use was merely a marker of severe coexisting illness, such as congestive heart failure, rather than the cause of excess mortality. Indeed, the Systolic Hypertension in the Elderly Study (SHEP) showed a 34% reduction in cardiovascular events in elderly hypertensive patients treated with diuretics.[106] However, studies in middle-aged men [107] and women [108], have shown an increased risk of diabetes in patients taking either thiazides or propranolol. Despite these adverse effects on glucose tolerance, however, beta blockers are thought to have beneficial effects on other determinants of cardiovascular disease, such as the coagulation system, arterial wall stress, and the uptake of LDL-cholesterol from blood into the vessel wall.[109] Therefore, the net effect of beta blockers on the atherosclerotic process is presently unclear, and trials such as the ALLHAT should help to determine whether agents that do not adversely effect glucose and lipid metabolism are associated with a greater degree of reduction in cardiovascular mortality per equivalent reduction in blood pressure.

In contrast to diuretics and beta blockers, the newer vasodilating antihypertensive agents have been shown to have either a beneficial effect on insulin sensitivity, or no effect at all. This has prompted some authorities to recommend ACE inhibitors, selective α_1-antagonists, and calcium channel blockers as better alternatives for individuals at high risk of CAD, especially diabetics or patients with the insulin resistance syndrome.[110] In the case of ACE inhibitors, a number of studies have documented their ability to improve insulin sensitivity in individuals with essential hypertension and/or NIDDM [100,111-118], while resulting in either no effect [100] or an improvement [112,119] in lipid metabolism. For instance, Pollare et al. studied a group of 50 patients with essential hypertension in a randomized, double-blind, crossover study comparing the effects on carbohydrate and lipid metabolism of either captopril or hydrochorothiazide, and found that captopril improved insulin sensitivity and did not alter plasma total cholesterol, LDL-cholesterol, or VLDL-triglyceride levels as compared to placebo.[100] These results were further confirmed at follow-up after 2 to 3 years of treatment.[103] The mechanism responsible for the improvement in glucose tolerance may be related to improvements in skeletal muscle blood flow [120], increased potassium levels [112,121], and/or an accumulation of bradykinin [113,122]. Finally, other investigators have addressed the issue of whether or not ACE inhibitors have similar effects in non-insulin resistant hypertensives, and they have found no appreciable effects on insulin sensitivity.[123-125] Thus, the benefits may be limited to those who are insulin resistant.

As in the case of ACE inhibitors, alpha-1 adrenergic antagonists have been extensively studied in hypertensives with or without NIDDM and subsequently shown to have beneficial effects on insulin sensitivity and either a beneficial or no effect on plasma lipids.[126-129] These agents appear to produce a decrease in total cholesterol, LDL-cholesterol, and triglycerides, and an increase in HDL-cholesterol.[130] A recent study by Maheux et al. compared the effects of doxazosin treatment on blood pressure reduction and lipid, insulin, and glucose metabolism in patients with or without NIDDM.[126] Interestingly, they found that while doxazosin significantly improved a number of CAD risk factors in the non-diabetic hypertensive group, the same benefit was not observed in the group with NIDDM and hypertension. In any case, the fact that adverse metabolic effects were not observed in either group and that improvement was demonstrated in one group still lends support to of alpha-1 blockers as a good choice for treating hypertensive individuals with the insulin resistance syndrome.

Calcium channel blockers are considered to be very effective agents for controlling blood pressure in diabetics and are generally neutral with regard to their effects on lipid metabolism. Total, LDL, and HDL-cholesterol, along with triglyceride levels are generally unaffected by calcium channel blockers.[131] In addition, several clinical trials utilizing a number of different representatives of the calcium antagonist class have shown no clinically important effects on glucose tolerance.[132-138] Recent interest has been generated by a new calcium antagonist, monatepil, which possesses alpha$_1$ adrenergic blocking activity and was shown in one study to improve glycemic control (as measured by HbA1c values), total cholesterol, and LDL-cholesterol levels when compared to nitrendipine.[139] Thus, it appears to be the first in a new class of calcium antagonists which may offer a favorable metabolic profile similar to that of the alpha$_1$ blocking agents.

Pharmacological treatment to directly improve insulin sensitivity

Thiazolidinediones are a new class of pharmacological agents that has recently emerged as a promising candidate for improving insulin sensitivity. One such agent, troglitazone (Rizulin), was approved for use in the U.S. in 1996 and is being widely utilized. This drug was evaluated by Nolan et al. in a study involving 18 nondiabetic, obese subjects, half of whom had impaired glucose tolerance.[140] They found that in both groups troglitazone improved insulin resistance, glucose intolerance, hyperinsulinemia, and hypertension. Troglitazone's mechanism of action is not fully understood, but appears to involve direct effects on skeletal muscle, liver, and adipose tissue which lead to an enhanced response to insulin action.[141-143] Reports in late 1997 of liver toxicity associated with its use (one fatal and one requiring liver transplant) prompted the U.S. Food and Drug Administration to recommend that "liver enzyme levels should be mesured in patients taking Rezulin at the start of therapy, every month for the first six months of treatment, every other month for the next six months, and periodiclly thereafter". Given the difficulty inherent in implementing weight reduction and exercise regimens, pharmacological intervention with agents such as troglitazone may soon offer a viable option for possibly preventing the development of overt NIDDM, essential hypertension, and dyslipidemia in individuals that are identified as having insulin resistance.

REFERENCES

1. Yki-Jarvinen H: Pathogenesis of non-insulin-dependent diabetes mellitus. Lancet 1994;343:91

2. Keen H: Insulin resistance and the prevention of diabetes mellitus. N Engl J Med 1994;331:1226

3. U.S.National Center for Health Statistics. Vital and Health Statistics 1992;10:

4. Flier JS: Lilly lecture: Syndromes of insulin resistance. From patient to gene and back again. Diabetes 1992;41:1207

5. Kahn CR: Causes of insulin resistance. Nature 1995;373:384

6. Moller DE: Insulin Resistance. Chichester, England, John Wiley & Sons, 1993, p 1

7. Shulman GI, Rothman DL, Jue T: Quantitation of muscle glycogen synthesis in normal subjects and in subjects with non-insulin-dependent diabetes by ^{13}C nuclear magnetic resonance spectroscopy. The New England Journal of Medicine 1990;322:223

8. DeFronzo RA, et al: Effects of insulin on peripheral and splanchnic glucose metabolism in non-insulin-dependent (type II) diabetes mellitus. J Clin Invest 1985;76:149

9. Reaven GM: Role of Insulin Resistance in Human Disease (Syndrome X): An Expanded Definition. Annual Review of Medicine 1993;44:121

10. Ferrannini E, et al: Insulin resistance in essential hypertension. N Engl J Med 1987;317:350

11. Modan M, et al: Hyperinsulinemia, sex and risk of atherosclerotic cardiovascular disease. Circulation 1991;84:1165

12. Haffner SM, et al: Prospective analysis of insulin-resistance syndrome (symdrome X). Diabetes 1992;41:715

13. Blaustein MP: Sodium ions, calcium ions, blood pressure regulation, hypertension: reassessment and a hypothesis. Am J Physiol 1977;232:C165

14. Alzaid A, Rizza RA: Insulin resistance and its role in the patogenesis of impaired glucose tolerance and non-insulin-dependent diabetes mellitus: perspectives gained from in vivo studies, in Moller DE (ed): Insulin Resistance. New York, Wiley, 1993, pp 143

15. Bonora E, et al: Normal inhibition by somatostatin of glucose-stimulated B-cell secretion in obese subjects. Hormonal and Metabolic Research 1990;22:584

16. Nestler JE: Assessment of insulin resistance. Scientific American 1994;12:58

17. Bergman RN, et al: Quantitative estimation of insulin sensitivity. Am J Physiol 1979;236:E667

18. Swan JW, Walton C, Godsland IF: Assessment of insulin sensitivity in man: a comparison of minimal model- and euglycaemic clamp-derived measures in health and heart failure. Clin Sci 1994;86:317

19. Saad MF, et al: A Comparison Between the Minimal Model and the Glucose Clamp in the Assessment of Insulin Sensitivity Across the Spectrum of Glucose Tolerance. Diabetes 1994;43:1114

20. Bergman RN, et al: Equivalence of the insulin sensitivity index in man derived by the minimal model method and the euglycemic glucose clamp. J Clin Invest 1987;79:790

21. DeFronzo RA, Tobin JD, Andres R: Glucose clamp technique: a method for quantifying insulin secretion and resistance. Am J Physiol 1979;237:E214

22. Sheu WHH, et al: Comparison of the effects of atenolol and nifedipine on glucose, insulin, and lipid metabolism in patients with hypertension. Am J Hypertens 1991;4:199

23. Eriksson J, et al: Early Metabolic Defects in Persons at Increased Risk for Non-Insulin-Dependent Diabetes Mellitus. The New England Journal of Medicine 1989;321:337

24. Welborn TA, et al: Serum insulin in essential hypertension and in peripheral vascular disease. Lance 1966;1:1336

25. Swislocki A, Hoffman BB, Reaven GM: Insulin resistance, glucose intolerance and hyperinsulinemia in patients with hypertension. Am J Hypertens 1989;2:419

26. Sechi LA, et al: Insulin resistance and beta-cell hypersecretion in essential hypertension. J Hypertens 1990;8:S87

27. Lind L, Lithell H, Pollare T: Is it hyperinsulinemia or insulin resistance that is related to hypertension and other metabolic cardiovascular risk factors. J Hypertens 1993;11 Suppl. 4:S11

28. Salomaa VV, et al: Glucose tolerance and blood pressure: long-term follow-up in middle-aged men. BMJ 1991;302:493

29. Resnick LM: Ionic basis of hypertension, insulin resistance, vascular disease, and related disorders: The mechanism of "syndrome X". Am J Hypertens 1993;6:123S

30. Draznin B: Cytosolic calcium: a new factor in insulin resistance? Diabetes Research in Clinical Practice 1991;11:141

31. Hellman B, Sehlin J, Taljedal JB: Calcium and secretion: distinction between two pools of glucose-sensitive calcium in pancreatic islets. Science 1976;194:1421

32. Altura B, Carella A: Mg++-Ca++ interaction in contractility of vascular smooth muscle: Mg++ versus organic calcium channel blockers on myogenic tone and agonist-induced responsiveness of blood vessels. Canadian Journal of Physiologic Pharmacology 1987;65:729

33. Skott P, et al: Effects of insulin on kidney function and sodium excretion in healthy subjects. Diabetologia 1989;32:694

34. DeFronzo RA, et al: The effect of insulin on renal handling of sodium, potassium, calcium, and phosphate in man. J Clin Invest 1975;55:845

35. Landsberg L, et al: Obesity, blood pressure, and the sympathetic nervous system. Annals of Epidemiology 1990;1:295

36. Abouchacra S, et al: Insulin Blunts the Natriuretic Action of Atrial Natriuretic Peptide in Hypertension. Hyper 1994;23:1054

37. Trevisan R, et al: Role of insulin and atrial natriuretic peptide in sodium retention in insulin-treated IDDM patients during isotonic volume expansion. Diabetes 1990;39:289

38. Phillips RA, et al: Hemodynamic and humoral correlates of insulin resistance in non-obese borderline hypertensives - A preliminary report Blood Pressure 1996;1:72

39. Scherrer U, et al: Nitric oxide release accounts for insulin's vascular effects in humans. J Clin Invest 1994;94:2511

40. Laasko M, et al: Decreased effect of insulin to stimulate skeletal muscle blood flow in obese man. J Clin Invest 1990;85:1844

41. Laakso M, et al: Impaired insulin-mediated skeletal muscle blood flow in patients with NIDDM. Diabetes 1992;41:1076

42. Baron AD, et al: Skeletal muscle blood flow: A possible link between insulin resistance and blood pressure. Hypertension 1993;21:129

43. Feldman RD, Bierbrier GS: Insulin-mediated vasodilation: Impairment with increased blood pressure and body mass. Lancet 1993;342:707

44. Baron AD, et al: Interactions between insulin and norepinephrine on blood pressure and insulin sensitivity. Studies in lean and obese men. J Clin Invest 1994;93:2453

45. Forte P, et al: Basal nitric oxide synthesis in essential hypertension [see comments]. Lancet 1997;349:837

46. Petrie JR, et al: Endothelial nitric oxide production and insulin sensitivity. A physiological link with implications for pathogenesis of cardiovascular disease. Circulation 1996;93:1331

47. Jansson PA, et al: Measurement by microdialysis of the insulin concentration in subcutaneous interstitial fluid. Importance of the endothelial barrier for insulin. Diabetes 1993;42:1469

48. Bergman RN, et al: The role of the transcapillary insulin transport in the efficiency of insulin action: studies with glucose clamps and the minimal model. Horm Metab Res Suppl 1990;24:49

49. Julius S, et al: The hemodynamic link between insulin resistance and hypertension. J Hypertens 1991;9:983

50. Pinkney JH, et al: Endothelial dysfunction: Cause of the insulin resistance syndrome. Diabetes 1997;46:S9

51. Jamerson KA, et al: Reflex sympathetic activation induces acute insulin resistance in the human forearm. Hypertension 1993;21:618

52. Jamerson KA, et al: Vasoconstriction With Norepinephrine Causes Less Forearm Insulin Resistance Than a Reflex Sympathetic Vasoconstriction. Hyper 1994;23:1006

53. Rowe JW, et al: Effects of insulin and glucose infusions on sympathetic nervous system activity in normal man. Diabetes 1981;30:219

54. Anderson EA, et al: Insulin increases sympathetic activity but not blood pressure in borderline hypertensive humans. Hypertension 1992;19:621

55. Supiano MA, et al: Hypertension and insulin resistance: role of sympathetic nervous system activity. Am J Physiol 1992;263:E935

56. Zavaroni I, et al: Risk factors for coronary artery disease in healthy persons with hyperinsulinemia and normal glucose tolerance. N Engl J Med 1989;320:702

57. Hollenbeck CB, et al: Relationship between the plasma insulin response to oral glucose and insulin-stimulated glucose utilization in normal subjects. Diabetes 1984;33:460

58. Ferrannini E: Syndrome X. Hormone Research 1993;39:107

59. Burke GL, et al: Fasting plasma glucose and insulin levels and their relationship to cardiovascular risk factors in children: the Bogalusa Heart Study. Metabolism 1986;35:441

60. Manolio TA, et al: Association of Fasting Insulin with Blood Pressure and Lipids in Young Adults - The CARDIA Study. Arteriosclerosis 1990;10:430

61. Pyorala K, et al: Plasma Insulin as Coronary Heart Disease Risk Factor: Relationship to other Risk Factors and Predictive Value during $9^1/_2$-year Follow-up of the Helsinki Policemen Study Population. Acta Med Scand 1985;701:38

62. Fontbonne AM, et al: Hyperinsulinemia as a predictor of coronary heart disease mortality in a healthy population: The Paris prospective study, 15 year follow-up. Diabetologia 1991;34:356

63. Welborn TA, Wearne K: Coronary heart disease incidence and cardiovascular mortality in Busselton with reference to glucose and insulin concentrations. Diabetes Care 1979;2:154

64. Cruz AB, et al: Effect of intra-arterial insulin on tissue cholesterol and fatty acids in alloxandiabetic dogs. Circulatory Research 1961;9:39

65. Bierman EL: Atherogenesis in Diabetes. George Lyman Duff Memorial Lecture. Ateriorscler-Thromb 1992;12:647

66. Oppenheimer MJ, Sundquist K, Bierman EL: Downregulation of high-density lipoprotein receptor in human fibroblasts by insulin and IGF-I. Diabetes 1989;38:117

67. Hu R-M, et al: Insulin stimulates production and secretion of endothelin from bovine endothelial cells. Diabetes 1993;42:351

68. Kurtz TW, Hamoudi AA, Morris RCJ: "Salt sensitive" essential hypertension in men: Is the sodium ion alone important? N Engl J Med 1987;317:1043

69. Dean JD, et al: Hyperinsulinemia and microvascular angina ("syndrome X"). Lancet 1991;337:456

70. Botker HE, et al: Insulin resistance in microvascular angina (syndrome X). Lancet 1993;342:136

71. Schunkert H, et al: Localization and regulation of c-fos and c-jun protooncogene induction by systolic wall stress in normal and hypertrophied rat hearts. Proc Natl Acad Sci USA 1991;88:11480

72. Ganau A, et al: Relation of left ventricular hemodynamic load and contractile performance to left ventricular mass in hypertension. Circulation 1990;81:25

73. Frohlich ED, Tarazi RC: Is arterial pressure the sole factor responsible for hypertensive cardiac hypertrophy? Am J Cardiol 1979;44:959

74. Phillips RA, Krakoff LR, Ardeljan M, Dunaif A, Finegood DT, Shimabukuro S, Gorlin R, Wilkenfeld C: Relation of left ventricular mass to insulin resistance and blood pressure in non-obese subjects. J Am Coll Cardiol 1994;23:48A(Abstract)

75. Lopes De Faria JB, et al: Sodium-lithium countertransport activity and insulin resistance in normotensive IDDM patients. Diabetes 1992;41:610

76. Grossman E, et al: Left ventricular mass in diabetes-hypertension. Arch Intern Med 1992;152:1001

77. Sharp SD, Williams RR: Fasting insulin and left ventricular mass in hypertensives and normotensive controls. Cardiology 1992;81:207

78. Sasson Z, et al: Insulin resistance is an important determinant of left ventricular mass in the obese. Circulation 1993;88:1431

79. Marcus R, et al: Sex-specific determinants of increased left ventricular mass in the Tecumseh blood pressure study. Circulation 1994;90:928

80. Lind L, et al: Left ventricular hypertrophy in hypertension is associated with the insulin resistance metabolic syndrome. J Hypertens 1995;13:433

81. Stein IF, Leventhal ML: Amenorrhea associated with bilateral polycystic ovaries. Am J Obstet Gynecol 1935;29:181

82. Dunaif A, et al: Profound peripheral insulin resistance, independent of obesity in polycystic ovary syndrome. Diabetes 1989;38:1165

83. Zimmerman S, et al: Polycystic ovary syndrome: Lack of hypertension despite profound insulin resistance. J Clin Endocrin Metab 1992;75:508

84. Birkeland KI, et al: Relationship Between Blood Pressure and In Vivo Action of Insulin in Type II (Non-Insulin-Dependent) Diabetic Subjects. Metabolism 1992;41:301

85. Ferrannini E, Haffner SM, Stern MP: Essential Hypertension: An Insulin-Resistant State. J Cardiovasc Pharmacol 1990;15:S18

86. Zavaroni I, et al: Hyperinsulinaemia, obesity, and syndrome X. J Int Med 1994;235:51

87. Evans DJ, et al: Relationship of androgenic activity to body fat topography, fat cell morphology, and metabolic abnormalities in pre-menopausal women. J Clin Endocrinol Metab 1983;57:304

88. Haffner SM, Dunn JF, Katz MS: Relationship of sex hormone binding globulin to lipid, lipoprotein, glucose, and insulin concentrations in post-menopausal women. Atherosclerosis 1992;41:278

89. Haffner SM, et al: Decreased Sex Hormone-Binding Globulin Predicts Noninsulin-Dependent Diabetes Mellitus in Women but not in Men. J Clin Endocrinol Metab 1993;77:56

90. Lindstedt G, et al: Low sex hormone binding globulin concentration as independent risk factor for development of NIDDM: 12-year follow-up of population study of women in Gothenburg, Sweden. Diabetes 1990;40:123

91. Haffner SM, et al: Insulin resistance, body fat distribution, and sex hormones in men. Diabetes 1994;43:212

92. Anonymous: The Fifth Report of the Joint National Committee on Detection, Evaluation, and Treatment of High Blood Pressure (JNC V). Arch Intern Med 1993;153:154

93. Veterans Administration Cooperative Study Group on Antihypertensive Agents: Effects of treatment on morbidity in hypertension: results in patients with diastolic blood pressures averaging 115 through 129 mm Hg. JAMA 1967;202:1028

94. Veterans Administration Cooperative Study Group on Antihypertensive Agents: Effects of treatment on morbidity in hypertension II. results in patients with diastolic blood pressure averaging 90 through 114 mm Hg. JAMA 1970;213:1143

95. Hypertension Detection and Follow-up Program Cooperative Group: Five-year findings of the Hypertension Detection and Follow-up Program. I. Reduction in mortality of persons with high blood pressure, including mild hypertension. JAMA 1979;242:2562

96. Multiple Risk Factor Intervention Trial Research Group: Multiple risk factor intervention trial: risk factor changes and mortality results. JAMA 1982;248:1465

97. Helgeland A: The treatment of mild hypertension: a five-year controlled drug trial; the Oslo study. Am J Med 1980;69:725

98. Medical Research Council Working Party: MRC trial of treatment of mild hypertension: principal results. Brit Med J 1985;291:97

99. Collins R, et al: Blood pressure, stroke, and coronary heart disease. Part 2, short-term reductions in blood pressure: overview of randomized drug trials in their epidemiological context. Lancet 1990;335:827

100. Pollare T, Lithell H, Berne C: A comparison of the effects of hydrochlorthiazide and captopril on glucose and lipid metabolism in patients with hypertension. N Engl J Med 1989;321:868

101. Ferrari P, Rosman J, Wiedmann P: Antihypertensive agents, serum lipoproteins, and glucose metabolism. Am J Cardiol 1991;67:26B

102. Wiedmann P, et al: Antihypertensive therapy in diabetic patients. J Hum Hypertens 1993;7:

103. Lind L, et al: Long-term metabolic effects of antihypertensive drugs. Am Heart J 1994;128:1177

104. Lithell HOL: Effect of antihypertensive drugs on insulin, glucose, and lipid metabolism. Diabetes Care 1991;14:203

105. Warram JH, et al: Excess mortality associated with diuretic therapy in diabets mellitus. Arch Intern Med 1991;151:1350

106. Curb JD, et al: Effect of diuretic-based antihypertensive treatment on cardiovascular disease risk in older diabetic patients with isolated systolic hypertension. Systolic Hypertension in the Elderly Program Cooperative Research Group. JAMA 1996;276:1886

107. Skarfors ET, et al: Do antihypertensive drugs precipitate diabetes in predisposed men? Brit Med J 1989;298:1147

108. Bengtsson C, et al: Do antihypertensive drugs precipitate diabetes? Brit Med J 1984;289:1495

109. Kendall MJ, et al: Beta blockers and sudden cardiac death. Ann Intern Med 1995;123:358

110. Moan A, et al: Hypertension therapy and risk of coronary heart disease: How do antihypertensives affect metabolic factors? Cardiology 1995;86:89

111. Helgeland A, et al: Enalapril, atenolol, and hydrochlorothiazide in mild to moderate hypertension. A comparative multicentre study in general practice in Norway. Lance 1986;328:872

112. Alkharouf J, et al: Long-term effects of the angiotensin converting enzyme inhibitor captopril on metabolic control in non-insulin-dependent diabetes mellitus. Am J Hypertens 1993;6:337

113. Jauch KW, et al: Captopril enhances insulin responsiveness of forearm muscle tissue in non-insulin-dependent diabetes mellitus. Europ J Clin Invest 1987;17:448

114. Torlone E, et al: ACE inhibition increases hepatic and extrahepatic sensitivity to insulin in patients with type 2 (non-insulin-dependent) diabetes mellitus and arterial hypertension. Diabetologia 1991;34:119

115. Bak JF, et al: Effects of perindopril on insulin sensitivity and plasma lipid profile in hypertensive non-insulin-dependent diabetic patients. Am J Med 1992;92:69S

116. Mattews DM, Wathen CG, Bell D: The effect of captopril on blood pressure and glucose tolerance in hypertensive non-insulin-dependent diabetes. Postgrad Med J 1986;62:73

117. Dominguez JR, et al: Effect of converting enzyme inhibitors in hypertensive patients with non-insulin-dependent diabetes mellitus. Postgrad Med J 1986;62:66

118. Lithell HO, Pollare T, Berne C: Insulin sensitivity in newly detected hypertensive patients: influence of captopril and other antihypertensive agents on insulin sensitivity and related biological parameters. J Cardiovasc Pharm 1990;15:S46

119. Paolisso G, et al: ACE inhibition improves insulin sensitivity in aged insulin-resistant hypertensive patients. J Hum Hyperten 1992;6:175

120. Kodama J, et al: Effect of captopril on glucose concentration: possible role of augmented postprandial forearm blood flow. Diabetes Care 1990;13:1109

121. Santoro D, et al: Effects of chronic angiotensin converting enzyme inhibition on glucose tolerance and insulin sensitivity in essential hypertension. Hypertension 1992;20:181

122. Tomiyama H, et al: Kinins contribute to the improvement of insulin sensitivity during treatment with angiotensin converting enzyme inhibitors. Hypertension 1994;23:450

123. Baba T, Kodama T, Ishizaki T: Effect of chronic treatment with enalapril on glucose tolerance and serum insulin responsen to glucose load in non-insulin-resistant Japanese patients with essential hypertension. Euro J Clin Pharm 1993;45:23

124. Allemann Y, et al: Insulin sensitivity in normotensive subjects during angiotensin converting enzyme inhibition with fosinopril. Euro J Clin Pharm 1992;42:275

125. Gans ROB, et al: The effect of angiotensin-1 converting enzyme inhibition on insulin action in healthy volunteers. Europ J Clin Invest 1991;21:527

126. Maheux P, et al: Changes in glucose, insulin, lipid, lipoprotein, and apoprotein concentrations and insulin action in doxazosin-treated patients with hypertension. Am J Hypertens 1994;7:416

127. Erman A, et al: Treatment with dexamethasone increases glomerular prostaglandin synthesis in rats. J Pharmacol Exp Ther 1986;239:296

128. Swislocki ALM, et al: Effect of prazosin treatment on carbohydrate and lipoprotein metabolism in patients with hypertension. Am J Med 1989;13:14

129. Giorda C, Appendino M: Effects of doxazosin, a selective a_1-inhibitor, on plasma insulin and blood glucose response to a glucose tolerance test in essential hypertension. Metabolism 1993;42:1440

130. Wilson MD, Weart CW: Hypertension: Are beta-blockers and diuretics appropriate first-line therapies? Ann Pharmacol 1994;28:617

131. Caldwell BV: Treating hypertension in the diabetic patient: therapeutic goals and the role of calcium channel blockers. Clinical Therapeutics 1993;15:618

132. Pollare T, et al: Metabolic effects of diltiazem and atenolol: results from a randomized, double-blind study with parallel groups. J Hypertens 1989;7:551

133. Morris AD, et al: Metabolic effects of lacidipine: a placebo-controlled study using the euglycaemic, hyperinsulinaemic clamp. Brit J Clin Pharm 1993;35:40

134. Collins WCJ, Cullen MJ, Feely J: Calcium channel blocker drugs and diabetic control. Clin Pharm Therapeut 1987;42:420

135. Faguer de Moustier B, Paoli V: The influence of nicardipine in type II diabetic patients with slight hypertension. J Cardiovasc Pharm 1990;16:S26

136. Hedner T, et al: Glucose tolerance in hypertensive patients during treatment with the calcium antagonist felodipine. Brit J Clin Pharm 1987;24:145

137. Kihara A: Effect of the calcium antagonist nicardipine hydrochloride on glucose tolerance and insulin secretion. Am Heart J 1991;122:363

138. Trost BN, Wiedmann P: Effect of calcium antagonists on glucose homeostasis and serum lipids in non-diabetic and diabetic subjects: a review. J Hypertens 1987;5:81

139. Sasaki J, et al: Comparative effects of monatepil, a novel calcium antagonist with alpha 1-adrenergic-blocking activity, and nitrendipine on lipoprotein and carbohydrate metabolism in patients with hypertension. Am J Hypertens 1994;7:161S

140. Griffing GT, et al: Plasma beta-endorphin levels in primary aldosteronsim. J Clin Endocrinol Metab 1985;60:315

141. Iwamoto Y, Kuzuya T, Matsuda A: Effects of new oral antidiabetic agent CS-045 on glucose tolerance and insulin secretion in patients with NIDDM. Diabetes Care 1991;14:1083

142. Fujiwara T, et al: Characterization of new oral antidiabetic agent CS-045: studies in KK and ob/ob mice and Zucker fatty rats. Diabetes 1988;37:1549

143. Ciaraldi TP, et al: In vitro studies on the action of CS-045, a new antidiabetic agent. Metabolism 1990;39:1056

144. Phillips RA: The cardiologist's approach to evaluation and management of the patient with essential hypertension. Am Heart J 1993;126:648

11 AMBULATORY BLOOD PRESSURE MONITORING

Peter A. Kringstein, Ethan D. Loeb, Robert A. Phillips

Diagnosis of hypertension with ambulatory blood pressure monitoring

Although it is well established that antihypertensive therapy is beneficial, it is still often difficult to determine whether a patient with borderline hypertension is in the range that requires treatment. Young adults may have a pattern of labile blood pressure, exhibiting occasional elevations >140/90 mm Hg on a casual screening. If only a few pressures are taken, a diagnosis of hypertension may be made before there is a clear-cut pattern of sustained elevation. As such, individual readings in the medical setting may not give one a true sense of a patient's typical pressure level.

To address this issue, we recently provided a statistically based graphical criteria *(Figure 11.1)* which greatly simplifies the diagnosis of hypertension in the borderline and "white coat" hypertensive patient.[1] We determined that if at least 40 ambulatory BP (ABP) measurements are obtained during the course of awake hours, if the systolic ABP is ≤137 mm Hg there is only a 10% probability that the patient's "true" average BP is actually in the hypertensive range. By contrast, if the systolic pressure is ≥143 mm Hg, there is a 90% probability that the patient is hypertensive. Similarly, if the diastolic is ≤88 mmHg, there is there is only a 10% probability that the patient's "true" average BP is actually in the hypertensive range. If the diastolic is ≥ 92, then there is a 90% probability that the patient is hypertensive.

Ambulatory blood pressure, end-organ damage and prognosis

Since the advent of ambulatory blood pressure monitoring (ABPM) in the 1960's, many studies have been performed to examine the prognostic value of this technique compared to office measured blood pressures. Most of these studies have examined the relationship between ambulatory blood pressure (ABP) and left ventricular hypertrophy (LVH).

A widely quoted study by Sokolow et al published in 1966[2], for instance, examined 124 patients with mild to moderate hypertension and evaluated the degree of hypertension-related organ damage in the heart and retinal vessels of each patient according to a grading system. They noted that ambulatory pressure correlated at a significantly higher level with the grade of organ damage (r=.63 for systolic pressure) than did office pressure (OBP) (r=.48). The incidental finding that many patients with persistently high office pressures had lower ambulatory levels, later to be recognized as the white coat effect, was merely pointed out as a research curiosity at the time. Gosse et al[3]. found that excercise blood pressure or 24 hour average ambulatory pressure levels correlated much more highly with echocardiographically measured LV mass than did resting office pressure. Another study by Devereux and colleagues[4] found that ambulatory pressure measured on a working day was better correlated with LV mass than either ambulatory pressure measured on a nonworking day or OBP.

Two studies, however, have prospectively evaluated the prognostic value of

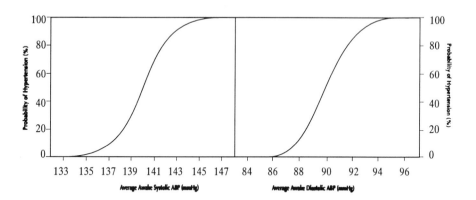

*Figure 11.1 **Left Panel:** Probability that average sysetolic blood pressusre is greater than 140 mm Hg. x axis, Average systolic ambulatory blood pressure (ABP); y axis, probability that the subject's average systolic blood pressure is in the hypertensive range (ie, ≥140 mm Hg). **Right Panel:** Probability that average diastolic blood pressusre is greater than 90 mm Hg. x axis, Average diastolic ambulatory blood pressure (ABP); y axis, probability that the subject's average diastolic blood pressure is in the hypertensive range (ie, ≥ 90 mm Hg).*

ambulatory blood pressure monitoring. Perloff et al.[5] studied a group of 1076 patients with essential hypertension as assessed by office blood pressure, and obtained an average ABP value for each patient. These data were used to create a scatter plot and generate a line of best fit from which linear regression was used to predict the ABP from a given patient's office blood pressure. They note that although the relationship was reasonably linear, there was "considerable deviation from the regression line in some patients." These patients were then separated into "high" and "low" groups depending on whether their systolic ABP was 10 mmHg greater or less than would have been predicted by regression from the office blood pressure. The "low" corresponded to the white coat hypertensives, although this phrase had not yet been coined. All patients were followed up in clinic and those with persistently high office blood pressures were treated with antihypertensives. It was found that those patients who had higher than predicted ABPs were significantly more likely to go on to develop a variety of cardiovascular events as compared to those with lower than predicted ABP's. Their conclusion was that for those patients with borderline hypertension in whom the decision to treat or not is often difficult, ABPM might provide a superior method over office blood pressure in terms of identifying high risk patients.

There were several weaknesses with regard to this study. The authors acknowledge that potential inadequacy of BP control in the group with high initial ABP values may have confounded the study. Inadequate control would magnify subsequent blood pressure differences between the two groups leading to a greater number of outcome events in the high ABP group. ABP monitoring subsequent to the initial measurement would have allowed for better assessment of control. In their defense, however, they claim that in those patients who had a high initial ABP and subsequently high office blood pressures, treatment was relatively aggressive - a policy that would have reduced the difference in the number of endpoints between the two groups instead of the opposite. Perhaps more significant than this shortcoming, however, is the fact that compared to those with low initial ABP's, patients with high initial ABP's were older, had a longer duration of previous hypertension and had more previous end-organ events. These differences cast some uncertainty on the issue of causality.

The other major prospective study of ABPM was published in 1994 by Verdecchia et al.[6] Similar to Perloff, they divided hypertensives into different groups based on their average ABP level. Verdecchia, however, defined a "normal" level of daytime BP as being below the 90th percentile of the daytime (waking) ABP distribution of the normotensive population. Office hypertensives whose daytime pressures fell below this cutoff were classified as white coat hypertensives. Those with persistently high daytime ABPs were subdivided into "dippers" and "nondippers" based on whether or not their sleeping ABPs dropped significantly below their waking ABPs. Follow up in clinic revealed that both the normotensive controls and the white coats went on to experience a relatively event-free survival as compared to both the dippers and the nondippers. The nondippers experienced the greatest subsequent accumulation of end-organ events. Not only did ABP predict end-organ damage better than office blood pressure, they also found that among patients with LVH, nondippers were more likely to have an event than dippers. This led them to the conclusion that ABP was a better predictor of a future event than simply the presence or absence of LVH.

This study had several advantages over that by Perloff. The development of automatically inflatable monitors allowed Verdecchia to obtain a full 24 hours of ambulatory data. Perloff was only able to obtain daytime levels since the devices used at that time were manually inflated. In addition, Verdecchia included a nor-motensive control group in his study and also attempted to adjust for covariates between groups such as age, prior cardiovascular events, LVH and diabetes by using the Cox regression model. The major disadvantage to the study is that only 30% of subjects had periodic follow-up visits so that subsequent assessment of BP control was difficult. There is also no indication as to whether the number of people who dropped out in each group was equal. In addition, as in the Perloff study, hyperten-sive management was based on office blood pressure and not subsequent ABP data since physicians generally considered the latter to be "investigational findings of unproven clinical utility."[5] The better prognosis in the white coats may have there-fore reflected a superior effect of treatment in this group. All in all, however, these two papers, in addition to numerous other cross-sectional studies, provide fairly strong evidence for the prognostic value of ABPM.

What is a normal ambulatory blood pressure?

One of the major problems with the research that has been done regarding the white coat phenomenon is the lack of agreement over what ambulatory cutoff value should be used to define who is a white coat hypertensive. This inconsistency makes it difficult to compare studies to one another. Although most investigators use an upper-normal value from the distribution of awake normotensives on ABPM, the cutoffs chosen still usually range from 130-135 systolic and 80-90 diastolic.[7-10] These values have resulted in reported prevalences ranging from 21% to as high as 61% *(Table 11.1)*. Some of the values used and the resulting prevalences are shown in the table below:

Verdecchia has pointed out that the ambulatory blood pressure cut-off chosen for the diagnosis of hypertension has a significant impact on the prevalence of the white coat effect. It was found that when four different cutoffs were applied to a single sample of 346 patients with untreated essential hypertension, prevalences of the white coat effect ranged from 12.1% to 53.2%. Essentially, the higher the cut-off, the higher the prevalence of white coat hypertensives. When the cutoff pro-posed by Staessen et al[15] is used (i.e. 146/91 mm Hg, which represents 2 standard deviations above the mean for daytime ambulatory pressure of normtensives), more patients are classified as white coat hypertensives than when a lower cut off is used (i.e. the 90th percentile of a normal distribution, or 136/87 for men and 131/86 for

Table 11.1   STUDIES OF ABP MONITORING

Author	ABP cutoff	Prevalence of WCH
Pickering[6]	134/90	21%
Baily[11]	diastolic ABP < 85	35.3%
Krakoff[12]	130/85	38%
Siege[19]	135/ 85	22%
Waeber[13]	140/90	61%

women as proposed by Verdecchia). Verdecchia notes that labelling patients as white coat when they are in fact truly hypertensive may lead to undertreatment. For example, when the higher cut-off is used (146/91 mm Hg), 9% of patients labelled as white coat will have LVH, whereas when the lower cut-off is used , then only 2-3% of the white coat hypertensives have LVH.14 Basing the choice of cutoff on the presence or absence of end-organ damage may be the most logical approach to the problem. For example, Phillips et al. determined that if the average awake BP was less than or equal to 130/85, then no LVH or diastolic dysfunction was noted, but ambulatory pressure above this level may be associated with early signs of cardiac involvement - i.e. left ventricular diastolic filling abnormalities.[16]

Gender and the white coat effect

Although much remains to be answered, many studies have attempted to character-ize the white coat effect in terms of prevalence and the types of people likely to exhibit the effect. Some of the more consistent findings in the literature concern the issue of gender.

Pickering found a prevalence of 21% white coat effect among a group of bor-derline hypertensives (69% male, diastolic BP 90-104 mmHg), with bivariate anal-ysis revealing that white coat patients tended to be female, younger, and weighed less. This study may have been complicated by the fact that some of the patients on antihypertensives stopped taking their medications only two weeks prior to the study. In addition, there were significant age differences between normotensive controls and borderline patients. The classification criteria used to identify white coat re-sponders (ABP < 134/90 and diastolic office blood pressure 90-105) may also have weakened the study by labelling some patients as white coats when their office blood pressures and ABPs were not substantially different.

Eison et al studied a group of 57 men and 30 women referred for mild hyper-tension (diastolic BP 90-104) and found a higher magnitude of white coat effect in women vs men (11 mmHg vs 6 mmHg).[17] The authors drew the conclusion that the better prognosis seen in hypertensive women for the same level of office pressure as men may in part be explained by the white coat effect. This is because office blood pressure in a woman is significantly higher than her ambulatory pressure, whereas a man's office pressure is a better reflection of his ambulatory pressure. As in the Pickering study, most subjects were Caucasian so that generalization to blacks and other ethnic groups can not be made. Disadvantages of this study include the fact that 75% of men worked on the day of ABPM vs only 68% of women. The latter was not a significant difference, but may have skewed the data in favor of the above findings since ABPM levels have been shown to be higher on working vs. nonworking days.[18]

In a group of 159 patients (86 women) with diastolic office blood pressure > 90 mmHg, Hoegholm also found a larger systolic white coat effect in women (16 vs 6 mmHg).[10] This study had the advantage that no patient had yet been started on therapy, but was weakened by the fact that many of the 24 hour records were not retrieved in their entirety.

Age, race and the white coat effect

Another characteristic of the white coat effect that has been investigated, although not in depth, is that of its existence in the very young and very elderly. Hornsby et al. studied a group of 159 children recruited on the basis of age (5-15 years old), sex (79 males, 80 female), race (65 black, 94 white), and a positive family history of essential hypertension.[19] Subjects who had office blood pressure greater than or equal to the 95th percentile for their age and sex were classified as hypertensive if their average ABP also exceeded this value. If the average ABP was below this level, they were considered white coat hypertensives. Those below the cutoff on both ABP and office blood pressure were considered normotensive. Of the 34 subjects considered to be hypertensive on the basis of office blood pressure, 44% were found to have the white coat effect. No differences across sex or race were found. A study by Trenkwalder et al. similarly found evidence for the effect in the elderly.[20]

The issue of race and potential differences in the white coat effect has been largely ignored. With the exception of the study noted above, we are aware of no others that draw any conclusions with regard to this characteristic. In those studies that do separate their patients in terms of race, there are not enough members in the minority groups to provide adequate statistical power for proper analysis.[7,21]

Etiology of the white coat effect

The etiology of the white coat effect remains a mystery. The simplest theory is that it is a stress-related phenomenon. Somewhat in support of this view is a study that showed an intraarterial rise in BP of hospitalized patients in response to a physician entering the room to take a cuff BP.[22] Another study of patients on ABPM on their way to clinic showed an increase in BP as the patient left home for the doctor's office.[23] Other studies have shown higher magnitudes of the white coat effect when office blood pressure is measured by a physician than by a nurse or technician.[24,25] The latter phenomenon is in line with greater anxiety and therefore greatest pressor response elicited by the figure perhaps perceived as most authoritative.

Despite these findings, numerous other studies looking to differentiate white coat responders from essential hypertensives and/or normotensives based on questionnaires or stress-related tasks have failed to discriminate between groups.[9,26,27] This lack of support for the stress-related theory may in part be due to the nature of these studies. As Pickering notes, the personality inventories used to measure traits such as "anxiety" are fraught with problems, the largest one being that people tend to portray themselves the way they would like to be perceived. There is also the fact that the correlation between different questionnaires claiming to measure the same characteristic is often low — simply because someone says their survey measures "anxiety" does not make this so.[28] "Stress-related tasks" performed by subjects in these studies such as video games, mental arithmetic, and forehead-icepack tests may also not be analogous enough to the kind of stress that may be elicited by a physician measuring one's BP. It is not unlikely that these studies simply have not yet tested the right measure of stress.

In light of the lack of findings for the stress-related theory, Pickering has proposed that the white coat effect may be a classically-conditioned response to the physician.[29] He draws an analogy to the Igvid syndrome in which the sight of the oncologist may induce nausea and vomiting in a patient's anticipation of the administration of chemotherapeutics. The problem with this theory is one of how the sight of the doctor becomes paired with the increase in BP. With the Igvid response, the relationship is much more obvious: chemotherapeutics (unconditioned stimulus) previously elicited an episode of nausea (unconditioned response) on their own, the doctor (conditioned stimulus) ultimately coming to elicit the response simply through the power of numerous reinforced pairings with the drug. Pickering's hypothesis that fear originally induces the increase in BP and the subsequent awareness of hypertension maintains sympathetic arousal to maintain BP over repeated visits is questionable in light of certain characteristics of the white coat effect. In particular is the fact that the white coat effect has been recognized in children[19] at an age when the risks and meaning of hypertension are not yet understood.[25]

Is the white coat effect an academic anomaly?

Almost all of the research concerning the white coat effect has been done in academic center clinics with only a few studies based in private practices. One of the important questions that comes to mind is that of generalizability from the research findings at these institutions to the community. Certainly it would be jumping to conclusions to assume that the findings in one setting will necessarily hold in another. For instance, a retrospective study of antihypertensive-related side effects found that cough induced by ACE inhibitors was prevalent in 25% of a private practice, but only 7% of a university-based clinic.[30] The authors ascribe these results to a number of possibilities. One of their arguments centers around the idea that although two populations may be demographically similar, there may also be unrecognized or unmeasured differences between groups causing some of the observed variability. This last point is relevant to any research finding from a referral center that one wishes to generalize to the larger patient population. Patients who come to the academic center are in many ways self-selected. They are a highly motivated group who have often been to several physicians seeking answers regarding their ailments. They may be more willing than the average patient to participate as subjects of medical research in exchange for what they perceive as high-quality health care. For instance, those who agree to undergo ABPM are allowing a medical instrument that has still not been widely accepted as a clinically useful tool to be used in the assessment and management of their health. How factors such as these might affect study outcomes is unclear, but the potential needs to be recognized.

One of the only studies of ABPM in a suburban private practice found evidence of the white coat effect in a group of 17 patients with no prior hypertension and also in a group of 43 established hypertensives.[31] All 60 patients had three office blood pressures > 140 mmHg systolic or 90 mmHg diastolic (Joint National Committee recommendations for the diagnosis of hypertension).[32] A white coat effect of 21 mmHg systolic and 20 mmHg diastolic was found in those with no prior history of hypertension and a similar effect was found in the established hypertensive group. Separate analyses were not carried out for each gender, and the racial makeup of the practice was not indicated. No cutoff values for ABP were used so that the prevalence of the effect could not be adequately determined. In addition, the results involving the hypertensive group may be confounded by the fact that many patients were on medication at the time of the study. A recent study, for instance, showed that calcium channel blockers may interact with the white coat effect in women.[33] Nevertheless, the importance of this community based study is that it shows that many patients in a private practice setting may be incorrectly diagnosed as being hypertensive according to standard guidelines. This surely would have resulted in unnecessary treatment if ABPM had not been performed.

In a study carried out by Khoury and colleagues, 131 patients were monitored in an attempt to define the prevalence of the white coat effect in a rural private practice.[34] All patients were white and had two previous diastolic office blood pressure readings between 90 and 115 mmHg. WCH was defined as diastolic ABP < 85 mmHg resulting in an overall prevalence of 34% and a magnitude of effect of 17 mmHg systolic and 8 mmHg diastolic. Women and men were found to have the same systolic ABP, but women had significantly higher office blood pressures (systolic white coat effect=12 mmHg in men, 22 mmHg in women). The white coat hypertensives were found to be younger, and predominantly female (59%), results generally in line with those of the Pickering et al. study6 done in an academic center.[7] There is not enough data reported in Pickering's article, however, to compare the magnitude of effect in women between the two settings. In addition, direct comparisons between these two studies should be made with caution. Pickering used a narrower range of diastolic office blood pressures to categorize his borderline hypertensive group and also a higher cutoff value of diastolic ABP to define the prevalence of WCH.

Khoury also concludes that the prevalence of the white coat effect is similar in the rural private practice and the academic center. In support of this, he cites several studies with the same diastolic ABP cutoff used to define the white coat effect. Examination of those studies, however, shows that they varied widely in their reported prevalences of white coat effect from 23% to 47%.[10,11,35,36] In addition, the similar diastolic cutoff used to group these studies oversimplifies the problem as there are surely many other subtle methodological variables that are not the same across these experiments.

Clinical recommendations

In summary, the white coat effect is a widely recognized and prevalent phenomenon. The most consistent findings relate to the issue of gender, and the evidence that those with lower ambulatory pressures are less likely to suffer cardiac end-organ events. In view of the latter, the white coat effect has important implications in terms of the misdiagnosis and unneccessary treatment of hypertension. For this reason, we have incorporated the reccommendations of the Fifth Report of the Joint National Committee on Detection, Evaluation and Treatment of High Blood Pressure[37] into our clinical practice with the following modifications:

1. In women with repeated office blood pressure between 90 and 110 diastolic or between 140 and 170 systolic, we often perform ambulatory blood pressure montoring. We make the diagnosis of definite hypertension ($>90\%$ liklihood of hypertension) if the awake systolic BP is $\geq$143 mm Hg, or the diastolic is $\geq$ 92 mm Hg.[1]

2. In men with persistently elevated office blood pressure (either on or off treatment) but normal blood pressure with home self-monitoring, we perform ambulatory blood pressure monitoring to assess whether there is a white coat effect or determine the efficacy of treatment.

3. In both men and women we alert the referring physician if sleep blood pressures decreases by $<10\%$ or if ambulatory blood pressure is higher than the office blood pressure.

4. Further studies are needed to determine whether patients with ambulatory blood pressure between 130/85 to 140/90 should have echocardiography to determine if they have left ventricular diastolic filling abnormalities, a condition which might warrant blood pressure lowering despite borderline levels of blood pressure[16].

REFERENCES

1. Moore, CR, Krakoff, LR, Phillips, RA. Confirmation or exclusion of stage I hypertension by ambulatory blood pressure monitoring. Hypertension, 1997;29:1109.

2. Sokolow M, et al. Relationship between level of blood pressure measured casually and by portable recorders and severity of complications in essential hypertension. Circulation 1966;34: 279.

3. Gosse P, et al. Left ventricular hypertrophy in hypertension: Correlation with rest, exercise and ambulatory systolic blood pressure. J Hypertension 19S6;4(85): S297.

4. Devereux RB, et al. Left ventricular hypertrophy in patients with hypertension: importance of blood pressure response to regularly recurring stress. Circulation 1983;68: 470.

5. Perloff D, Sokolow M, Cowan R. The prognostic value of ambulatory blood prqssure monitoring. JAMA 1983;249: 2792.

6. Verdecchia P, et al. Ambulatory blood pressure - an independent predictor of prognosis in essential hypertension. Hypertension 1994;24: 793.

7. Pickering TG et al: How common is white coat hypertension? JAMA 1988;259: 225.

8. White WB, Schulman P, McCabe EJ. Average daily blood pressure, not office blood pressure, determines cardiac function in patients with hypertension. JAMA 1989;261: 873.

9. Siegel WC, Blumenthal JA, Divine GW. Physiological, psychological, and behavioral factors and white coat hypertension. Hypertension 1990;16: 140.

10. Hoegholm A et al. White coat hypertension diagnosed by 24-hour ambulatory monitoring: Examination of 159 newly diagnosed hypertensive patients. Am J Hypertens 1992;5: 64.

11. Baily GB, et al. Comparison of office, home and 24 hour ambulatory blood pressures in borderline and mild hypertension. Angiology 1988;2: 752.

12. Krakoff LR, Eison H, Phillips RA. Effect of ambulatory blood pressure monitoring on the diagnosis and cost of treatment for mild hypertension. Am Heart J 1988;116: 1152.

13. Waeber B, et al. Ambulatory blood pressure recording to identify hypertensive patients who truly need therapy. J Chron Dis 1984;37:55.

14 Verdecchia P, et al. Variability between current definitions of 'normal' ambulatory blood pressure - Implications in the assessment of white coat hypertension. Hypertension 1992;20: 555.

15. Staessen J, et al. Mean and range of the ambulatory pressure in normotensive subjects from a meta-analysis of 23 studies. Am J Cardiol 1991; 67: 723.

16. Phillips RA, et al. Determinants of abnormal left ventricular filling in early hypertension. J Am Coll Cardiol 1989;14:979.

17. Eison H, et al. Differences in ambulatory blood pressure between men and women with mild hypertension. J Hum Hypertens 1990;4: 400.

18. Pickering T, et al. Comparisons of blood pressure during normal daily activities, sleep, and exercise in normal and hypertensive subjects. JAMA 1982;247: 992.

19. Hornsby LJ, et al. 'White coat' hypertension in children. J Fam Pract 1991;33: 617.

20. Trenkwalder P, et al. "White Coat" hypertension and alerting reaction in elderly and very elderly hypertensive patients. Blood Press 1993;2(4): 262.

21. Lerman CE, et al. The white coat hypertension response: prevalence and predictors. J Gen Int Med 1989;4: 226.

22. Mancia 0, Grassi 6, Pomidossi G et al: Effects of blood pressure measurement by the doctor on patient's blood pressure and heart rate. Lancet 1983;2: 695.

23. Elijovich F, Laffer CL: Magnitude, reproducibility, and components of the pressor response to the clinic. 1990;15: I-161.

24. Mancia G, et al. Alerting reaction and rise in blood pressure during measurement by physician and nurse. Hypertension 1987;6: 375.

25. Richardson JF, Robinson D. Variations in the measurement of blood pressure between doctors and nurses. J R Coll Gen Pract 1977;21: 69S.

26. Cardillo C, et al. Psychophysiological reactivity and cardiac end- organ changes in white coat hypertension. Hypertension 1993;21: 836.

27. Julius S, et al: White coat hypertension: a follow-up. Clin and Exper Hyper.- Theory and Practice 1992;A14: 45.

28. Pickering TG: Tension and Hypertension. JAMA 1993;270: 2494.

29. Pickering TG, et al. The role of behavioral factors in white coat nnd sustained hypertension. J Hypertension 1990;8(S7): S141.

30. Simon SR, Black HR, Moser M, Berland WE: Cough and ACE inhibitors. Arch Int Med 1992;152: 1698.

31. Ferguson JH, Shaar CJ. The effective diagnosis and treatment of hypertension by the primary care physician: Impact of ambulatory blood pressure monitoring. J Am Board Fam Pract 1992;5: 457.

32. The 1988 report of the Joint National Committee on Detection, Evaluation and Treatment of High Blood Pressure. Arch Intern Med 1988;148: 1023.

33. Loeb ED, et al. Real versus apparent gender differences in blood pressure response to calcium channel blocker in the treatment of hypertension. [Abstract] Circulation 1994;90:I-566.

34. Khoury S, et al. Ambulatory blood pressure monitoring in a nonacademic setting - effects of age and sex. Am J Hypert 1992;5: 616.

35. " Schnall PL, et al: The relationship between "job strain," workplace, diastolic blood pressure, and left ventricular mass index. JAMA 1990;263: 1929.

36. Gradman AH, et al. Lack of correlation between clinic and-24 hour ambulatory blood pressures in subjects participating in a therapeutic drug trial. J Clin Epidemiol 1989;42: 1049.

37. Anonymous: The Fifth Report of the Joint National Committee on Detection, Evaluation, and Treatment of High Blood Pressure (JNC V). Arc Intern Med 1993; 153:154.

12 ANGIOTENSIN CONVERTING ENZYME INHIBITORS

Theodore D. Mountokalakis

The synthesis of the first orally active angiotensin converting enzyme (ACE) inhibitor in the 1977, heralded one of the major therapeutic advances of the last decades. Initially designed to be a pathophysiologically meaningful tool for the treatment of severe malignant hypertension, ACE inhibitors are now widely accepted as first line approach to the treatment of mild to moderate essential hypertension and of congestive heart failure. In addition to the clinical importance of the results of clinical trials, studies aiming to elucidate the precise mode of action of these agents have led to the concept of tissue renin-angiotensin systems, and have clarified several aspects of the pathophysiology of hypertension and heart failure.

Mechanism of action of ACE inhibitors

ACE is a monomeric zinc dipeptidyl carboxypeptidase. It cleaves the carboxyl-terminal peptide of angiotensin I, generating the active vasopressor hormone angiotensin II; and it removes two carboxyl-terminal peptides from bradykinin, inactivating this vasodepressor hormone (kininase II).[1] ACE is a membrane-bound enzyme oriented in a way that permits exposure of its catalytic sites on the extracellular surface of the cell. ACE of human endothelial cells contains one amino and one carboxyl sites. Both of them seem to be catalytically active but it is not known whether they display different substrate specifities.[2]

Due to its binding to the plasma membrane of vascular endothelial cells, ACE is characterized by an ubiquitous tissue distribution. High levels of the enzyme have also been found in the absorptive epithelium of the small intestine, the epithelial cells of the proximal convoluted tubule[3], the choroid plexus and other structures of the brain[4], the prostate and the epididymis of the male genital tract, and in mononuclear cells.[5] A secreted form of ACE occurs also in biological fluids such as plasma, cerebrospinal fluid, amniotic fluid, and semen. In addition to the *somatic* isoform, a smaller *germinal* isoform of the enzyme occurs in the testis.[2] Molecular cloning of the somatic and germinal ACE has demonstrated that: [(a)] both isoforms are transcribed from a unique gene, (b) the endothelial form consists of two highly homologous domains, suggesting a gene duplication during evolution, and (c) the germinal isomer contains only one of the two putative catalytic sites identified in the endothelial isomer.[6]

Based on the x-ray crystal structure of a related enzyme, carboxypeptidase A, a large number of specific and potent compounds which bind to the active sites of the enzyme, has been synthetized since 1977. The first orally active ACE inhibitor, captopril, was designed to possess a sulphydryl group capable of interacting with the zinc ion and a polar ketone moiety attached to the aminoacid site.[7] Because of some side-effects attributed to the sulphydryl moiety, newer compounds, such as enalapril and lisinopril, have been designed which possessed a carboxyl group in the place of the sulphydryl group. Finally, potential pharmacological disadvantages related to existence of biologically inactive *cis* isomers of captopril, enalapril, and lisinopril, have led to the design of structurally modified forms of ACE inhibitors which are not isomerized during preparation. Recent studies suggest that various ACE inhibitors interact with both the amino and the carboxyl active sites of the enzyme, showing, however, a difference in potency towards each of them.[8]

The classic concept concerning the mechanism underlying the therapeutic efficacy of ACE inhibitors has as follows: Renin, an enzyme secreted by the kidney, acts on angiotensinogen, its substrate produced by the liver and circulating in the plasma, to release angiotensin I; angiotensin I is then converted to the biologically active angiotensin II by ACE, mainly in the pulmonary circulation; by inhibiting the action of the enzyme, ACE inhibitors prevent the formation of angiotensin II. In recent years, this concept has been challenged by several observations suggesting that all the components of the RAS may be *synthesized locally in tissues.* Such locally synthesized components may interact with components derived from the circulation and determine the amount of angiotensin II generated in tissues. The therapeutic efficacy of ACE inhibitors is, therefore, likely to depend on the action of these agents not only in the circulation but also in critical tissue sites.[9]

Recent studies has revealed a new role for the ACE; the cloning of the *ACE* gene had made possible the identification of a deletion (D)-insertion (I) polymorphism of the ACE gene as a molecular genetic marker associated with an elevated risk of left ventricular hypertrophy in normotensive adults.[10] Thus, left ventricular hypertrophy, a major independent cardiovascular risk factor, seems to be at least partially determined by genetic disposition associated with ACE.

In addition to the inhibition of angiotensin II formation, *other mechanisms* have been postulated to operate when ACE is inhibited. Among them the most likely appears to be the potentiation of bradykinin. Indeed, several studies using specific antibodies to bradykinin or specific bradykinin antagonists, have indicated that bradykinin plays a contributory role in the blood-lowering effects of ACE inhibition.[11] On the other hand, prostacyclin, vasopressin and endothelin are agents closely interrelated to the RAS and the final response to ACE inhibition may reflect its effects on their interdependent functions.[12,13]

Antihypertensive efficacy of ACE inhibitors

Since hyperactivity of the rerin-angiotensin system (RAS) has been known to be associated with severe and malignant hypertension, the first orally active ACE inhibitor, captopril, was initially introduced for the treatment of severe or resistant forms of hypertension. In early studies, captopril was administered in daily doses up to 1000mg Subsequently, the agent was found to be effective in much lower doses given two or three times daily in patients with mild and moderate essential hypertension. Newer ACE inhibitors with longer half-lives permitted the use of these agents at a single daily dose.[14] It is now generally accepted that ACE inhibitors exert antihypertensive effects comparable to those of thiazides, beta-blockers and calcium antagonists.[15]

The efficacy of ACE inhibitors is enhanced when these agents are combined with diuretics, This is presumably due to the increase of the activity of the RAS caused by diuretics. In fact, in large groups of patients, the magnitude of blood pressure response to ACE inhibition has been found to be related to baseline renin levels. However, some patients with low-renin hypertension show considerable response to ACE inhibitors. Furthermore, although in hypertension plasma renin tends to fall with increasing age, severed studies have shown that the administration of ACE inhibitors in the elderly is as effective as in younger hypertensives. The explanation of this phenomenon may lie on the fact that ACE inhibition acts not only on circulating angiotensin II levels but also on local angiotensin II generation within the vascular wall.[16]

In recent years, a controversy evolved as to whether ACE inhibitors and calcium antagonists, the other major class of newer antihypertensive agents, should be considered in the selection of *initial antihypertensive therapy*.[17] According to the fifth report of the Joint National Committee on Detection, Evaluation, and Treatment of High Blood Pressure published in January 1993, diuretics and beta-blockers should be preferred for initial drug therapy mainly because they are the only classes of drugs that have been used in long-term controlled clinical trials. The newer drugs although equally effective in reducing blood pressure, they have not been used in long-term controlled trials to demonstrate their efficacy in reducing cardiovascular morbidity and mortality and "should be reserved for special indications or when diuretics and beta-blockers have proved unacceptable or ineffective".[18]

On the other hand, there is now growing evidence that when compared with diuretics and beta-blockers, antihypertensive therapy with ACE inhibitors may provide additional benefit. By inhibiting rend angiotensin II formation, ACE inhibitors increase renal blood flow and reduce glomerular hydrostatic pressure while preserving glomerular filtration rate.[19] They may, therefore, exert a favourable effect on renal hemodynamics both in the presence and in the absence of renal insufficiency. Furthermore, they decrease proteinuria more than any other class of antihypertensive drugs.[20] On the basis of the above evidence, some investigators proposed the hypothesis that due to their effects on intrarenal formation of angiotensin II and therefore glomerular hemodynamics, ACE inhibitors are *renoprotective* independently of their effect on blood pressure. Large randomised controlled trials are expected to answer this important question.

In addition to their potential renoprotective properties, ACE inhibitors may prevent coronary atherosclerosis and fatal cardiac arrhythmias. Indeed, ACE inhibitors are known to have no adverse effect on lipids or glucose tolerance and may reduce insulin resistance.[21] They neither activate sympathetic nervous system nor cause potassium depletion. ACE inhibitors may also reduce myocardial oxygen demand and increase oxygen supply. Finally, recent studies have shown that angiotensin II stimulates the growth in culture of vascular muscle cells, possibly through induction of proto-oncogene expression, suggesting that local generation of angiotensin II in the vascular wall and heart may contribute to the development of vascular and cardiac hypertrophy.[22] Taken together these experimental data suggest that ACE inhibitors may offer primary *cardioprotection* and may exert beneficial effects in hypertensive patients with ischemic heart disease. However, this suggestion also waits confirmation by large prospective trials. At present, the only antihypertensive agents that have been shown to reduce the risk of secondary event and sudden death in patients who have had a myocardial infarction are beta-blockers without intrinsic sympathomimetic activity.

When first introduced, antihypertensive therapy with captopril was found to be associated with the development of membranous glomerulonephritis. This adverse effect was attributed to the sulphydryl group in captopril, and to the very high doses of the drug used at that time. Indeed, membranous glomerulonephritis has not been reported to occur with either ACE inhibitors without this specific group, or the currently used doses of captopril. In renal artery stenosis, intrarenal renin increases to sustain the renal artery pressure distal to the stenosis. By blunting this compensatory mechanism, ACE inhibitors can cause severe and progressive -although often reversible- renal failure. However, renal failure develops only in patients with bilateral renal artery stenosis or those with tight stenosis of the artery supplying a solitary kidney.[23]

On the basis of the results of a study which campopril with methyldopa propranolol, treatment with ACE inhibitors has been suggested to be associated with a better *quality of life* than treatment with other antihypertensive agents. Subsequent studies have shown that this is only partly true. ACE inhibitors seem to be as well tolerated as thiazides and beta-blockers, but are better tolerated than calcium antagonists.[16] In any case, it is generally accepted that ACE inhibitors are relative free of common or troublesome side-effects. Persistent and bothersome *dry cough* is the most common and important subjective side-effect of these agents. Prospective studies has shown that its incidence is as high as 15%.[24] It is generally believed that its mechanism is related to inhibition of kininases. The only potentially life threatening side-effect of ACE inhibitors, also attributed to the accumulation of kinins, is *angio-edema,* This is a rare reaction, which in most instances occurs shortly after the initiation of treatment.[25] Rash and loss of taste are uncommon and not severe side-effects.

First dose hypotension is a reaction known to occur when starting treatment with ACE inhibitors, especially in patients who have already been treated with high doses of diuretics or those with high plasma renin activity associated with renovascula disease. Its duration is shorter with drugs with a short half-life, such as captopril, and such a drug is preferred for the initiation of therapy in patients at risk. Syncope, ischemic stroke or myocardial infarction may occur when the fall in systolic blood pressure is more than 50 mm Hg. When ACE inhibitors are started it is wise to ask the patient to omit diuretic therapy for one or two days and to take the first dose while recumbent. Patients at high risk are elderly patients receiving high doses of loop diuretics for heart failure. These patients may need to be admitted in hospital for the initiation of ACE inhibitors. Hyperkalemia can develop in patients treated with ACE inhibitors, and potassium supplements or potassium-sparing diuretic should be stopped when ACE inhibitors are started. ACE inhibitors are absolutely contraindicated in the second and trimesters of pregnancy because of a high incidence of intrauterine death in animal studies, as well as oligohydramnios and fetal anuria when used in humans.[14]

ACE inhibitors in the treatment of chronic heart failure

Both hemodynamic and neurohormonal factors contribute to the development and progression of chronic heart failure. Several therapeutic approaches that antagonize hemodynamic factors may activate endogenous neurohormonal systems and as a result, their efficacy may be restricted. Thus, vasodilator drugs produce favourable short-term hemodynamic effects by alleviating peripheral vasoconstriction, but many of these agents have limited long-term efficacy because they activate sympathetic nervous system Also, many patients whose symptoms are rapidly relieved with the initiation of diuretic treatment, deteriorate clinically during long-term follow-up when diuretics are used as monotherapy, probably because of the activation of the RAS by the diuretics.[26]

In patients with moderate heart failure, the administration of captopril results in a fall of systemic vascular resistance by 20-40%, a fall of right atrial and pulmonary wedge pressures by around 40%, and a rise of cardiac output by 15-30%, while mean arterial pressure falls by about 20%. The hemodynamic responses to enalapril, lisinopril and other ACE inhibitors have generally been found to be more modest, with reductions in systemic vascular resistance and atrial pressures of about 25-30%, and little or no increase in cardiac output. In addition to their hemodynamic effects ACE inhibitors have been found to modify structural remodelling of the enlarging heart, and to prevent the development of replacement fibrosis and disease progression.[27]

Several controlled clinical trials have indicated that in patients with chronic heart failure, ACE inhibitors relieve dyspnea and improved exercise performance to greater extent than other agents, and that tolerance rarely develop during treatment. More importantly, ACE inhibitors (and in particular enalapril) have been found to increase survival of patients with mild, moderate or severe chronic heart failure more than other therapeutic interventions.[28,29] In addition, ACE inhibitors given shortly after a myocardial infarction improved prognosis in patients with low ejection fraction.[29] These beneficial effects of ACE inhibitors are believed to be related to the dual action of ACE inhibitors on both the hemodynamic and the neurohormonal mechanisms of heart failure.

It should be noted, however, that treatment of chronic heart failure with an ACE inhibitor *alone* is not particularly effective. In most clinical trials, ACE inhibitors were added to the treatment of patients with chronic heart failure after their condition had been stabilized with a diuretic.[30] On the other hand ACE inhibitors exert hemodynamic and clinical benefits similar or superior to digitalis and in addition, they extend life. Some investigators have suggested that digitalis treatment can be discontinued in patients with chronic cardiac failure receiving diuretics and an ACE inhibitor. Recent observations, however, indicate that this is not true, and that in patients with chronic heart failure and impaired systolic function who have remained stable while receiving digoxin, diuretics, and an ACE inhibitor (captopril or enalapril), the withdrawal of digitalis often results in clinical deterioration.[31]

As already mentioned, the first dose of an ACE inhibitor may induce abrupt fall in blood pressure severe enough to cause syncope. First-dose hypotension is more of a problem in heart failure than in hypertension. In one study designed to evaluate the effect of enalapril on survival in patients with mild-to-moderate heart failure (SOLVD study), the incidence of symptomatic hypotension was found to be around 2.2%.[29] Older patients, with more severe forms of heart failure, or treated with high doses of diuretics were found to be at greater risk.[32] Specifically in patients with severe heart failure, treatment with ACE inhibitors should always start with small doses (e.g., captopril 6.25mg) and under close hospital supervision. There is no evidence that the incidence of syncope is different among the various ACE inhibitors. However, longer-acting agents are likely to produce symptomatic hypotension of greater duration.

REFERENCES

1. Erdos EG. Angiotensin I converting enzyme and the changes in our concepts through the years. Lewis K. Dahl memorial lecture. Hypertension 1990: 16:368.

2. Soubrier F, et al. Molecular biology of the angiotensin I converting enzyme : I. Biochemistry and structure of the gene. J Hypertens 1993, 11: 471.

3. Bruneval P, et al. Angiotensin I converting enzyme in human intestine and kidney. Ultrastructure and immunohistochemical localization. Histochemistry 1986, 85 : 73.

4. Arregin A, Iversen LL. Angiotensin - converting enzyme: presence of high activity in choroid plexus of mammalian brain. Eur J Pharmacol 1978 : 52 : 27.

5. Costerousse O, et al. Angiotensin I - converting enzyme in human circulating mononuclear cells. Genetic polymorphism of expression in T-lymphocytes. Biochem J 1993, 290 : 33.

6. Soubrier F, et al. Molecular biology of the angiotensin I converting enzyme : II. Structure - function . Gene polymorphism and clinical implications. J Hypertens 1993, 11: 599.

7. Ondetti MA, Rubin B, Cushman DW. Design of specific inhibitors of angiotensin-converting enzyme : New class of orally active antihypertensive agents. Science 1977, 196: 441.

8. Wei L, et al. The two homologous domains of human angiotensin I - converting enzyme interact differently with competitive inhibitors. J Biol Chem 1992, 267 : 13398.

9. Samani NJ. New developments in renin and hypertension. Tissue generation of angiotensin I and II changes the picture. Br Med J 1991, 302 : 981.

10. Schunkert H, et al. Riegger GA.J. Association between a deletion polymorphism of the angiotesin-converting enzyme gene and left ventricular hypertrophy. N Engl J Med 1994, 330 : 1637.

11. Carbonell LF, et al. Effect of a kinin antagonists on the acute antihypertensive activity of enalapril in severe hypertension. Hypertension 1988, 11 : 239.

12. Spertini F, et al. Opposing effects of chronic angiotensin-converting enzyme blockade by captopril on the responses to exogenous angiotensin II and vasopressin vs norepinephrine in rats. Circ Res 1981, 48 : 621.

13. Oparil S, et al. Antihypertensive effect of enalapril in essential hypertension : role of prostacyclin. Am J Med Sci 1987, 294 : 395.

14. McInnes GT, Stergiou GS. Clinical pharmacology of ACE inhibitors. In : Cleland JGF (ed.) The clinician's guide to ACE inhibition. Edinburgh, London, Churchill Livingstone 1993 : 23.

15. Yeo WW, Ramsey LE, Jackson PR. ACE inhibitors and hypertension. In : Cleland JGF (ed.) The clinician's guide to ACE inhibition. Edinburgh, London, Churchill Livingstone 1993 : 37.

16. Sambhi MP, et al. Long-range safety and protective benefits of angiotensin-converting enzyme inhibitors for hypertension - do we need more clinical trials? West J Med 1993, 158 : 286.

17. Weber MA, Laragh JH. Hypertension : Steps forward and steps backward. Arch Intern Med 1993, 153 : 149.

18. The Joint National Committee on Detection, Evaluation, and Treatment og High Blood Pressure. The fifth report on the Joint National Committee on Detection, Evaluation, and Treatment og High Blood Pressure. Arch Intern Med 1993, 153 : 154.

19. Brunner HR, Waeber B, Nussberger J. Angiotensin converting enzyme inhibition and the normal kidney. Kidney Int 1987, 31 (Suppl 20) : 5104.

20. Mogensen CE. Angiotensin converting enzyme inhibitors and diabetic nephropathy. Their effects on proteinuria may be independent of their effects on blood pressure. Br Med J 1992, 304 : 327.

21. Pollare T, Lithell H, Berne C. A comparison of the effects of hydrochlorothiazide and captopril on glucose and lipid metabolism in patients with hypertension. N Engl J Med 1989, 321 : 868.

22. Dzau VJ, Gibbons G. Cell biology of vascular hypertrophy in hypertension. Am J Cardiol 1988, 62 : 30G.

23. Anderson WP, Woods RL. Intrarenal effects of angiotension II in renal artery stenosis. Kidney Int 1987, 31 (Suppl 20) : 5157.

24. Yeo WW, Foster G, Ramsay LE. Prevalence of cough in patients taking enalapril : controlled study versus nifedipine. Quart J Med 1991, 239 : 763.

25. Hedner T, et al. Angioedema in relation to angiotensin converting enzyme inhibitors. Br Med J 1992, 304 : 941.

26. Packer M. Treatment of chronic heart failure. Lancet 1992, 340 : 92.

27. Cleeland JGF. The haemodynamic effects of ACE inhibitors. In : Cleland JGF (ed.) The clinician's guide to ACE inhibition. Edingurgh, London, Churchill Livingstone 1993: 76.

28. CONSENSUS Trial Study Group. Effects of enalapril on mortality in severe congestive heart failure. Results of the cooperative north Scandinavian enalapril survival study (CONSENSUS). N Engl J Med 1987, 316 : 1429.

29. SOLVD Investigators. Effect of enalapril on survival in patients with reduced left ventricular ejection fractions and congestive heart failure. N Engl J Med 1991, 325:293.

30. Poole-Wilson PA, Lindsay D. Advances in the treatment of chronic heart failure. Br Med J 1992, 304 : 1069.

31. Packer M, et al. for the RADIANCE study. Withdrawal of digoxin from patients with chronic heart failure treated with angiotensin-converting-enzyme inhibitors. N Engl J Med 1993, 329:1.

32. Hood WB, Youngblood M, Ghali JK, et al for the SOLVD investigators. Initial blood pressure response to enalapril in hospitalized patients (studies of left ventricular dysfunction [SOLVD]). Am J Cardiol 1991, 68:1465.

13 HYPERTENSION AND AORTIC MECHANICS

Christos Pitsavos, Christodoulos I. Stefanadis,
Pavlos K. Toutouzas

Structural changes of the aortic wall in hypertension

Significant structural alterations have been shown to develop within the aortic wall in hypertensive states, both in humans and in animal models.[1-4] These alterations represent the local manifestations of a generalized remodeling process involving all parts of the vasculature,[5] i.e. large conduit arteries, peripheral resistance arteries as well as veins. Adaptation of the design of the vascular wall is induced as a response to increased functional load, imposed on the vessels by pressure elevation. Through the building of a large muscle bulk, that being the predominant characteristic of the procedure, and subsequent readjustment of the wall to lumen ratio, avoidance of increase in wall tension or stress is aimed at, according to Laplace's law. When the onset of the hypertensive stimulus is prompt, mural changes evolve quite rapidly. They seem to spare no component of the aortic wall, being particularly pronounced in the tunica media and tunica intima.

The characteristic feature of the hypertensive media is diffuse thickening,[1,3] resulting from a substantial increase of the total mass of vascular smooth muscle. A combination of smooth muscle cell hyperplasia, hypertrophy and polyploidy produces this effect.[6] The contribution of each of the three processes most likely differs among different vascular beds, with hypertrophy and polyploidy prevailing, in the aorta, and hyperplasia characterizing, the response in peripheral arteries.[4,6] Hernias of medical smooth muscle into the intima are often demonstrated.[7] Accumulation of fibrous proteins - collagen and elastin - as well as of mucopolysaccharide-rich, ground substance further add to medial thickening.[2,4] It should be noted, however, that the increase of the amount of medial components does not result in the formation of new distinct structural - functional layers (lamellar tinits) within the vascular wall.[3,8]

Widening of the subendothelial space is among the earliest discernible alterations regarding the tunica intima, being the result of increased synthesis and deposition of extracellular matrix by the endothelium.[9] Endothelial cell shape changes, hypertrophy and hyperplasia, as well as an increase of homocellular tight junctions also occur. Blood-borne mononuclear cells adhere on to the endothelial surface and subsequently migrate and colonize the subendothelial space. The latter is also invaded by migrating medial smooth muscle cells.[7,10] Participation of the aortic adventitia in the remodeling process consists mainly of an increase of its collagen content.

The distinct vascular network of the vasa vasorum, which contributes significantly to the nutrition of the outer half of the thoracic aortic wall, is also influenced by the hypertensive stimulus. A decrease in the capacity of these vessels has been demonstrated in chronic hypertensive states, possibly due to wall thickening and narrowing of their lumen.[11] Diminished flow through the vasa vasorum, combined with the impaired diffusion of blood-borne nutrients within the thickened aortic wall and the increased metabolic needs of the hypertrophied aortic smooth muscle, may well predispose to medial ischemia and necrosis.[12] Such a predisposition would be expected, and indeed seems to be, even more pronounced in the abdominal aorta, which is normally avascular.[13]

Marked qualitative similarities between the mural changes induced by hypertension and the ones encountered with advancing age, [14] have led to the description of the former as results of an accelerated form of aging.

There is an increasing amount of evidence suggesting that genetic mechanisms[5,15-16] play an important role in the growth processes of the hypertensive vessel wall, particularly in some variants of essential hypertension (such as in the spontaneously hypertensive rat model - SHR - or in certain human variants). Not far from this concept lies the intriguing assumption that some of the earliest morphologic changes may represent steps of the very pathogenesis of hypertension, rather than mere consequences of the elevated blood pressure stimulus. Conceptualization of the vasculature as an active synthetic and secretary organ has handed the key to resolution of relevant issues in the future. Exploration of autocrine and paracrine pathways[17-19] regulating arterial wall function and relation of morphologic changes to functional alterations of the involved cellular populations, is expected to provide insight on the overall significance of hypertensive arterial wall remodeling.

The functional aspect:
aortic elastic properties are altered

The aortic media is the principal determinant of the vessel's physical properties.[20-21] Given the magnitude of changes described above, resultant alterations of the mechanical behavior of the aorta come as no surprise. Indeed, as various investigational approaches confirm, hypertension results in a reduction of aortic distensibility (in other words, the aorta becomes stiffer in hypertension). Apart from diffuse medial thickenning, several other mechanisms have been postulated to contribute to this effect.

Increased arterial pressure per se interferes with the aortic elastic properties, in a way predicted by the function of the aortic media as a " two-phase" material.[22] While at low distending pressure wall tension is bome by the elastin fibers, as pressure increases and the artery is distended further, most of the stressing force is transferred to the far less extensible collagen fibers, rendering the vascular wall considerably more rigid. This phenomenon is reflected in the non-linear appearance of the aortic pressure-volume curve.[23, 24]

Increased smooth muscle tension[25] is yet another possible contributor to aortic wall stiffening in hypertension. This may result from increased levels of, or increased sensitivity to vasoactive substances reaching the arterial wall by the circulation or through nerve endings, or even synthesized locally.[26] Hypertension-induced endothelial cell dysfunction 27 seems to contribute to alterations of arterial wall tone, most likely through impairment of nitric oxide-mediated vascular smooth muscle relaxation.

Finally, the role of vasa vasorum in alterations of the aortic elastic properties is also attracting attention. As demonstrated recently in our laboratory,[28] removal of the vasa vasorum in a group of experimental animals led to an acute and significant decrease of the ascending aortic distensibility. The findings were attributed to a lack of blood supply to the outer layers of the vascular wall. As previously noted, blood flow through the vasa vasorum may be diminished in hypertension, thus leading to similar effects of aortic wall stiffening.

Role of decreased aortic distensibility in the hemodynamics of hypertension

Advances in cardiovascular research have made clear that the spectrum of pathophysiologic consequenses of decreased aortic distensibility exceeds the local scale of the vessel itself, affecting profoundly cardiac function and structure. It now seems likely that the role of this feature in the overall hemodynamics of hypertension and its contribution to the induction of certain complications, notably left ventricular hypertrophy and heart failure,[29-30] are important enough to deserve much of the attention monopolized for long, by the other common denominator of established hypertensive states, i.e. increased peripheral resistance.

Decreased aortic distensibility exerts its effects on cardiac performance both directly and indirectly,[31-33] through the ecceleration of propagation of the pulse wave, which causes inappropriately early return of reflected waves from the arterial periphery. Combined, these two pathophysiolocical pathways result in the disturbance of left ventricular-vascular coupling throughout the cardiac cycle, thereby gravely off balancing myocardial oxygen demand and supply.

Produced changes are reflected in alterations of the amplitude and contour of the ascending aortic pressure wave, as well as in alterations of the characteristics of the ascending aortic impedance pattern.

During ejection, the ability of the rigid to function as a Windkessel and to cushion pulsations produced by the cardiac pump is compromised. Aortic stiffness per se causes a disproportionate increase of systolic aortic (and left venticular) pressure. This precise effect is further intensified by early wave reflection.[34]

In the ascending aortic impedance spectrum, aortic rigidity is manifested as an increase of the impedance modulus over high frequencies (the characteristic impedance). On the other hand, early wave reflection shifts the whole impedance curve to the right; the resultant left venticular-vascular mismatch evident from the fact that the minimal values of impedance no longer correspond to the highest values of the ventricular ejection flow wave, as is the case under normal circumstances.[32,35]

The net result of the described phenomena is an increase of left ventricular afterload, accompanied by an increase of left ventricular systolic wall stress and myocardial metabolic requirements.[36-40] In the long run, elevated systolic pressure and stress are believed to contribute significantly to an increase of left ventricular mass.[29,41]

Damaging effects expand over diastole, where impaired recoil of the rigid aortic wall seems to contribute to a reduction or misdirection of the normal aortic retrograde blood flow.[42] In addition, early wave reflection causes a new exponential decline of the aortic pressure, without interruption by any diastolic wave.[32] Both these alterations are believed to have a deleterious effect on coronary artery perfusion, thus further disrupting myocardial metabolic equilibrium. Indeed,[43] experimental decrease of aortic distensibility in animals was shown to impair subendocardial perfusion during increased ventricular contraction, even in the absence of coronary artery stenoses.

Finally, as far as the local scale is regarded, elevation of peak systolic pressure and pulse pressure, together with the increase in the rate of change of pressure, are expected, according to the principles of material fatigue, to predispose to further degeneration of the aortic wall.

Evaluating aortic mechanics in hypertensive humans: Issues regarding methodology

The presence of decreased aortic distensibility in hypertensive patients has been demonstrated by employment of various techniques. The velocity of the pulse wave this effect[29,44-45] has been used quite extensively, nevertheless providing only an indirect estimation of the elastic properties of lengthy aortic segments or even of the entire vessel. In contrast, methods relating radial aortic expansion to the pulse pressure[45-55] have enabled direct determination of the aortic distensibility at any given level from the aortic root to the aortic bifurcation.

In view of the increasing interest about aortic elastic behavior in hypertension, a comment regarding methodology seems appropriate at this point. As concerns accurate evaluation of the regional aortic elastic properties, regardless of clinical setting, invasive techniques are considered to represent the optimal approach. [46-48] In the catheterization laboratory, aortic diameters in systole and diastole can be measured by contrast angiography;[47-48] accuracy of distensibility calculations is ensured by the simultaneous recording of aortic pressure at the same precise level of the vessel, ideally by means of sensitive catheter-tip micromanometers.[49]

Application of these techniques, however, in the study of large patient populations meets with obvious ethical and practical problems. As a result, attention has been shifted toward the development and assessment of non-invasive alternatives. Thus, two-dimensional echocardiography[45,50-54] as well as magnetic resonance imaging techniques[55-56] have been shown to provide reliable data on aortic diameter; the same seems to stand for the determination of the pulse pressure sphygmomanometry at the brachial artery, despite the well-known differences of the pressure wave between the aorta and peripheral arterial sites. By combining transcutaneous echocardiography, in particular, with cuff pressure measurements, [45,49-51] patient discomfort is obviously minimal.

Invasive and non-invasive techniques were compared by Stefanadis et al[57] in 46 male patients (30 with coronary artery disease and 16 age-matched normal controls) who were evaluated by both approaches. Aortic systolic and diastolic diameters were measured both angiographically and by 2D-guided M-mode transthoracic echocardiography. The pulse pressure was recorded by means of an intraaortic fluid-filled catheter and by the auscultatory method at the brachial artery. The systolic and diastolic, aortic diameters obtained by echocardiography correlated well with those measured angiographically (r=0.847, SEE=0.214, P= 0.001 and r= 0.852, SEE=0.206, P=0.001 for systolic, and diastolic diameters respectively). The same stood for the mean chance in aortic diameter (r= 0.939, SEE=0.025, P=0.001). The pulse pressure obtained sphygmomanometrically was lower than that measured by direct catheterization, mainly because the former approach overestimated diastolic pressure. This discrepancy however did not prevent invasive and noninvasive results from correlating well (r=0.913, SEE=2.82, P=0.001). Aortic distensibility calculated from non-invasive data was slightly greater than aortic distensibility calculated invasively (2.78± 1.58 cm2 dyn-1 vs 2.42± 1.37 cm2 dyn-1 respectively, P< 0.001). Still, an excellent correlation between the two methods was found (r= 0.949, SEE= 0.501, P< 0.001).

Emergence of a new therapeutic target: pharmacological manipulation of aortic elastic behavior in hypertension

Appreciation of the pathophysiological importance of hypertensive aortic disease stimulated interest about potential therapeutic intervention in this particular field. Identification and use of antihypertensive agents that are capable of improving aortic elastic properties, in addition to their blood pressure lowering capability, should be expected to render antihypertensive treatment more efficient in the avoidance of cardiac functional compromise and cardiac hyper-trophy. However, as indicated by the increasing inflow of information, the new, area of research could prove to be much vaster than might have been expected initially. Thus, [58-59] even drugs that belong to the same category appear to have slightly or markedly different effects on aortic mechanics, as well as on left ventricular function and mass. Moreover, the possibility of the same agent exhibiting different actions in different models of hypertension cannot be excluded. Generalizations and issuing of therapeutic guidelines do not seem, therefore, to be close at hand. Up to date, relatively, clear-cut conclusions have been drawn in only, a few selected cases.

In the case of nitroglycerin, there has been no demonstration of any improvement in aortic distensibility. Studies[60-63] of the aortic impedance spectrum and of the aortic pressure wave revealed that a decrease in the magnitude of reflected waves, as well as a delay[61] of their return to the ascending aorta are the responsible mechanisms for the drug's beneficial effect on the pulsatile component of left ventricular afterload, in a state of unaltered aortic elastic behavior. Chances in wave reflection are the result of dilatation of small systemic arteries by nitroglycerin.[60]

In contrast, the calcium channel blocker nifedipine influences aortic distensibility. Evidence of such action was provided after intravenous infusion of this agent in experimental animals.[64] In our institution, Stratos et al., [65] studied the effect of sublingually administered nifedipine on the distensibility of the ascending aorta in 22 hypertensive humans and 12 age-matched normotensive controls.In this study, a combination of invasive and noninvasive techniques was employed for distensibility measurements; aortic pressure was monitored by direct catheterizabon of the ascending aorta, whereas aortic diameters were measured simultaneously by transthoracic 2D-guided M-mode echocardiography. Ascending aortic distensibility was calculated by the formula: **Ao dist = 2 x Dd / d x DP**, where Dd =pulsatile change in aortic diameter, DP=pulse pressure and d= diastolic aortic diameter. In basal conditions, as expected, aortic distensibility was significantly lower in hypertensive patients than in normotensive controls (1.326 ± 0.393 vs 2.457 ± 0.588 cm^2 dyn^{-1} 10^{-6}, p= 0.001). A strong, inverse correlation was demonstrated between the ascending, aortic distensibility, and the mean aortic pressure (r= -0.81). Ten minutes after 10 mg of nifedipine were administered sublingually, aortic distensibility increased significantly in both groups. Improvement of distensibility was, in absolute values, less in hypertensives patients than in normotensive controls (0.339 ± 0.273 vs 0.812 ± 0.316 cm^2 dyn^{-1} 10^{-6} respectively, p = 0.001), although the percentage change in aortic distensibility from the basal state was not statistically different between the two groups. Increase in distensibility was associated with a decrease of aortic pressure but no change of the diastolic aortic diameter; this led investigators to postulate the contribution of non-passive mechanisms (ie, independent of the decrease in blood pressure) in the action of nifedipine on the elastic properties of aortic wall. Similar conclusions were drawn during a second study conducted by Stefanadis et al.[66], with the same methodology, in patients with coronary artery disease. A direct relaxing, effect on aortic smooth muscle, possibly combined with an increase in blood flow via the vasa vasorum (due to their decompression in the relaxed aortic wall or even due to relaxation of their own wall muscle layer) are examples of such potential non-passive effects of nifedipine. However, in order to definitely, differentiate between passive and non passive effects of drugs on the elastic properties of the aortic wall, study of the pressure-diameter relation of the vessel and of its changes after each intervention is necessary.

Studies with angiotensin-converting enzyme inhibitors received considerable thrust after the identification of the well-developed and fully operational renin-angiotensin system in the vascular wall and its contribution to local growth processes. [26,67] In animal models, as well as in humans (the former being as yet the source of the vast majority of available data), results have been pointing at the same direction. With most of the studied agents, an improvement in aortic distensibility was demonstrated. Quite often, ACE-inhibitor activity was shown to be characterized by prevention, or regression of already developed aortic medial hypertrophy.

It is clear that much has yet to be done for the determination of the effects of different antihypertensives on the mechanics of the hypertensive aorta. The original expectations, however, for the establishment of an additional criterion in selecting drugs for efficient antihypertensive treatment, seem justified. The employment of noninvasive techniques for the determination of aortic distensibility will enable evaluation of pharmacological manipulations in large populations of hypertensive humans and will hopefully accelerate gain of knowledge and subsequent reorientation of therapeutic strategies.

Acknowledgment

The contribution of Dr. Spiros Lambrou to this work is gratefully acknowledged.

REFERENCES

1. Karsner HT. Thickness of aortic media in hypertension. Ass Amer Physicians 1938: 53:54.

2. Wolinski H. Response of the rat aortic media to hypertension. Morphological and chemical studies. Circ Res 1970: 26: 507.

3. Wolinski H. Effects of hypertension and its reversal on the thoracic aorta of male and female rats. Circ Res 1971: 28: 622.

4. Olivetti G, et al. Quantitative structural changes of the rat thoracic aorta in early spontaneous hypertension. Tissue composition, and hypertrophy and hyperplasia of smooth muscle cells. Circ Res 1982: 51 : 19.

5. Folkow B. Structure and function of the arteries in hypertension. Am Heart J 1987: 114: 938.

6. Chobanian A. The arterial smooth muscle cell in systemic hypertension. Am J Cardiol 1987:60:941.

7. Kowala MC, et al. Cellular changes during hypertension: a quantitative study of the rat aorta. Exp Mol Pathol 1986: 45: 323.

8. Wolinski H, Glagov S. A lamellar unit of aortic medial structure and function in mammals. Circ Res 1967: 20: 99.

9. McGuire PG, et al. Increased deposition of basement membrane macromolecules in specific vessels in the spontaneously hypertensive rat. Am J Pathol 1989: 135: 291.

10. Todd ME. Hypertensive structural changes in blood vessels: do endothelial cells hold the key? Can J Physiol Pharmacol 1992: 70: 536.

11. Marcus ML, et al. Effects of chronic hypertension on vasa vasorum in the thoracic aorta. Cardiovasc Res 1985: 19: 777.

12. Wilens SL, Malcolm JA, Vazquez JM. Experimental infarction and medial necrosis of the dog's aorta. Am J Pathol 1965: 47: 695.

13. Wolinski H. Comparison of medial growth of human thoracic and abdominal aortas. Circ Res 1970: 27: 531.

14. Wolinski H. Long-term effects of hypertension on the rat aortic wall and their relation to concurrent aging changes. Circ Res 1972: 30: 301.

15. Kanbe T, et al. Studies of hypertension-induced vascular hypertrophy in cultured smooth muscle cells from spontaneously hypertensive rats. Hypertension 1983: 5: 887.

16. Scott-Burden T, Resink TJ, Buhler FR. Growth regulation in smooth muscle cells from normal and hypertensive rats. J Cardiovasc Pharmacol 1988: 12(suppl 5) : S124.

17. Luscher TF, Vanhoutte PM. The endothelium: Modulator of cardiovascular function. Boca Raton, FL, CRC Press, 1990.

18. Dzau V, Gibbons G. Autocrine - paracrine mechanisms of vascular myocytes in systemic hypertension. Am J Cardiol 1987: 60: 991.

19. Yamori Y, et al. Humoral trophic influence on cardiovascular structural changes in hypertension. Hypertension 1984: 6 (suppl III): 11127.

20. Dobrin PB. Mechanical properties of arteries. Physiol Rev 1978: 58: 397.

21. Milnor WR. Hemodynamics. Baltimore, Md: Williams & Wilkins, 1989: 90.

22. Bergel DH. The static elastic properties of the arterial wall. J Physiol 1961: 156: 445.

23. Wolinski H, Glagov S. Structural basis for the static mechanical properties of the aortic media. Circ Res 1963: 24: 400.

24. Luscher TF. Heterogeneity of endothelial dysfunction in hypertension. Circulation 1988: 77: 949.

25. Roach MR, Burton AC. The reason for the shape of the distensibility, curve of arteries. Can J Biochem Physiol 1957: 35: 681.

26. Dobrin P, Rovick, A. Influence of vascular smooth muscle on contractile mechanics and elasticity of arteries. Am J Physiol 1969: 217: 1644.

27. Dzau VJ, Safar ME. Large conduit arteries: Role of the vascular renin-angiotensin system. Eur Heart J 1992 13 (suppl D) i50.

28. Stefanadis Cl, et al. Medial necrosis and acute deteriorations in aortic distensibility following removal of the vasa vasorum of canine descending aorta. Cardiovasc Res 1993: 27: 951.

29. Bouthier JD, et al. Cardiac hypertrophy and arterial distensibility in essential hypertension. Am Heart J 1985: 100: 1345.

30. Merillon JP, et al. Relationship between physical properties of the arterial system and left ventricular performance in the course of aging and arterial hypertension. Eur Heart J 1985: 3: 95.

31. Nichols CR, et al. lnput impedance of the systemic circulation in man. Circ Res 1977: 40: 451.

32. O'Rourke MF. Arterial stiffness, systolic blood pressure and logical treatment of arterial hypertension. Hypertension 1990: 15:339.

33. Boudoulas H, Toutouzas P, Wooley C. Functional Abnormalities of the Aorta. Futura Publishing. Armonk, NY. 1996: 333.

34. O'Rourke MF. The arterial pulse in health and disease. Am Heart J 1971: 82: 687.

35. Niurgo JP, et al. Aortic input impedance in normal man: Relationship to pressure- wave forms. Circulation 1980: 69: 105.

36. Ting CT, et al. Arterial hemodynamics in human hypertension. J Clin Invest 1986: 1462.

37. Milnor WR. Arterial impedance as ventricular afterload. Circ Res 1975:36:565.

38. Urschel CW, et al. Effects of decreased aortic compliance on performance of the left ventricle. Am J Physiol 1968:214:198.

39. Nichols WW, et al. Ventricular/vascular interaction in patients with mild systemic hypertension and normal peripheral resistance. Circulation 1986: 74: 455.

40. Binkley PF, Boudoulas H. Measurement of myocardial inotropy. In: Leier CV, ed. Cardiotonic drugs: A clinical review. Marcel Dekker 1991.

41. Nichols WL, O'Rourke MF. Biology in arteries, 3rd ed. London, London, 1990.

42. Safar ME, et al. Arterial dynamics, cardiac hypertrophy and antihypertensive treatment. Circulation 1987: 75 (suppl I): I156.

43. Bogren HG, et al. The function of the aorta in ischemic heart disease: A magnetic resonance and angiographic study of aortic compliance and blood flow patterns. Am Heart J 1989: 118: 234.

44. Matsuka S, et al. Chronically decreased aortic distensibility deterioration of coronary, perfusion during increased left ventricular contraction. J Am Coll Cardiol 1994: 24: 1406.

45. Avolio AP, et al. Effects of aging on arterial distensibility in populations with high and low prevalence of hypertension: comparison between urban and rural communities in China. Circulation 1985: 71: 202.

46. Isnard RN, et al. Pulsatile diameter and elastic modulus of the aortic arch in essential hypertension: a noninvasive study. J Am Coll Cardiol 1989: 13: 399.

47. Greenfield JC, Patel DJ. Relation between pressure and diameter in the ascending aorta of man. Circ Res 1962: 10: 778.

48. Merillon JP, et al. Evaluation of the elasticity and characteristic image of the ascending aorta in man. Cardiovasc Res 1978: 12: 401.

49. Boudoulas H, et al : Functional Abnormalities of the Aorta Futura Publishing Company, Inc. Armonk, NY, 1996, 121.

50. Stefanadis C, et al. Aortic distensibility abnormalities in coronary artery disease. Am J Cardiol 1987: 59:1300.

51. Dart A, et al. Aortic distensibility and left ventricular structure and function in isolated systolic hypertension. Eur Heart J 1993:14:1465.

52. Imura T, et al. Non-invasive ultrasonic measurement of the elastic properties of the human abdominal aorta. Cardiovascular Res 1986:20:208.

53. Hirai T, et al. Stiffness of systemic arteries in patients with myocardial infarction. A noninvasive method to predict severity of coronary atherosclerosis. Circulation 1989: 80:78.

54. Lang RM, et al. Measurement of regional elastic properties of the human aorta. A new application of transesophageal echocardiography with automated border detection and calibrated subclavian pulse tracings. Circulation 1994: 90: 1875.

55. Mohiaddin RH, et al. Regional aortic compliance studied by magnetic resonance imaging: the effects of age, training and coronary artery disease. Br Heart J 1989: 62: 90.

56. Honda T, et al. Evaluation of aortic distensibility in patients with essential hypertension by using cine magnetic resonance imaging. Angiology 1994: 13: 207.

57. Stefanadis C, et al. Distensibihty of the descending aorta: comparison of invasive and non-invasive techniques in healthy men and in men with coronary artery disease. Eur Heart J 1990: 11: 990.

58. Safar ME, et al. Cardiac mass and aortic distensibility following calcium blockade in hypertension. J Cardiovasc Pharmacol 1991: 17(suppl 2): 575.

59. Frohlich ED, et al. Changes in cardiovascular mass, left ventricular pumping ability and aortic distensibility after calcium antagonists in Wistar-Kyoto and spontaneously hypertensive rats. J Hypertens 1992: 10: 1369.

60. Michel JB, et al. Effect of the dihydropyridine isradipine on the large arterial walls of spontaneously hypertensive rats. Circulation 1994: 90: 3024.

61. Yaginuma T, et al. Effect of glyceryl trinitrate on peripheral arteries alters left ventricular load in man. Cardlovasc Res 1986: 20: 153.

62. Latson TW, et al. Effect of nitroglycerin on aortic impulce, diameter and pulse-wave velocity. Circ Res 1988: 62: 884.

63. Fitchett DH, et al. Reflected pressure waves in the ascending aorta: effect of glyceryl trinitrate. Cardlovasc Res 1988: 22: 494.

64. Kelly RP, et al. Nitroglycerin has more favourable effects on left ventricular afterload than apparent from measurement of pressure in a peripheral artery. Eur Heart J 1990: 11: 138.

65. Kohno M, et al. Evaluation of aortic wall distensibility by aortic pressure-dimension relation: Effects of nifedipine on aortic wall. Cardiovasc Res 1987: 21: 305.

66. Stratos C, et al. Ascending aorta distensibility abnormalities in hypertensive patients and response to nifedipine administration. Am J Med. 1992: 93: 505.

67. Stefanadis C, et al. Distensibility of the ascending aorta in coronary artery disease and changes after nifedipine administration. Chest 1994: 105: 1017.

Section C
CARDIOMYOPATHIES

14 PATHOPHYSIOLOGY AND MANAGEMENT OF HEART FAILURE

Daniel K. Levy, George Dangas, Richard Gorlin

Heart failure affects an estimated 1% of the population in the western world and results in an average mortality rate of 10% at 1 year and 50% after 5 years [1]. The incidence of heart failure rises substantially beyond age 65, therefore, the prevalence of this condition is likely to increase as the population ages. In fact, in the elderly the incidence approaches 1 in 10 [2]. Consequently, heart failure places a significant economic burden on society [1].

Pathophysiology of heart failure: neurohormonal model

Until recently, heart failure was viewed in mechanical terms. This mechanical view of heart failure regarded the failing heart as "too weak" to perfuse the peripheral organs. The kidney would then retain sodium which led to pulmonary edema and peripheral edema. The therapeutic focus when treating "congestive heart failure", in this model was the use of diuretics and digoxin, in an attempt to get rid of the excess fluid and improve the pump. The modern view is that heart failure is a disease of the circulation, not merely the heart. The bodies own compensatory mechanisms can offset clinical heart failure even though the systolic or diastolic function of the left ventricle is poor. It is only when these endogenous compensatory mechanisms become overwhelmed that clinical heart failure develops. Initially these hemodynamic and neurohormonal mechanisms increase inotropic support for the injured heart. However, these compensatory mechanisms can become detrimental, when there is "excessive compensation".[3]

The clinical appearance of heart failure is preceded by an insult to and/or a loss of myocardial cells. Acute myocardial infarction, alcohol, cytotoxic drugs, viral infections, Chagas disease, or prolonged myocardial pressure or volume loading stress such as hypertension or valvular heart disease all can cause cellular injury to the myocardium. Often the cause of the injury is unknown. Furthermore, metabolic heart disease such as vitamin B1 defficiency, hypophosphatemia and hypothyroidism may lead to heart failure as well. After such injury occurs, both hemodynamic and neurohormonal mechanisms are activated to enhance the contractile force of non-injured myocardium. For instance, the Frank-Starling principle leads to enhanced contraction of the non-injured portion of the heart, in response to increasing diastolic tensions. Also, in response to myocardial injury, the sympathetic nervous system becomes active and stimulates the -adrenergic receptors of the non-injured myocardium which initially increases both inotropy and chronotropy. Endogenous catecholamines also lead to stimulation of the renin-angiotensin system with subsequent vasoconstriction. Both of these mechanisms lead to increased angiotensin-II activity and increase in the contractile force of the non-injured myocardium via pathways that involve intracellular calcium. The sympathetic activation increases the delivery of calcium to myofilament, whereas ventricular dilatation (Frank-Starling principle) enhances sensitivity of the myofilament to calcium.[4]

The increase in diastolic wall stress of the non-injured portion of the ventricle after an injury, leads to an increase in ventricular wall thickness of the non-injured portion of the ventricle. The mechanism by which this occurs may be via the induction of proto-oncogenes (*c-fos* and *c-myc*) which trigger synthesis of proteins increasing the wall thickness of that portion of the ventricle.[5] This increase in wall thickness reduces ventricular strain by distributing the excess stress among an increased number of sarcomeres. Also, the proteins synthesized during hemodynamic stress have the biochemical characteristics of fetal myocardium and are more efficient than their adult isoforms.[5]

When diastolic wall stress becomes excessive, counterbalancing mechanisms are activated to reduce the hemodynamic load to the heart. Atrial stretch, in response to diastolic wall stress, stimulates atrial baroreceptor that inhibit sympathetic outflow from the vasomotor center in the central nervous system.[6] Atrial stretch also leads to the secretion of atrial natriuretic peptide, which inhibits the release of noradrenaline and also inhibits the actions of noradrenaline on peripheral blood vessels.[7] The atrial natriuretic peptide has both a natriuretic and a direct vasodilator effect. Thus, the release of this peptide in response to atrial stretch reduces the hemodynamic load to the heart using a variety of mechanisms. There is increased sodium and water excretion by a direct effect of the atrial natriuretic peptide on glomerular and tubular function, as well as by an inhibitory effect on the release and actions of renin and vasopressin.

However, patients with heart failure, have an attenuated response to atrial natriuretic peptide.[8] This attenuated response may be caused by a decrease in renal blood flow, which leads to intra-renal release of vasoconstrictors.[9] In the normal situation, the actions of these endogenous vasoconstrictor factors are counterbalanced by endogenous vasodilators.[10] The attenuated response in heart failure may be due to structural changes in the atrial receptor endings secondary to prolonged atrial distension.[11] Also, after prolonged atrial distension, the release of atrial natriuretic peptide becomes blunted[12], and eventually depleted.[11] At a certain point of ventricular dilatation, further compensatory mechanisms are lost. The Frank Starling principle is no longer operative and the ventricle loses its ability to enhance its inotropic state. As a result, the Frank-Starling curve becomes both depressed and flattened. The mechanism of this is not entirely understood

In severe heart failure, normal cardiac output cannot be maintained and in order to guarantee an acceptable perfusion pressure, especially for the brain and the kidneys, and the heart, peripheral vasoconstriction occurs. With this elevated resistance, perfusion pressure can be maintained at an acceptable level, but at the cost of an increased work load on the failing heart. Volume retention occurs, and left ventricular end-diastolic pressure increases, leading finally to pulmonary congestion and to peripheral edema (if the right heart fails). Peripheral vasoconstriction and sodium retention in heart failure is maintained by several neurohormonal systems such as, the sympathetic nervous system, the renin-angiotensin system, and vasopressin. In addition to these circulating factors, endothelin produced by the vascular endothelium is released locally and contributes to the peripheral vasoconstriction in heart failure. Recent evidence has shown endothelin concentrations to be increased in heart failure in proportion to the severity of the disease.[13] Because of these factors, vasoconstriction in heart failure, is left relatively unopposed.

A variety of symptoms may result from low cardiac output to the gastrointestinal tract and peripheral muscle. Dilatation and hypertrophy of the heart, as well as enhanced ventricular ectopic activity can cause arrhythmias, which may become symptomatic.[14] Ventricular arrhythmias have been found up to 70-80% of patients with heart failure, and the presence of ventricular arrhythmias on holter monitor is associated with a higher mortality.[15]

After prolonged adrenergic stimulation, there is an attenuation to the positive inotropic effects of both endogenous and exogenous catecholamines. This results from changes in the cardiac adrenergic pathway, which include down-regulation of receptors and uncoupling of $_1$-receptors from adenylate cyclase.[16] Such uncoupling of the receptors from adenylate cyclase, seems to be related to an alteration in guanine nucleotide binding proteins that stimulate (Gs) or inhibit (Gi) the interaction between the receptor and the enzyme. Both a decrease in Gs and an increase in Gi have been reported in patients with heart failure.[17]

The high levels of sympathetic hormones, renin/angiotensin, and vasopressin eventually becomes detrimental. The activation of neurohormonal systems eventually exacerbates salt and water retention in patients with heart failure.[18] This alteration in fluid balance results from the direct and indirect effects of the renin-angiotensin system on glomerular and tubular function. Angiotensin augments sodium reabsorption directly and indirectly by stimulating the release of aldosterone and, in a respond to falling renal blood flow, it also causes water retention. The latter effect is caused by stimulation of the thirst center in the brain and the release of vasopressin from the pituitary.

In a comparison of neuroendocrine activation in patients with left ventricular dysfunction both with and without congestive heart failure, a substudy of SOLVD showed the neuroendocrine activation to be highest in patients with overt signs and symptoms of heart failure. Furthermore, the addition of diuretics was associated with increased neuroendocrine activation.[19].

Thus, the development of peripheral vasoconstriction and sodium retention in a patient with heart failure represents a shift in the balance of compensatory mechanisms.

Another contributing factor may be the direct toxic effects of high concentrations of noradrenaline and angiotensin on myocardial cells. Although the precise mechanism of how this occurs is unknown [20], some investigators have suggested that these neurohormones cause a state of calcium overload. Other investigators have suggested that exposure to high concentrations of neurohormones may induce free radical production leading to direct tissue damage.[3]

An additional source of myocardial damage in heart failure may be the release of cytokines which may contribute to the development of the anorexia and cachexia often associated with long standing decompensated heart failure. There is also evidence to show that cytokines enhance the production of free radicals which can cause tissue damage. The increased levels of cytokines in heart failure may also be responsible for the attenuated myocardial response to endothelium-mediated vasodilator.[3] Tumor necrosis factor (TNF-α) is a cytokine produced by inflammatory cells, and has been found to be elevated in severe heart failure.[3] It is not known whether this elevation is beneficial or detrimental to the patient with severe heart failure.[21] TNF-α leads to the increase of nitric oxide in the endothelial cells which may lead to vasodilatation, a potential beneficial effect in heart failure. However, TNF- is a negative inotrope, and is also believed to be involved in the apoptosis (programmed cell death) in heart failure [21]. TNF-α (previously named "cachectin") may also have a role in the cachexia seen in severe chronic heart failure.[22]

Other factors that lead to progression of heart failure include presence of associated mitral regurgitation. Also, in some patients with significant coronary disease, the hypertrophic response to myocardial stress may further increase energy demands while reducing energy supply, since wall thickening may impair oxygen diffusion. This could ultimately lead to significant myocardial ischemia and further damage to previously non-injured portions of the heart in decompensated heart failure.

Thus, all the above hemodynamic, circulatory and local factors appear to form a complex web of pathophysiologic mechanisms that lead to the onset and progression of clinical heart failure. Many exciting opportunities for pharmacologic intervention of one or more of the above pathways may further improve the quality and quantity of life for patients with heart failure in the future.

Current conventional therapy

Angiotensin-converting enzyme inhibitors

According to the neurohormonal view of pathophysiology of heart failure, prevention or slowing of the progression of disease should be the primary goal of therapy. There is considerable evidence to show that angiotensin-converting enzyme (ACE) inhibitors prevent the progression of disease in the asymptomatic patient with heart failure. It is therefore recommended that asymptomatic patients who are found to have moderately or severely reduced left-ventricular systolic function (ejection fraction, EF < 35-40%) should be treated with an ACE inhibitor to reduce the chance of developing clinical heart failure or to delay the onset of the disease.[23]

In the Survival and Ventricular Enlargement (SAVE) trial, patients with an MI in the preceding 3-16 days and EF's of 40% of less were treated with captopril titrated to 50 mg TID as tolerated.[24] Overall mortality during the 2-5 year period was reduced by 20% in the captopril group compared to placebo. The proportion of patients developing heart failure that require open-label treatment with ACE inhibitors was reduced from 16% to 11%, and the proportion of patients hospitalized for heart failure was reduced from 17% to 14%.

Not only have ACE inhibitors been found to prevent the progression of heart failure in asymptomatic patients, but major clinical trials have demonstrated a mortality benefit as well. In the CONSENSUS trial, which studied only patients with NYHA Class IV heart failure, one-year mortality was reduced from 52% with placebo to 36% with enalapril.[25] The SOLVD treatment trial found that enalapril reduced overall 4-year morality from 40% to 35%.[26] The survival curves indicated that median survival in patients receiving enalapril was increased by approximately 6 months. ACE inhibitors have been shown to enhance functional status in patients with heart failure.[27,28] The SOLVD treatment trial also found that enalapril decreased the total number of patients hospitalized from 74% to 69% and the number of patients hospitalized for cardiovascular reasons decreased from 63% to 75%.[29]

ACE inhibitors are known to decrease blood pressure and increase serum creatinine and potassium. However, the average changes in blood pressure and serum chemistries in the SOLVD trial were actually quite small, with an average systolic blood pressure decrease of 5 mmHg and a diastolic blood pressure decrease of 4 mmHg. The study also found a 0.1 mg/dL increase in creatinine, and 0.2 mEq/L increase in serum potassium.[29] Even in the CONSENSUS trial, which enrolled only patients with NYHA class IV heart failure, only 5.5% of those treated with enalapril were withdrawn because of symptomatic hypotension, and there was only a 1.5% increase in withdrawals due to renal insufficiency compared with patients receiving placebo.[29] Thus, relatively low blood pressure, moderate renal insufficiency, and mild hyperkalemia are not contraindications to ACE inhibitors, as demonstrated by the major clinical trials.

Although the exact mechanism of how ACE inhibitors exert their beneficial effects in heart failure patients is not entirely known, this is most likely related to the action of ACE inhibitors on both the hemodynamic and neurohormonal mechanisms of heart failure. In CONSENSUS enalapril reduced mortality primarily in patients who had the most marked neurohormonal activation [30] prior to therapy. ACE inhibitors are thought to prevent the structural remodeling that develops after prolonged increases in ventricular wall stress.[31] ACE inhibitors also may reduce the direct toxic effects of angiotensin on myocardial cells, which may lead to cell necrosis, replacement fibrosis, and disease progression.[32] In an echocardiographic substudy of SOLVD, echocardiograms were performed at baseline, 4 and 6 months. Left ventricular end diastolic and end-systolic volumes increased in the placebo groups but not in the enalapril treated group. Also, left ventricular mass tended to increase in the placebo group and to be reduced in enalapril treated group, and these differences were highly significant. This evidence suggests that treatment with enalapril attenuates progressive increases in ventricular dilatation and hypertrophy in patients with left ventricular dysfunction. This is believed to be related to ACE-inhibitors effect on remodeling.[33] Long-term treatment with enalapril was associated with a decrease in neurohormonal levels. An analysis of a substudy of the SOLVD trial showed that enalapril was associated with lower levels of plasma norepinephrine as compared to controls.[34]

Recent post MI trials with ACE inhibitors indicate that delayed initiations of therapy (such as 24 hours post suspected MI) and maintenance of ACE inhibitor treatment, such as ramapril used in the AIRE, trandolapril used in TRACE [35], or captopril used in ISIS-4 result in significant reductions in mortality.[36] In consideration of the results of CONSENSUS II, it is not recommended to give ACE-inhibitors immediately after infarction, especially using an intravenous route of administration.[37] In The Survival of Myocardial Infarction Long-term Evaluation (SMILE), the ACE inhibitor zofenopril was compared to placebo in patients who presented within 24 hours of an anterior wall MI and were started on therapy in the first day (low dose, titrated carefully). The incidence of death and severe congestive heart failure at 6 weeks was significantly reduced in the zofenopril group compared to placebo and the cumulative reduction in the risk of death or severe congestive heart failure was 34 %. The one-year mortality rate was significantly lower in the zofenopril group in comparison to placebo (10% vs. 14.1%).[38]

Therefore, major clinical trials have demonstrated that the benefits of ACE inhibitors in heart failure are three fold: prevention of disease progression, symptomatic improvement, and lower mortality rates. Doses of ACE inhibitors should be titrated upwards over 2-3 weeks with the goal of reaching the doses used in large-scale clinical trials; for example captopril 50 mg TID or enalapril 10 mg BID.[1] According to the AHCPR panel, in patients with creatinine clearance of 30 ml/min or less, ACE inhibitors should be used with caution and uptitrated slowly, as tolerated, to a maximum of half the usual maintenance dose.[1] In our opinion, higher doses can be administered after careful follow-up of the serum creatinine values.

Digoxin

Cardiac glycosides have been used to treat heart failure for more than 200 years. However, the effect of this drug on exercise tolerance and mortality in heart failure patients has only recently been tested in randomized trials.

The RADIANCE trial showed withdrawal of digoxin therapy from patients previously taking "triple" therapy with digoxin, ACE inhibitor and diuretics, led to a sixfold increase in the patients' likelihood to deteriorate clinically compared to patients who were continued on "triple" therapy.[39] When digoxin was withdrawn from patients in the RADIANCE trial, exercise tolerance, NYHA class, and quality-of-life scores deteriorated [39]. However, "withdrawal" trials may not address whether digoxin should be initiated to a stable patient with heart failure who was never started on digoxin.

There are some experimental data on isolated myocardial tissue to support the use of digoxin in heart failure. Usually an increase in the frequency of stimulation of myocardial tissue results in an increase of force of contraction (the Bowditch effect). Feldman et al.[40] have shown that patients with heart failure do not exhibit this increase in contractility after rapid stimulation. In fact, explanted hearts from patients with class IV heart failure show a decrease force of contraction with rapid stimulation.[41] Erdmann found that digitalis, when added to these cardiac tissue specimens, restores the normal force frequency relationship [42]. There is also experimental evidence on isolated cardiac tissue from patients with heart failure to show that cardiac glycosides tend to restore the normal preload force relationship (Frank-Starling mechanism).

In addition, special interest has been focused recently in the potential role of digoxin in the modulation of the neurohormonal system in patients with heart failure. The apparent benefit of digoxin over the cAMP-dependent inotropic drugs (see below) may be related to the fact that digitalis reduces activation of both the sympathetic nervous system and the renin-angiotensin system by correcting the baroreflex dysfunction of heart failure, thereby restoring the inhibitory effect of the cardiac baroreceptors on sympathetic outflow from the central nervous system.[43]

The unclear (or unproven) benefit of digoxin therapy in heart failure is currently considered a paradox of medical research, in view of the wide spectrum of the potentially beneficial mechanisms of the action of digoxin in heart failure patients. The recently completed DIG trial[44] addressed the issue of the use of digoxin in heart failure in utilizing a prospective, multicenter, placebo-controlled methodology with an average period of observation of 37 months in a total of 7888 patients across a wide range of ejection fractions, including 987 patients with normal values. The effect of digoxin in all-cause mortality was found to be neutral. There was a significant decrease in heart failure-related deaths, which was counterbalanced by an insignificant increase in the "presumed arrhythmic" deaths and deaths attributed to other cardiac causes. Patients on digoxin were less often hospitalized for worsening heart failure than those on placebo (RR=0.73, p=0.0001). There was no difference in hospitalizations for ventricular arrhythmias between the two groups and supraventricular arrhythmias as a cause of hospitalization appeared to be less frequent in the digoxin group. Patients in the ancillary trial with normal ejection fraction were more often female, older and hypertensive. Contrary to expectations, they responded to digoxin and ACE inhibitors.[44] Whether this is related to the neurohormonal inhibitory actions of Digoxin seems logical but is only conjectural at this time.

Thus, digoxin would appear to have complementary role in the management of heart failure and this role is not predicted solely on the need to improve myocardial contractility. The optimal dosage of digoxin has been debated for long; the DIG trial actually showed that the drug can be administered to a predictable blood level of 0.75-1.0 g/ml utilizing a nomogram which takes into account the body size and gender.[44]

Diuretics

According to the AHCPR panel recommendations, patients with heart failure and signs of significant volume overload should be started immediately on a diuretic. Patients with mild volume overload can be managed adequately on thiazide diuretics whereas, those with more severe volume overload should be started on a loop diuretic.

Loop diuretics are used clinically in patients with pulmonary or peripheral congestion. These drugs rapidly relieve dyspnea and edema, and have natriuretic action. Although diuretics are extremely effective in treating heart failure patients with pulmonary and peripheral edema, controlled clinical trials show that many heart failure patients deteriorate if they are treated with diuretics alone.[45] Diuretic therapy is known to be somewhat problematic when used in the out patient setting because, diuretic use is associated with the risk of potassium and magnesium depletion which may predispose the patient to life threatening ventricular arrhythmias. The most commonly used drugs of this category are furosemide and bumetanide. Combination therapy with the new thiazide metolazone administered before the daily dose of loop diuretic provides more effective diuresis. However, more profound electrolyte and creatinine changes occur as well. Therefore, this type of therapy should prompt close clinical and laboratory follow-up. Newer loop diuretics may further improve this form of heart failure therapy.

Diuretics are known to increase plasma renin activity in patients with heart failure. This increase plasma renin activity could have a deleterious effect. However, the increased renin activity from diuretic therapy is successfully reduced with the addition of an ACE inhibitor.[45]

Other important management issues

Vasodilators

Although β-adrenergic blockers have been used in patients with heart failure and in some studies have produce short-term hemodynamic improvements, larger clinical trials have shown that their long-term use does not favorably affect symptoms, exercise tolerance, or survival.[46] The pharmacodynamic explanation for this finding is thought to be due to the development of tolerance to β-adrenergic receptors). It is known that direct vasodilators like α-blockers can activate the renin-angiotensin system inducing vasoconstriction and this may relate to their lack of efficacy in heart failure over the long term.[47]

In addition to α-blockers, there are three classes of vasodilators: 1) those that act mainly on peripheral veins (nitrates and molsidomine), 2) those that act mainly on peripheral arteries (hydralazine, minoxidil, and calcium channel blockers) and 3) those with combined actions on both arteries and veins (flosequinan).[48]

Several controlled trials have been unable to show a favorable effect of nitrates or hydralazine on symptoms and exercise tolerance when added to conventional therapy [49]. This lack of efficacy has been attributed to development of tolerance to the vasodilator effects of these drugs during their long term use.[50] In the Veterans Administration Cooperative Study [51] however, which used a combination of hydralazine and nitrates, this type of medical therapy showed an improvement in mortality and in exercise tolerance[52], but their use was associated with a high frequency of adverse reactions.

In the Veterans Affairs Vasodilator-Heart Failure Trial (VHeFT) II, which compared enalapril with the combination hydralazine/isosorbide, the average daily doses of hydralazine and isosorbide dinitrate were 200 mg and 100 mg respectively.[51] The VHeFT II trial demonstrated that ACE inhibitors show an even greater effect than the vasodilator combination.

Several studies show that patients treated with minoxidil or calcium channel blockers (verapamil, nifedipine, and diltiazem) were at higher risk of worsening heart failure and cardiovascular death than patients not treated with these drugs [53]. However, additional studies are currently evaluating the role of calcium channel blockers with mild negative inotropism (e.g. diltiazem or amlodipine in IDC and PRAISE studies) in the management of heart failure.

As in the case of diuretics, both the limited efficacy and potential toxicity of direct-acting vasodilator may be related to the predilection of these drugs to activate endogenous neurohormonal systems. Nitrates and hydralazine both increase the activity of the sympathetic nervous system and renin-angiotensin system, which may blunt these hemodynamic effects of the drugs and contribute to tolerance.[49] Like nitrates, long-term calcium channel blocker therapy can cause an increase in neurohormonal activity. The detrimental effects of an increased neurohormonal activity in heart failure may explain the poor clinical results with these agents in patients with heart failure.[53]

Systemic anticoagulation

Routine anticoagulation for patients with heart failure is not recommended by the AHCPR panel. However, heart failure patients with a history of systemic or pulmonary embolism, recent atrial fibrillation, or mobile left-ventricular thrombi should be anticoagulated to a prothrombin time ratio of 1.2-1.8 times control (International Normalization Ratio 2.0-3.0), according to the panel recommendations.

In the SOLVD trial, which included patients with NYHA class II or III heart failure, the incidence of fatal stroke was only 0.24 per 100 patient-years.[29] The CONSENSUS trial included only patients with NYHA Class IV heart failure.[25] Half of those enrolled had atrial fibrillation, but only one-third of all patients were receiving anticoagulation at the start of the trial. Of 253 patients, 3 suffered a stroke over the average follow up period of 6 months, and the cumulative incidence was 2.3 strokes per 100 patient-years.

The observed incidence of strokes in patients with heart failure should be compared with the reported incidence of major and minor bleeding complication resulting from anticoagulation. In recent randomized clinical trials, the risk of serious bleeding complications ranged from 0.8 to 2.5 percent per year in patients anticoagulated to prothrombin time ratios of 1.2-1.8 [54], which is equivalent to INR 2.0-3.0. However, the incidence of serious or fatal bleeding was not different from that observed in the controls. It is important that the INR should be closely monitored, particularly during periods of exacerbations of heart failure when hepatic congestion may occur. The INR and not the prothrombin time ratio alone is the gold standard for the accurate measurement of the anticoagulation level.

Myocardial revascularization

Coronary artery disease is currently the most common cause of heart failure in the United States. Heart failure patients without contraindications to revascularization who have exercise-limiting angina, angina that occurs frequently at rest, or recurrent episodes of acute pulmonary edema should be advised to undergo coronary angiography as the initial test for identification of coronary lesions, according to the AHCPR recommendation.

Patients without significant angina, but with a history of MI, should be advised to undergo first a physiologic test for myocardial viability (such as PET or SPECT scanning or dobutamine echocardiography) followed by coronary angiography, if warranted. Available evidence suggests that about 40-45% of patients who suffer an MI have clinically important myocardial ischemia in areas supplied by other coronary arteries. There are no data, however, to show that revascularization of these areas is beneficial (in terms of increased life expectancy or enhanced quality of life) if angina or anginal equivalent is not present. Furthermore, no data are available to address the question of the extent of viability necessary to improve the risk/benefit ratio of the revascularization procedure, thereby leading to improved survival.[1]

Coronary artery bypass grafting (CABG) is the only revascularization procedure that has been shown to prolong life in patients with heart failure and angina. Percutaneous revascularization may be an alternative revascularization procedure for some patients, however no large scale clinical trial has demonstrated a survival benefit with angioplasty.

For patients with ischemic cardiomyopathy, the goal of myocardial revascularization is to prevent further ischemic injury to remaining functional myocardium or to restore function in areas of hibernating myocardium. Most cohort studies that have evaluated the effect of surgical revascularization on survival in patients with both left-ventricular dysfunction (at least moderate) and severe or limiting angina have shown positive results.[1]

However, CABG has not been shown to improve survival in patients with heart failure who do not have angina. An analysis of the Coronary Artery Surgery Study by Alderman et al.[55] showed that patients with dyspnea on exertion or fatigue as their predominant complaint had the same 3-year mortality and symptom-free survival with either CABG or medical therapy. Mortality rates from CABG increase significantly when the ejection fraction is <20% or with severe heart failure symptoms (NYHA class IV) prior to surgery.[56]

Positive inotropic agents

Augmenting the contractility of the heart can be accomplished pharmacologically by several mechanisms. Drugs that increase the concentration of intracellular cAMP, either by augmenting its synthesis (β-adrenergic agonists) or by inhibiting its degradation (phosphodiesterase inhibitors) will potentiate cardiac contraction. Drugs like digoxin which cause Na/K ATPase inhibition also augment cardiac contraction. Of the different types of mechanisms, cAMP-dependent agents produce a greater reduction in wall stress because they dilate peripheral blood vessels in addition to enhancing contractile force.

Dobutamine is an excellent intravenous β-adrenergic agonist, but its proarrhythmic properties have limited its use to the intensive care setting for acute exacerbations of heart failure. This drug has also been administered intermittently in outpatients with short-term symptomatic improvement in certain patients. There have been several clinical trials that have shown an increase in cardiovascular morbidity and mortality with β-agonists and phosphodiesterase inhibitors.[52] For instance, the PROMISE trial was stopped early secondary to oral milrinone causing a higher mortality rate in the patients treated with active drug. For the time being, intravenous dobutamine and intravenous milrinone (a phosphodiesterase inhibitor) are the most used inotropes. Active research is ongoing in the area.

Other management issues

The AHCPR suggested that a T4 and thyroid-stimulating hormone (TSH) level should also be checked in all patients over the age or 65 with heart failure and no obvious etiology, and in patients who have atrial fibrillation or other signs or symptoms of thyroid disease. Additionally, regular exercise with post-exercise rest period periods, a 2g Na diet, and limitation of alcohol intake should be stressed in patients with stable heart failure. Daily weight monitoring is an effective way to follow outpatient fluid status and the effects of diuretic therapy. Patients should be instructed to call their physicians with an unexplained weight gain greater than 2Kg since their most recent clinical evaluation. Indications for cardiac transplantation in patients with refractory heart failure will be discussed in the respective chapter.

New therapeutic approaches

β-adrenergic antagonists

Aiming to directly counteract the overstimulation of the sympathetic nervous system in chronic heart failure, β-adrenergic antagonists have been used and studied in patients with heart failure. Initial studies have shown favorable effects on the symptoms of patients with idiopathic dilated cardiomyopathy and a survival benefit of patients with heart failure secondary to ischemic heart disease.[57] The first β-blocker used successfully in heart failure was metoprolol.[58] Therapy was initiated at 6.25 mg twice a day and was increased to 100 mg BID over a period of 6 weeks; it was reasonably well tolerated, but 6-15% of patients could not tolerate it even at the low dose.[59] Controlled clinical trials have shown that the long-term administration of β-blockers can improve ventricular function and clinical status in selected patients with idiopathic dilated cardiomyopathy.[59] Long-term therapy with propranolol should reduce mortality in patients with left ventricular dysfunction after a myocardial infarction.[59] These preliminary studies were in patients with relatively mild heart failure. In the early reports of patients with severe heart failure, patients treated with β-blockers failed to show improvement, and many tolerated the drugs poorly.[59] All β-blockers have negative inotropic action and their administration in patients with heart failure is associated with a substantial risk (5-20%) of worsening heart failure. This occurs if the standard dosage of β-blockers for hypertension or angina is used in heart failure patients. Therefore, β-blockers should be initiated in small doses and up-titrated slowly with careful clinical observation. Another strategy to minimize the initial unfavorable effects of β-blockade in heart failure is the use of β-blockers with either direct or indirect peripheral vasodilatory effects. Bucindolol is a potent, nonselective β-blocking agent with mild vasodilator activity by virtue of a direct effect on vascular smooth muscle cells [59] and is currently being studied in the BEST trial.

Carvedilol is a non-selective, vasodilating β-blocker which also has α-adrenergic blocking properties which has been shown to be relatively well tolerated [60]. It has also been shown to be a potent antihypertensive and anti-anginal agent. Carvedilol is also a potent antioxidant. The novel antioxidant activity of carvedilol resides in the carbazole moiety.[61] Carvedilol has been shown to protect cultured cells from oxygen radical-induced damage and to prevent the depletion of the endogenous antioxidants, vitamin E and glutathione from tissues subjected to oxidative stress.[62]

Several metabolites of carvedilol found in human plasma and urine exhibit even more potent antioxidant activity than does carvedilol itself. [61] Carvedilol has been shown to reduce infarct size in different animal models of acute infarction, an action that has also been linked to the drug's antioxidant properties.[63] The role of myocardial oxygen free radicals in precipitating further myocardial events in patients with heart failure is still an open question, although there is an increasing body of evidence to suggest that drugs with anti-oxidative properties may have adjuvant benefits in preventing myocardial necrosis in areas of ischemia.[2]

Clinical studies have shown significant increase in exercise capacity, resting ejection fraction and stroke volume index associated with reduction in pulmonary artery wedge pressure, systemic vascular resistance, and rest and exercise heart rate and blood pressure with carvedilol.[63] Krum et al. showed that the addition of carvedilol to conventional therapy in severe heart failure led to an improvement in symptoms, functional capacity, and exercise tolerance. Hemodynamic improvement was also demonstrated.[64] The same investigators further showed that in patients with severe heart failure who could tolerate carvedilol, the combined risk of death, worsening heart failure, and life-threatening ventricular arrhythmias was significantly lower in patients treated with carvedilol than those treated with placebo.[64] However, the study did not show unequivocal total mortality benefit in the treated patients compared to placebo.

The favorable response to the β-blockade with carvedilol may be related to the drug's ability to attenuate the adverse effects of prolonged sympathetic stimulation on the failing heart .[65] Perhaps the favorable responses to β-blockers may be related to their to their ability to reverse the β-receptor downregulation, a characteristic of patients with heart failure. The resulting increase in β-receptor density in the cell membrane may provide hemodynamic benefits by sensitizing the heart to the inotropic effects of endogenous catecholamines.[64] Although no study has directly investigated the type of -receptors that are affected, the β_1 type is thought to be primarily involved in this process.

In a recent study, 60 patients with NYHA class II-IV and ejection fractions <35% were randomized to receive carvedilol or placebo (after an initial challenge with carvedilol), and the study was continued for three months. Carvedilol therapy resulted in a significant reduction in heart rate and mean pulmonary artery and pulmonary capillary wedge pressure and a significant increase in stroke volume and left ventricular stroke work. Left ventricular ejection fraction increased from 21% to 32% in the carvedilol group and carvedilol treated patients reported a significant decrease in heart failure symptoms.[66]

Angiotensin-II receptor inhibitors

ACE inhibitor induced cough can be a limiting side effect in patients taking this class of agents and is thought to be due to the release of bradykinin. In the SOLVD treatment trial, 37% of patients receiving enalapril reported cough, compared with 31 percent of those receiving placebo.[29] Cohn et al. reported similar figures, but only 1 percent of patients receiving enalapril and 1 percent of those receiving isosorbide dinitrates and hydralazine stopped medication because of cough.[51] Patients who can not tolerate ACE inhibitors, should be placed on hydralazine and isosorbide dinitrate, or perhaps on direct angiotensin II (A-II) inhibitors, which are now under active clinical investigation.

The potential advantage that the A-II inhibitors may have over ACE inhibitors is that these new agents do not produce the accumulation of kinins, and therefore should not produce the side-effects such as cough and angioedema attributed to high levels of kinins. In a clinical comparison between a direct A-II inhibitor (losartan) and a conventional ACE inhibitor (enalapril) no significant difference was found in exercise capacity, clinical status and neurohumoral activation between the two medication groups.[67]

Data do not currently exist on the long-term effects of angiotensin-II inhibitors on mortality in patients who have congestive heart failure. A large-scale clinical trial known as the Losartan Intervention for Endpoint (LIFE) Study has been initiated to evaluate the long-term effects of losartan, an A-II inhibitor, on reducing cardiovascular morbidity and mortality.

Flosequinan and Vesnarinone

Flosequinan is a positive inotropic with peripheral vasodilator effects which initially showed positive results in heart failure hemodynamics. However, when the drug was tested in larger clinical trials, it was associated with increased mortality in heart failure patients.[68]

Vesnarinone is a weak positive inotropic agent.[69] It has been shown not to activate neurohormonal activity when given to patients with heart failure.[69] Vesnarinone has effects on phosphodiesterase inhibition, blockade of the sodium and potassium channel, and blocking effects on the cytokine system.[70] In an initial mortality trial, the higher dose arm of the trial (120 mg) was terminated due to a higher mortality rate. However, in the lower dose arm of the trial (60 mg) there was a 62% reduction in the risk of dying from all cause mortality. Ongoing trials will further elucidate the use of vesnarinone in the treatment of heart failure.

Future perspectives

At present, the neurohormonal model of the pathophysiology of heart failure has yielded several beneficial therapies for heart failure patients. Following the same directions future research on the pathogenesis of heart failure should yield promising new treatments. These may include novel vasomotor antagonists (e.g. vasopressin or endothelin) and cytoprotective agents (e.g. free radical scavengers or cytokine inhibitors), or drug that inhibit the enzyme that metabolizes the atrial natriuretic peptide.[71] Direct inhibitors of renin have also been studied and specifically enalkiren (administered intravenously) increased cardiac index while decreasing right sided filling pressures among other hemodynamic benefits.[72]

Apart from the pharmacologic approaches to treating heart failure, there are exciting developments being made in the mechanical approach for treating patients with heart failure. These developments are being made in a variety of areas, such as cardiomyoplasty (the use of skeletal muscle to assist the heart), left ventricular assist devices (as a bridge to cardiac transplantation or as a permanent support) and cardiac transplantation, xenotransplantation, and the possibilities for a implantable mechanical heart. The hope is that as our knowledge of this complex disease increases, future therapeutic strategies will benefit the heart failure patients in both the quantity and the quality of life.

REFERENCES

1. Agenct for Health Care Policy and Research (AHCPR) panel for Heart failure 1995.

2. Taylor SH. The heart failure syndrome - from prevention to treatment. Eur Heart J 1995: 16: 1.

3. Packer M. Pathophysiology of chronic heart failure. Lancet 1992: 340: 88.

4. Kentish JC, et al. Comparison between the sarcomere length-force relations of intact and skinned trabeculae from rat right ventricle. Circ Res 1986: 58: 755.

5. Nadal-Ginard B, et al. Molecular basis of cardiac performance: Plasticity of the myocardium generated through protein isoform switches. J Clin Invest 1989: 84: 1693.

6. Hirsch AT, Dzau VJ, Creager MA. Baroreceptors function is congestive heart failure: effect on neurohormonal activation and regional vascular resistance. Circulation 1987: 75 (suppl IV): 36.

7. Floras JS. Sympathoinhibitory effect of atrial natriuetic factor in normal humans. Circulation 1990: 81: 1860.

8. Cody RJ, et al. Atrial Natriuretic factor in normal subjects and heart failure patients: plasma levels and renal, hormonal, and hemodynamic responses to peptide infusion. J Clin Invest 1986: 78: 1362.

9. Abassi Z, et al. Effect of converting-enzyme inhibition on renal response to ANF in rats with experimental heart failure. Am J Physiol 1990: 259: R84.

10. Kimura K, et al. Effects of atrial natiuretic peptide on renal arterioles: morphologic analysis using microvaswculr cells. Am J Physiol 1990:259:F939.

11. Moe GW, et al. Response of atrial natriuretic factor to acute and chronic increases of atrial pressure in experimental heart failure in dogs: role of changes in heart rate, atrial dimensions, and cardiac tissue concentration. Circulation 1991: 83: 1780.

12. Hirooka Y, et al. Attenuated forearm vasodilative response to intra-arterial arterial natriuretic peptide in heart failure. Circulation 1990: 82: 147.

13. Margulies KB, Hildebrand FL, Lerman A, Perrella MA, Burnett JC Jr. Increased endothelin in experimental heart failure. Circulation 1990: 82: 2226.

14. Burkart F. Rationale for current drug treatment. Eur Heart J 1995: 16F: 2.

15. Pitt B, et al. The effect of treatment on survival in congestive heart failure. Clinical Cardiology 1992: 15: 323.

16. Neumann J, et al. Increase in myocardial Gi-proteins in heart failure. Lancet 1988:ii:936.

17. Horn EM, et al. Reduced lymphocyte stimulatory guanine nucleotide regulatory protein and beta-adrenergic receptors in congestive heart failure and reversal with angiotensin converting-enzyme-inhibitor therapy. Circulation 1988: 78: 1373.

18. Eiskjaer H, et al. Mechanisms of sodium retention in heart failure: relation to the renin-angiotensin-aldosterone system. Am J Physiol 1991: 260: F883.

19. Francis GS, et al. Comparison of neuroendocrine activation in patients with left ventricular dysfunstion with and without congestive heart failure. A substudy of the studies of left ventricular dysfunstion (SOLVD). Circulation 1990: 82: 1724.

20. Pettersson A, Hedner J, Hedner T. Renal interaction between the sympathetic and ANP in rats with chronic ischemic heart failure. Acta Physiol Scand 1989: 135: 487.

21. Ferrari R, Corti A, Bachetti T. Tumor necrosis factor alpha in heart failure. Heart Failure 1995: 11: 142.

22. McMurray J, et al. Increased concentrationsof tumor necrosis factor in "cachectic" patients with severe chronic heart failure. Br Heart J 1991: 66: 356.

23. Riegger GA. Lessons from recent randomized controlled trials for the management of congestive heart failure. Am Journal Cardiol 1993: 71: E38.

24. Pfeffer MA, et al. Effect of captopril on mortality and morbidity in patients with left-ventricular dysfuction after myocardial infarction: results of the survival and ventricular enlargement trial. N Engl J Med 1992: 327: 669.

25. CONSENSUS Trial Study Group. Effects of enalapril on mortality in severe congestive heart failure. N Engl J Med 1987: 316: 1429.

26. SOLVD Investigators. Effect of enalapril on mortality and the development of heart failure in asymptomatic patients with reduced left-ventricular ejection fractions. N Engl J Med 1992: 327: 685.

27. Lewis GR. Comparison of lisinopril versus placebo for congestive heart failure. Am J Cardiol 1989: 63:12D.

28. Harlan WR, et al. Chronic congestive heart failure in coronary artery disease: clinical critera. Ann Intern Med 1977: 86: 133.

29. SOLVD Investigators. Effect of enalapril on survival in patients with reduced left-ventricular ejection fractions and congestive heart failure. N Engl J Med 1991: 325: 293.

30. Packer M. Evolution of the neurohormonal hypothesis to explain the progression of chronic heart failure. Eur Heart J1995: 16: F4.

31. Pfeffer MA, et al. Effect of captopril on progressive ventricular dialtation after anterior myocardial infarction. N Engl J Med 1988: 319: 80.

32. Tan LB, et al. Cardiac myocyte necrosis induced by angiotensin II. Circulation Research 1991: 69: 1185.

33. Greenberg B, et al. Effects of long-term enalapril therapy on cardiac structure and function in patients with left ventricular dysfunction. Results of the SOLVD echocardiography sudstudy. Circulation 1995: 91: 2573.

34. Benedict CR, et al. Effect of long-term enelapril therapy on neurohormones in patients with left ventricular dysfunction. SOLVD Investigators. Am J Cardiol 1995 : 75: 115.

35. The TRACE Study Group. The TRAndolapril Cardiac Evaluation (TRACE) study: rationale, design, and baseline characterists of the screened population. Am J Cardiol 1994: 73: C44.

36. Ball SG, Hall AS, Murray GD. ACE inhibition, atherosclerosis and myocardial infarction-The Acute Infarction Ramipril Efficacy Study (AIRE). Eur Heart J 1994: 15: B20.

37. Swedberg K, et al. Effects of the early administration of enalapril on mortality in patients with acute myocardial infarction: results of the Cooperative New Scandinavian Enalapril Survival Study II (CONSENSUS II). N Engl J Med 1992: 327: 678.

38. Ambrosiano E, Borghi C, Magnani B. The effect of the angiotensin-converting-enzyme inhibitor zofenopril on mortality and mobibidity after anterior myocardial infarction. The Survival of Myocardial Infarction Long-Term Evaluation (SMILE) Study Investigators. N Engl J Med 1995: 332: 80.

39. Packer M, et al. Withdrawal of digoxin from pateints with chronic heart failure treated with angiotensin-converting-enzyme inhibitors. N Engl J Med 1993: 329: 1.

40. Feldman MD, et al. Depression of systolic and diastolic myocardial reserve during atrial pacing tachycardia in pateints with dilated cardiomyopathy. J Clin Invest 1988:82:1661.

41. Scwinger RHG, et al. Force-frequency-relation in human atrial and ventricular myocardium. Mol Cell Biochem 1993: 119: 73.

42. Erdmann E. Digitalis-friend or foe? Eur Heart J 1995: 16: F16.

43. Ferguson DW, et al. Sympatho-inhibitory responses to digitalis glycosides in heart failure patients: direct evidence from sympathetic neural recordings. Circulation 1989: 80: 65.

44. The Digitalis Investigation Group. The effect of digoxin on mortality and morbidity in patients with heart failure. N Engl J Med 1997:336:525.

45. The Captopril-Digoxin Multicenter Reseach Group. Comparative effects of captopril and digoxin in patients with mild to moderate heart failure. JAMA 1988: 259: 539.

46. Cohn JN, et al. Effect of vasodilator therapy on mortality in chronic congestive heart failure: results of a Veterans Administration Cooperative Study. N Engl J Med 1986: 314: 1547.

47. Agostoni PG, et al. Afterload reduction: a comparison of captopril and nifedipine in dilated cardiomyopathy. Br Heart J 1986: 55: 391.

48. Packer M. Treatment of chronic heart failure. Lancet 1992: 340: 92.

49. Packer M. Vasodilator and inotropic drugs for chronic heart failure: Distinguishing hype from hope. Journal American College of Cardiology 1988:12:1299.

50. Packer M, et al. Prevention and reversal of nitrate tolerance in patients with congestive heart failure. New England Journal of Medicine 1987: 317: 799.

51. Cohn JN, et al. A comparison of enalapril with hydralazine-isosorbide dinitrate in the treatment of chronic congestive heart failure. N Engl J Med 1991: 325: 303.

52. Packer M, et al. Effect of milrinone on mortality in severe chronic heart failure. N Engl J Med 1991: 325: 1468.

53. Packer M. Pathophysiologic mechanisms underlying the adverse effects of calcium channel blocking drugs in patients with chronic heart failure. Circulation 1989: 80(S. IV): 59.

54. The Stroke Prevention in Atrial Fibrillation Investigators. Stoke prevention in atrial fibrillation. Final results. Circulation 1991: 84: 527.

55. Alderman EL, et al. Results of coronary artery surgery in patients with poor left ventricular function (CASS). Circulation 1983: 68: 785.

56. Higgins TL, et al. Stratification of morbidity and mortality outcome by preoperative risk factors in coronary artery bypass patients: A clinical severity score. JAMA 1992: 267: 2344.

57. Englemeier RS, et al. Improvement in symptoms and exercise tolerance by metoprolol in patients with dilated cardiomyopathy: a double-blind, randomized, placebo-controlled trial. Circulation 1985: 72: 536.

58. Waagstein F, et al. Beta-Blockers in cardiomyopathies: They work. Eur Heart J 1983: 4: 173.

59. Bristow MR. Pathophysiologic and pharmacologic rationales for clinical management of chronic heart failure with beta-blocking agents. Am J Cardiol 1993: 71: C12.

60. Gilbert EM, et al. Long-term beta-blocker vasodilator theray impoves cardiac function in idiopathic dialated cardiomyopathy: a double-blind, randomized study of bucindolol versus placebo. Am J Med 1990: 88: 223.

61. Feuerstein GZ, Ruffolo Jr. Carvedilol, a novel multiple action antihypertensive agent with antioxidant activity and the potential for myocardial and vascular protection. Eur Heart J 1995: 16: F38.

62. Yue TL, et al. Carvedilol, a new beta-adrenergic antagonist and vasodilator antihypertensive drug, inhibits superpoxide release from human neutrophils. Eur J Pharmacol 1992: 214: 277.

63. Yue TL, et al. Carvedilol, a new vasodilator and beta adrenoreceptor antagonist, is an antioxidant and free radical scavenger. J Pharmacol Exper Ther 1992: June: 92.

64. Raftery EB. Vasodilating beta-blockers in heart failure. Eur Heart J 1995: 16: F32.

65. Packer M. Long-term stategies in the management of heart failure: Looking beyond ventricular function and symptoms. Am J Cardiol 1992: 69: G150.

66. Olsen SL, et al. Carvedilol improves left ventricular function and symptoms in chronic heart failure: a double-blind randomized study. J Am Coll Cardiol 1995: 25: 1225.

67. Dickstein K, et al. Comparison of the effects of losartan and enalapril on clinical status and exercise performace in patients with moderate or severe chronic heart failure. J Am Coll Cardiol 1995: 26: 438.

68. Binkley PF, et al. Flosequinan augements parasympathetic tone and attenuates sympathetic drive in congestive heart failure demonstration by analysis of heart rate variability. J Am Coll Cardiol 1992: 19: 147A.

69. Feldman AM, et al for the Vesnarinone Study Group. Effects of vesnarinone on morbidity and mortality in patients with heart failure. N Engl J Med 1993: 329: 149.

70. Matsumori A, et al. Vesnarinoe, an inotropic agent, inhibits cytokine production by stimualted human blood from patients with heart failure. Circulation 1994: 89: 955.

71. Northridge DB, et al. Inhibition of the metabolism of atrial natriuretic factor cause diuresis and natriuresis in chronic heart failure. Am J Hypert 1990: 3: 682.

72. Neuberg GW, et al. Hemodynamic effects of renin inhibtion by enalkiren in chronic congestive heart failure. Am J Cardiol 1991: 67: 63.

15 HYPERTROPHIC CARDIOMYOPATHY

David P. Dutka, Celia M. Oakley

Hypertrophic cardiomyopathy has intrigued clinicians since the condition was first described in eight patients by Donald Teare almost 40 years ago.[1] The classic morphology of asymmetrical septal hypertrophy remains the most common form of the condition, but the increased availability of echocardiography, together with family and routine screening has demonstrated a diversity of cardiac phenotype.[2-5] Patients may be profoundly disabled or asymptomatic,6 and presentation may occur at any age.[7-9] Although the early studies focused on the classic form of the disease, the heterogeneity of the cardiac phenotype precludes a satisfactory definition, and diagnostic difficulty is relatively common. A working definition is to regard hypertrophic cardiomyopathy as an idiopathic condition characterised by a hypertrophied and non-dilated left and/or right ventricle in the absence of an identified cause such as hypertension or valvular heart disease.[10,11] A positive family history greatly strengthens the diagnosis in uncertain cases.[12,13]

The implication is that familial hypertrophic cardiomyopathy (FHC) is secondary to an intrinsic abnormality of the myocardium, although a number of other conditions may mimic it. The phenotypic expression of other genetic diseases may resemble familial hypertrophic cardiomyopathy although a common genetic link has not yet been identified. In patients with Friedreich's ataxia, for example, the genetic abnormality lies on chromosome 9, unrelated to the chromosomal abnormalities so far identified with familial hypertrophic cardiomyopathy. The gene for Noonan's syndrome has been tentatively placed on chromosome 15 so providing a possible theoretical link with one form of familial hypertrophic cardiomyopathy.[14] Some individuals develop an exaggerated response to a physiological stimulus such as exercise. Athletic training may provoke myocardial hypertrophy which is difficult to distinguish from, or may become, familial hypertrophic cardiomyopathy. There are no genetic studies yet of athletes with seemingly "excessive" myocardial hypertrophy. Hypertrophy may simply reflect the considerable increase in stroke volume which athletes in training are able to mount, but such hypertrophy should not be diagnosed as adaptive and physiological in the occasional jogger or past competitor. Athletic training reduces the sympathetic response for a given level of exercise[15] and this adaptation may protect against high catecholamine surges which have been documented to invoke large potassium fluxes during sustained exercise above the lactate threshold.[16] Some athletes who suffer sudden cardiac death may undoubtedly have genetic hypertrophic cardiomyopathy but others may possess a susceptibility to catecholamine induced arrthymias during extreme competitive physical effort.[17]

Considerable progress in our understanding of hypertrophic cardiomyopathy has come with advances in molecular genetic techniques facilitating detection of mutations which may eventually allow diagnostic testing.[18-21] The number of identified mutations (which continues to increase) has so far limited the adoption of genetic techniques for confirmation of the diagnosis and assessment of prognosis, and at present a mutation can still only be identified in about 30% of families. As hypertrophic cardiomyopathy remains the most prevalent cause of sudden cardiac death in apparently healthy people under 35 years of age and of athletes, considerable effort has been directed towards identifying individuals who are at risk. Many have been asymptomatic until the sudden death episode and their identification continues to pose a challenge.[22]

Pathogenesis

The considerable variation in cardiac phenotype and prognosis in affected individuals is not yet fully understood.[23,24] The multiple different mutations within the · cardiac myosin gene may indicate allelic heterogeneity which determines phenotypic variation in unrelated families. Phenotype/genotype studies have not demonstrated clear prognostically important echocardiographic features of hypertrophy, but important differences in the prognosis of families with certain · myosin missense mutations have been reported.[23,25,26] The influence of a specific mutation may be determined in such families in which prognosis and outcome are more likely to relate to the family genetic abnormality than to other genetic or environmental factors,[19,20,26] but other genes as yet unknown may modify both expression and progression in FHC families.

The amount of myocardial hypertrophy is often variable within members of one family. The histological features of unexplained ventricular hypertrophy with extensive myocardial disarray are regarded as specific, together with an excess of connective tissue which is quantitatively different from the changes which occur in secondary hypertrophy.[27] The myocardial muscle bundles are disorganised in a characteristic whorled pattern, the individual myocytes are distinctly short and fat, sometimes with nuclear polyploidy and with ultrastructural abnormalities including disorganisation of the myofibrils within individual cells. Myocardial changes in the ageing process, "apical hypertrophic cardiomyopathy" and myocyte disarray in the absence of wall thickening pose additional classification difficulties in sporadic cases.

There is no proven relationship between prognosis and cardiac phenotype or symptoms. Syncope and a positive family history of sudden cardiac death are weak specific predictors of sudden death. Electrical instability accompanying myocyte disarray may be one factor in the pathogenesis of sudden death in this condition, with the degree and extent of the disarray being related to prognosis. The disarray has been found to be less in patients with hypertrophic cardiomyopathy who die from other causes and greatest in those patients who suffer sudden cardiac death.[28] Conventional electrophysiological studies, whilst demonstrating abnormalities, have not indicated any specific finding predictive of sudden death. Asymptomatic abnormalities of sinus node function (66% of cases) and His-Purkinje conduction (30%) are relatively common in hypertrophic cardiomyopathy, with accessory pathways being present in 5% of cases. Re-entrant tachycardia via these pathways offers an explanation for sudden death in rare cases, but programmed ventricular stimulation is unrewarding in predicting ventricular arrythmias.[29-31]

An alternative electrophysiological technique has been developed with the object of assessing the degree of myocyte disarray on the basis that the electrical signal is conducted at differing speeds through the abnormal myocardium. Such non-homogeneous conduction may promote re-entrant dysrythymias and the technique appears to hold promise for stratification of the risk of sudden cardiac death but prospective evaluation is still awaited.[32]

Diagnosis

The diagnosis of hypertrophic cardiomyopathy is not challenging in classic cases or in first degree relatives of the proband. The clinical features of hyperkinetic systolic ventricular function and outflow tract gradients (with associated late systolic ejection murmur at the left sternal edge) are hallmarks of the condition, but only a quarter of cases recognised today have a resting outflow tract gradient.[4] Diagnosis may be difficult in patients with seemingly mild hypertension, the serious athlete or in mild valvular disease with dis-proportionate myocardial hypertrophy. The disorder is missed in many asymptomatic people who do not consult their doctors. It is also over-diagnosed, usually as a result of mis-interpretation of the echocardiogram; common errors include joining the moderator band with the septum or measuring at the point of septal curvature in the elderly with resultant false-positive septal hypertrophy. The prevalence of genetic abnormalities which might predispose to the development of myocardial hypertrophy in response to a relatively minor physiological stimulus remain unknown.

Only a minority of patients present with classical symptoms of syncope, chest pain and dyspnoea. In approximately 50% of cases the diagnosis is made following family screening or incidental medical examination. Breathlessness on exertion is the most common limiting symptom and is usually attributed to increased left atrial pressure secondary to impaired left ventricular diastolic function. The main haemodynamic limitation is caused by a low stroke volume which does not increase in a normal fashion with exercise. Haemodynamic monitoring yields little additional information. Changes in peripheral vascular resistance, together with heightened sympathetic nervous system activity, may play a more dominant role in symptomatic exercise limitation. Chest pain is also a common symptom and may be typical angina pectoris secondary to increased oxygen demand or atypical due to increased capillary myocyte distance or to changes in the microvasculature. Cardiopulmonary exercise testing shows wide variability ranging from a normal (or even supernormal) VO_2 max down to severe limitation which is often increased by unfitness and chronic hyperventilation.

Syncope is an ominous prognostic sign experienced by approximately one sixth of patients, manifest by a fall in stroke volume and blood pressure without loss of sinus rhythm and often with a striking increase in outflow tract gradient, "the empty heart", usually after exercise or stress (which may implicate the sympathetic system and catecholamines[33,34]). Atrial fibrillation is common in older patients who usually deteriorate symptomatically following its onset. Patients with hypertrophic cardiomyopathy rely on atrial systole to achieve adequate diastolic filling of the hypertrophied and stiffened left ventricle. The onset of atrial fibrillation also reduces the time available for passive diastolic filling when the ventricular response is uncontrolled. Varying diastolic intervals determine loss of minute output in addition to the loss of atrial contribution and the irregularity is indeed probably more contributory to the fall in cardiac output because atrial fibrillation sometimes reflects left atrial mechanical failure.

Investigations

The ECG is rarely normal in hypertrophic cardiomyopathy and this makes it a most important diagnostic tool despite the wide variety of electrocardiographic changes seen. Flamboyant criteria of left ventricular hypertrophy or inappropriate Q waves may be pathognomic in the context of the patient being seen. Voltage criteria of left ventricular hypertrophy (with deep septal S waves), ST-segment and T-wave changes are the most common abnormalities. An abnormal ECG in a member of an affected family is a more sensitive indicator than echocardiography.[35,36] The echocardiogram is the most available and therefore the standard diagnostic test to delineate the extent and distribution of ventricular hypertrophy. M-mode measurements are made at mitral valve level to quantify septal and posterior left ventricular wall thickness but hypertrophy may be largely apical or in rare cases confined to the lateral wall of the left ventricle. Cardiac catheterisation is usually not necessary although patients with hypertrophic cardiomyopathy are not immune from coronary artery disease. As patients with hypertrophic cardiomyopathy may have ischaemic chest pain despite widely patent epicardial arteries and the abnormal electrocardiogram (such as resting J point depression) renders interpretation of an exercise test difficult, coronary angiography may be required.

Natural history

The natural history of hypertrophic cardiomyopathy has not yet been adequately defined, due to the heterogeneity of the condition, differing genetic abnormalities which are only just beginning to be realised and the absence of sufficiently long-term studies. In recent years it has been found that remodelling of the myocardium plays an important role in the adaptive processes which follow an insult such as myocardial infarction, and it is now apparent that substantial remodelling of left ventricular morphology occurs in patients with hypertrophic cardiomyopathy. In children, rapid progression of myocardial hypertrophy has been noted, particularly in association with the pubertal growth spurt.[37,38] These children usually remain asymptomatic although a left ventricular outflow tract gradient (with murmur) may develop. Similar progression has not been found in adults[39] and indeed the changes which occur in adulthood are eventually in the opposite direction with progressive wall thinning and relative cavity dilatation.[40] Absolute ventricular dilatation is rare, probably limited by the fibrosis which accompanies the myocardial disarray. Longitudinal studies are required to confirm whether the majority of surviving patients with hypertrophic cardiomyopathy develop thinning of the ventricular walls with age, although there is increasing anecdotal evidence to support this hypothesis.[7,8,41]

It is not known whether older people first diagnosed perhaps in their sixth or later decade have had a cardiac disorder since adolescence and all through their healthy active adult lives or whether the onset occurred later. These patients appear to have a more benign course, although the fact that they have survived introduces bias. The changes in the myocardium with age can be very similar to those of hypertrophic cardiomyopathy with septal angulation, narrowing of the outflow tract with turbulence (even a gradient in some cases) and mitral regurgitation.

A degree of natural selection and subsequent bias may also play a role as certain cardiac phenotypes (and hence genetic mutations, some of which have been found to be associated with an increased risk of sudden cardiac death) may predispose a patient to a more adverse prognosis. Wall thinning and fibrosis are probably secondary to myocyte drop-out either due to advance of the myopathy with apoptosis or from ischaemia. The benefits of angiotensin converting enzyme inhibitors in limiting remodelling following myocardial infarction are now well established, and have focused attention on the close inter-relationship between the components of the renin-angiotensin system and cardiac hypertrophy and myocyte growth. A number of these peptides, kinins and enzymes are putative growth factors and are expressed in human myocardium. The influence of polymorphism of genes encoding components of the renin angiotensin system and cardiac morbidity and mortality are now being recognised,[42-45] and the interaction of racial origin and environmental factors merits close attention. In the small studies undertaken to date, no benefit was demonstrated following the use of angiotensin converting enzyme inhibitors in hypertrophic cardiomyopathy, and indeed in the same manner as there is no relationship between prognosis and cardiac morphology, there is currently no evidence that an adverse prognosis might be favourably changed by pharmacologically inducing regression of the hypertrophy.

As the clinical course of hypertrophic cardiomyopathy is so variable, caution should be exercised in the counselling of patients regarding the natural history of their condition.[34] There is increasing evidence that the prognosis of many patients with the condition is not as grave as had been thought. Some patients have a strong family history of sudden cardiac death, and may carry one of the genetic mutations associated with a poor prognosis. These patients are at greater risk. Other patients are, and will remain, relatively asymptomatic with perhaps only mild reduction in maximal exercise tolerance and oxygen consumption. The mortality of these patients appears to be substantially lower than the frequently quoted figure of 3-4% per annum,[46] and they may have a normal prognosis.

Management

Once the diagnosis of hypertrophic cardiomyopathy has been made, there are a number of aspects of management which merit attention. Firstly, the patient must be given a full explanation to the limits of our current knowledge, the pedigree must be obtained in as much detail as possible (including sight of death/autopsy certificates if possible) and arrthymias sought. With the wide publicity of this high-profile disease and development of patient support groups many patients are greatly concerned about their risk of sudden death. They should be told that there is a risk of sudden death in all forms of heart disease but that the bad reputation of hypertrophic cardiomyopathy is caused by sudden death in young, asymptomatic and often previously undiagnosed people. In older patients (and many young ones too) this risk is much less than in coronary artery disease for example.

The identification of patients at risk of sudden death is difficult as the mechanism(s) that singly or in combination might be responsible have not been elucidated. Some of these mechanisms appear to be arrhythmic, others haemodynamic.[22,47] Holter monitoring may demonstrate short bursts of ventricular tachycardia, paroxysmal atrial fibrillation, other supraventricular tachycardias (with or without an accessory pathway) leading to accelerated atrioventricular conduction, and conduction abnormalities including sinoatrial node dysfunction and complete heart block.[48] Ambulatory monitoring has a number of limitations, but the absence of ventricular tachycardia places the adult patient (but not the child) in a low risk category for sudden death. Those patients with dysrthymias during Holter monitoring should be treated with amiodarone in low dose to minimise the potential adverse effects whilst retaining the drug's efficacy. Such low dose treatment has not yet been proven to be efficacious.

The patient should undergo exercise testing to assess the haemodynamic response. Many patients demonstrate haemodynamic instability with an inappropriate fall in systemic vascular resistance and blood pressure on exercise.[49,50] Patients who are young with haemodynamic instability on exercise and a family history of sudden death are at increased risk. Other haemodynamic variables do not appear to offer predictive information.[49,51]

Dyspnoea is the commonest symptom of patient with hypertrophic cardiomyopathy. The cause is probably multifactorial with the low cardiac output, reduced left ventricular compliance, unfitness and often chronic hyperventilation all contributing.[52] Some workers have claimed improvement in both symptoms and exercise tolerance following pharmacological therapy which includes the use of beta-adrenergic blocking drugs and calcium antagonists.[53-55] The beta blockers reduce heart rate and thereby prolong diastole to optimise ventricular filling and coronary blood flow, blunt the chronotropic response to exercise and improve ventricular compliance. The negative inotropic effect of these drugs may also reduce the outflow tract gradient and mitral regurgitation enhancing stroke volume. The effects of calcium antagonists (of which the greatest experience is with verapamil) are similar to those of the β-blockers, via a different mechanism of action.[56] Verapamil appears to carry a greater risk of inducing brady-arrthymias which in association with the negative inotropic effect may induce pulmonary oedema. Diltiazem may be preferable but nifedipine should not be used due to its vasodilating properties with loss of central blood volume, a fall in left ventricular filling and size and a paradoxical increase in outflow tract gradient. Drug therapy should be tailored to the individual patient and diastole prolonged if this enhances ventricular filling (as assessed by transmitral Doppler).[57,58] Dyspnoeic patients with a high outflow tract gradient may benefit from high dose verapamil.

Surgery in the form of myomectomy to try and restore more normal cardiac morphology offers another therapeutic option. It is effective in some patients (as is mitral valve replacement which relieves outflow tract obstruction and corrects mitral regurgitation due to cavity distortion) but the 5-10% mortality in even the most experienced hands necessitates very careful patient selection and the onset of left ventricular failure is hastened.

Patients with hypertrophic cardiomyopathy should be maintained in sinus rhythm. If atrial fibrillation develops the patient should be anticoagulated and a therapeutic trial of amiodarone may be successful (with careful monitoring of the INR in view of the interaction between warfarin and amiodarone). If not, DC cardioversion should be undertaken and efforts should be made to maintain the patient in sinus rhythm for as long as possible using amiodarone and repeated DC cardioversion as necessary.

A recently re-developed alternative therapeutic strategy utilises atrioventricular pacing with a short programmed AV delay.[59-61] This has been reported to reduce outflow tract gradients, decrease filling pressures and improve exercise tolerance.[62] The short AV delay ensures that the ventricle is always paced and we have found optimisation of transmitral left ventricular filling using Doppler to be helpful in ensuring maximal priming of the ventricle during diastole. There have been more recent reports in a small series of patients that symptomatic benefit is greatest using extremely short AV intervals. The synchronisation of atrial contraction with apical right ventricular stimulation appears to produce optimal haemodynamics in this group's experience but diastolic filling must be suboptimal except in patients who are in an advanced restrictive phase of the disease. Repeated adjustment of pacing parameters may be required and a multi-programmable device, including rate-responsive ability for those patients in atrial fibrillation or with atrial chronotropic incompetence, is a prerequisite. The precise mode of action of pacing remains unclear, with the dyskinesia and paradoxical septal motion induced by pacing the apex of the right ventricle thought to widen the outflow tract, reduce the gradient and improve stroke volume but figures comparing exercise capacity before and after pacing have not been convincing.

Chronotropic incompetence is also a factor limiting exercise tolerance of some patients with hypertrophic cardiomyopathy. The inability of the sino-atrial node to increase the heart rate and thereby increase cardiac output in response to exercise is exacerbated by drugs such as verapamil and propanolol. Restoring the chronotropic capacity by rate responsive pacing may offer advantages for some patients but not to all - depending on the stage of the disease. As diastolic dysfunction progresses patients develop a restrictive pattern of ventricular filling (with E>A on Doppler, cf the enhanced A seen earlier) and these patients may have better performance with a more rapid heart rate.

The use of automatic implantable cardioverter defibrillator (AICD) remains controversial. Most units with expertise in this area reserve their use for those patients with sustained ventricular tachycardia or who have survived an episode of ventricular fibrillation. Haemodynamic instability may be a more frequent cause of syncope than arrhythmia in hypertrophic cardiomyopathy. Patients have been documented to suffer loss of consciousness during sinus rhythm, with asymptomatic ventricular tachycardia documented during the same episode of Holter monitoring. Improvements in implantable defibrillator technology may facilitate a prospective trial of their use in patients at high risk of sudden cardiac death.

Conclusion

There is no algorithm which one can apply to all patients with hypertrophic cardiomyopathy. The most important initial point is to try to ensure that the diagnosis is beyond doubt. Risk assessment should be undertaken and those patients at low risk should be strongly reassured of this. Patients with a high risk of sudden cardiac death (including those who have survived such an episode, suffer repeated syncope or have a strong family history of sudden cardiac death) should be treated with amiodarone and some will need an implanted defibrillator. It is important for patients at low risk , with no arrthymias on ambulatory monitoring and who can perform a satisfactory exercise test to remain under continuing review for evidence of change so that treatment can be instigated or new information transmitted and in order to learn the natural history of different forms of the disease which at present remain unknown.

REFERENCES

1. Teare RD. Asymmetrical hypertrophy of the heart in young adults. Brit Heart J 1958:20:1.

2. Maron BJ, et al. Patterns and significance of left ventricular hypertrophy in hypertrophic cardiomyopathy. A wide angle, two dimensional echocardiographic study of 125 patients. Am J Cardiol 1981:48: 418.

3. Shapiro LM, McKenna WJ. Distribution of left ventricular hypertrophy in hypertrophic cardiomuopathy : a two dimensional echocardiographic study. J Am Coll Cardiol 1983:2:437.

4. McKenna W, et al. Prognosis in hypertrophic cardiomyopathy : role of age and clinical, electrocardiographic and hemodynamic features. Am J Cardiol 1981:47:532.

5. Maron BJ, et al. How common is hypertrophic cardiomyopathy? Echocardiographically identified prevalance in a general population of young adults. (The CARDIA Study). Circulation 1993: 88:211.

6. Spirito P, et al. Severe functional limitation in patients with hypertrophic cardiomyopathy and only mild localised left ventricular hypertrophy. J Am Coll Cardiol 1986:8:537.

7. Spirito P, Maron BJ. realtion between of left ventricular hypertrophy and age in hypertrophic cardiomyopathy. J Am Coll Cardiol 1989: 13:820.

8. Lewis JF, Maron BJ. clinical and morphologic expression of hypertrophic cardiomyopathy in patients> or = 65 years of age. Am J Cardiol 1994: 73:1105.

9. Pomerance A, Davies MJ. Patholical features of hypertrophic obstructive cardiomyopathy (HOCM) in the elderly. Brit Heart J 1975:37:305.

10. Maron BJ, Epstein SE. Hypertrophic cardiomyopathy : a discussion of nomenclature. Am J Cardiol 1979: 43:1242.

11. Report of the WHO/IFSC task force on the definition and classification of cardiomyopathies. Brit Heart J 1980:44:672.

12. Greaves SC, et al. Inheritance of hypertrophic cardiomyopathy: a cross-sectional and M-mode study of 50 families. Brit Heart J 1987:58:259.

13. Maron BJ, et al. Patterns of inheritance in hypertrophic cardiomyopathy: assessment by M-mode and two-dimensional echocardiography. Am J Cardiol 1984: 53:1087.

14. Lewis JF, et al. Usefulness of Doppler echocardiographic assessment of diastolic filling in distinguishing "athlete's heart" from hypertrophic cardiomyopathy. Br Heart J 1992:68:296.

15. Cousineau D, et al. Catecholamines in coronary sinus during exrecise in man before and after training. J Appl Physiol 1977:43:801.

16. Coplan NL, et al. Exercise-related changes in serum catecholamines and potassium: effect of sustained exercise above and below lactate threshold. Am Heart J 1989: 117:1070.

17. Lehman M, et al. Plasma catecholamines in trained and untrained volunteers during graduated exercise. Int J Sports Med 1981: 2:143.

18. McKenna WJ, et al. Hypertrophic cardiomyopathy without hypertrophy : two families with myocardial disarray in the absence of increased myocardial mass. Br Heart J 1990:63:287.

19. Watkins H, et al. Characteristics and prognostic implications of myosin missense mutations in familial hypertrophic cardiomyopathy. N Engl J Med 1992:326:1108.

20. Epstein ND, et al. Differences in clinical expression of hypertrophic cardiomyopathy associated with two distinct mutations in the beta-myosin heavy chain gene. A 908Leu − >Val mutation and a 403Arg − >Gln mutation. Circulation 1992:86:345.

21. Hengstenberg C, Schwartz K. Molecular genetics of familial hypertrophic cardiomyopathy. J Mol Cell Cardiol 1994: 26:3.

22. McKenna WJ, et al. Sudden death in hypertrophic cardiomyopathy: Identification and management of high risk patients. In : Advances in cardiomyopathies. Baroldi G, Camerini F, Goodwin JF. eds. Springer-Verlag, Berlin, 1990:72.

23. Fananapazir L, Epstein ND. Genotype-phenotype correlations in hypertrophic cardiomyopathy. Insights provided by comparisons of kindreds with distinct and identical beta-myosin heavy chain gene mutations. Circulation 1994:89:22.

24. Hengstenberg C, et al. Clinical and genetical heterogeneity of familial hypertrophic cardiomyopathy. Herz 1994:19:84.

25. Solomon SD, et al. Left ventricular hypertrophy and morphology in familial hypertrophic cardiomyopathy associated with mutations of the beta-myosin heavy chain gene. J Am Coll Cardiol 1993:22:498.

26. Anan R, et al. Prognostic implications of novel beta cardiac myosin heavy chain gene mutations that cause familial hypertrophic cardiomyopathy. J Clin Invest 1994: 93:280.

27. Davies MJ. the current status of myocardial disarray in hypertrophic cardiomyopathy. Brit Heart J 1984:51:361.

28. Maron BJ, et al. Realtion between extent of cardiac muscle cell disorganization and left ventricular wall thickness in hypertrophic cardiomyopathy. Am J Cardiol 1192:70:785.

29. Kuck KH, et al. Programmed electrical stilmulation in hypertrophic cardiomyopathy. Results in patients with and without cardiac arrest or synopse. Eur Heart J 1988:9:177.

30. Fananapazir L, et al. Prognostic determinants in hypertrophic cardiomyopathy. Prospective evaluation of a therapeutic strategy based on clinical, Holter, hemodynamic and electrophysiological findings. Circulation 1992:86:730.

31. Fananapazir L, Epstein SE. value of electrophysiologic studies in hypertrophic cardiomyopathy. Am J Cardiol 1191:67:175.

32. Saumarez RC, et al. Ventricular fibrillation in hypertrophic cardiomyopathy is associated with increased fractionation of paced right ventricular electrograms. Circulation 1992:86:467.

33. Lefroy DC, et al. Diffuse reduction of myocardial beta-adrenoceptors in hypertrophic cardiomyopathy : a study with positron emission tomography. J Am Coll Cardiol 1993:22:1653.

34. Davies MJ, Krikler DM. Genetic investigation and counselling of families with hypertrophic cardiomyopathy. Br Heart J 1994, 72:99.

35. Al Mahdawi S, et al. The electrogram is a more sensitive indicator than echocardiography of hypertrophic cardiomyopathy in families with a mutation in the MYH7 gene. Br Heart J 1994:72:105.

36. Ryan MP, et al. The standard electrocardiogram as a screening test for hypertrophic cardiomyopathy. Am J Cardiol 1995:17:452.

37. Maron BJ, et al. Development or progression of left ventricular hypertrophy in children with hypertrophic cardiomyopathy: identification by two-dimensional echocardiography. New Engl J Med 1986:315:610.

38. Panza JA, et al. Development and determinants of dynamic obstructions to left ventricular outflow in young patients with hypertrophic cardiomyopathy. J Am Coll Cardiol 1989:13:820.

39. Spirito P, Maron BJ. Absence of progression of left ventricular hypertrophy in adult patients with hypertrophic cardiomyopathy. Am J Cardiol 1987:9:1013.

40. Spirito P, et al. Occurence and significance of progressive left ventricular wall thinning and relative cavity dilatation in patients with hypertrophic cardiomyopathy. Am J Cardiol 1987:60:123.

41. Maron BJ, et al. Prevalence of hypertrophic cardiomyopathy in an outpatient population referred for echocardiographic study. Am J Cardiol 1994: 73:577.

42. Bohn M, et al. Insertion/deletion (I/D) polymorphism at the locus for angiotensin I-converting enzyme and parental history of myocardial infarction. Clin Genet 44:298.

43. Schunkert H, et al. Association between a deletion polymorphism of the angiotensin-converting enzyme gene and left ventricular hypertrophy. N Engl J Med 1994: 330:1634.

44. Marian AJ, et al. Angiotensin-converting enzyme polymorphism in hypertrophic cardiomyopathy and sudden cardiac death. Lancet 1993:342:1085.

45. Schunkert H, Paul M. Cardiac angiotensin converting enzyme and diastolic function of the heart. Agents Actions Suppl 38:119.

46. Kofflard MJ, et al. Prognosis in hypertrophic cardiomyopathy observed in a large clinic population. Am J Cardiol 1993: 72: 939.

47. Maron BJ, Fananapazir L. Sudden cardiac death in hypertrophic cardiomyopathy. Circulation 1992: 85: 157.

48. Maron BJ, et al. Prognostic significance of 24-hour ambulatory monitoring in patients with hypertrophic cardiomyopathy. Am J Cardiol 1981: 48:252.

49. Frenneaux P, et al. Abnormal blood pressure response during exercise in hypertrophic cardiomyopathy. Circulation 1991: 82:1995.

50. McKenna WJ, et al. Syncope in hypertrophic cardiomyopathy. Brit Heart J 1982: 47:177.

51. Counihan PJ, et al. Abnormal vascular responses to supine exercise in hypertrophic cardiomyopathy. Circulation 1991: 84:686.

52. Nihoyannopoulos P, et al. Diastolic function in hypertrophic cardiomyopathy : relation to exercise capacity. J Am Coll Cardiol 1992: 19: 536.

53. Messmer BJ. Extended myectomy for hypertrophic obstructive cardiomyopathy. Am Thorac Surg 1994: 58:575.

54. Delahaye F, et al. Postoperative and long-term prognosis of myotomy-myomectomy for obstructive hypertrophic cardiomyopathy : influence of associated mitral valve replacement. Eur Heart J 1993: 14: 1229.

55. Stone CD, et al. Operative treatment of pediatric obstructive hypertrophic cardiomyopathy : a 26-year experience. Ann thorac Surg 1993: 56: 1308.

56. Wagner JA, et al. Calcium-antagonist receptors in the atrial tissue of patients with hypertrophic cardiomyopathy. N Engl J Med 1989: 320:755.

57. Doiuchi J, et al. Comparative effects of calcium-channel blockers and beta-adrenergic blocker on early diastolic time intervals and A-wave ratio in patients with hypertrophic cardiomyopathy. Clin Cardiol 1987:10:26.

58. Gilligan DM, et al. A double-blind, placebo-controlled crossover trial of nadolol and verapamil in mild and moderately symptomatic hypertrophic cardiomyopathy. J Am Coll Cardiol 1993: 21:1672.

59. Fananapazir L, et al. Impact of dual-chamber permanent pacing in patients with obstructive hypertrophic cardiomyopathy with symproms refractory to verapamil and beta-adrenergic blocker therapy. Circulation 1992: 85:2149.

60. Jeanrenaud X, et al. Effects of dual-chamber pacing in hypertrophic obstructive cardiomyopathy. Lancet 1992:339:1318.

61. McAreavey D, Fananapazir L. Altered cardiac hemodynamic and electrical state in normal sinus rhythm after chronic dual-chamber pacing for relief of left ventricular outflow obstruction in hypertrophic cardiomyopathy. Am J Cardiol 70: 651.

62. Cannon RO, et al. Results of permanent dual-chamber pacing in sympromatic nonobstructive hypertrophic cardiomyopathy. Am J Cardiol 1994: 73: 571.

16 DILATED CARDIOMYOPATHY

Philip J. Keeling, William J. McKenna

Idiopathic dilated cardiomyopathy is a chronic heart muscle disease characterised by ventricular dilatation and impaired systolic function.[1] The prevalence and incidence of dilated cardiomyopathy is increasing and now represents the commonest indication for cardiac transplantation worldwide. In recent years the increasing clinical and economic importance of dilated cardiomyopathy and the lack of information on pathogenesis and prognosis has stimulated a considerable amount of research on dilated cardiomyopathy.

Epidemiology

Dilated cardiomyopathy occurs throughout the world but estimates of frequency are available only for a few countries and vary considerably depending on the diagnostic criteria employed. In the United States of America clinical studies suggest a prevalence of 36.5 per 100 000 with an annual incidence of 8 per 100 000.[2] Autopsy studies from Sweden report a incidence of 5 per 100 000.[3] Although similar estimates have been proposed for England precise data are not available. These figures are likely to be an underestimate because dilated cardiomyopathy has a long preclinical phase during which the patient is asymptomatic and remains undiagnosed. Of concern, the frequency of dilated cardiomyopathy appears to have doubled from 1975-9 to 1980-4 but it is unclear if this reflects a real increase in frequency or improved case ascertainment.[2] Dilated cardiomyopathy most commonly affects young men but may occur from infancy to old age[4-6] and appears to be particularly common in negroes who demonstrate a 2.5-fold risk.[7]

Natural History

Dilated cardiomyopathy often presents at a late stage and is associated with a poor long term prognosis. Early studies demonstrated that patients with dilated cardiomyopathy had a one and two year mortality of approximately 30% and 50%, respectively.[8-10] More recent studies have shown little temporal improvement in survival.[11-14] Death usually occurs from progressive heart failure but sudden death accounts for 25-50% of deaths.[15] The major determinants of all-cause mortality in patients with dilated cardiomyopathy are left ventricular ejection fraction, exercise capacity, ventricular arrhythmic activity, increased plasma levels of noradrenaline.[16-22] However these standard prognostic indices fail to distinguish between patients at risk of sudden death and progressive heart failure.[23] Although a number of additional prognostic variables have been described in dilated cardiomyopathy [24-32] these have not proved to be clinically useful. In our own experience patients with progressive heart failure are best identified and monitored by serial assessment over time.

The mechanism of sudden death in dilated cardiomyopathy remains controversial [33] but has always been assumed to be tachyarrhythmic in origin. This is supported by the successful use of implantable cardioverter defibrillator therapy in patients with dilated cardiomyopathy and ventricular tachyarrhythmias.[34] However the recent identification of bradyarrhythmic death in the majority of patients with dilated cardiomyopathy [35] and the high elective implantation rate for permanent pacemaker have renewed interest in other causes of sudden death in dilated cardiomyopathy. In particular our attention has been drawn to the frequent occurrence of pulmonary and systemic emboli in this condition.[8,12] Autopsy studies have demonstrated an annual incidence of between 3.5 and 5.5% and have confirmed that these were largely unsuspected during life and a relatively frequent cause of death in these patients.

Etiology

The pathogenesis of dilated cardiomyopathy has become increasingly controversial over recent years. Assessment of pathogenesis in human dilated cardiomyopathy is limited by the late presentation of the condition and by its multicausal aetiology with different aetiologies operating in different patients to produce the same clinical syndrome. Many different aetiologies have been proposed for dilated cardiomyopathy; these include enteroviral infection, autoimmunity, familial factors, systemic hypertension, excessive alcohol consumption, pregnancy, drugs and toxins, dietary deficiencies, tropical infections, metabolic abnormalities and intractable tachycardias. However the following have emerged as major pathogenic hypotheses in dilated cardiomyopathy;

Persistent enteroviral infection

Although there is clear experimental evidence implicating enterovirus, and particularly Coxsackie B viruses, in the pathogenesis of murine myocarditis and dilated cardiomyopathy[36-38], the evidence in man is much less convincing. Whilst it seems clear that a proportion of patients (10-20%) develop clinical dilated cardiomyopathy following an episode of acute viral myocarditis[39-43], precise data are lacking because of the uncertainty surrounding the diagnosis of both myocarditis and active viral infection.[44,45] Until recently the principal supportive evidence linking enteroviruses to dilated cardiomyopathy was its association with antibodies against enteroviruses.[46,47,41] The recent detection of enteroviral genome within a significant proportion (approximately 50%) of dilated cardiomyopathic hearts[49] promised to provide direct evidence of enteroviral involvement in dilated cardiomyopathy. Unfortunately subsequent studies using more sensitive and specific assays have failed to confirm this finding with enteroviral genome being detected in 0-20% dilated cardiomyopathic hearts [50-57] and also in normal and pathological hearts.[53, 55, 57, 58]

Autoimmunity

There is now an increasing body of evidence from experimental models of acute and chronic heart disease that dilated cardiomyopathy can be caused by cardiac autoimmunity.[59, 60] In man similar evidence has begun to accumulate; this includes the demonstration of an association with a specific HLA phenotype (DR4)[61] inappropriate expression of major histocompatability complex class II antigens on endocardium and cardiac endothelium[62], and the identification of autoantibodies against the heart. A number of putative autoantigens has been reported and include the β1 adrenergic receptor [63, 64], M7 mitochondrial antigen[65], adenine nucleotide translocator [66] and other myofibrillar and sarcolemmal components.[67] Unfortunately these antibodies are not restricted to patients with dilated cardiomyopathy and their pathogenic relevance remains unclear. Caforio et al have recently described a novel organ-specific cardiac antibody in more than a quarter of patients with dilated cardiomyopathy and have shown that this antibody is rare in healthy subjects and in patients with other forms of heart disease (<3.5%).[68] The principal autoantigen recognised by this antibody is heavy chain myosin.[69] Of course, the viral and autoimmune hypothesis are not mutually exclusive and it is quite conceivable that a viral infection within the heart can initiate a self perpetuating autoimmune response as has been described in an experimental model of dilated cardiomyopathy.[70]

Familial factors

The familial nature of dilated cardiomyopathy was first noted by William Evans in 1947 [71] who reported to the British Cardiac Society in that year. Since this time there have been many anecdotal reports of families with dilated cardiomyopathy in more than one family member.[72-77] Until recently familial dilated cardiomyopathy was considered but recent studies have shown that dilated cardiomyopathy is familial in at least 20% of families and is consistent with autosomal dominant inheritance.[78-80] For this reason it is now our policy to offer screening to all first degree relatives of patients with dilated cardiomyopathy. Several groups are currently engaged in linkage analysis in order to determine the molecular basis of familial dilated cardiomyopathy.

Alcoholic dilated cardiomyopathy

Chronic excessive consumption has a variety of cardiotoxic effects and has long been associated with dilated cardiomyopathy.[27] However a direct cause-and-effect relationship has not been clearly established and its importance in pathogenesis of dilated cardiomyopathy remains unclear.[81] In an attempt to identify alcoholic dilated cardiomyopathy several workers have reported distinct biochemical[82, 83] and histological[84] markers of alcoholic cardiomyopathy. Unfortunately these laboratory markers do not reliably identify patients with an alcoholic pathogenesis and the diagnosis of alcoholic dilated cardiomyopathy usually remains inferential.[85] Abstinence from alcohol is now accepted as a pre-requisite for recovery from alcoholic dilated cardiomyopathy[86] and full recovery is possible.

Hypertensive dilated cardiomyopathy

The importance of systemic arterial hypertension in the pathogenesis of dilated cardiomyopathy is unclear.[87] A proportion of patients (approximately 5%) with persistent hypertension develop clinical dilated cardiomyopathy and become normotensive and have normal left ventricular wall thickness.[88] Identification of an aetiology is problematic because many patients presenting with dilated cardiomyopathy have not had their blood pressure assessed or only report mildly elevated blood pressure readings which are often unsustained and considered unimportant.[89] This difficulty is further illustrated by the observation that a proportion of patients who recover from with dilated cardiomyopathy develop clear sustained systemic arterial hypertension.[87]

Clinical features and investigations

Non-invasive assessment

There are no specific physical findings in dilated cardiomyopathy and the signs are those of low-output biventricular failure. The electrocardiogram is almost invariably abnormal but has no specific features; common findings include the presence of atrial fibrillation, widespread ST/T changes, ventricular hypertrophy, pathological Q waves, bundle branch block, or degrees of conduction disturbance.[90, 91] Chest x-ray shows an increased cardiothoracic ratio and often features of pulmonary venous hypertension. Echocardiography confirms the diagnosis demonstrating the presence of left ventricular dilatation and impaired systolic function, and excludes organic valvular disease. Left ventricular wall thickness is usually normal although ventricular mass is often increased and correlates with voltage hypertrophy on the electro-cardiogram.[92] Echocardiographic assessment of the right ventricle is technically more difficult and less reliable. Radionuclide imaging may show biventricular dilatation and impaired contractility and thallium-201 scintography demonstrates the presence of both fixed and reversible defects.[29]

The role of exercise testing in heart failure has been the subject of much debate. Exercise duration suffers from problems in reproducibility in patients with moderate to severe failure[93] and cardiopulmonary exercise testing with respiratory gas analysis is now an essential part of the assessment[94,95] and monitoring of patients with chronic heart failure.[96,97] Measurements made during cardiopulmonary exercise testing have been shown to be reliable parameters for evaluation of the severity of heart failure and are sensitive enough to determine the efficacy of therapeutic intervention.[98]

More recently analysis of the signal-averaged electrocardiogram has shown that late potentials are present in 13-44% patients with dilated cardiomyopathy using conventional time-domain criteria.[99-101] Some authors have suggested that the presence of late potentials in these patients is associated with ventricular arrhythmias[102] and sudden death[103] but others have failed to confirm these findings.[101,104] The application of new frequency domain techniques such as 2-dimensional frequency domain analysis and spectral turbulence analysis promises to help with the identification of patients with clinically important ventricular tachycardia.[101]

Invasive assessment

Cardiac catheterisation allows angiographic and haemodynamic confirmation of left ventricular dysfunction and demonstrates an absence of obstructive coronary disease. Difficulties are however encountered when severe left ventricular dysfunction is documented in association with minor degrees of coronary artery disease (eg <50% coronary stenoses), particularly when the left anterior descending coronary artery is spared. The role of endomyocardial biopsy in dilated cardiomyopathy remains controversial. Although an endomyocardial biopsy may be useful in excluding specific heart muscle diseases[105], the histopathological findings are non-specific and include myocyte damage, myofiber loss, and patchy interstitial fibrosis.[106] Characteristic features of myocarditis should not be present and this accounts for a large part of the diagnostic dilemma in dilated cardiomyopathy.[107-109]

There has been considerable debate as to the usefulness of electrophysiological assessment in patients with sustained ventricular tachycardia and dilated cardiomyopathy. Some workers report that ventricular arrhythmias are often provoked by programmed electrical stimulation[110, 111] the suppression of which by antiarrhythmic therapy leads to improved survival.[112,113] However other studies have shown that sustained ventricular arrhythmias are difficult to reproduce by programmed electrical stimulation[114, 115], usually remain inducible despite antiarrhythmic therapy and even if suppressed do not reduce the occurrence of sudden death during follow-up.[110]

Diagnostic criteria

The diagnosis of dilated cardiomyopathy is based on World Health Organisation criteria.[116] This requires the demonstration of a dilated and poorly contracting left and/or right ventricle in the absence of systemic arterial hypertension, systemic disorders known to affect the heart, obstructive coronary heart disease, valvular or pericardial disorders and specific heart muscle diseases including myocarditis. The use of such extensive exclusion criteria and the lack of clear guide-lines as to what constitutes a "dilated" and "poorly contracting" ventricle accounts for the difficulties encountered in making a diagnosis of dilated cardiomyopathy and in interpreting the literature.

Recognising these difficulties the National Heart, Lung and Blood Institute convened a workshop during which standardised diagnostic criteria were developed[117]; these include a left ventricular ejection fraction of <45% or fractional shortening <30%, an end-diastolic diameter >2.7 cm/m^2, and an absence of coronary heart disease or previous myocardial infarction, active myocarditis, significant persistent untreated hypertension or isolated right ventricular dilatation. In addition it was proposed that patients with dilated cardiomyopathy who consumed excessive amounts of alcohol (>100 g/day) over the previous 12 months, and those who presented during the peripartum period should be included but clearly distinguished from other patients.

Although these criteria will help to standardise epidemiological and interventional studies in dilated cardiomyopathy a number of difficulties still remain. Endomyocardial biopsy, although recommended, was not considered mandatory and even when performed is limited by the inconsistencies surrounding the diagnosis of active myocarditis. In addition these recommendations do not identify patients with early dilated cardiomyopathy in which there may be less pronounced ventricular dilatation/dysfunction.[118] This is particularly relevant considering the recent demonstration of the effectiveness of early treatment of heart failure[119] and that study of these individuals is likely to be helpful in further assessing pathogenesis.[120]

Treatment

Treatment is principally that of chronic heart failure and has three primary aims; 1) to relieve symptoms, 2) to retard disease progression and 3) to improve survival. In addition patients with dilated cardiomyopathy may suffer from a number of complications which require specific management. Although medical therapy improves symptoms in most patients with dilated cardiomyopathy, long term survival remains poor, and despite the use of angiotensin converting enzyme inhibitors, cardiac transplantation provides the only effective treatment in those patients with refractory heart failure.

Medical treatment

Patients with dilated cardiomyopathy should be placed on a no added salt diet and if they are overweight this should be reduced. Avoidance of alcohol is recommended as is a flu vaccination. Mild physical exercise can be undertaken as long as it does not produce undue symptoms and has been shown to be beneficial in patients with heart failure. Driving is usually permitted unless symptoms are severe.

Diuretics. Although diuretics are highly effective at relieving dyspnea and peripheral edema there is no evidence that they provide survival benefit in chronic heart failure. Care must be taken to avoid hypokalaemia as this may be arrhythmogenic.

Angiotensin converting enzyme inhibitors. The mainstay of treatment in chronic heart failure is now vasodilator drug therapy particularly with angiotensin converting enzyme inhibitors. Angiotensin converting enzyme inhibitors act predominantly on the angiotensin-renin-angiotensin system and alter the neurohumoral events that exaggerate heart failure. In combination with diuretics they have been shown to provide marked symptomatic and survival benefit in patients with severe[121], mild-moderate [122, 123] and asymptomatic heart failure.[119] Care should be taken as first dose hypotension and deterioration in renal function are recognised complications, particularly in patients with severe heart failure on large doses of diuretics. It is our current practice to introduce ACE inhibitor therapy at an early stage in patients with dilated cardiomyopathy and with appropriate patient selection this can usually be achieved as an outpatient

Other vasodilators. The first drugs shown to improve survival in patients with chronic heart failure were the combination of oral hydralazine and nitrates.[124] Subsequent work has shown that this combination of drugs is as effective as enalapril with regard to symptomatic improvement but that they do not provide as marked a survival benefit.[125] For these reasons it is our policy to prescribe this combination only in patients intolerant of angiotensin converting enzyme inhibitors. The improved mortality conferred by afterload reducing agents has stimulated development of novel vasodilator agents. One such drug, flosequinan, has been shown to provide effective symptoms relief in patients with chronic heart failure [126] but has recently been withdrawn because of worsened mortality.[127]

Anticoagulants. The use of long-term anticoagulation in patients with dilated cardiomyopathy has been the subject of controversy over the years. Retrospective studies have suggested that prophylactic anticoagulation in patients with dilated cardiomyopathy reduces the risk of venous and arterial thromboembolism[8] however other studies have failed to support such a claim.[128] Of interest, several recent large studies in patients with chronic heart failure and atrial fibrillation[129, 130,131] have confirmed the benefit of long-term anticoagulation and included significant numbers of patients with dilated cardiomyopathy. It is not currently known if patients with dilated cardiomyopathy and intra-cardiac thrombus, or those with spontaneous echocardiographic contrast and increased risk of clot formation should be anticoagulated. It is our current policy not to routinely anticoagulate all patients with dilated cardiomyopathy but to restrict this to those patients with established or paoxysmal atrial fibrillation, previous thromboembolism or clear evidence of intra-cardiac thrombus. The timing and duration of such therapy, and the optimal level of anti-coagulation are unknown and await formal prospective evaluation.[132]

Anti-arrhythmic therapy. Anti-arrhythmic treatment is often indicated because atrial fibrillation and ventricular arrhythmias are common in dilated cardiomyopathy. Anti-arrhythmic drug therapy has been disappointing in dilated cardiomyopathy in that it is often unsuccessful and has made little or no impact on survival.[133, 134] One exception is the treatment of established atrial fibrillation which can usually be controlled by digoxin (with or without adjunctive β-blocker therapy). More recently a number of uncontrolled retrospective studies have suggested that amiodarone is effective in the treatment of ventricular tachycardia and improves survival [111, 136], however other studies have not confirmed these findings [137] and we await the results of current prospective studies. The use of internal cardioverter-defibrillator devices appears to be effective in reducing sudden death mortality in patients with dilated cardiomyopathy who have survived an out of hospital cardiac arrest or syncopal episodes.[34]

β-blockers. Since Waagsein et al[138] pioneering report in 1975 numerous groups have investigated the effects of β blocker therapy in patients with chronic heart failure. Early non-randomised studies showed that chronic β blocker therapy improved symptoms in patients with dilated cardiomyopathy[139] and has since been confirmed in randomised controlled trials.[140,141] Though none of the studies performed so far have had sufficient power to study its effect on survival most studies report a trend towards improved survival in patients receiving chronic β blocker therapy.[142] A number of large multicentre trials are currently underway and should provide definitive data on this subject but until this has been confirmed, and we are better able to identify patients at risk of clinical deterioration[143], we do not advise the routine use of β blocker therapy in patients with dilated cardiomyopathy.

Inotropic agents. Following much controversy the long held conviction that digoxin therapy improves symptoms and exercise capacity in patients with dilated cardiomyopathy who remain in sinus rhythm has been confirmed.[144] Digoxin therapy however does not confer improvement in mortality and although its withdrawl from patients receiving angiotensin converting enzyme inhibitors is associated with clinical deterioration [145] its use as adjunctive therapy requires confirmation. Many different inotropes have been developed for use in cardiac failure. While some are useful in the management of acute refractory heart failure[146,147] their use in chronic stable heart failure has been disappointing and often associated with a worsened prognosis.[148, 149, 150]

Others treatment strategies: There are a number of anecdotal reports which suggest that patients with dilated cardiomyopathy benefit from immunosuppressive drug treatment. However in a recent prospective, randomised, placebo-controlled trial patients treated with prednisolone failed to show any clinical benefit.[45] Until we can reliably identify immune-mediated dilated cardiomyopathy and distinguish this from virus-mediated disease the use of immunosuppression cannot be recommended. Two groups have recently reported that patients with dilated cardiomyopathy and refractory heart failure benefit from dual chamber pacing with non-physiological atrio-ventricular delay.[151-153] The mechanism of this response is unclear but may result from improvement in mechanical factors which limit ventricular filling.[151]

Surgical treatment

In recent years there have been a number of new surgical approaches to the management of patients with chronic heart failure. Although cardiac transplantation has received most attention there is a growing acceptance of the need for other surgical techniques in the management of patients with severe refractory heart failure. Surgical techniques include intra-aortic balloon counterpulsation, dynamic cardiomyoplasty, and mitral and tricuspid annuloplasty.[154]

Cardiac transplantation. Since its introduction over 20 years ago there has been a progressive improvement in long-term survival following cardiac transplantation.[155] As a result cardiac transplantation remains the only treatment modality to markedly improve survival figures in patients with refractory heart failure. However the effectiveness of cardiac transplantation is limited by the availability of donor organs [155] and our inability to predict the time at which mortality with medical therapy exceeds that achieved by transplantation.[13] This has been highlighted by a recent retrospective analysis [156] of 528 consecutive patients (49% dilated cardiomyopathy) hospitalised for management of refractory heart failure and transplantation assessment, of whom 11% died suddenly and 9% died from progressive heart failure within the first year of follow-up.

Future developments

Over the last decade there have been significant advances in our understanding and management of patients with dilated cardiomyopathy. Despite these advances many important questions remain unanswered concerning aetiology, identification of individuals with early disease, prognostic stratification, and the development of new and effective treatments for dilated cardiomyopathy.

REFERENCES

1. Goodwin JF, Oakley CM. The Cardiomyopathies. Br Heart J 1972: 34 : 545.
2. Godd MB, et al. Epidemiology of idiopathic dilated cardiomyopathy : a population based study in Olmstead County, Mn, 1975-84. Circulation 1989 : 80 : 564.
3. Torp A. Incidence of congestive cardiomyopathy. Postgrad Me J 1978 : 54 : 435.
4. Taliercio CP, et al. Idiopathic dilated cardiomyopathy in the young : clinical profile and natural history. J Am Coll Cardiol 1985 : 6 : 1126.
5. Tripp ME. Congestive cardiomyopathy of childhood. Adv Pediatr 1984 : 31 : 179-206.

6. Akagi T, et al. Natural history of dilated cardiomyopathy in children. Am Heart J 1991: 121: 1502.

7. Gillium RF. Idiopathic dilated cardiomyopathy in the United States. Am Heart J 1986 111: 752.

8. Fuster V, et al. The natural history of idiopathic dilated cardiomyopathy. Am J Cardiol 1981: 47 : 525.

9. Franciosa JA, et al. Survival in men with severe chronic left ventricular failure due to either coronary heart disease or idiopathic dilated cardiomyopathy. Am J Cardiol 1983: 51 : 831.

10. Unverferth DV, et al. Factors influencing one-year mortality of dilated cardiomyopathy. Am J Cardiol 1984 : 54 : 147.

11. Diaz RA, Obasohan A, Oakley CM. Prediction of outcome in dilated cardiomyopathy. Br Heart J 1987: 58:393.

12. Roberts WC, Siegel RJ, McManus BM. Idiopathic dilated cardiomyopathy : analysis of 152 necropsy patients. Am J Cardiol 1987: 60 : 1340.

13. Keogh AM, et al. Timing of transplantation in idiopathic dilated cardiomyopathy. Am J Cardiol 1988: 61: 418.

14. Hofman T, et al. Mode of death in idiopathic dilated cardiomyopathy : a multivariate analysis of prognostic determinants. Am Heart J 1988;133:250.

15. Francis GS, Boosalis PJ. Mechanism of death in patients with congestive cardiac failure: the change in plasma norepinephrine and its relation to sudden death. Cardioscience 1990: 1 : 29.

16. Kao W, et al. Relation between plasma norepinephrine and response to medical therapy in men with congestive heart failure secondary to coronary artery disease or idiopathic dilated cardiomyopathy. Am J Cardiol 1989: 64 : 609.

17. Goldrach S, Haissaguerre M, Broustet JP. Prognostic value of the hemodynamic study at rest and during the exercise test in 103 cases of primary dilated cardiomyopathies. Arch Mal Coeur 1987: 80: 1333.

18. Hagege A, et al. Prognostic factors in dilated cardiomyopathies. Arch Mal Coeur 1988: 81: 1473.

19. Julliere Y, et al. Dilated cardiomyopathy : long - term follow-up and predictors of survival. Int J Cardiol 1988: 21 : 269.

20. Komajda M, et al. Factors predicting mortality in idiopathic dilated cardiomyopathy. Eur Heart J 1990: 11: 824.

21. Romeo F, et al. Determinants of end-stage idiopathic dilated cardiomyopathy : a multivariate analysis of 104 patients. Clin Cardiol 1989: 12 : 387.

22. Zanchetta M, et al. Dilated cardiomyopathy. Multivariate discriminant analysis of main hemodynamic-angiographic indices. G Ital Cardiol 1990: 20:15.

23. Olshausen KV, et al. Long-term prognostic significance of ventricular arrhythmias in idiopathic dilated cardiomyopathy. Am J Cardiol 1988: 61: 146.

24. Gallo P, et al. Predictive value of myocellular hypertrophy in idiopathic dilated cardiomyopathy. Cardiologia 1989: 34: 53.

25. Kahler M, et al. Mitochondria number as a prognostic parameter in dilated cardiomyopathy. A long-term follow-up study. Z Kardiol 1990: 79: 748.

26. Hammond EH, Menlove RL, Anderson JL. Predictive value of immunofluorescence and electron microscopic evaluation of endomuocardial biopsies in the diagnosis and prognosis of myocarditis and idiopathic dilated cardiomyopathy. Alcohol 1986: 21: 185.

27. Dancy M, Maxwell JD. Alcohol and dilated cardiomyopathy. Alcohol Alcohol 1986: 21: 185.

28. Archard LC, et al. Molecular probes for detection of persisting enterovirus infection of human heart and their prognostic value. Eur Heart J 1991: 12: 56.

29. Takata J, et al. Prognostic significance of large perfusion defects on thallium - 201 myocardial scintigraphy in dilated cardiomyopathy. J Cardiol 1989: 19 : 1081.

30. Blondheim DS, et al. Dilated cardiomyopathy with mitral regurgitation : decreased survival despite a low frequency of left ventricular thrombus. Am Heart J 1991: 122: 763.

31. Hayakawa M, Inoh T, Fukuzaki H. Dilated cardiomyopathy. An echocardiographic follow-up of 50 patients. Jpn Heart J 1984: 25: 955.

32. Mestoni L, Neri R, Camerini F. The electrocardiogram in dilated cardiomyopathy. G Ital Cardiol 1986: 16: 1009.

33. Packer M. Sudden unexpected death in patients with congestive heart failure : a second frontier. Circulation 1985: 72: 681.

34. Fazio G, et al. Long-term follow.up of patients with nonischemic dilated cardiomyopathy and ventricular tachyarrhythmias treated with implantable cardioverter defibrillators. PACE 1991;17:310.

35. Bayes dLA, Coumel P, Leclercq JF. Ambulatory sudden cardiac death : mechanisms of production of fatal arrhythmia on the basis of data from 157 cases. Am Heart J 1989: 117: 151.

36. Wilson FM, et al. Residual pathologic changes following murine coxsackie virus A and B myocarditis. Am J Pathol 1969: 55: 253.

37. Woodruff JF. Viral myocarditis : A Review. Am J Pathol 1980: 101: 425.

38. Reyes MP, Lerner AM. Coxsackievirus Myocarditis- With special reference to acute and chronic effects. Prog Cardiovasc Dis 1985; 27: 373.

39. Sainani GS, Krompotic E, Slodki SJ. Adult heart disease due to coxsackie virus B infection. Medicine Baltimore 1968; 47: 133.

40. Smith WG. Adult heart disease due to the Coxsackie virus B infection. Am Heart J 1970; 80: 34.

41. Daly K, et al. Acute myocarditis. Role of histological and virological examination in the diagnosis and assessment of immunosuppressive treatment. Br Heart J 1984; 51: 30.

42. Das SK, Colfer HT, Pitt B. Long-term follow-up of patients with previous myocarditis using radionuclide venticulography. Heart Vessels 1985 Suppl; 1: 195.

43. Billingham ME, Tazelaar HD. The morphological progression of viral myocarditis. Postgrad Med J 1986; 62: 581.

44. Peters NS, Pool-Wilson PA. Myocarditis: a controversial disease. J R Soc Med 1991; 84: 1.

45. Parrillo JE, et al. A prospective, randomized, controlled trial of prednisone for dilated cardiomyopathy. N Engl J Med 1989; 321: 1061.

46. Cambridge et al. Antibodies to Coxsackie B viruses in congestive cardiomyopathy. Br Heart J 1979; 41: 692.

47. Muir P, et al. Chronic relapsing pericarditis and dilated cardiomyopathy: serological evidence of persistent Enterovirus infection. Lancet 1989; 1: 804.

48. Keeling PJ, et al. A prospective case-control study of antibodies to Coxsackie B virus in idiopathic dilated cariomyopathy. J Am Coll Cardiol, in press.

49. Bowles NE, et al. Detection of Coxsackie B-virus-specific RNA sequences in myocardial biopsy samples from patients with myocarditis and dilated cardiomyopathy. Lancet 1986; 1: 1120.

50. Tracy S, et al. Molecular approaches to enteroviral diagnosis in idiopathic cardiomyopathy and myocarditis. J Am Coll Cardiol 1990; 15: 1688.

51. Jin O, et al. Detection of Enterovirus RNA in myocardial biopsies from patients with myocarditis and cardiomyopathy using gene amplification by polymerase chain reaction. Circulation 1990; 82: 8.

52. Kandolf R. Molecular studies on enteroviral heart disease. In Brinton MA and Heinz FX, eds, New Aspects of Positive Strand RNA Viruses. 1990; American Society Microbiology: 340.

53. Keeling PJ, et al. Similar prevalence of enteroviral genome in myocardium from patients with idiopathic dilated cardiomyopathy and controls by the polymerase chain reaction. Br Heart J 1991; 68: 554.

54. Grasso M, et al. Search for coxsackievirus B3 RNA in idiopathic dilated cardiomyopathy using gene amplification by polymerase chain reaction. Am J Cardiol 1992; 69: 658.

55. Weiss LM, et al. Detection of enteroviral RNA in idiopathic dilated cardiomyopathy and other human cardiac tissues. J Clin Invest 1992; 90: 156.

56. Liljeqvist JA, et al. Failure to demonstrate enterovirus aetiology in Swedish patients with dilated cardiomyopathy. J Gen Virol 1993; 39: 6.

57. Muir P, et al. Rapid diagnosis of enterovirus infection by magnetic bead extraction and polymerase chain reaction detection of enterovirus RNA in clinical specimens. J Clin Micro 1993; 31: 31.

58. Petitjean J, et al. Detection of enteroviruses on endomyocardial biopsy by molecular approach. J Med Virol 1992; 37: 76.

59. Huber S, et al. Immunopathogenetic mechanisms in experimental Picornavirus induced autoimmunity. Pathol Immunopathol Res 1988; 7: 279.

60. Neu N, et al. Cardiac myosin-induced myocarditis as a model of postinfectious autoimmunity. Eur Heart J 1991; II: 260.

61. Anderson JL, et al. HLA A B C and DR typing in idiopathic dilated cardiomyopathy: a search for imune response factors. Am J Cardiol 1984; 53: 1326.

62. Caforio AL, et al. Class II major histocompability complex antigens on cardiac endothelium: an early marker of rejection in the trasnplanted human heart. Transplant Proc 1990; 22: 1830.

63. Limas CJ, et al. Anti-beta-receptor antibodies in human dilated cardiomyopathy and correlation with HLA-DR antigens. Am J Cardiol 1990; 65: 483.

64. Magnusson Y, et al. Mapping of a functional autoimmune epitope on the beta 1-adrenergic receptor in patients with idiopathic dilated cardiomyopathy. J Clin Invest 1990; 86: 1658.

65. Kliein R, et al. Demonstration of organ-specific antibodies against heart mitochondria (anti-M7) in sera from patients with some forms of heart disease. Clin Exp Immunol 1984; 58: 283.

66. Schultheiss HP, Bolte HD. Immunological analysis of auto-antibodies against the adenine nucleotide translocator in dilated cardiomyopathy. J Mol Cell Cardiol 1985; 17: 603.

67. Maisch B, et al. Diagnostic relevance of humoral and cytotocix immune reactions in primary and secondary dilated cardiomyopathy. Am J Cardiol 1983; 52: 1072.

68. Caforio A, et al. Novel Organ-Specific circulating autoantibodies in dilated cardiomyopathy. J Am Coll Cardiol 1990; 15: 1527.

69. Caforio ALP, et al. Identification of the α and β Cardiac Myosin Heavy Chain Isoforms as Major Autoantigens in Dilated Cardiomyopathy. Circulation 1992; 85: 1734.

70. Neu N, et al. Coxsackievirus induced myocarditis in mice: cardiac myosin autoantibodies do not cross-react with the virus. Clin Exp Immunol 1987; 69: 566.

71. Evans W. Familial cardiomegaly. Br Heart J 1949; 11: 68.

72. Ross RS, et al. Idiopathic familial myocardiopathy in three generations: A clinical and pathological study. Am Heart J 1978; 96: 170.

73. Gardner RJ, et al. Dominantly inherited dilated cardiomyopathy. Am J Med Genet 1987; 27: 61.

74. MacLenna BA, et al. Familial idiopathic congestive cardiomyopathy in three generations: a family study with eight affected members. Q J Med 1987; 63: 335.

75. Emanuel R, Withers R, O'Brian K. Dominant and recessive modes of inheritance in idiopathic cardiomyopathy. Lancet 1971; 13: 1065.

76. Goldblatt J, Melmed J, Rose AG. Autosomal recessive inheritance of idiopathic dilated cardiomyopathy in a Madeira Portuguese kindred. Clin Genet 1987; 31: 249.

77. Berko BA, Swift M. X-linked dilated cardiomyopathy. N Engl J Med 1987; 316: 1186.

78. Mestroni L, et al. Clinical and pathologic study of familiar dilated cardiomyopathy. Am J Cardiol 1990; 65: 1449.

79. Michels VV, et al. The frequency of familial dilated cardiomyopathy in a series of patients with idiopathic dilated cardiomyopathy. N. Eng J Med. 1992; 326: 77.

80. Zachara E, et al. Familial aggregation of idiopathic dilated cardiomyopathy: clinical features and pedigree analysis in 14 families. Br Heart J 1993; 69: 129.

81. Walsh TK, Vacek JL. Ethanol and heart disease. An understimated contributing factor. Postgrad Med 1986; 79: 60.

82. Richardson PJ, Atkinson L, Wodak A. The measurement of enzyme activities in endomyocardial biopsies from patients with congestive (dilated) cardiomyopathy and specific heart muscle disease. Z Kardiol 1982; 71: 522.

83. Richardson PJ, et al. Relation between alcohol intake, myocardial enzyme activity, and myocardial function in dilated cardiomyopathy. Evidence for the concept of alcohol induced heart muscle disease. Br Heart J 1986; 56: 165.

84. Ferriere M, et al. Histological aspects of congestive cardiomyopathy caused by alcohol. Comparison with so-called primary cardiomyopathies. Ann Cardiol Angeiol Paris 1983; 32: 225.

85. Wang RY, et al. Alcohol abuse in patients with dilated cardiomyopathy. Laboratory vs clinical detection. Arch Intern Med 1990; 150: 1079.

86. Juilliere Y, et al. Abstention from alcohol in dilated cardiomyopathy: complete regression of the clinical disease but persistence of myocardial perfusion defects on exercise thallium 201 tomography. Eur J Nucl Med 1990; 17: 279.

87. Oakley C. Diagnosis and natural history of congested (dilated) cardiomyopathies. Postgrad Med J 1978; 54: 440.

88. Takarada A, et al. Hypertensive heart disease simulating dilated cardiomyopathy. J Cardiogr 1985; 15: 1015.

89. Lawal SO, Osotimehin BO, Falase AO. Mild hypertension in patients with suspected dilated cardiomyopathy: cause or consequence? Afr J Med Med Sci 1988; 17: 101.

90. Soria R, et al. Dilated cardiomyopathy: electrocardiographic forms. Arch Mal Coeur 1987; 80: 581.

91. Wilensky RL, et al. Serial electrocardiographic changes in idiopathic dilated cardiomyopathy confirmed at necropsy. Am J Cardiol 1988; 62: 276.

92. Brohet C, et al. Electrovectorcardiographic diagnosis of left ventricular hypertrophy in complete left bundle-brandh block. Ann Cardiol Angeiol Paris 1990; 39: 207.

93. Janicki JS, et al. Long-term reproducibility of respiratory gas exchange measurements during exercise in patients with stable cardiac failure. Chest 1990; 97: 12.

94. Weber KT, et al. Oxygen utilization and ventilation during exercise in patients with chronic cardiac failure. Circulation 1982; 65: 1213.

95. Van den Brock SA, et al. Comparison between New York Heart Association classification and peak oxygen consumption in the assessment of functional status and prognosis in patients with mild to moderate chronic congestive heart failure secondary to either ischemic or idiopathic dilated cardiomyopathy. Am J Cardiol 1992; 70: 359.

96. Willens HJ, et al. The prognostic value of functional capacity in patients with mild to moderate heart failure. Am Heart J 1987; 114: 377.

97. Likoff MJ, Chandler SL, Kay HR. Clinical determinants of mortality in chronic congestive heart failure secondary to idiopathic dilated or to ischemic cardiomyopathy. Am J Cardiol 1987; 59: 634.

98. Itoh H, et al. Severity and pathophysiology of heart failure on the basis of anaerobic threshold (AT) and related parameters. Jpn Circulation J 1989; 53: 146.

99. Iannucci G, et al. Late potentials in idiopathic dilated cardiomyopathy. G Ital Cardiol 1990; 20: 549.

100. Fauchier JP, et al. Late ventricular potentials and spontaneous and induced ventricular ar-

rhythmias in dilated or hypertrophic cardiomyopathies. A prospective study about 83 patients. Pace 1988; 11: 1974.

101. Keeling PJ, et al. Usefulness of signal-averaged electrocardiogram in idiopathic dilated cardiomyopathy for identifying patients with ventricular arrhythmias. Am J Cardiol 1993; 71: 78.

102. Poll DS, et al. Abnormal signal-averaged electrocardiograms in patients with nonischemic congestive cardiomyopathy: relationship to sustained ventricular tachyarrhythmias. Circulation 1985; 72: 1308.

103. Ohnishi Y, Inoue T, Fukuzaki H. Value of the signal-averaged electrocardiogram as a predictor of sudden death in myocardial infarction and dilated cardiomyopathy. Jpn Circulation J 1990; 54: 127.

104. Middlekauf HR, et al. Comparison of frequency of late potentials in idiopathic dilated cardiomyopathy and ischemic cardiomyopathy with advanced congestive heart failure and their usefulness in predicting sudden death. Am J Cardiol 1990; 66: 1113.

105. Unverferth DV, Baker PB. Value of endomyoardial biopsy. Am J Med 1986; 57: 321.

106. Davies MJ. The cardiomyopathies: a review of terminology, pathology and pathogenesis. Histopath 1984; 8: 363.

107. Vasiljevic JD, et al. The incidence of myocarditis in endomyocardial biopsy samples from patients with congestive heart failure. Am Heart J 1990; 120: 845.

108. Billingham ME. The diagnostic criteria of myocarditis by endomyocardial biopsy. Heart Vessels 1985 Suppl; 1: 133.

109. Zee Cheng CS, et al. High incidence of myocarditis by endomyocardial biopsy in patients with idiopathic congestive cardiomyopathy. J Am Coll Cardiol 1984; 3: 63.

110. Poll DS, et al. Usefulness of programmed stimulation in idiopathic dilated cardiomyopathy. Am J Cardiol 1986; 58: 992.

111. Brembilla-Perrot B, et al. Diagnostic value of ventricular stimulation in patients with idiopathic dilated cardiomyopathy. Am Heart J 1991; 121: 1124.

112. Rae AP, et al. Electrophysiologic assessment of antiarrhythmic drug efficacy for ventricular tachyarrhythmias associated with dilated cardiomyopathy. Aj J Cardiol 1987; 59: 291.

113. Constantin L, et al. Induced sustained ventricular tachycardia in nonischemic dilated cardiomyopathy: dependence on clinical presentation and response to antiarrhythmic agents. Pace Pacing Clin Electrophysiol 1989; 12: 776.

114. Das SK, et al. Prognostic usefulness of programmed ventricular stimulation in idiopathic dilated cardiomyopathy without symptomatic ventricular arrhythmias. Am J Cardiol 1986; 58: 998.

115. Gonska BD, Bethge KP, Kreuzer H. Programmed ventricular stimulation in coronary artery disease and dilated cardiomyopathy: influence of the underlying heart disease on the results of electrophysiologic testing. Clin Cardiol 1987; 10: 294.

116. Brandenberg RO, et al. Report of the WHO/ISFC task force on definition and classification of the cardiomyopathies. Circulation 1981; 64: 1397.

117. Manolio TA, et al. Prevalence and etiology of idiopathic dilated cardiomyopathy (summary of National Heart, Lung, and Blood Institute workshop). Am J Cardiol 1992; 69: 1458.

118. Keren A, et al. Mildly dilated congestive cardiomyopathy. Circulation 1985; 72: 302.

119. The SOLVD Investigators. Effect of enalapril on mortality and the develpment of heart failure in asymptomatic patients with reduced left ventricular ejection fractions. N Eng J Med 1992; 327: 685.

120. Caforio ALP, Stewart J, McKenna WJ. Idiopathic dilated cardiomyopathy. Brit J Med. 1990; 300: 890.

121. The CONSENSUS Trial Study Group. Effects of enalapril on mortality in severe congestive heart failure. Results of the Cooperative North Scandinavian Enalapril Survival Study. N Engl J Med 1987; 316: 1429.

122. The SOLVD Investigators. The effect of enalapril on survival in patients with reduced left ventricular ejection fractions and congestive heart failure. N Eng J Med 1991; 325: 293.

123. Kleber FX, et al. Influence of the severity of heart failure on the efficacy of angiotensin-converting enzyme inhibition. Munich mild heart failure trial (MMHFT). Am J Cardiol 1991; 88 (Suppl D): 121.

124. Cohn JN, et al. Effect of vasodilator therapy on mortality in chronic congestive heart failure. Results of a Veterans Adminitration Cooperative Study. N Engl J Med 1986; 314: 1547.

125. Cohn JN, et al. A comparison of enalapril with hydralazine-isosorbide dinitrate in the treatment of chronic congestive heart failure. N Engl J Med 1991; 325: 303.

126. Packer M, et al. Double-blind, placebo-controlled study of the efficacy of flosequinan in patients with chronic heart failure. Principal Investigators of the REFLECT Study. J Am Coll Cardiol 1993; 22: 65.

127. Letter. Flosequinan withdrawn, Lancet 1993; 342 (8865): 235.

128. Tobin R, Slutsky RA, Higgins CB. Serial echocardiograms in patients with congestive cardiomyopathies: lack of evidence for thrombus formation. Clin Cardiol 1984; 7: 99.

129. Petersen P, et al. Placebo-controlled, randomised trial of warfarin and aspirin for prevention of thromboembolic complications in chronic atrial fibrilation. The Copenhage AFASAK Study. Lancet 1989; 8631: 75.

130. The Boston Area Anticoagulation Trial for Atrial Fibrillation Investigators. The effect of low dose warfarin on the risk of stroke in patients with nonrheumatic atrial fibrillation. N Eng J Med 1990; 323: 1505.

131. Chesebro JH, Fuster V, Halperin JL. Atrial fibrilation - risk marker for stroke. N Eng J Med 1990; 22: 1556.

132. Falk RH. A plea for a clinical trial of anticoagulation in dilated cardiomyopathy. Am J Cardiol 1990; 65: 914.

133. Oakley C. Genesis of arrhythmias in the failing heart and therapeutic implications. Am J Cardiol 1991; 67: 421.

134. Poll DS, et al. Sustained ventricular tachycardia in patients with idiopathic dilated cardiomyopathy: electrophysiologic testing and lack of response to antiarrhythmic drug therapy. Circulation 1984; 70: 451.

135. Dargie HJ, Cleland JO. Arrhythmias in heart failure - the role of amiodarone. Clin Cardiol 1988; 12: 78.

136. Neri R, et al. Ventricular arrhythmias in dilated cardiomyopathy: efficacy of amiodarone. Am Heart J 1987; 113: 707.

137. Keogh AM, Baron DW, Hickie JB. Prognostic guides in patients with idiopathic or ischemic dilated cardiomyopathy assessed for cardiac transplantation. Am J Cardiol 1990; 65: 903.

138. Waagstein F, et al. Effect of chronic beta-adrenergic receptor blockade in congestive cardiomyopathy. Br Heart J 1975; 37: 1022.

139. Swedberg K, et al. Beneficial effects of long-term beta-blockade in congestive cardiomyopathy. Br Heart J 1980; 44: 117.

140. Anderson JL, et al. Long-term (2 year) beneficial effects of beta-adrenergic blockade with bucindolol in patients with idiopathic dilated cardiomyopathy. J Am Coll Cardiol 1991; 17: 1373.

141. Engelmeier RS, et al. Improvement in symptoms and exercise capacity by metoprolol in patients with dilated cardiomyopathy: a double-blind, randomised, placebo-controlled trial. Circulation 1985; 72: 536.

142. Bashir Y, McKenna WJ, Camm AJ. β blockers and the failing heart: is it time for a U-turn. Br Heart J 1993; 70: 8.

143. Fisher ML, Plotnick GD, Peters RW, Carliner NH. Beta-blockers in congestive cardiomyopathy. Conceptual advance for contraindication? Am J Med 1986; 42: 116.

144. Diabanco R, et al. A comparison of oral milrinone, digoxin and their comination in the treatment of patients with chronic heart failure. N Eng J Med 1989; 320: 677.

145. Packer M, et al Withdrawal of digoxin from patients with chronic heart failure treated with angiotensin-converting-enzyme inhibitors. RADIANCE Study. N Engl J Med 1993; 329: 1.

146. Bonelli J, Jancuska M. Comparison of digoxin and dobutamine in patients with severe dilatative cardiomyopathy. Int J Clin Pharmacol Ther Toxicol 1989; 27: 120.

147. Dec GW, et al. Long-term outcome of enoximone therapy in patients with refractory heart failure. Am Heart J 1993: 123: 526.

148. Wilmshurst P. Why inotropes continue to disappoint in heart failure. Br Heart J 1993; 70: 4.

149. Om A, Hess ML. Inotropic therapy of the failing myocardium. Clin Cardiol 1993; 16: 5.

150. Packer M, et al. Effect of oral milrinone on mortality in severe chronic heart failure. The PROMISE Study Research Group. N Engl J Med 1991; 325: 1468.

151. Brecker SJD, et al. Effects of dual-chamber pacing with short atrioventricular delay in dilated cardiomyopathy. Lancet 1992; 340: 1308.

152. Hochleitner M, et al. Usefulness of physiologic dual-chamber pacing in drug-resistant idiopathic dilated cardiomyopathy. Am J Cardiol 1990; 66: 198.

153. Hochleitner M, et al. Long-term efficacy of physiologic dual-chamber pacing in the treatmen of end-stage idiopathic cardiomyopathy. Am J Cardiol 1992; 70: 1320.

154. Spodick DH. Effective management of congestive cardiomyopathy. Relation to ventricular structure and function. Arch Intern Med 1982; 142: 680.

155. Kriett JM, Kaye MP. The Registry of the International Society for Heart Transplantation: seventh official report 1990. J Heart Transplant 1990; 9: 323.

156. Saxon LA, Stevenson WG, et al. Predicting death from progressive heart failure secondary to ischemic or idiopathic dilated cardiomyopathy. Am J Cardiol 1993; 71: 62.

17 AUTOIMMUNE CARDIAC DISEASES

Manousos M. Konstadoulakis, George D. Kymionis,
Marina G. Toutouza, Emanuel Leandros

The human body has the immune system to recognize substances which do not belong to it and produces against them, compounds called "antibodies". People may form antibodies against substances of their own ("autoantibodies"), giving birth to various clinical syndromes. Although the mechanisms are not yet clearly understood, clinical and experimental data support the suggestion that autoimmune mechanisms play a significant role in the pathogenesis of heart diseases as myocarditis and dilated cardiomyopathy.

Autoantibodies directed against a wide spectrum of myocardial antigens (myosin, actin, tropomyosin, adenosine nucleotide translocator -ANT) are found in patients with idiopathic dilated cardiomyopathy, myocarditis, rheumatic heart disease, post myocardial infarction and post perimyocardiotomy syndrome.

Immunopathologic basis of cardiac disease

Myocarditis and dilated cardiomyopathy

Dilated cardiomyopathy is a chronic heart muscle disorder of unknown etiology, characterised by ventricular dilatation and poorly contracting left ventricle.[1] Clinical[2] and experimental[3] data provide enough evidence that viral myocarditis may lead to dilated cardiomyopathy, or, in other words, that myocarditis is a precursor of dilated cardiomyopathy. It is now known that viral myocarditis can progress to idiopathic dilated cardiomyopathy, as a consequence of an autoimmune reaction.[4,5] This is supported by the identification of coxsackie virus B-specific RNA sequences and infiltrating lymphocytes among damaged myocytes, in heart muscle biopsy specimens from patients with idiopathic dilated cardiomyopathy.[6,7]

This autoimmune though to be initiated by a coxsackie B3 (CB3) virus infection. Experiments in mice were able to reproduce autoimmune myocarditis by infecting susceptible strains with coxsackie B3 virus[8,9] or by immunization with cardiac myosin.

Schwimmbeck et al[10] identified regions of high homology between coxsackie B3 virus and rabbit cardiac myosin and demonstrated an immunologic cross reactivity between coxsackie B3 virus peptides and the myosin peptide. Other animal studies with CB3 virus which induces muring myocarditis demonstrated the appearance of circulating autoantibodies against cardiac tissue after the viral infection.[11] These antibodies (IgG type) react with the heavy chain of cardiac myosin and are equally directed to ventricular and skeletal myosin because the β-myosin heavy chain of human cardiac muscle and the myosin heavy chain of skeletal muscle are products of the same gene.[12,13]

Lauer et al[14] have also demonstrated the presence of autoantibodies against human ventricular myosin in patients with myocarditis. They identified low titres (1/40), of antibodies against the human B-myosin in 42% of patients with acute myocarditis and in a 21% of a heterogeneous group of cardiac patients who mainly had coronary disease. Anti-myosin antibodies can be used as a marker of myocardial injury but their pathogenic role is debuted.

Caforio et al[15] showed that patients with heart failure have anti-myosin antibodies while Konstadoulakis et al[16] showed a high incidence of antibodies against tropomyosin, actin and myosin in patients with dilated cardiomyopathy.

Damage to the myocardium is associated with the induction of antibodies to mitochondria adenine nucleotide translocator (ANT) branched chain ketoacid dehydrogenase (BCKD) proteins and myosin. The degree of injury in CB3-infected mice is correlated with the amount of myosin and BCKD antibody found in the systemic circulation. It is also correlated the amount of ANT and BCKD antibody concentration found in the heart.[17]

Autoantibodies to a and b myosin heavy chain, have also been identified in dilated cardiomyopathy patients.[18,19] Elevated values of these autoantibodies were found in a high percentage of people suffering from dilated cardiomyopathy, leading to the suggestion that autoimmunity plays an important role in the initiation and progression of myocardial injury in dilated cardiomyopathy.

Goldman et al[19] identified anti-a-myosin antibodies in 20% of patients with dilated cardiomyopathy and in 16% of their asymptomatic relatives. The presence of anti-myosin antibodies in patients with dilated cardiomyopathy (familiar and non-familiar) does not support a primary pathogenic role of this antibody which is more likely to be a marker of disease predisposition[20].

Cardiac antigens other than myosin may also be important in the pathogenesis of dilated cardiomyopathy. Limas et al[21] documented a high prevalence of β-receptor autoantibodies in familiar cardiomyopathy. He suggested that their presence is under genetic control of the human leukocyte antigen (HLA) class II genes. These antibodies inhibit adenylate cyclase activity and may, as a result, contribute to the downregulation of b-adrenergic pathways. They have a positive chronotropic effect on isolated rat heart myocytes and they are also able to induce an agonist-like stimulation of the cardiac myocytes. The therapeutic efficacy of selective β_1-blockers in some patients with dilated cardiomyopathy may be partly explained by their ability to dissociate the β-adrenoreceptor-antibody complex and to block the continuous adrenergic stimulation.[22] Therefore, a more favourable response to long-term β-blockade in patients with circulating antireceptor autoanitbodies might be expected compared with patients where these antibodies are not present in their serum.

In both viral myocarditis and dilated cardiomyopathy antimitochondrial antibodies are directed against the ADP/ATP translocator of the inner mitochondrial membrane, inhibiting nucleotide transport in vitro.[23] These antibodies as well as rabbit antibodies against the ADP/ATP translocator, cross react with proteins located within the plasma membrane of cardiac myocytes. After the neutralization of antibodies with the purified ADP/ATP translocator, neither intracellular binding to mitochondria nor cell surface binding is detected. This indicates that anti-mitochondrial antibodies bind to cross-reacting antigenic determinants. Holzinger et al[24] demonstrates that all types of infiltrating cells (T cells, B cells, macrophages and granulocytes) are increased in the tissue compartments of hearts with idiopathic dilated cardiomyopathy. The CD8 T cells and macrophages are also increased in number when compared with the other leukocyte subpopulations. The quantitative increase of leukocytes in idiopathic dilated cardiomyopathy is associated with an activation stated increased number of activated T cells within the heart. This suggests a direct role of infiltrating leukocytes in the pathogenesis of idiopathic dilated cardiomyopathy and favours the theory of an ongoing, chronic immune process in responsible for the pathogenesis of IDC.

Anderson et al[25] published a pilot study from six medical centres in the United States, examining the role of immunosuppresive therapy in biopsy-proven myocarditis. In this pilot study, immunosuppression offered no clear advantage over conventional therapy. We should not overlook the fact that the number of patients was very small and the period of treatment was brief. There are reports that have shown, in a subset of patients with viral myocarditis and/or dilated cardiomyopathy a clear benefit from immunosuppressive therapy. Still only prospective study could demonstrate the benefit or not of immune manipulation, in the study of patients with IDM.

Rheumatic heart disease (RHD)

Group A streptococci contain antigens that are immunologically cross-reactive with human antigens like myosin. Heart reactive antibodies have been reported in sera after infection of humans with group A streptococci and subsequent development of acute rheumatic fever. Studies of hearts at autopsy from individuals with acute rheumatic fever have demonstrated the presence of antibody and complement bound to the heart tissue.

Immunization with *Streptococcus pyogenes* type SM protein produces type-specific M protein antibodies that cross-react with a high molecular weight antigen from cardiac sarcolemma. M protein is a major component of the streptococcal cell surface. It has antiphagocytic properties, shares structural homology and antibody cross-reactivity with "a helical coiled-coil" proteins like myosin and tropomyosin in the heart muscle.[26] Murine monoclonal antibodies cross-reactive with the M protein and myosin recognize epitopes located in the S2 and light meromyosin (LMM) subfragment of the heavy chain.[27] Antibodies that cross-react with heart tissue and *S.pyogenes* and *S.mutans* have also been produced in animals after immunization with these micro-orga-nisms but direct evidence between the antibodies and the disease process has not been documented.

The presence of CD4+ T cells at lesion sites in the heart of patients with RHD has been demonstrated, suggesting a direct role of these cells in the pathogenesis of rheumatic heart disease. In favour of this role for T cells, M-protein-stimulated peripheral blood T cells display a cytotoxic activity toward immortalized human heart cells. It has also been shown that streptococcal M protein may be a superantigen, i.e., a protein capable of stimulation a large number of T cells that share a T-cell antigen receptor variable region element[28], a fact that can have important immunopathological consequences. Recently Gullherme et al[29] have isolated T-cell clones from heart lesions of rheumatic heart disease patients. These T-cell clones recognize both streptococcal M-protein synthetic peptides and heart tissue protein fractions.

Myocardial infarction

In patients with ischemic heart disease (IHD), autoantibodies (anti-nuclear, anti-smooth muscle, antimitochondrial, antithyroid) are more common than in healthy subjects.[30]

Oxidation of low-density lipoproteins (LDL) plays a role in the pathogenesis of atherosclerosis. Elevated title of these antibodies are predictive of myocardial infarction. Antibodies against oxidized low-density lipoprotein, are associated with nonfatal myocardial infarction.[31]

Antiphospholipid syndrome has been defined as venous or arterial thrombosis, recurrent fetal loss and/or thromocytopenia associated with an increased level of antiphospholipid antibodies (aPLAs). This syndrome can be either primary or secondary to an underlying condition, most commonly the systemic lupus erythematosus (SLE). Alder et al[32] have demonstrated that there is an association between increased titles of five different aPLAs (antibodies to anticardiolipin, antiphosphatidylcholine, antiphosphatidylserine, antiphosphatidylethanol and antiphosphatidylinositol) in young patients' sera and acute myocardial infarction. They have significantly elevated title of different aPLAs at the early presentation of patients with acute myocardial infarction, suggesting that these antibodies are present before the infarction secondary to them. Antiphospholipid antibodies may represent a risk factor for the acute development of myocardial infarction, in specially patients at a younger age group without cardiovascular risk factors.

Post-cardiac injury syndrome

During local necrosis of the cardiac muscle there is cell lysis and appearance of intracellular proteins in the circulation. These proteins can "fool" the immune system into producing autoantibodies. The presence of these antibodies has been linked to the development of fever, leucocytosis and signs of pericardial and often pleural reaction (post-cardiac injury syndrome). The clinical observation that this syndrome appears seven or more days after the acute injury and responds to corticosteroid therapy suggests that immunology factors are involved in its pathogenesis. Patients with acute myocardial infarction and patients who underwent cardiac surgery, have been shown to have antiheart antibodies, that may be involved in the pathogenesis of post-cardiac injury syndrome. Anti-heart antibodies (AHA) and circulating immune complexes in sera are found in the majority of these patients. Post-cardiac injury syndrome is most frequently seen in patients who underwent cardiac surgery compared with patients with acute myocardial infarction. Actin and myosin are the major constituents of the heart cellular proteins. High levels of autoantibodies against these proteins were found in patients with post-cardiac injury syndrome.[33] Whether these antibodies play a role in the pathogenesis of post-operative complications remains unclear.

De Scheerder et al[33] have also demonstrated a correlation between post-pericardiotomy syndrome, anti-heart antibodies and circulatory immune complexes, suggesting a possible role of these immune complexes in the pathogenesis of the post-pericardiotomy syndrome.

Hypertensive disease

There is growing evidence that hypertension is associated with immunological dysfunction. Hypertensive patients have increased concentrations of immunoglobulins increased numbers of autoantibodies against the nuclear membrane and increased number of activated T lymphocytes. Autoantibodies against the a1-adrenergic receptor are present in patients with malignant hypertension.[34] Experimental studies have also demonstrated that autoantibodies directed against the β_1-adrenoreceptor are able to induce a positive chronotropic effect.[35]

Electrical cardiac abnormalities

Primary electrical cardiac abnormalities (atrial arrhythmia's, ventricular arrhythmia's and conduction disturbances) are associated with a high prevalence of antibodies interacting with functional epitopes mapped to the second extracellular loop of the beta-adrenoreceptors. These seem to be interested through a similar abnormal immunoregulatory process involving the beta-adrenoreceptors. These cardiac abnormalities seem to be interrelated through a similar abnormal immunoregulatory process involving the beta-adrenoreceptors. These antibodies exert agonist- or catecholamine-like effect that facilitate the occurrence of ventricular arrhythmia's and play a role in the development of dilated cardiomyopathy.[36]

Heart block children has been associated with maternal systemic lupus erythematous, the so-called neonatal lupus syndrome. Two types of heart block can be recognized: The congenital heart block which is associated with maternal anti-Ro/

SSA antibodies and the acquired heart block which is seen in older children and is not associated with maternal autoimmunity.[37,38]

The congenital heart block is the result from the transplacental passage of maternal autoantibodies into the fetal circulation resulting in damage to the otherwise normally developing heart. Major cardiac anatomic abnormalities rarely occur in autoimmune-associated congenital heart block. Ro/SSA and La/SSB are polypeptides associated with small RNA species known as the hYRNAs and RNA polymerase III products. Antibodies against the 52-kd, the 60-kd SSA/Ro and to the 48-kd SSB/La proteins. These polypeptides identified in the fetal cardiac tissue, compose the major conducting system.[39] The functional role of the Ro peptides is still unknown, but the La particle is a transcription termination factor of RNA polymerase III. Although the target antigens of anti-SSA/Ro and anti-SSB/La antibodies are ribonucleoproteins normally sequestered intracellularly, there is evidence from immunohistochemical studies to support the hypothesis that heart fetal tissue damage is mediated by these antibodies.

Cardiac transplantation

In our days the detection of panel reaction antibodies is the most reliable-pretransplantation test to identify patients likely to have a donor-specific positive crossmatch. Patients with a panel-reactive antibodies less than 15% are accepted for heart transplantation. The presence of IgM anti-heart antibodies greater than 15% in the sera of patients waiting heart transplantation predisposes them to a significantly greater number of rejection episodes and more severe rejection episodes as assessed by the immunosuppressory therapy required.[40]

Conclusions

The presence of autoantibodies against a variety of cardiac antigens has been shown in a broad spectrum of cardiac diseases. It is still unclear what triggers the production of these autoantibodies. Bacterial and viral infections have been shown to induce their production through a cross-reactive mechanism. Antibodies produced against the intruding bacteria and/or virus cross-react with "self" antigens, causing direct tissue destruction. A hypothesis which is further strengthened by the known similarities between bacterial and/or viral antigens and the molecules of actin and myosin. Furthermore the process of myofibre necrosis known to be associated with various cardiac diseases and the liberation of heart antigens into the systemic circulation could also trigger the liberation of heart antigens into the systemic circulation. The presence of these antigens in high quantities into the systemic circulation could lead to the production of autoantibodies against heart constituents. No matter what is the mechanism for the production of these autoantibodies the correlation between their presence and several functional heart parameters observed by many researchers strongly advocates their participation in the pathogenesis of various cardiac diseases. Several recent reports have been able to find alterations in cell-mediated immune mechanisms in cardiac diseases like Chaga's disease, post myocardial infarction syndrome and dilated cardiomyopathy. These reports support the hypothesis that cell-mediated immunity has a role in myocyte degeneration or destruction and argue in favour of an ongoing, chronic immune process in its pathogenesis.

It is clear that with the existing knowledge one cannot support a definitive explanation of the etiology of the cardiac diseases analysed previously, though there are many indications that the immune system has a key role in their clinical course.

REFERENCES

1. Manolio TA, et al. Prevalence and etiology of idiopathic dilated cardiomyopathy. Am J Cardiol 1992: 69:1458.

2. MacArthur CGC, et al. The relationship of myocarditis to dilated cardiomyopathy. Eur Heart J 1984:5:1023.

3. Huber SA, Lyden DC, Lodge PA. Myocarditis. Herz 1985:10:1.

4. McManus BM, Gauntt CJ, Cassling RS. Immunopathologic basis of myocardial injury. Cardiovasc Clin 1988:18:163.

5. Zee-Cheng CS, et al. High incidence of myocarditis by endomyocardial biopsy in patients with idiopathic congestive cardiomyopathy. J Am Coll Cardiol 1984:3:63.

6. Bowles NE, et al. Detection of coxsackie B virus specific TNA sequences in myocardial biopsy samples from patients with myocarditis and dilated cardiomyopathy. Lancet 1988:1:1120.

7. Tazelaar HD, Billingham ME. Leukocytic infiltrates in idiopathic dilated cardiomyopathy. Am J Surg Pathol 1986:10:405.

8. Grodums EL, Dempster G. Myocarditis in experimental coxsackie B3 infection. Con J Microbiol 1959:5:605.

9. Wolfgram LJ, et al. Variation in the susceptibility to coxsackie virus B3-induced myocarditis among different strains of mice. J Immunol 1986:136:1846.

10. Schwimmbeck PL, Shyltheiss HP, Strauer BE. Isolation of myocardial antibodies using imunoabsorption with synthetic peptides as antigens. Eur Heart J 1990:280:463.

11. Wolfgram LJ, Beisel KW, Rose NR. Heart specific autoantibodies following murine coxsackie B3 myocarditis. J Exp Med 1985:161: 112.

12. Alvarez FL, et al. Heart specific autoantibodies induced by coxsackie-virus B3 identification of heart autoantigens. Clin Immunol Immunopathol 1987:43:129.

13. Neu N, et al. Autoantibodies specific for the cardiac myosin isoform are found in mice susceptible to coxsackievirus B3-induced myocarditis. J Immunol 1987:138:2488.

14. Lauer B, et al. Autoantibodies against human ventricular myosin in sera of patients with acute and chronic myocarditis. J Am Coll Cardiol 1994:23:146.

15. Caforio ALP, et al. Identification of a and b cardiac myosin heavy chain isoforms as major autoantigens. Circulation 1992:85:1734.

16. Konstadoulakis MM, et al. Clinical significance of antibodies against tropomyosin, actin and myosin in patients with dilated cardiomyopathy. J Clin Lab Immunol 1993:40:61.

17. Neumann DA, et al. Induction of multiple heart autoantibodies in mice with coxsackievirus B3 and cardiac myosin induced autoimmune myocarditis. J Immunol 1994: 152:343.

18. Limas CJ, Goldenberg IF, Limas C. Autoantibodies against b-adrenoreceptors in human idiopathic dilated cardiomyopathy. Circ Res 1989:64:97.

19. Goldman JH, et al. Autoimmunity to a-myosin in a subset of patients with idiopathic dilated cardiomyopathy. Br Heart J 1995:74:598.

20. Herskowitz A, Neumann DA, Ansari AA. Concepts of autoimmunity applied to dilate cardi-omyopathy. J Am Coll Cardiol 1993:22: 1385.

21. Limas Cath, et al. Anti-b-receptor antibodies in familiar cardiomyopathy: Correlation with HLA-DR and HLA-DQ gene polymorphisms. Am Heart J 1994:127:382.

22. Magnusson Y, et al. Autoimmunity in idiopathic dilated cardiomyopathy. Circulation 1994:89:2760.

23. Kuhl U, Ulrich G, Schultheib H-P. Cross-reactivity of antibodies to the ADP/ATP translo-cator to the inner mitochondrial membrane with the cell surface of cardiac myocytes. Eur Heart J 1987:8 (Suppl.1):219.

24. Holzinger C, et al. Phenotypic patterns of mononuclear cells in dilated cardiomyopathy. Circulation 1995: 92:2876.

25. Anderson JL, et al. Immunosuppressive therapy of myocardial inflammatory disease. Initial experience and future trials to define indications for therapy. Eur Heart J 1987:8(Suppl.):263.

26. Robinson JH, Kehor MA. Group A streptococcal M proteins: virulence factors and protec-tive antigens. Immunol. Today 1992:13:362.

27. Dell A, et al. Autoimmune determinants of rheumatic carditis localization of epitopes in human cardiac myosin. Eur Heart J 1991:12(Suppl.D):158.

28. Watanabe-Ohnishi R, et al. Characterization of unique human TCR specifies for a family of streptococcal superantigens represented by rheumatogenic serotypes of M protein. J Immu-nol 1994:152:2026.

29. Guilherme L, et al. Human heart-infiltrating T-cell clones from rheumatic heart disease patients recognize both streptococcal and cardiac proteins. Circulation 1995:92:415.

30. Potocka-Plazak K, Noworolska A, Kocemba J Prevalence of autoantibodies in the very eld-erly association with symptoms ischemic heart disease. Aging Milano 1995:7:218.

31. Maggi E, et al. Autoantibodies against oxidised low density lipoproteins in patients with coronary disease. Presse Med 1994:9:1158.

32. Alder Y, et al. The presence of antiphospholipid antibodies in acute myocardial infarction. Lupus 1995:4:309.

33. Scheerder I, et al. Post cardiac injury syndrome and an increased humoral immune response against the major contractile proteins (actin and myosin). Am J Cardiol 1985:56:631.

34. Fu M, et al. Functional autoimmune epitope on a1-adrenergic receptors in patients with malignant hypertension. Lancet 1994:344:1660.

35. Wallukat G, et al. The sera of spontaneously hypertensive rats contain agonistic auto-anti-bodies against the beta 1-adrenoceptor. J Hypertens 1995:13:1031.

36. Chiale P, et al. High prevalence of antibodies against beta1-beta2 adrenoceptors in patients with primary electrical cardiac abnormalities. J Am Coll Cardiol 1995:26:864.

37. Frohn-Mulder I, et al. Clinical significance of maternal anti-Ro/SSA antibodies in children with isolated heart block. J Am Coll Card 1994:23:1677.

38. Garcia S, et al. Cellular mechanism of the conduction abnormalities induced by serum from anti-Ro/SSA positive patients in rabbit hearts. J Clin Invst 1994:93:718.

39. Waltuck J, Buyon JP. Autoantibody-associated congenital heart block: outcome in mothers and children. Ann Intern Med 1994: 120:544.

40. Maisch B, et al. Value of immunohistological and immunoserological monitoring in cardiac transplantation. Eur Heart J 1987:8(Suppl.J):29.

18 CARDIAC TRANSPLANTATION

Ronald S. Freudenberger, Alan Gass

The National Heart Lung, and Blood Institute estimates that over 2,000,000 Americans have heart failure and about 400,00 new cases are diagnosed each year. Over 200,000 people in the United States die each year from congestive heart failure. In addition there are over I million hospitalizations at a cost over 7 million dollars. Total treatment costs for heart failure were over 10 million dollars in 1990.

Drug therapy for the treatment of congestive heart failure has improved with the widespread use of angiotensin converting enzyme inhibitors (ACE). Nevertheless, the one year mortality for hospitalized patients with congestive heart failure New York Heart Association Class IV approaches 50 %.

Since the first successful human cardiac transplant performed by Christian Bernard in 1967, public interest in cardiac transplantation has increased dramatically. With improvement of technique in the 1970's and the development of cyclosporine, for prevention of rejection, in the 1980's professional and public interest has increased dramatically. Approximately 20,000 cardiac transplants have been performed, there are 3,500 patients on a waiting list for heart transplantation and approximately 4,000 more will be fisted this year.

Indications

The number of heart transplants performed has reached a plateau over the last several years. Because of the limited availability, it is therefore, imperative that we optimally identify patients who will do well with transplantation and exclude those who dare not optimal candidates.

In general patients with advanced heart failure, on maximal medical therapy including vasodilators, particularly angiotensin-corverting enzyme (ACE) inhibitors, digoxin and diuretics. Those patients with increasing medication requirements, frequent hospitalizations or overall deterioration of clinical status should be considered for evaluation for cardiac transplantation.

In addition to these clinical parameters, ejection fraction and hemodynamic parameters are generally obtained to further risk stratify patients. Patients with low ejection fractions tend to have a poor prognosis. However, among patients with ejection fractions less than 20 % there is limited ability to further determine prognostic information. The use of bicycle ergometry with gas exchange to determine the oxygen consumption at maximal exercise has proven to be a very useful tool. Data from Mancini et al, demonstrates that a maximal oxygen consumption greater than 14 milliliters (ml)/ kilogram (kg)/ minute (min) predicts a good prognosis. On the other hand, patients with maximal oxygen consumption less than 14 mm/kg/min have a poor prognosis and should be considered for cardiac transplantation.[1]

The etiologies of congestive heart failure that result in cardiac transplantation are; primary cardiomyopathy, coronary artery disease with either resultant ischemic cardiomyopathy and symptoms of congestive heart failure or inoperable ischemic coronary disease with refractive chest discomfort. A small percentage of patients who undergo cardiac transplantation do so for valvular heart disease with severe left ventricular dysfunction and congenital heart disease. Other underlying etiologies in patients who have undergone cardiac transplantation include inoperable hypertrophic cardiomyopathy, sarcoidosis and amyloidosis although these two latter entities have been reported to recur post transplantation and are considered a contraindications by many centers.

Exclusion criteria

In 1992 a group of transplantation cardiologists, surgeons, nurses and representatives from the United Network of Organ Sharing (UNOS) met to discuss various aspects of cardiac transplantation including criteria for exclusion.

Irreversible pulmonary hypertension that is irreversible, creates a high risk of postoperative right ventricular failure. Pulmonary vascular resistance index higher than 6-8 Woods units/meter^2, a pulmonary artery systolic pressure greater than 50-60 millimeters (mm) of mercury (Hg), a transpulmonic gradient of > 15 mm, hg, that do not decrease by 50% with use of vasodilators is a contraindication to cardiac transplantation. Various pharmacological agents including, dobutamine, nitroglycerine, prostacyclin and nitic oxide have been used to assess reversibility of these pressures.[2,3]

Coexistent medical illness with a poor prognosis remains a contraindication to transplantation, since the patient is likely to have a poor short term survival or a difficult postoperative course. Patients with irreversible pulmonary parenchymal disease are poor operative candidates. Irreversible pulmonary disease is defined as those with a forced expiratory volume 1 min /forced vital capacity (FEVI/FVC) of less than 50% of the predicted value or patients with restrictive lung disease with a FEV<50% Patients with obstructive lung disease are at higher risk of perioperative lung infection adding to the risk of perioperative complications.

Irreversible renal dysfunction defined as a creatinine greater than 2 mg/dL or a creatinine clearance less than 50 ml/min. All attempts to determine the degree of prerenal azotemia to determine the degree of renal dysfunction that is reversible from that which is intrinsic and irreversible. Preexisting renal dysfunction is likely to worsen with postoperative fluid shifts and the introduction of cyclosporine an agent with a high degree of nephrotoxicity.

Primary hepatic dysfunction such as cirrhosis or any hepatic dysfunction with resultant coagulopathy increases the risk of perioperative complications and is therefore considered a contraindication to cardiac transplantation. Also, the primary immunosupressant agents, cyclosporine and tacrolimus (FK 506) are hepatically metabolized.An attempts to differentiate between primary hepatic dysfunction and passive congestion should be made, including liver biopsy when necessary.

Significant peripheral and cerebrovascular disease are considered contraindications to transplantation. The presence of cerebrovascular disease increases the risk of neurological complications perioperatively. The use of steroids postoperatively may cause rapid progression of vascular disease.

Insulin dependent diabetes mellitus with end organ damage or high insulin requirements without end organ damage is a contraindication to cardiac transplantation. Patients with orally controlled diabetes without end organ damage have successfully undergone cardiac transplantation with similar outcome as those without diabetes. However, with steroid use borderline diabetics develop overt diabetes, orally controlled diabetics usually tend to require insulin therapy.

Transplantation should be deferred in patients with active infection, peptic ulcer disease and diverticulosis or diverticulitis. These entities, when active, pose a higher perioperative risk. Deferment of transplantation until these problems have been effectively treated is prudent.

Patients with coexisting neoplasm should not undergo cardiac transplantation. However, those who have a history of localized malignancy that was successfully treated may be a candidate for transplantation. Disease free interval of at least one year and a negative evaluation for metastatic disease is required prior to consideration for cardiac transplantation.

Acute pulmonary embolism or infarction increases the perioperative risk of lung infection. It is generally recommended to defer cardiac transplantation until at least 6 weeks have passed.[4]

Myocardial infiltrative or inflammatory diseases such as sarcoidosis and amyloidosis, results in positive intermediate term prognosis but have been reported to recur in the transplanted organ[5]. For these reasons presence of these conditions are considered a contraindication to cardiac transplantation in most centers.

Severe osteoporosis is likely to worsen with steroid administration postoperatively and is considered a contraindication in many transplant centers.

Psychosocial instability and substance abuse are risk factors for patient noncompliance. Craft loss secondary to noncompliance is well described. Risk factors for noncompliance include previous substance abuse, mood and personality disorders, history of previous noncompliance and inadequate family support.[6]

Physiology of the transplanted heart

Soon after transplantation, the cardiac output is often depressed and maintenance of high central venous pressure is important to maintain the cardiac output.[7] This is likely due to an early restrictive type of physiology and abnormal atrial dynamics. Because of the mid atrial anastomosis between the donor and recipient hearts, varying proportions of the donor and recipient are present. Furthermore, the recipient atria do not contract synchronously with donor atria because recipient sinus node electrical activity does not pass through the anastomotic sutures lines. This results in approximately 20 % of normal atrial contribution to the total stroke volume of the heart.[8]

Many patients have normal resting intra-cardiac pressures after transplantation that can increase with exercise. This is due to an early restrictive hemodynamic pattern. When present early after transplantation it usually resolves. More recently, it is recognized that there is a subclinical, latent, restrictive component that is present and unmasked by volume challenge. This may be confounded by post-transplantation hypertension with resultant hypertrophy and by bouts of rejection.[9]

The transplanted heart demonstrates a unique response to exercise. During early exercise the cardiac output increases by augmentation of end-diastolic volume and stroke volume. At more intense exercise levels, heart rate and contractility are increased by circulating catecholamines.[10,11] The heart rate response is blunted in these individuals. The maximal cardiac output achieved is generally lower than that of normal people, because of a blunted heart rate response and a lower peak stroke volume.[2]

Denervation of the heart leads to a resting tachycardia (95-115 beats per minute) due to loss of vagal input. Also, the rate does not respond to carotid sinus massage or to drugs that are dependent on intact innervation to the heart, such as atropine. As mentioned above, there is a blunted heart rate response to exercise because of the denervation that occurs the increased heart rate that occurs relatively late in exercise is due to high levels of circulating catecholamines. Administration of beta blocking agents eliminates this response and should therefore be avoided. Because of dennervation the administration of digoxin in patents who have undergone cardiac transplantation has little electrophysiological effect on the heart. Administration of quinidine and disopyramide, agents that have vagolytic effects in the innervated heart, tend to increase AV conduction time due to its direct AV nodal affects.[13]

Life after transplantation

Psychosocial aspects

Given 1 year survival rates of 80% to 90% and 5 year survival rates of 60%-70%, patients who have undergone cardiac transplantation have an improvement in survival and longer life expectancy. Several studies have addressed the quality of life in addition to the quantity of life. The National Transplantation Study [14] examined quality of life in detail. This study examined data from 85 % of transplantation programs in the United States. This study found that 80-85 % of the patients were physically active. 90 % of the patients analyzed referred to themselves as normal or stared that they had minimal signs or symptoms of disease. Only 7.2 % rate their health status as poor. 9 % of patients needed assistance in traveling around their community and only 1 % needed assistance in eating, dressing, bathing or using the toilet. Patients rated their life satisfaction, well-being and psychological affect as equal to that of the general population.

In spite of these good ratings of physical activity and well being, only 32-50 % of patients are employed after transplantation. Reasons for this surprising number is thought to be multifactorial. Employers may be reluctant to hire people who have undergone transplantation because of fear of absenteeism and increase in group health insurance rates. Patients may be less motivated to work following a serious illness.

Routine follow-up

The most common causes of death in the first year post transplantation is rejection and infection. Both of these complications occur most frequently in the first two months after transplantation. Therefore the most intensive follow up post-transplantation is within this initial period. During this period patients are required to live in close proximity to the medical center. Patients are seen twice weekly as an outpatient to examine for evidence of infection, rejection or graft dysfunction. Patient undergo frequent EKG analysis, Chest-X-Ray analysis and blood chemistries to monitor renal and hepatic function as well as serum levels of the pharmacological agents used. In addition patients undergo endomyocardial biopsy i.e. weekly during the first 6-8 weeks and gradually at lower frequencies.

After the first six months, barring any significant complications patients are usually followed every month for the first 1-2 years. Patients undergo endomyocardial biopsy, serum chemistries complete blood counts, EKG and other evaluations as necessary. Follow up after this time period is adjusted to the individual patient and the individual transplant center.

Routine immunosupression

Immunosupression is often begun with preoperative administration of azathioprine and intraoperative administration of corticosteroids. On day one post-transplantation cyclosporine is initiated. Some centers routinely use anti T-cell antibodies, either monoclonal (OKT3) or polyclonal (antithymocyte globulin) as induction therapy in lieu of cyclosporine. Some centers use antilymphocyte preparations as induction therapy only when the patient has renal insufficiency or hemodynamic instability, to delay the use of cyclosporine until after the immediate postoperative period.

Routine immunosupression for most patients includes cyclosporine, a drug that inhibits lymphokine production by T lymphocytes, azathioprine which inhibits purine synthesis and cell proliferation and corticosteroids which inhibit gene transcription for the production of cytokines.

In addition to these agents, patients also receive oral nystatin or clortrimazole to prevent candidal infections. Oral acyclovir is often administered to prevent herpes zoster infection. Trimethoprim-sulfamethoxazole or pentamidine is administered to prevent infection with pneumocystis carinii. Pyrimethamine and sulfadiazine is given to toxoplasma gondii seronegative patients who receive organs from seropositive donors.

Complications

Early postoperative. Right ventricular failure due to high pulmonary vascular resistance in the recipient remains one of the leading causes of early mortality. With careful screening of the potential recipient and re-evaluafion while on the waiting list this problem can potentially be avoided.

2-10 % of the recipients will require permanent pacing because of dysfunction or block of the atrioventricular node. The use of terbutafine or theophylline may enhance sinus activity and delay or obviate the need for permanent pacing.

Infection. One third of all transplant patients develop an infection that requires intravenous antibiotics during the first year following transplantation. Infection is the most common cause of death in the first year after transplantation. 46 % of infections in the first year are bacterial infection, with the peak incidence is during the first postoperative week. The majority of bacterial infections are lung infections, line infections and rarely sternal wound infections. A patient who was on a mechanical ventilator prior to transplantation is at highest risk for developing a bacterial lung infection. Sternal wound infections account for 6 % of serious wound infections but result in 22 % mortality rate. Opportunistic bacterial infections such as legionella and listeria also occur. However these infections generally occur in the later postoperative period.

Viral infections occur with a peak incidence of 30-60 days post transplantation. Cytomegalovirus (CMV) is the most common pathogen responsible for serious infection in the post-transplant population. The majority of transplant recipients are seropositive for CMV and harbor dormant viral organisms. With induction immunosupressant therapy reactivation of this dormant virus may occur or reinfection with another CMV strain may occur. If the recipient is seronegative for CMV and the donor is seropositive there is a risk of transmission of this virus and appearance of primary CMV infection.

Infection with CMV is most commonly localized to the lung where it presents as pneumonia, with the appearance of fever, dyspnea, hypoxemia and a diffuse infiltrate. The next most common area of localized CMV infection is the gastrointestinal tract.

Gastrointestinal CMV infection can present as fever, diarrhea and massive gastrointestinal bleeding. Hepatic involvement manifested as hepatitis and eye involvement manifested as chorioretinitis and papillitis also occur. General or non-localized infection, manifested as malaise and lethargy with positive blood or urine cultures may also occur. Treatment is with 2-4 weeks of intravenous ganciclovir.

Fungal infections account for approximately 7% of infections post-transplantation. The peak incidence of these infections are within weeks 2-6. The most common is candidal infection that is present in blood or as a sternal wound infection. Pulmonary aspergilosis, nocardia and cryptococcal infections also occur.

Protozoal infections peak at months 3-4. The most common protozoal infection is Pneumocystus Carinii pneumonia. Patients present with diffuse pulmonary infiltrate, dyspnea and hypoxemia. Prophylaxis with trimethoprim-sulfamethoxazole has resulted in a lower incidence of this infectious process. However, on discontinuation of this agent infection with this pathogen may occur. Toxoplasmosis often occurs as a donor transmitted disease. Prophylaxis with pyrimethamine and sulfadiazine is effective in preventing active disease.

Rejection. Cell mediated rejection is the most common form of acute rejection, whereas antibody mediated rejection is far less common however, it is much more resistant to treatment.

The Cardiac Transplant Research Database indicates that at the end of one year post-transplantation 37 % of patients were free from rejection, 40 % of patients had one episode of rejection and 23 % had more than one rejection. The majority of all rejections occurred within the first six months after transplantation and rejection accounted for 17 % of all deaths within the first year.[15]

Symptoms associated with rejection are non-specific and include malaise, lethargy, fatigue and low grade fevers. If the rejection episode is severe and associated with graft dysfunction, dyspnea, an S_3 gallop and lower blood pressure may be seen. However, most cases of rejection are associated with few specific symptoms or physical signs. Therefore, diagnosis of rejection is on the basis of endomyocardial biopsy. In 1989 the International Society for Heart Lung Transplantation standardized the grading system for endomyocardial biopsy [16] allowing transplant physicians a uniform way of diagnosing and treating rejection. Surveillance biopsies are performed frequently within the first six months. Since endomyocardial biopsy is an invasive procedure, there has been much effort to develop an noninvasive method to detect rejection. Various forms of electrocardiography, echocardiography and immunologic markers have been investigated to allow a non-invasive means to detect ejection. However, none have proven to be sensitive or specific enough to replace endomyocardial biopsy.

Treatment of rejection is generally reserved for higher grades of rejection. Generally, patients with mild rejection are not actively treated but are followed closely for worsening rejection. Those with higher grade rejection are treated with high dose oral or intravenous steriods. Doses range from 1,500-3000 mgs. of methylprednisolone divided over three days. Alternatively, 300-1000 mgs of oral prednisone tapered over 7-14 days. Rejection that is associated with hemodynamic compromise or graft dysfunction or rejection episodes resistant to the second course of steroid therapy are usually treated with monoclonal or polyclonal antibodies in addition to high dose steroids.

Humoral rejection is diagnosed by immunoflorescent staining of the biopsy specimens.[17] Antibody and complement deposition is seen on the vascular endothelium. Humoral rejection is associated with a higher incidence of fatality and decreased long term survival. In general no treatment is recommended for humoral rejection unless there is concomitant graft dysfunction. In this case high dose steroids, antihympcyte globulin, cyclophosphamide and plasmapharesis have been used with variable success.

Hyperacute rejection is a form of humoral rejection that causes immediate graft dysfunction at time of implantation and is due to preformed antibodies in the recipient. Those with hyperacute rejection have a poor prognosis.

Malignancy. Immunosupressed transplant recipients have a 1-2 % risk per year of developing a malignancy. This risk may become higher as patients survive longer following their transplant. Also, this risk may be higher in those with a history of previous malignancy.[18] The overall risk is approximately 6%, about 100 times that of the general population. Solid organ transplant patients are not at higher risk for developing the common tumors such as lung, prostate, breast and colon. rather they are at higher risk of developing squamous cell carcinoma of the skin, lymphoma, Kaposi's sarcoma, carcinoma of the vulva, perineun, carcinoma of the kidney and hepatobiliary tumors. Cutaneous malignancy is the most common malignancy and is associated with the use of azathioprine.[19] The high incidence of skin carcinoma is believed to be due to the photosensitizing effects of the azathioprine metabolite, nitroimidazole.

A unique type of lymphoma, referred to as post transplant lymphoproliferative disease is a non-Hodgkins B-cell lymphoma. the mean time to presentation of these tumors is 12 to 18 months post-transplantation. The tumor appears to be induced by the Epstein-Barr virus. Data from the Cincinnati Transplant Tumor Registry suggest that up to 40 % of the patients with this disease may respond to reduction in immunosupressant therapy.[20] Presentation of this type of lymphoma is similar to that of lymphomas in the non-transplant population and may present with lymphadenopathy, abdominal mass, gastrointestinal ulceration, seizures and fever of unknown origin. Chemotherapy, radiation therapy and surgical excision when possible should be considered, however long term survival is poor.

Cardiac allograft vasculopathy (CAV). The leading cause of death after the first year post-transplantation is CAV. This is an unusual form of accelerated coronary artery disease. This phenomenon is detected angiographically in 30-500/o of patients by five years after transplantation and can be detected as early as six months after transplantation.[21] This process differs from native coronary atherosclerotic disease in several important ways; this disease is diffuse, concentric, longitudinal and develops rapid pruning and obliteration of distal branch vessels.[22] Focal stenosis of these vessels may occur however, this is less common than the diffuse type of stenoses that occur. Because of the diffuse narrowing that is found, coronary angiography, which relies on the adjacent "normal" vessel caliber to diagnose stenotic lesions, coronary angiography is a relatively insensitive way to diagnose CAV. More recently, intravascular ultrasound was shown to be a more sensitive way to diagnose this disease[23]. Histologically, this disease reveals hyperplasia of the smooth muscle cells and macrophages that migrate into the intima which results in lumenal narrowing. These changes are almost identical to that seen in patients who develop restenosis following percutaneous transluminal coronary angioplasty.

Because of denervation that occurs with the transplanted heart, patients usually do not present with angina. Presenting signs of this disease include; graft failure, acute myocardial infarction and sudden death. Angiographic changes may occur as early as one year after transplantation. Therefore, most transplant centers perform baseline coronary angiography at 1 month after transplantation and at yearly intervals.

CAV is thought to be multifactorial in origin but is believed to be immune mediated, injury to the vascular endothelium. Development of methods to prevent this entity from occurring has been difficult. The relationship between this disease and known risk factors for coronary artery disease such as: hypertension, hyperlipidemia and smoking have not been firmly established. Links between CAV and the number and severity of rejection episodes and the use of corticosteroids and cyclosporine, as well as, infection with CMV, have been suggested but are not firmly established.

Treatment for CAV, has include the use of calcium channel blockers which may increase luminal diameter, PTCA, atherectomy and coronary artery bypass grafting for focal lesions have been used with varying success. However, the only definitive treatment for this progressive disease, is retransplantation. This remains a controversial area with due to the shortage of donor organs and the relatively poor survival post-transplantation.

Survival

In spite of these potential complications, as indicated earlier, the patients experience a general improvement in quality of life and in survival. Data from the Cardiac Transplant Research Database indicates that one year survival in major North American transplant centers is 85 %. It is estimated that 5 year survival in the average transplant patient is 75%. Thus, in spite of its' limitations, cardiac transplantation offers a viable option to improve both quality and quantity of life in the selected patient.

REFERENCES

1. Mancini D, et al. Value of peak oxugen consumption for optimal timing of cardiac transplatation in ambulatory patients with heart failure. Circulation 1991:83:778.

2. Costard-Jackle A, Fowler M. Influence of preoperative pulmonary artery pressure on mortality after heart transplatation: testing of potential reversibility of pulmonary hypertension with nitroprusside is useful in defining a high risk group. J Am Coll Cardiol 1992:19:48.

3. Murali S, Uretsky B, Armitage J. Utility of prostaglandin E1 in the pretranplant evaluation of cardiac failure patients with significant pulmonary hypertension. J Heart Lung Transplant 1992:11:716.

4. Carvarocchi N, et al. Successful heart transplatation in recipients with recent perioperative pulmonary emboli. J Heart Lung Transplant 1989:8:494.

5. Hosenpud J, et al. Successful intermediate term outcome for patients with cardiac amyloidosis undergoing heart transplatation: results of a multicenter survey. J of Heart and Lung Transplant 1990:9:346.

6. Mai F, McKenzie F, Kostuk W. Psychiatric aspects of heart transplatation: preoperative evaluation and postoperative sequelae. Br Med J 1986:292:311.

7. Stinson E, et al. Initial clinical experience with heart transplatation. Am J Cardiol 1968:22:791.

8. Young J, et al. Evolution of hemodynamics after orthotopic heart and heart/lung transplatation: early restrictive patterns rersisting in occult fashion. J Heart Transplatation 1987:6:34.

9. Tischler M, et al. Serial assessment of left ventricular function and mass after orthotopic heart transplatation: a four year longitudinal study. J Am Coll Cardiol 1992:19:60.

10. Mc Laughlin P, et al. The effect of exercise and atrial pacing on left ventricular volume and contractility in patients with intervated and denervated hearts. Circulation 1978:58:476.

11. Ingels N, et al. Relation between longitudinal, circumferential, and oblique shortening and torisional deformation in the left ventricle of the transplated human heart. Circ Res 1989:64:915.

12. Plugfelder P, et al. Cardiac hemodynamics during supine exercise in cyclosporine treated orthotopic heart transplant recipients: Assessment by radionuclide angiography. J Am Coll Cardio 1987:10:336.

13. Bexton R, et al. The direct electrophysilogical effects of dsopyramide phosphate in the transplated human heart. Circulation 1983:67:38.

14. Evans R. Executive summary: The National Cooperative Transplantatino Study. BHARC-100-91-020 1991.

15. Kobashigawa J, et al. Prentransplant risk factors for acute rejection after cardiac transplatation: a multiinstitutional study. J Heart Lung Transplant 1993:12:303

16. Billingham M, et al. A working formulation for the standardizatino of nomenclature in the diagnosis of heart and lung rejection: Heart Rejection Study Group. J Heart Transplamt 1990:9:587.

17. Hammond E, et al. Vascular rejection of human cardiac allografts and the role of humoral immunity in chronic allograft rejection. Transplant Proc 1991:23:26.

18. Armitage J, et al. Heart transplatation in patients with previous malignant disease. J Heart Lung Transplant 1990:627.

19. Penn I. Cancers after cyclosporine therapy. Tranplsant Proc 1988:20:276.

20. Hanto D, et al. The Ebstein-Bar virus in the epathogenesis of post-transplant lymphoproliferative disorders. Surgery 1981:90:204.

21. O'Neil et al. Frequency of angiographic detection and quantitative assessment of coronary arterial disease one and three years after cardiac transplatation. Am J Cardiol 1989:63:1211.

22. Gao S, et al. Accelerated coronary vascular disease in the heart transplant patient: Coronary arteriographic findings. J Am Coll Cardiol 1988:12:34.

23. St Goar F, et al. Intracoronary ultrasound in cardiac trasnplant recipients. In vivo evidence of angiographically "silent" intimal thickening. Circulation 1992:85:979.

Section D

CARDIAC GENETICS

19 DIFFERENTIAL GENE EXPRESSION IN MUSCLE

R.Sanders Williams

Anatomy of a gene switch

Genes that encode proteins are transcribed by RNA polymerase II (Pol II), and primary RNA transcripts are processed and exported to the cytoplasm as mature RNA messengers (mRNA). These are translated on cytoplasmic ribosomes to generate polypeptides, which are folded, assembled with cofactors, and partitioned to the correct subcellular location to generate mature, functional proteins. The process of "gene expression" includes all of these steps, any one or all of which can be regulated to control the abundance of the ultimate product of the pathway *(Figure19.1)*. In addition, both the final and intermediate components of this pathway are degraded at a certain rate, such that the stability, as well as the rate of synthesis, of RNA and polypeptide gene products determine the level of gene expression. For many genes, however, expression is controlled predominately at the first step — transcription — and this chapter will focus on biochemical and molecular regulation of this event, as it relates to normal development and physiology of the heart, and to cardiac disease states.

Transcriptional control of gene expression can be envisioned as a switch mechanism that the cell sets in the "OFF" or "ON" position. In the "ON" position, transcription can be modulated quantitatively over a broad range (at least 1000-fold), though much smaller changes (e.g. 2-fold) may be physiologically relevant in some situations. The number of mRNA molecules synthesized per unit time is determined primarily by the rate at which new transcripts are initiated, though the rate of elongation of nascent transcripts also may be regulated.

Transcription of protein-coding genes by Pol II is initiated by formation of an aggregate of several proteins (transcription factors) that directs the polymerase to the site at which the first two ribonucleotides are joined to begin the RNA chain *(Figure19.2)*. Some of these transcription factors are common to most genes transcribed by Pol II, and are termed "core" or "basal" transcription factors. An important basal transcription factor is TBP (TATA Binding Protein), which binds to a DNA sequence (TATA box) containing the nucleotide bases TATAAAA (or close variants thereof) and serves as the nidus around which other essential basal transcription factors join to form the complex.[1] Many of these additional basal transcription factors do not directly contact DNA but are retained in the initiation complex by protein-protein interactions.

In most mammalian genes, transcription is initiated approximately 30 nucleotides "downstream" (5' to 3' with respect to polarity of the coding strand of the DNA double helix) from the TATA box. The region of the gene immediately "upstream" from the site at which transcription is initiated is called a promoter. While most promoters include a TATA box, some do not. In these TATA-less promoters, the initiation complex still includes TBP, but other proteins that recognize different nucleotide sequences provide the starting point around which the complex forms.

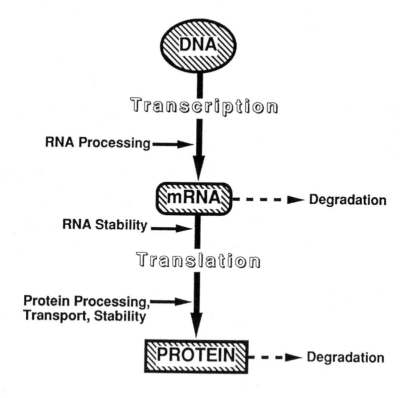

Figure 19.1 Steps in gene expression.

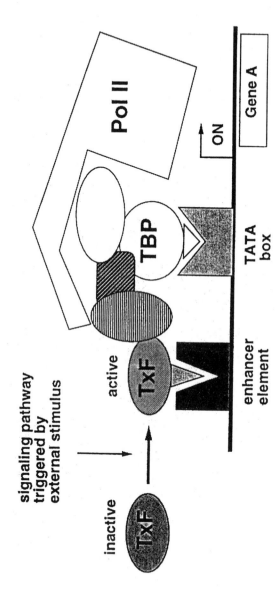

Figure 19.2 Schematic representation of a gene switch. The initial portion of the transcribed region of a representative gene (Gene A) is boxed and the transcriptional start site is illustrated by an arrow. The gene is switched "ON" and RNA transcription by RNA Polymerase II(Pol II) begins when a basal initiation complex containing multiple proteins (shown as ovals) forms on a basal promoter element (TATA box) near to the transcriptional start site. The rate at which transcriptional initiation occurs is controlled by regulatory transcription factors (TxF) that bind to other DNA sequences (enhancer element). The functional activity of regulatory transcription factors can be modulated by a variety of mechanisms, in response to specific stimuli.

If a promoter cannot form a transcriptional initiation complex, it is functionally in the "OFF" position, and the gene linked to that promoter will not be transcribed. In fact, of the approximately 100,000 genes estimated to be present in the human genome, only a few thousand are active in any given cell at any given time. A variety of situations can prevent formation of the initiation complex and hold a gene in the "OFF" state. DNA in chromosomes in packaged with proteins as chromatin, and interacts with cytoskeletal components within the nucleus (nuclear matrix). For genes to be transcribed, the chromatin structure must be disrupted to open the DNA such that the transcriptional initiation complex can form. Chemical modification of the DNA itself (methylation), chromatin condensation, or matrix effects can render certain chromosomal regions inert with respect to transcription.[2-4] In addition, genes can be held in the "OFF" state either because of repressor factors that disrupt or prevent transcriptional initiation [5], or because essential positively acting transcription factors are not available.

A gene promoter is switched "ON" when the components of the basal transcriptional apparatus assemble and Pol II becomes engaged. In the absence of other inputs, however, the rate at which this process occurs may be so low as to be physiologically insignificant. To modulate the rate of transcriptional initiation, and ultimately the level of gene expression, assembly of the active transcriptional complex is controlled by the action of other "regulatory" (as opposed to "basal") transcription factors *(Figure19.2)*.

Regulatory transcription factors bind to specific DNA sequence motifs consisting of 6 to 15 nucleotide bases that are located on the same chromosome as the basal promoter and gene. The binding sites for regulatory transcription factors are sometimes termed "upstream activation sequences" since they are commonly found adjacent to the basal promoter in a position 5 '("upstream") of the TATA box. Activation elements are not uniformly located in this position, however, and may reside 3' ("downstream") of the site of transcriptional initiation within the gene itself or distal to the point of transcriptional termination (polyadenylation site). The binding sites for several different types of regulatory transcription factors often occur in clusters that comprise an "enhancer": a segment of DNA that exercises a regulatory function (by virtue of binding specific proteins) over a basal promoter. Enhancers may be found very close to the TATA box, or in remote locations many thousands of base pairs distant from the transcriptional start site. When regulatory transcription factors bind to enhancers in such remote sites, the intervening DNA is looped out to form contacts with the transcriptional complex that forms on the basal promoter.

Regulatory transcription factors come in many varieties and often function in a combinatorial manner to impart fine control of gene expression in response to developmental cues or other physiological stimuli. These proteins can be grouped into several categories or families based on shared structural characteristics. Prominent families (and superfamilies) of transcription factors are listed in *Table 19.1*. Individual members of a given family of transcription factors, however, may serve very diverse functions.

Most transcription factors have a modular nature *(Figure19.3)*, meaning that

TABLE 19.1   *TRANSCRIPTION FACTOR FAMILIES*

Family	Representative members
basic helix-loop-helix	MyoD,myogenin,E12*,c-myc*
leucine zipper	c-fos*,c-jun*
homeodomain	Csx*
MADS	MEF-2*,SRF*
winged helix	HNF-3,MNF*
GATA	GATA-1,GATA-4*
steroid receptor	thyroid receptors*

*expressed in the myocardium and implicated in cardiac gene regulation

discrete and separable regions of the protein have defined functions with respect to DNA binding, transcriptional activation, and interactions with other proteins or signaling molecules. This feature of transcription factors permits engineering of chimeric proteins with unique properties from components derived from several different native proteins. For example, it is possible to make a given transcription factor a more potent transactivator, or to place it under a new form of regulation (e.g. hormone responsiveness), and thereby to manipulate expression of target genes for experimental (and ultimately clinical) purposes.

Each type of cell expresses a unique complement of regulatory transcription factors to activate only those genes necessary to determine the specialized properties of that cell. Because transcription factors function in a combinatorial manner, variations in the concentration or the activity of a relatively small number of transcription factors can result in a huge number of possible regulatory states, thereby permitting fine control of expression of single genes or groups of coordinately regulated genes.

The functional activity of transcription factors can be regulated in several ways such that stimuli acting upon a pre-existing pool of transcription factors can produce rapid responses that do not require new protein synthesis *(Figure19.2)*. Several important varieties of transcription factors are held in an inactive state by binding to other proteins that prevent access of the factor to its binding site on DNA.[6] The activating stimulus releases the transcription factor such that it becomes competent for DNA binding and subsequent transcriptional activation of its target genes. Binding to other proteins (co-activators or dimerization partners), conversely, may be essential for the function of certain transcription factors.[7, 8] Finally, transcription factors may be controlled by covalent modifications: phosphorylation at certain critical residues within the transcription factor protein may either activate or inactivate its DNA binding or transcriptional activation functions.[9]

Gene switching during cardiac development

Cells acquire specialized characteristics by virtue of differences in gene expression.

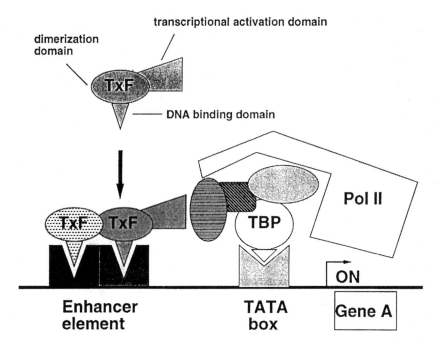

*Figure 19.3 **Modular nature of transcription factors**. The schematic model shown in Figure 2 is repeated, but with an additional degree of complexity to illustrate a transcription factor (TxF) that forms a heterodimer with another factor, each member of which recognizes half sites within an enhancer element. Three functionally discrete domains of this transcription factor monomer are illustrated. The DNA binding domain is the region of the molecule that contacts the DNA recognition site. The dimerization domain is the portion of the protein required to form the heterodimeric complex, and increase the affinity for binding DNA. The transcriptional activation domain is the region of the protein that communicates with the basal transcription complex.*

During embryonic and early post-natal development, terminally differentiated cell types, such as cardiac or skeletal myocytes, are derived from pluripotent progenitor cells through a series of steps outlined in *Figure19.4*. Each of these transitional steps is governed (and to some degree defined) by the expression and/or activity of specific transcription factors. Our understanding of the molecular controls over these events is more complete with respect to development of skeletal muscle than cardiac muscle, though certain similarities in the process of differentiation make it useful to discuss these cell types in parallel.

Both skeletal and cardiac myocytes are derived from mesodermal precursors, but they arise from entirely different regions of the early embryo. Skeletal muscles of both the axial skeleton and the limbs originate within the somites, while the earliest identifiable cardiomyocyte precursors are found within the lateral plate mesoderm. In either case, premyogenic cells at some point undergo a process called

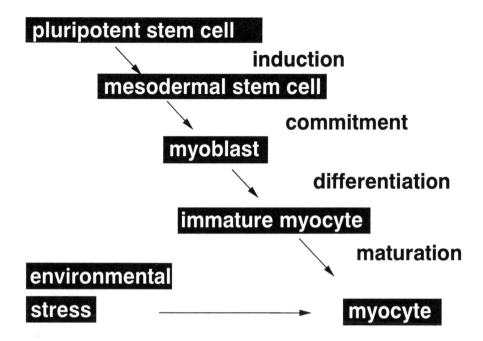

*Figure 19.4 **Stages of myocyte development**. Pluripotent embryonic stem cells undergo a process called **induction** to form mesodermal stem cells, one of three general classes of cells in the early embryo. Myoblasts are mesodermally derived cells in which a number of irreversible genetic switches have been activated in a process called **commitment**, such that these cells have a restricted fate. Under the proper conditions, myoblasts then undergo **differentiation** and begin to manifest the distinctive morphological and functional characteristics of skeletal or cardiac myocytes. Additional gene switching events, some of which occur only after birth, promote **maturation** of myocytes so that they acquire adult properties. The **adaptation** of fully differentiated, mature myocytes to stresses such as work overload or ischemia permits the heart and skeletal muscles to respond to changing environmental conditions.*

commitment, resulting in myoblasts: cells that do not yet express markers of terminal differentiation (e.g. contractile proteins), but are competent to do so when conditions are right, and are restricted from differentiation into other cell types (e.g. adipocytes or fibroblasts). In the cell lineage that gives rise to skeletal myocytes, commitment to the myoblast stage is closely associated with the appearance of one or more of four types of myogenic determination factors (MyoD, myogenin, myf5, and MRF4) that are members of the basic helix-loop-helix (bHLH) family of transcription factors.[10-12] Myogenin and related proteins, though present in myoblasts, are largely inactive at this stage. Their activity is suppressed by one or more of several mechanisms *(Figure 19.5)* that include: competition for a cofactor (EI2) by an inhibitor of differentiation (Id); phosphorylation of a critical threonine residue within the DNA binding domain (basic region) by protein kinase C under the control of peptide growth factors; or suppressive interactions with proto-oncogenes.[9]

During terminal differentiation of skeletal myocytes, these brakes on the activity of myogenin and other myogenic determination factors of this class are released and these proteins bind to sites within enhancer regions of target genes *(Figure 19.5)*. Genes activated by myogenic bHLH proteins include terminal differentiation markers such as the muscle-specific isoform of creatine kinase, as well as other transcription factors that, in turn, activate other terminal differentiation markers in a cascading fashion.[13]

We presume that a similar process takes place during development of cardiac myocytes, but the essential regulatory molecules have not yet been defined so clearly. The myogenic bHLH proteins, which are essential for skeletal muscle differentiation, are not found in cardiac myocytes at any stage. It is intriguing, however, that many of the same genes activated by myogenin and related bHLH proteins in skeletal myocytes also are switched on during cardiac development. Apparently, other transcription factors serve to activate these genes in the heart.

Figure 19.5 *Myogenic bHLH proteins in skeletal muscle development.*   ➡

(A)   *Regulation by heterodimer formation. MyoD and myogenin activate muscle-specific genes by binding to enhancer elements characterized by the nucleotide sequence CAnnTG (where n = any nucleotide). Binding is most efficient when MyoD forms a heterodimeric complex with another bHLH protein called E12. In non-muscle cells E12 is complexed with yet another bHLH protein termed Id (Inhibitor of differentiation), but this complex does not bind DNA, and muscle-specific genes are not expressed. In the committed myoblast, MyoD is present, but most muscle-specific genes continue to be inactive (i.e. transcription is "OFF"). When conditions are right for differentiation, Id disappears, MyoD can now form the active complex with E12, and genes that encode markers of terminal differentiation are actively transcribed.*

(B)   *Multiple mechanisms by which the activity of myogenic bHLH proteins can be regulated by growth factors. Several peptide growth factors (e.g. FGF) suppress differentiation of skeletal myoblasts. At least four independent mechanisms of this suppressive effect of growth factors have been described. Growth factors stimulate expression of Id (see Figure 5A) and prevent formation of active heterodimers between E12 and myogenic bHLH proteins (illustrated here as myogenin: MG). Growth factors also induce expression of immediate early genes such as c-fos, which form inactive complexes with myogenin. Signaling cascades triggered by growth factors activate protein kinase C (PKC), leading to phosphorylation of myogenin on a critical threonine residue in the DNA binding domain, and inactivation of the protein. Finally, growth factors promote hyperphosphorylation of the product of the retinoblastoma (Rb) tumor suppressor gene. The hypophosphorylated form of Rb protein enhances assembly of myogenin or MyoD into active transcriptional complexes, such that this effect of growth factors restrains myogenesis.*

(A)

Non-muscle cell

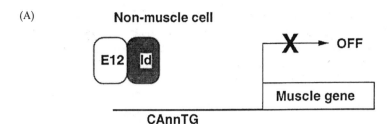

Committed myoblast

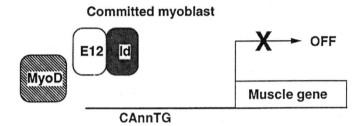

Differentiated myotube

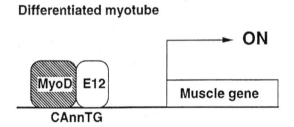

(B)

+ Growth factors

induce Id

induce fos/jun

activate PKC

inactivate Rb

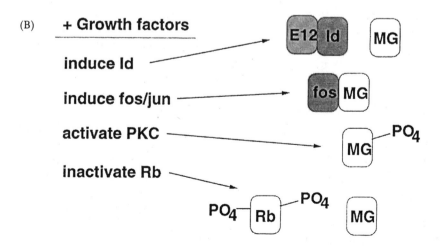

Which transcription factors are involved in gene regulation during development of cardiomyocytes? At least three families of proteins currently appear to have important roles and others are under investigation in this regard *(Table 19.1)*. Myocyte Enhancer Factor-2 (MEF-2) is expressed in both skeletal and cardiac myocytes and binds to regulatory elements essential for transcription of certain genes in both cell types.[14] MEF-2 has several isoforms, all of which are included as member of the MADS box family of transcription factors. Homeodomain proteins represent an extensive gene family with members important for pattern formation in many cell types at several stages of embryonic development. Certain members of this class (e.g. Csx or Nkx2.5) are expressed in the early heart and may exert important regulatory functions.[15] Mutations in a gene called *tinman* of the fruit fly *Drosophila melanogaster,* which encodes a protein closely related to mammalian Csx, prevent development of the insect heart.[16] Recent data indicate that homeodomain proteins may activate certain muscle-specific genes in conjunction with SRF (Serum Response Factor).[17, 18] The GATA family of transcription factors includes proteins essential for transcription of hemoglobin genes in erythrocytes, but one member, GATA-4, is implicated in control of gene expressed selectively in cardiac muscle.[19] Other transcription factors characterized by zinc fingers, winged helix, or bHLH domains also have been identified in cardiac myocytes[20, 21] and also may have important functions in differentiation of these cells.

An issue important to the developmental biology of cardiac and skeletal muscles, as well as to clinical disease states associated with cell death in these tissues (such as myocardial infarction), is the relationship between cellular differentiation and cell proliferation. In the embryonic heart, terminal differentiation of cardiomyocytes occurs very early and the heart begins to beat at a time when development of other organs is quite rudimentary. Throughout fetal life, cardiomyocytes continue to replicate, and the increase in cardiac mass that occurs throughout this period is based on a large increase in the number of myocytes within the heart. After birth, however, cardiac myocytes lose the capacity for mitotic replication, and further growth, impressive as it is, is based almost solely on hypertrophy of a fixed number of cardiomyocytes. In the adult heart, no pool of myoblast precursors remains, and injury associated with myocardial infarction or other stresses cannot be repaired.

Skeletal myoblasts, in contrast, permanently withdraw from the cell cycle coincident with differentiation and fusion to form multinucleated myotubes. Recent work, in fact, suggests that molecular interactions between MyoD and tumor suppressor gene products like the retinoblastoma (Rb) protein may coordinate terminal differentiation with the loss of mitotic capacity.[22] After differentiation, skeletal myocytes cannot divide and, like cardiomyocytes, grow during post-natal life only by hypertrophy. There is, however, a critical difference between adult skeletal and cardiac muscle relating to its capacity for regeneration. Adult skeletal muscles retain a population of stem cells — myoblasts, called satellite cells — that can be stimulated to proliferate, and ultimately to reconstruct functional myofibers, following muscle injury. This capacity is maximal in young animals, but persists to some degree throughout adult life.

Finally, terminal differentiation of both skeletal and cardiac myocytes is followed by a maturation stage. This final stage of development is associated with additional gene switching events that result in specialized characteristics of various myocyte subtypes (i.e. fast vs. slow skeletal fibers, atrial vs. ventricular cardiomyocytes vs. specialized cardiac conduction and pacemaker cells), and that match myocyte phenotype to changing conditions (e.g. mitochondrial proliferation in the heart during the transition from the hypoxic fetal environment to the actively respiring neonate).

Gene switching in adults:
hormones, physiological stresses, cardiac diseases

Pressure overload and cardiac hypertrophy

Also noted in *Figure 19.4*, the expression of many genes continues to be modulated by external stimuli even after terminal differentiation and maturation of cardiac and skeletal myocytes is complete. In this way, myocytes can adapt to changing physiological demands. The adaptive capabilities of cardiomyocytes, and the limits thereof, are pertinent to several forms of cardiac disease. For example, pressure overload of the left ventricle resulting from systemic hypertension or aortic stenosis induces myocyte hypertrophy and thickening of the ventricular wall. This process, at least initially, is compensatory in nature, and permits the heart to generate sufficient contractile force to support the circulation in the face of increased afterload. Ultimately, however, the hypertrophic process reaches or exceeds an adaptive limit such that further modulation of gene expression either is inadequate to meet physiologic demands or becomes frankly maladaptive.

In animal and cell culture models, a number of gene switching events are characteristic of both early and late stages of cardiac hypertrophy. Mechanical stretch of cardiac myocytes triggers a rapid and massive induction of several so-called "immediate early" genes such as c-fos and egr- 1.[23, 24] This up-regulation of c-fos gene transcription has been shown recently to result from mechanically stimulated release of angiotensin II from cardiac myocytes, which acts in an autocrine manner on myocyte A-II receptors.[25] Agonist occupancy of this receptor results in activation of both protein kinase C and tyrosine kinases, which lead to activation of MAP kinase, and ultimately stimulates DNA binding and activity of a transcription factor complex consisting of Serum Response Factor and other proteins binding to an enhancer element of the c-fos promoter.[25,26]

The precise consequences of stretch induced activation of c-fos and other immediate early genes are not known at this time. c-fos dimerizes with another protein called c-jun to form a transcription factor termed AP-1, but the target genes regulated by AP- I that are critical to the hypertrophic process have not yet been identified. Immediate early genes are similarly activated by peptide growth factors in other cell types, such as fibroblasts, in which they contribute to mechanisms that promote re-entry into the cell cycle. In cardiac myocytes, however, activation of immediate early genes does not promote mitotic replication, but appears to contribute in some way to the development of hypertrophy.

In cultured neonatal cardiac myocytes the catecholamine hormone norepine-phrine, acting via alpha adrenergic receptors, promotes cellular hypetrophy. Nore-pinephrine activates protein kinase C in these cells, and triggers a cascade that converges on a transcription factor called TEF-1.[27-29] Binding sites for TEF-1 are present in enhancers from several genes that encode proteins of the contractile apparatus, such that norepinephrine-induced activation of TEF-1 stimulates tran-scription of these genes, which contributes to the hypertrophic process.

In laboratory rodents, the major isoform of myosin heavy chain expressed in the adult heart is the alpha subtype (αMHC), which forms sarcomeres with rapid ATPase activity and fast contractile properties (fast myosin). Pressure overload, however, promotes down-regulation of transcription of the αMHC gene, and up-regulation of the beta subtype (βMHC).[30,31] Sarcomeres comprised of βMHC con-sume ATP at a slower rate relative to the force generated and have slower contrac-tile properties (slow myosin). Since βMHC is the predominant myosin heavy chain isoform expressed in the fetal heart, the stress of pressure overload reinduces the fetal pattern, a theme that recurs with respect to several other genes. Several tran-scription factors that regulate the αMHC and βMHC genes have been identified, but the molecular basis for the gene switching events associated with pressure overload has not yet been fully established. Cardiac hypertrophy in larger mam-mals that express βMHC in the adult heart, including humans, is not associated with isomyosin switching in the left ventricle, though myosin isoform patterns in atrial myocytes may be altered.

Reactivation of fetal genes, induction of immediate early genes and isoform switching are interesting and important features of the hypertrophic process, but the central feature of the response to pressure overload — increased myocyte mass — is based on an increase in global rates of protein synthesis. For some genes, as we have seen, increased transcription contributes to the increase in abundance of the protein products of those genes. The protein products of many other genes, howev-er, increase in absolute terms within the hypertrophic heart without demonstrable changes in transcription. The synthetic machinery for protein translation is aug-mented in response to work overload, in part due to increased synthesis of ribosom-al RNA and ribosomal proteins. Ribosomal RNA (rRNA) genes are transcribed by RNA Polymerase I (Pol I), and are regulated, at least in part, by the activity of UBFI (Upstream Binding Factor), a DNA binding protein that increases transcrip-tional initiation by Pol I.[32] DNA binding activity of UBF1 has been reported to be stimulated in models of pressure overload.[33]

Hyper- and hypothyroidism

The effects of thyroid hormone on αMHC and βMHC gene expression have been studied in some detail, and are mediated by binding of thyroid hormone receptors to transcriptional control elements adjacent to these genes. Thyroid hormone re-ceptors, of which there are several isoforms, are members of the steroid receptor superfamily, and exhibit properties shared with other transcription factors of this class. In the absence of the physiological ligand, in this case triiodothyronine, thyroid hormone receptors assume a protein conformation in which the DNA binding domain is masked, and the receptors do not bind DNA. Binding of agonist (triiodothyronine) opens the DNA binding domain of the receptor so that it binds with high affinity to a specific recognition sequence (thyroid hormone response element; TRE) within promoter/enhancer regions of target genes, including αMHC and βMHC. The subsequent effects on these two genes are, however, diametrically opposed: in hyperthyroidism the αMHC gene is activated while the βMHC gene is suppressed, and vice versa in the hypothyroid state.[34, 35] Enhanced binding of thyroid hormone receptors to the αMHC gene functions synergistically with other factors to stimulate transcription.[36-38] Several mechanisms have been proposed to account for suppression of βMHC gene transcription.[39]

Myocardial ischemia and infarction

Transcriptional control of specific genes is pertinent to ischemic heart disease in both chronic and acute stages. Within the weeks and months following a myocardial infarction, the remaining viable cardiomyocytes hypertrophy, and the shape of the ventricular wall becomes altered. Gene switching events like those described in previous sections are likely to have a role in this remodeling process.

In the acutely ischemic or hypoxic heart, a number of genes are activated to generate products that may influence the outcome of the ischemic event. Synthesis of the heat shock protein, hsp70, is increased within minutes following a fall in oxygen supply to myocardial cells, through mechanisms that include transcriptional activation of the hsp70 gene.[40-42] In the normoxic, well-perfused cell, the hsp70 gene is transcribed only at low, basal rates. Ischemic stress, however, activates a pre-existing cellular pool of a transcription factor called HSF (Heat Shock Factor) so that it binds (as a trimer) with high affinity to a DNA sequence (Heat Shock Element) within the hsp70 promoter and dramatically up-regulates transcription.[43] The common denominator for activation of HSF, irrespective of the inducing stimulus, appears to be an increase in the concentration of unfolded or malfolded proteins within the cell.[44] Thermal denaturation of cytosolic and nuclear proteins is a potent trigger for this response but, apparently, depletion of high energy phosphate stores in ischemic or hypoxic cells also leads to protein denaturation and activation of hsp70 gene transcription mediated by HSF.

The concentration of hsp70 within the cell is a determinant of survival during metabolic stress, as shown in cell culture models[45,46], in animal models[47], and more recently in intact hearts of transgenic animals.[48] The molecular mechanisms by which hsp70 protects myocardial cells from ischemic injury remain to be defined, but presumably relate to the known functions of hsp70 and related proteins in facilitating folding of nascent or denatured proteins to correct, enzymatically functional conformations.[49, 50] Other genes besides hsp70 are activated during hypoxia or ischemia[51, 52] and may contribute to the ability of myocardial cells to recover from a transient ischemic episode.[53] These include genes encoding enzymes to detoxify free radicals generated during reperfusion (catalase) as well as enzymes of the glycolytic pathway. The mechanisms by which these other genes are induced in the ischemic heart have not yet been defined, but may involve a signaling cascade triggered directly by low oxygen tension. Transcription of the erythropoietin gene is stimulated by a factor called HIF-I (Hypoxia Inducible Factor-1) that binds an oxygen response element within a 3'enhancer region.[54] DNA binding activity of HIF-I cannot be detected in normoxic cells, but appears rapidly when cells are made hypoxic. Importantly, HIF-I is present in many cell types, including myocytes, that do not express erythropoietin and presumably has other targets in these cells.

Prospects for therapeutic advances from the study of gene expression

Drugs to modify gene expression

Current therapeutics in cardiovascular medicine are based primarily on administration of drugs that produce acute effects on the physiology of the heart and/or blood vessels. It has become increasingly clear, however, that clinical benefits resulting from chronic administration of some drugs may arise from long term effects that are distinct from acute physiological responses produced by that drug. For example, angiotensin converting enzyme inhibitors improve long term survival of patients with poor left ventricular function following myocardial infarction.[55,56] Other drugs that are equally potent in reducing afterload and improving cardiac output on an acute basis do not confer the same survival advantage. Changes in gene expression triggered by angiotensin II that alter cardiac structure are diminished by ACE inhibition, and presumably this contributes to the improved prognosis.

The inhibitors of 3-hydroxy-3-methylglutaryl coenzyme A (HMG CoA) reductase used to treat hypercholesterolemia (e.g. lovastatin) for prevention of atherosclerotic cardiovascular disease also exert their therapeutic effects in large measure by altering transcription. By lowering intracellular sterol concentrations, these drugs activate a transcription factor that binds an enhancer element in the gene encoding the low density lipoprotein (LDL) receptor.[57] Enhanced transcription of this gene leads to an increased abundance of LDL receptors on hepatocyte cell membranes, and this secondary response exerts the predominant cholesterol lowering effect of lovastatin and related agents.

Very few, if any, cardiovascular drugs have been developed explicitly because of their ability to modulate expression of specific genes. In the examples given in the previous paragraphs, the effects of these drugs on gene expression became apparent only after the compounds had been developed for other reasons. This situation is likely to change, however, as we learn more about the molecular mechanisms by which gene expression is controlled. It may prove possible to develop drugs that modulate the activity of some of the transcription factors that have already been mentioned in this chapter, and such drugs may have quite different therapeutic ratios than current medications. A drug that would activate transcription of the

LDL receptor gene without modifying intracellular cholesterol synthesis may, for example, be more effective or produce fewer side effects than current HMG CoA reductase inhibitors.

Genes as medicines

We have already entered an era of medicine in which DNA itself is administered to human patients as a drug. This era remains in its infancy, but the direct use of genes as medicines is certain to grow. Our understanding of gene regulation assumes vital importance in this effort for two reasons. First, any foreign gene introduced into a patient must be controlled. It must be expressed in the proper cell at the proper time and in the proper amount so as to exert optimal therapeutic benefits. Information gained from the study of gene switches that are controlled during muscle development or activated by hormones has already been incorporated into the design of genetic medicines, and even more sophisticated approaches can be expected in the future. Second, some of the foreign genes one may wish to insert to treat certain diseases encode transcription factors. In this way it may be possible to manipulate expression of large sets of endogenous genes though expression on only one foreign protein. This approach could be employed, for example, to modify the natural history of diseases associated with cardiac hypertrophy or perhaps to regenerate functional cardiomyocytes in areas damaged by myocardial infarction. This latter general strategy for gene therapy of cardiovascular diseases is farther from current application, but may become feasible as knowledge in this field advances.

REFERENCES

1. Weinzierl ROJ, et al. Largest subunit of drosophila transcription factor IID directs assembly of a complex containing TBP and a coactivator. Nature 1993: 362: 511.

2. Prioleau MN, et al. Competition between chromatin and transcription complex assembly regulates gene expression during early development. Cell 1994: 77: 439.

3. Garrad WT. Histone H1 and the conformation of transcriptionally active chromatin. BioEssays 1991: 13: 87.

4. Kornberg RD, Lorch Y. Chromatin structure and transcription. Annu. Rev. Cell Biol. 1992; 8: 563.

5. Saha S, et al. New eukaryotic transcriptional repressors. Nature 1993: 363: 648.

6. Liou HC, Baltimore D. Regulation of the NF-kappa B/rel transcription factor and I kappa B inhibitor system. Curr Opin Cell Biol 1993: 5: 477.

7. Hoey T, et al. Molecular cloning and functional analysis of drosophila TAF110 reveal properties expected of coactivators. Cell 1993: 72: 247.

8. Olson EN. Regulation of muscle transcription by the MyoD family. Circ Res 1993: 72: 1.

9. Li L, et al. FGF inactivates myogenic helix-loop-helix proteins through phosphorylation of a conserved protein kinase C site in their DNA-binding domains. Cell 1992: 71: 1181.

10. Edmondson DG, Olson EN. Helix-loop-helix proteins as regulatiors of muscle-specific transcription. J Biol Chem 1993; 268: 755.

11. Hasty P, et al. Muscle deficiency and neonatal death in mice with a targeted mutation in thw myogenic gene. Nature 1993; 364: 501.

12. Olson EN, Klein WH. BHLH factors in muscle development : dead lines and commitments, what to leave in and what to leave out. Genes & Devel. 1994: 8: 1.

13. Cserjesi P, Olson EN. Myogenin induces the myocyte-specific enhancer binding factor MEF-2 independently of other muscle-specific gene products. Mol Cell Biol 1991: 11: 4854.

14. Yu Y-T, et al. Human myocyte-specific enhancer factor 2 comprises a group of tissue-restricted MADS box transcriptional factors. Genes Dev. 1992: 6: 1783.

15. Komuro I, Izumo S. Csx : A murine homeobox-containing gene specifically expressed in the developing heart. Proc Natl Acad Sci USA 1993: 90: 8145.

16. Bodmer R, et al. A new homeobox-containing gene, msh-2, is transiently expressed early during mesoderm formation of Drosophila. Development 1990: 110: 661.

17. Grueneberg DA, et al. Human and drosophila homeodomain proteins that enhance the DNA-binding activity of serum response. Science 1992: 257: 1089.

18. Moss JB, et al. The avian cardiac alpha-actin promoter is regulated through a pair of complex elements composed of E boxes and serum response elements that bind both positive- and negative-active factors. J Biol Chem 1994: 269: 12731.

19. Arceci RJ, et al. Mouse GATA-4: a retinoic acid-inductible GATA-binding transcription factor expressed in endodermally derived tissues and heart. Mol Cell Biol 1993: 13: 2235.

20. Bassel-Duby R, et al. Myocyte nuclear factor, a novel winged helix transcription factor under both developmental and neural regulation in striated myocytes. Mol. Cell: Biol. 1994: 14: 4596.

21. Navankasattusas S, et al. A ubiquitous factor (HF-1a) and a distinct muscle factor (HF-1b/MEF-2) form an E-box-independent pathway for cardia muscle gene expression. Mol Cell. Biol. 1992: 1469.

22. Gu W, et al. Interaction of myogenic factors and the retinoblastoma protein mediates muscle cell commitment and differentiation. 1993: 72: 309.

23. Izumo S, et al. Protooncogene induction and reprogramming of cardiac gene expression produced by pressure overload. Proc. Nat. Acad. Sci. 1988: 85: 339.

24. Neyses L, et al. Induction of immediate-early genes by angiotensin II and endothelium-1 in adult rat cardiomyocytes. J Hypertens 1993: 11: 927.

25. Sadoshima J, et al. Autocrine release of angiotensin II mediates stretch-induced hypertrophy of cardiac myocytes in vitro. Cell 1993: 75: 977.

26. Sadoshima J, Izumo S. Mechanical stretch rapidly activates multiple signal transduction pathways in cardiac myocytes : potential involvement of an autocrine/paracrine mechanism. Embo J 1993: 12: 1681.

27. Farrance IKG, et al. M-CAT binding factor is related to the SV40 enhancer binding factor, TEF-1. J. Bio. Chem. 1992: 267: 17234.

28. Kariya K, et al. An enhancer core element mediates stimulation of the rat beta-myosin heavy chain promoter by an alpha 1-adrenergic agonist and activated beta-protein kinase C in hypertrophy of cardiac myocytes. J Biol Chem 1994: 269: 3775.

29. Stewart A, et al. Muscle-enriched TEF-1 isoforms bind M-CAT elements from muscle-specific promoter and differentially activate transcription. J Biol Chem 1994: 269: 3147.

30. Umeda PK, et al. Control of myosin heavy chain expression in cardiac hypertrophy. Am J Cardiol 1987: 59:543.

31. Everett AW, et al. Expression of myosin heavy chains during thyroid hormone-induced cardiac growth. Fed Proc 1986: 45: 2568.

32. O' Mahony DJ, et al. Analysis of the polysphorylation, DNA-binding and dimerization properties of the RNA polymerase I transcription factors UBF1 and UBF2. Nucleic Acids Res. 1992: 20: 1301.

33. Xie W, Rothblum LI. RDNA transcription and cardiac hypertrophy. Trends in Cardiovascular Sciences 1993: 3: 7.

34. Gustafson TA, et al. Effects of thyroid hormone on alpha-actin and myosin heavy chain gene expression in cardiac and skeletal muscles of the rat : measurement of mRNA content using synthetic oligonucleotide probes. Cirv Res 1986: 59: 194.

35. Izumo S, et al. All members of the MHC multigene family respond to thyroid hormone in a highly tissue-specific manner. Science 1986: 231: 597.

36. Izumo S, Mahdavi V. Thyroid hormone receptor alpha isoforms generated by alternative splicing differnetially activate myosin HC gene transcription. Nature 1988: 334: 539.

37. Subramaniam A, et al. Transgenic analysis of the thyroid-responsive elements in the alpha-cardiac myosin heavy chain gene promoter. J Biol Chem 1993: 268: 4331.

38. Kitsis RN, et al. Hormonal modulation of a gene injected into rat heart in vivo. Proc Natl Acad Sci USA 1991: 88: 4138.

39. Mahdavi V, Izumo S, et al. Developmental and hormonal regulation of sarcomeric myosin heavy chain gene family. Circ Res 1987: 60: 804.

40. Benjamin IJ, Kroger B, et al. Activation of the heat shock transcription factor by hypoxia in mammalian cells. Proc Natl Acad Sci USA 1990: 87: 6263.

41. Knowlton AA, et al. Rapid expression of heat shock protein in the rabbit after brief cardiac ischemia. J Clin Invest 1991: 87: 139.

42. Iwaki K, et al. Induction of HSP70 in cultured rat neonatal cardiomyocytes by hypoxia and metabolic stress. Circulation 1993: 87: 2023.

43. Benjamin IJ, et al. Induction of stress proteins in cultured myogenic cells. Molecular signals for the activation of heat shock transcription factor during ischemia. J Clin Invest 1992: 89: 1685.

44. Morimoto RI, et al. Transcriptional regulation of heat shock genes. A paradigm for inductible genomic responses. J Biol Chem 1992: 267: 21987.

45. Williams RS, et al. Human heat shock protein 70 (hsp70) protects murine cells from injury during metabolic stress. J clin Invest 1993: 92: 503.

46. Mestril R, et al. Expression of inductible stress protein 70 in rat heart myogenic cells confers protection against simulated ischemia-induced injury. J Clin Invest 1994: 93: 759.

47. Currie RW, et al. Heat-shock response and limitation of tissue necrosis during occlusion/reperfusion in rabbit hearts. Circulation 1993: 87: 963.

48. Radford NB, et al. Cardioprotective effects of hsp70 in transgenic mice. (Submitted).

49. Craig EA, et al. Heat shock proteins: Molecular chaperones of protein biogenesis. Microbiol. Rev 1993: 57402.

50. Georgopoulos C, Welch WJ. Role of the major heat shock proteins as molecular chaperones. Annu. Rev. Cell Biol. 1993: 9: 601.

51. Zimmerman LH, et al. Hypoxia induces a specific set of stress proteins in cultured endothelial cells. J Clin Invest 1991: 87: 908.

52. Webster KA, et al. Regulation of fos and jun immediate-early genes by redox or metabolic stress in cardiac myocytes. Circ Res 1994: 74: 679.

53. Wall SR, et al. Role of catalase in myocardial protection against ischemia in heat shocked rats. Mol Cell Biochem 1993: 129: 187.

54. Semenza GL, Wang GL. A nuclear factor induced by hypoxia via de novo protein synthesis binds to the human erythroprotein gene enhancer at a site required for transcriptional activation. Mol Cell Biol 1992: 12: 5447.

55. Mitchell GF, et al. Ventricular remodeling after myocardial infarction. Adv Exp Med Biol 1993: 346: 265.

56. Vaughan DE, Pfeffer MA. Angiotensin converting enzyme inhibitors and cardiovascular remodelling. Cardiovasc Res 1994: 28: 159.

57. Yokohama C, et al. SREBP-1, a basic-helix-loop-helix-leucine zipper protein that controls transcription of the low density lipoprotein receptor gene. Cell 1993: 75: 187.

20 GENETIC ANALYSIS OF CARDIOVASCULAR DISEASE

Ralph V. Shohet

We all recognize the importance of a familial predisposition to cardiovascular disease as a substantial risk factor in the clinical evaluation of patients. In atherosclerotic syndromes it carries predictive value similar to tobacco use or hypertension Many relatively rare cardiovascular syndromes have been explained by single gene defects and many others, including the most common, clearly have a familial component. A comprehensive description of these genetic influences is beyond the scope of a brief chapter but several excellent reviews are available.[1,2] Here I will describe the progress made recently in the explication of three cardiovascular diseases, each of which illustrates different strengths and weaknesses of genetic analysis.

Marfan Syndrome is a generalized disorder of connective tissue with a clear set of diagnostic characteristics (phenotype), autosomal dominant inheritance pattern, varying degrees of cardiac involvement, and known molecular etiology. The Long QT Syndrome exclusively affects the conduction system of the heart, has a relatively clear electrocardiographic appearance, varying degrees of symptomatology and is caused by mutations in several different cardiac ion channels. Dilated cardiomyopathy is a common, multifactorial illness clearly resulting from an interplay of many environmental and genetic factors. It has many precipitants, and little genetic description other than a familial predisposition in a minority of patients. These three disorders exemplify the range of challenges and opportunities found in cardiovascular genetics today.

The reasons for trying to decipher the molecular causes of cardiovascular disease are clear. Only with such information can drug development be intelligently guided to more effective therapies. Molecular biology has become a potent tool to better understand the physiology and biochemistry of disease. Ultimately, gene therapy to correct molecular defects requires an understanding of disease at the molecular level. In the intervening period genetic markers of disease also provide an important prognostic tool in families.

Marfan syndrome

The Marfan syndrome (MFS) is a relatively common autosomal dominant disorder of connective tissue that affects the skeletal, ocular and cardiovascular systems. It occurs in approximately 1 in 10,000 and demonstrates high penetrance (affects all of those carrying the mutated allele) and variable expressivity (with differing severity of organ system dysfunction). Over the past ten years genetic linkage, biochemical analysis and candidate gene strategies have combined to reveal the molecular etiology of this disease.

Skeletal abnormalities are the most obvious manifestation of the Marfan phenotype. These include a tall, narrow frame, pectus deformities, arachnodactyly and hypermobile joints. Myopia is caused by dislocations of the lens. The cardiovascular abnormalities that shorten the lives of Marfan patients are due to decay of the aortic media with subsequent dilation, dissection and valvular insufficiency. During the 1980s an international consortium of geneticists examined a large panel of anonymous polymorphic markers looking for linkage of a specific allele to the disease in various large families, (this method is described in greater detail below and elsewhere in this volume; excellent reviews are available[3]). Meanwhile, histological and biochemical analysis of the aortas of these patients demonstrated a marked decrease in the amount of elastic fibers and focused attention on the components of that fiber. Initial interest focused on elastin, the principal protein of the elastic lamina (and a protein subsequently implicated in supravalvular aortic stenosis[4]). However, no linkage to this gene was found in MFS families. The other component of the elastic fiber was a more productive target. Around an amorphous core of elastin is a matrix of microfibrils, 10 nm fibers that also appear in the suspensory ligament that holds the lens in place. When this coincidence was recognized the major protein of the microfibril - fibrillin - became a prime candidate in Marfan syndrome.

The genetic linkage project showed that the gene for MFS was on a small portion of chromosome 15. Fibrillin was subsequently mapped to the same location. Final proof of the role of fibrillin included the demonstration of mutations in the coding region of the fibrillin gene in MFS patients, as well as biochemical evidence of dysfunctional fibrillin. The demonstration of the clinical importance of fibrillin generated enthusiasm for understanding its regulation and function.

Salient observations include the findings that:

1. Almost all of the families studied have different fibrillin mutations, although most seem to disrupt the structure of the repetitive epidermal growth factor like domains of the molecule.[5]

2. There seems to be little correlation of a given mutation with a specific phenotype of MFS, and the severity of disease with the same mutation can vary substantially.

3. A small amount of mutant protein exerts a disruptive effect over the entire elastic fiber.

4. Other syndromes may be caused by fibrillin mutations, including isolated ectopia lentis, adolescent idiopathic scoliosis, and Neonatal Marfan syndrome. The later is a particularly severe form of the disease with other associated problems such as facial deformity and emphysema.[6]

Most of these observations are probably due to the wide tissue distribution of microfibrils (which are found to some extent in many connective tissues) as well as the varying types of molecular dysfunction which result from the large number of distinct mutations. It is also likely that other genetic and environmental influences affect the characteristics and severity of the disease.

Now that the principal molecular cause of MFS has been identified the work of determining appropriate therapies to ameliorate or eliminate the disease can begin. The traditional approaches of pharmacology have been inconsistently successful in treating genetic disorders. For example, inhibitors of mevalonic acid synthase have been helpful in the management of familial hypercholesterolemia. However, no therapy has been found for sickle cell disease, although the single amino acid mutation in hemoglobin has been known for over forty years. Replacement of genetically defective or missing proteins has been useful in rare syndromes such as Gaucher's disease or Adenosine Deaminase deficiency where small amounts of humoral activity are sufficient to treat the problem. However, this approach will not work in a disease where the normal protein must be delivered to, or perhaps even produced in, a specific anatomic location. Furthermore, the dominant negative character of the Marfan mutation might interfere with any direct replacement therapy. The abnormality, in at least some cases, is caused by the presence of abnormal fibrillin rather than simply the absence of sufficient normal protein. Eventually a more detailed understanding of the function and regulation of fibrillin may produce useful pharmacological approaches. In the short term only existing palliative measures such as beta blockade (to reduce the shear forces on the aortic intima) are likely to work.

Two other therapeutic interventions offer substantial promise. More than half of MFS patients have a family history of disease. The demonstration of the specific mutations causing Marfan syndrome allows prenatal diagnosis and subsequent consideration of abortion of severely affected progeny. It is theoretically possible to substantially decrease the incidence of this disease very rapidly in this manner. In our society this presents significant ethical concerns, especially since this is a disease that has variable expressivity, ranging from incapacitating anatomical deformities to correctable myopia. As more is learned about the correlation of specific mutations with the degree of disability we will be in a better position to address these concerns. Furthermore, as methods for the selection of unaffected progeny improve, such decisions may be made at an earlier stage.

One limitation of genetic screening in MFS is the large number of different mutations in the fibrillin gene that cause disease. Careful analysis of the fibrillin gene in an affected member of each family would be required to determine which allele carries the mutation. Multiple polymorphic markers within the fibrillin gene have been developed which allow identification of the disease causing allele in individual families.[7] This is a requirement until an assay of the gene can be developed which directly detects the mutation. All of these methods have been used in the analysis of diseases such as myotonic dystrophy and cystic fibrosis and are undergoing rapid evolution and improvement.

Even if genetic selection becomes simple and accepted there would still be many Marfan patients born every year. This is because spontaneous, new fibrillin mutations are estimated to account for about 25% of patients. A second more theoretical but broadly applicable approach to therapy of genetic disease is direct genetic manipulation of the affected tissues. Gene transfer technologies can potentially augment production of the normal gene product, in this case in the elastic lamina of the aorta. The crucial prerequisite for such therapy is an intimate knowledge of the biochemistry and metabolism of the defective protein as well as an understanding of the regulation of the mutated gene. The systems for delivery of replacement genes to specific locations and the regulation of such "transgenes" are still primitive. However, this is an area of rapid progress combining disciplines of virology, vascular biology, molecular biology and bioengineering.[8] It is theoretically possible that even the problem of abnormal fibrillin causing disease could be addressed by strategies that turned off the mutated gene while introducing a normal one, or increased production from the endogenous normal gene. For example, an antisense strategy that turned off translation of abnormal messenger RNA in aortic cells by tightly binding only to the mutated messenger might restore the microfibrils and aortic integrity. Such therapies are presently being evaluated in laboratories around the country for other proteins and will enter clinical practice within ten years.

Long QT syndrome

Prolongation of the QT interval is an important electrocardiographic clue to abnormalities of ventricular repolarization. It is often seen as a secondary manifestation of myocardial ischemia, cardiomyopathy, electrolyte abnormalities, antidysrhythmic drugs and tricyclic antidepressants. A prolonged QT interval is associated with life-threatening dysrhythmias, particularly torsade de points, and suggests dangerously disturbed ventricular electrophysiology. If we could better understand the mechanism of QT prolongation we could more successfully manage this common clinical problem.

There are two recognized familial Long QT syndromes. Jervell Lange-Nielsen disease is an autosomal recessive disorder associated with deafness. The Romano-Ward syndrome is more common, inherited in an autosomal dominant manner and has been the subject of elegant linkage analysis. Substantial preliminary work on Long QT syndrome (LQT) included an ongoing multinational registry of over 300 affected families from which valuable information about the epidemiology and inheritance of the disorder was gleaned.[9] The limitations of the electrocardiographic diagnosis of the disease have been revealed by clinical studies. For example, syncope occurs even in those members of these families who have a QTc in the normal range, and there is no clear linear association of QT prolongation and the severity or frequency of symptoms. Furthermore, there is variation in the measurement of QT in any individual depending on heart rate, age, emotion and other factors. The genetic markers that have been developed now allow a much more precise identification of affected patients and have recently led to the specific cause of the disease.

A large family with LQT and symptoms (sudden death or syncope) was the first prerequisite for this study. A significant task in this linkage analysis was the segregation of affected and unaffected family members into two distinct groups. Such identification defines a trait as dichotomous and facilitates all subsequent analysis. In the case of LQT, the large amount of overlap between affected and unaffected family members made the distinction difficult. It was necessary to remove from consideration those subjects with intermediate (QTc between 0.42 and 0.46 s), and thus indeterminate phenotype. This allowed the reliable identification of affected subjects on clinical grounds in a large enough family for statistically significant linkage analysis. A comprehensive screening of polymorphic genetic loci throughout the genome then revealed tight linkage of a marker in the Harvey ras-1 locus to the trait.[10] Briefly, sequence variations (polymorphisms) are used to identify a small region of genomic DNA. One then looks for a greater than expected association of a specific version of that polymorphism (an allele) with the disease in affected family members.

It is worth noting that initial efforts to screen candidate genes thought to be associated with the physiology of long QT, such as potassium channels, were unsuccessful and that 245 different markers were examined before linkage was established to H ras-1. These markers were screened by Southern hybridization. Radioactively labeled fragments of DNA derived from polymorphic loci were hybridized to genomic DNA that had been digested with a restriction enzyme that revealed the polymorphism.

Such restriction fragment length polymorphism (RFLP) analysis was state-of-the-art 5 years ago and has now been almost entirely replaced by polymerase chain reaction (PCR) based strategies *(Figure 20.1, 20.2)*. These take advantage of the frequent occurrence in the genome of microsatellites. These are highly variable stretches of a short, repeated block of nucleotides. They can be amplified by unique oligonucleotides that bracket the variable sequence and thereby identify both a specific location in the genome and a specific allele of that site.

Once a specific site in the chromosomal DNA is genetically linked to the disease, a shift in the search for the causative gene must take place. Genetic linkage, even at its most refined, can only localize the cause of a disorder to about a million bases of DNA (out of the total of about three billion). This is a substantial help but such a fragment of the genome could still contain more than fifty genes and the subsequent physical mapping of those genes and the search for a causative mutation is often an even more challenging task. Some of the obstacles involved are yielding to modern technology. New vectors such as Yeast Artificial Chromosomes allow manipulation of large pieces of DNA. New screening techniques allow the identification of the small portion of genomic DNA that is eventually processed into messenger RNA and then protein. Automated sequencing machines and computer programs also help to identify the important genes in the sea of uninvolved data. As the Human Genome project progresses more markers and genes will be identified and the genetic map will become more refined. Eventually the tissue localization and timing of expression of all human genes will be known and the identification of disease genes will be relatively simple. However, presently this is one of the most difficult problems facing those seeking to convert linkage information into useful biological insights.

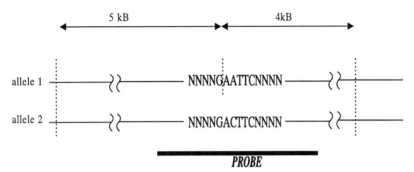

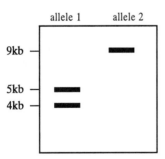

Figure 20.1 An example of Restriction Fragment Length Polymorphism (RFLP) Analysis is outlined in this sketch. A specific site (GAATTC) in allele 1 is changed in allele 2 so that it is no longer cleaved by a certain restriction enzyme. (Cleavage is rendered as a vertical dotted line.) As a result the two smaller fragments revealed by the probe for allele 1 now appear as the larger, single band on Southern analysis.

Prior to the identification of specific genes, linkage data can be of great value in clarifying pathophysiology. For it provides a way of definitively identifying those carrying the defective gene. This improved diagnostic capability allows more accurate predictions of prognosis. Potentially, one might offer treatment even to those who have not developed symptoms (if this is shown to be useful) and avoid inappropriate diagnosis of those in affected families who do not carry the presumed mutated gene. For example, using the genotype as the gold standard for diagnosis, the previous criterion of a QTc greater than 0.44s produced false positive diagnoses in 11% of the family members. Similarly a QTc greater than 0.47, although not generating any false positives, would have missed the diagnosis in 40% of the men and 20% of the women affected.[11] This is important because there is still a substantial risk of sudden death even in carriers with QTc in the previously recognized normal range. Therapies such as beta blocker treatment or defibrillator placement may be considered for these patients, and avoided in those without the implicated allele.

Two problems prevent the general application of genetic linkage information to the majority of patients. One is the need for large families, with DNA samples available from affected and unaffected subjects, in order to establish the specific

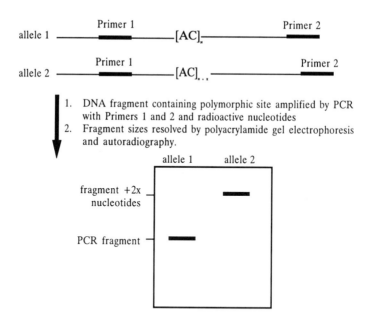

Figure 20.2 An example of Microsatellite Analysis is outlined in this sketch. The dinucleotide repeat (CA) occurs a variable number of times (N+x). It thus produces several possible size alleles in a population when amplified. One generic example is shown.

allele of the locus that is associated with disease. Essentially, a small linkage study has to be performed on each new family studied, as the marker identifies the region of DNA associated with the disease and not the specific mutation. Many patients do not have many family members available or they may have new mutations that do not allow genetic predictions. A second problem that limits the application of linkage data is locus heterogeneity of many diseases.[12] In families with the Long QT syndrome linked to chromosome 3 or 7, or yet another locus[13] on chromosome 4, the markers used to identify the disease-containing fragment of DNA would not segregate with the locus on chromosome 11. The affected patients in these families have subtly different phenotypes from the typical LQT syndrome - for example sudden death occurred at rest or upon awakening rather than with exertion - and thus might have been thought to have a different mechanism as well as genetic locus responsible.

In families with LQT a candidate gene approach did lead to the identification of two of the rarer mutations causing the disorder. A potassium channel[14] on chromosome 7 and a sodium channel[15] on chromosome 3 were suspected because of their proximity to the genetically linked loci and were found to contain mutations in affected patients. These findings tell us much about the mechanism of the repolarization abnormality, but a substantial physical cloning project was required to discover the gene causing the more common chromosome 11 linked disease.[16]

With the identification of the ion channels on chromosome 3 and 7 causing the disorder it became clear that endogenous ventricular repolarization defects were causing the QT prolongation, rather than the previously considered involvement of sympathetic input. However, a straight-forward candidate gene approach did not demonstrate an ion channel in the linked region of chromosome 11. Thus further physical mapping was required. Using refined genetic mapping the involved portion of chromosome 11 was narrowed down to two markers that were indistinguishable by genetic analysis. These markers were then used to isolate fragments of chromosome 11 that included all of the DNA between them. Thus the genetic map, with a resolution of about a million bases of DNA, was converted into a series of overlapping fragments of DNA that could be physically mapped to any resolution required. This 700 kilobases of DNA was then subjected to tests that revealed the fragments encoding exons, the portions of genes that are eventually processed into messenger RNA. These were sequenced and one included sequence similar to that seen in known potassium channels. This fragment was then used to isolate the complete messenger RNA coding for a previously unknown potassium channel. When the sequence of this gene was examined in families with LQT linked to chromosome 11, mutations were seen in all, and only, affected members. Furthermore, the messenger RNA for this gene is most abundant in heart

Now that the genes causing Long QT syndrome are known, the biochemistry of the mutations can be explored and specific therapies directed at each defect. For example, the sodium channel defect has been explored by expression of the mutant protein on the surface of frog eggs for electrophysiological study.[17] Perhaps sodium channel blockers would reverse the prolonged inward current seen in these studies.

The most exciting potential use of the data generated from the hereditary forms of QT prolongation will be its application to those with the far more common QT prolongation of exogenous etiology. Eventually the insights garnered from a full understanding of the mutated genes in this syndrome will clarify the molecular mechanisms of ventricular repolarization abnormalities in general. This, in turn, should produce novel therapeutic interventions for the ventricular irritability that is a principal cause of death in developed societies. For example, appropriate pharmacological manipulation of potassium channels might effectively treat the common form of Long QT, and deserves consideration in the far more common repolarization abnormalities associated with ischemia.

Dilated cardiomyopathy

Dilated cardiomyopathy (DCM) is a major public health problem causing one million hospitalizations and 200,000 deaths annually at a price to the United States of at least eight billion dollars in direct medical costs alone. The broad spectrum of clinical presentations of DCM suggests a polygenic, multifactorial etiology of this disorder. The genetic analysis of dilated cardiomyopathy is presently in its earliest stage. A few, rare syndromes in the pediatric population have been explained by mutations in genes important in cardiac energetics. In this subset of infants and children, DCM is caused by monogenic lesions that give rise to defects in fatty-acid oxidation. Although these are single gene defects the phenotype is still modulated by exogenous factors. For example, increased cardiac metabolism of fatty acids, resulting from malnutrition, may increase the pathologic effect of deficiencies of medium-chain and short-chain acyl-CoA dehydrogenases.

Another heritable cause of DCM also affects cardiac energy metabolism, specifically mitochondrial oxidative phosphorylation. Mitochondrial disorders such as the MELAS syndrome or Kearns-Sayre syndrome have prominent cardiomyopathic components, probably because the heart is one of the organs most dependent on oxidative phosphorylation. Another example would be the dystrophin related muscular dystrophies that are characterized by progressive muscle wasting and varying degrees of cardiomyopathy. Recently, in a large kindred with only cardiomyopathy, the disorder was localized to the dystrophin locus,.

In the much more common adult forms of DCM, focal or extensive necrosis of cardiomyocytes is often caused by exogenous insults. The definition of DCM has been complicated by the heterogeneous nature of the initiating events. When a specific insult is obvious as in the case of myocardial infarction, hypertension or toxins, the disease is usually subdivided as, for example, "ischemic cardiomyopathy" or "hypertensive cardiomyopathy" leaving "primary" or "idiopathic" DCM for those cases where the cause is occult. However, all of these disorders share a common pathophysiology with ventricular dilation and predominant systolic dysfunction. Histologically all reveal fibrosis and cardiomyocyte hypertrophy. At a biochemical level it is impossible to differentiate the biological responses of the cardiomyopathic heart, (for example adrenergic receptor down-regulation), among different etiologies. It thus seems reasonable to consider DCM as a final common result of many cardiac insults. One of these is certainly the genetic predisposition (or resistance) to the panoply of possible precipitants. Wide variation in susceptibility to myocardial dysfunction induced by toxins such as ethanol or adriamycin is indicative of modifying factors. Similarly, equivalent amounts of necrosis secondary to an acute myocardial infarction do not lead predictably to equivalent degrees of systolic dysfunction or ventricular remodeling. These insults induce compensatory reparative processes intended to maintain cardiac function that may ultimately lead to further functional and pathological deterioration. Progress has been made over the last ten years in exploring the molecular biology of hypertrophied and failing myocardium but these efforts have focused on relatively few metabolic, structural, and signaling components.

There is epidemiological evidence for a familial predilection to DCM in at least 20% of cases. In a prospective study of the relatives of patients with ejection fractions less than 50%, diastolic dimensions above the 95th percentile and no coronary disease or hypertension, similar evidence of DCM was seen in first order relatives in 12 of 59 families. Remarkably, most of the relatives of the index cases had not previously been recognized to have ventricular dysfunction. Furthermore, an additional 9% of the relatives had ventricular dilation (without systolic dysfunction).

As discussed above, most recent progress in cardiovascular genetics has focused on single gene disorders that are amenable to linkage analysis. Linkage analysis is most successful in cohorts of large kindreds with well-defined phenotypes and modes of inheritance. None of the characteristics of DCM lend themselves to such linkage analysis. What is the role for genetic analysis in elucidating the cause or precipitating factors of DCM?

One possible application of genetic analysis to DCM would be the use of association studies of candidate genes to confirm or reject their importance as risk factors for the disease. In one analysis of a specific candidate gene, a polymorphism in the angiotensin-converting enzyme (ACE) gene has been associated with a variety of cardiovascular disorders, including both ischemic and idiopathic Dilated Cardiomyopathy. Although this is a provocative result, it may be that this allele is in linkage disequilibrium with some other mutation, either in the ACE gene or a neighboring gene that contributes to the pathology. This study supports the concept that different types of cardiomyopathy may share a common pathophysiology. Moreover, if the suggestion of ACE involvement is borne out, this work will provide genetic support to the biological role of ACE and refine our understanding of the role of ACE inhibition in the treatment of heart failure.

Hybrid amalgams of linkage analysis and association studies are another approach to demonstrating the importance of a given candidate gene, or anonymous locus, with a disease. The angiotensinogen gene has been analyzed in this manner in patients with primary hypertension. First, using a type of linkage called sibship analysis, a highly polymorphic marker near the angiotensinogen gene was examined in affected patients and their unaffected siblings. A greater than expected frequency of a shared allele between siblings with hypertension suggested genetic linkage. A direct search for mutations in the gene revealed a molecular variant that was significantly more frequent in hypertensive subjects. Further evidence of an etiologic role included the demonstration of elevated plasma concentrations of angiotensinogen in those subjects with the variant protein. As the technology for genotypic evaluation of large numbers of people advances it is likely that less focused association studies will become possible. For example, within the next twenty years, it will become possible to efficiently search the entire genome in large numbers of patients for alleles of cardiac genes that are associated with heart failure.

Many factors may contribute to the genotypic milieu in which DCM develops. In addition to the relatively rare single gene disorders described above there may be a general deterioration of oxidative capacity with age due to decay of the mitochondrial genome (postulated to result from favored replication of deleted forms) which would be particularly evident in the myocardium. The frequency of a common mitochondrial deletion increases with age and coronary artery disease. Depletion of components of pathways of oxidative metabolism might exacerbate the myopathic influence of ischemia or viral infection and may become targets for genetic manipulation.

Even lacking genetic evidence for an etiological role of a given gene it is likely that genetic manipulation of the heart will become a useful therapeutic option. Recently, in a dramatic demonstration of genetic engineering, an expression construct for the beta-2 adrenergic receptor was introduced into the germline of transgenic mice. The overexpression of this receptor augmented cardiac contractility and adrenergic responsiveness.

Conclusion

We have reviewed the recent progress in understanding the genetic etiology of three important cardiovascular disorders. In Marfan syndrome, the specific gene is known and current efforts are directed at determining how mutations affect the function of fibrillin and how that dysfunction produces the typical features of the disease. In the Long QT syndrome three genes, all encoding ion channels, cause the disease, and other loci have been implicated. As the mutant proteins encoded by these genes are investigated, we expect to learn more about the mechanism of electrical instability that predisposes these patients to sudden death. These insights may be applied to the much larger group of patients who suffer sudden cardiac death from more common precipitants. Finally, we have briefly described the outline of how a search for genetic factors may proceed for Dilated Cardiomyopathy. Much of this work will depend on the continued progress and support of the Human Genome Project and basic genetic research. However, the future can be glimpsed in the current batch of successful linkage studies. We have also tried to suggest how the various levels of genetic understanding can lead to new diagnostic and therapeutic approaches, many of which will follow closely upon a basic molecular and genetic understanding of cardiovascular disease.

REFERENCES

1. Pierpont MEM and Moller JH (eds). Genetics of Cardiovascular Disease. Martinus Nijhoff Publishing; Boston,MA, 1987.

2. Pyeritz RE. Genetics and cardiovascular disease. In Braunwald E (ed.) Heart Disease W. B. Saunders Company, Philadelphia, 1992 p. 1622.

3. Keating M. Linkage analysis and long QT syndrome. Using genetics to study cardiovascular disease.Circulation 1992: 85:1973.

4. Ewart AK, et al. Supravalvular aortic stenosis associated with a deletion disrupting the elastin gene. J Clin Invest 1994: 93:1071.

5. Ramirez F, et al. The fibrillin-Marfan syndrome connection. Bioessays 1993 15:589.

6. Milewicz DM. Identification of defects in the fibrillin gene and protein. Texas Heart Inst J 1994: 21:22.

7. Pereira L, et al. A molecular approach to the stratification of cardiovascular risk in families with Marfan's syndrome. N Engl J Med 1994: 331:148.

8. Nabel EG, et al. Gene transfer and vascular disease. Cardiovasc Res 1994: 28:445.

9. Moss AJ, et al. The long QT syndrome. Prospective longitudinal study of 328 families. Circulation 1991: 84:1136.

10. Keating M, et al. Linkage of a cardiac arrythmia, the long QT syndrome, and the Harvey ras-1 gene. Science 1991: 252: 704.

11. Vincent GM, et al. The spectrum of symptoms and QT intervals in carriers of the gene for the long-QT syndrome. N Engl J Med 1992: 327:846.

12. Curran M, et al. Locus heterogeneity of autosomal dominant long QT syndrome. J Clin Invest 1993: 92:799.

13. Schott J, et al. Mapping of a gene for long QT syndrome to chromosome 4q25-27. Am J Hum Genet 1995; 57:1114.

14. Curran ME, et al. A molecular basis for cardiac arrhythmia: HERG mutations cause long QT syndrome. Cell 1995: 80:795.

15. Wang Q, et al. SCN5A mutations associated with an inherited cardiac arrythmia, long QT syndrome. Cell 1995: 80:805.

16. Wang Q, et al. Positional cloning of a novel potassium channel gene: KVLQT1 mutations cause cardiac arrythmias. Nature Genetics 1996: 12:17-23.

17. Bennett PB, et al. Nature 1995: 376:683.

18. Garg R, et al. Heart failure in the 1990's: Evolution of a major public health problem in cardiovascular medicine. J Amer Coll Cardiol 1993: 22(suppl. A):3A.

19. Kelly DP and Strauss AW. Inherited Cardiomyopathies. N Engl J Med 1994: 330:913.

20. Wallace DC. Diseases of the mitochondrial DNA. Ann Rev Biochem 1992: 61:1175.

21. Berko BA, Swift M. X-linked dilated cardiomyopathy. N Engl J Med 1987: 316:1186.

22. Towbin JA, et al. X-linked dilated cardiomyopathy. Molecular genetic evidence of linkage to the Duchenne muscular dystrophy (dystrophin) gene at the Xp21 locus. Circulation 1993: 87:1854.

23. Moushmoush B, Abi-Mansour P. Alcohol and the heart: The long-term effects of alcohol on the cardiovascular system. Arch Int Med 1991: 151:36.

24. LeJemtel T, Sonnenblick EH. Heart failure: Adaptive and maladaptive processes. Circulation 1993; 87:VII-1.

25. Sadoshima J-I, et al. Autocrine Release of Angiotensin II Mediates Stretch-Induced Hypertrophy of Cardiac Myocytes In Vivo. Cell 1993: 75:977-984.

26. Michels VV, et al. The frequency of familial dilated cardiomyopathy in a series of patients with idiopathic dilated cardiomyopathy. N Engl J Med 1992: 326:77.

27. Raynolds MV, et al. Angiotensin-converting enzyme DD genotype in patients with ischemic or idiopathic dilated cardiomyopathy. Lancet 1993; 342:1073.

28. Jeunemaitre X, et al. Molecular basis of human hypertension: role of angiotensinogen. Cell (1992): 71:169.

29. Corral-Debrinski M, et al. Association of mitochondrial damage with aging and coronary atherosclerotic disease. Mut Res 1992: 275:169.

30. Milano CA, et al. Enhanced myocardial function in transgenic mice overexpressing the β_2-adrenergic receptor. Science 1994: 264:582.

21 GENETICS OF HYPERTROPHIC CARDIOMYOPATHY

Calum MacRae

Hypertrophic cardiomyopathy (HC) is one of the most common causes of sudden death in the young, yet until recently its etiology was unknown. The earliest descriptions of HC recognized its familial nature. Subsequent studies demonstrated a pattern of inheritance consistent with a single autosomal dominant trait in up to 90% of kindreds. Genetic linkage analysis and positional cloning have enabled the identification of the causative mutations in many such single gene disorders. The power of these molecular genetic techniques is that the gene defect can be identified without making any prior assumptions regarding the pathophysiological mechanisms of the disease. In the last 5 years the familial hypertrophic cardiomyopathy (HC) syndrome has been shown to be an heterogeneous group of disorders and mutations have been identified in four different genes. This review will discuss these recent advances highlighting those points which are of relevance to clinical practice.

Clinical genetics

The basis for any genetic study must be a precise definition of the phenotype. As improvements in echocardiographic technology led to more complete ascertainment, it became clear that in the vast majority of pedigrees HC is transmitted as an autosomal dominant Mendelian trait. The syndrome has a high adult penetrance in most families when assessed by both ECG and 2-D echocardiography [1,2]. That is most adults carrying a disease-causing mutation who have completed the adolescent growth spurt will have evidence of the disease. Evolving clinical understanding and detailed pathological studies defined subsets of familial HC before molecular tools became available. Mitral valve abnormalities, resting outflow tract "obstruction" and ventricular prexcitation identified possible heterogeneity within HC. The extent of the ventricular hypertrophy itself may also vary markedly. Kindreds in which myocyte and myofibrillar disarray are present without hypertrophy have been described.[1]

Simple segregation analysis has demonstrated kindreds with possible autosomal recessive or sex-linked inheritance. There are also reports of HC in association with a variety of other genetic disorders and chromosomal anomalies (table 21.1).[1]

Myosin

Early linkage studies suggested tentative genetic loci for HC on chromosome 6 and on chromosome 2p. These loci have not been substantiated by subsequent investigation. In 1989 Jarcho et al demonstrated definitive evidence of linkage, that is tight cosegregation between disease and an anonymous genetic marker, on chromosome 14 (with the marker D 14S26) in a large French-Canadian kindred. This linkage was confirmed in another unrelated family.[2] The cardiac β-myosin heavy chain (MHC) gene which encodes the dominant adult ventricular myosin isoform was known to be located close to the marker D 14S26. In both kindreds mutations were found in the β-MHC gene of affected individuals.[3]

Several lines of evidence support the hypothesis that β-MHC gene mutations cause HC at the CMH- I (Cardiomyopathy,Hypertrophic - 1) locus on chromosome 14. First, these abnormalities segregate perfectly with disease in the respective families and were not found on over 100 normal chromosomes. Second, comparison of the human β-MHC gene sequence with the sequence of all other known myosin genes confirms that the mutations alter amino acid residues which are remarkably conserved in multiple myosin isoforms across many species and can thus be inferred to be functionally important. The most robust support comes from the observation of HC in an individual whose parents were normal. Neither parent had any abnormalities in the sequence of their β-MHC genes but a germ-

Table 21.1 SYNDROMES ASSOCIATED WITH HC

Syndrome	Cardiac phenotype	Chromosomal localization
Hypertrophic cardiomyopathy	Typical HC	Ch16q-fragile site
Freidreich's ataxia	Hypertrophy and dilation	Ch9ql-Frataxin
Noonan's	FHC and Pulm Stenosis	Ch12q
Leopard	FHC and Pulm Stenosis	Unknown
SCD and myopathy	FHC	Unknown
Cardioauditory	Hypertrophy	Unknown
Spherocytosis	Typical FHC	Unknown

line mutation in the paternal copy of the β-MHC gene was found in the affected offspring. Thus, this single base change when inherited in the germline is apparently sufficient to cause FHC [4] Importantly this result also implies that a proportion of so-called sporadic HC is actually *de novo* familial HC.

Subsequently more than 30 discrete missense mutations have been described in the β-MHC gene in families with HC.[5] More detailed analysis of the CMH-1 locus has also found evidence of a high rate of new mutations in the β-MHC gene.[6] The same mutation has arisen independently on a variety of different genetic backgrounds or so-called haplotypes. Some nucleotides within the gene may be particularly susceptible to mutation or may be more likely to result in clinical disease.[7] These findings, taken together, imply that simply screening probands for previously described mutations will not suffice as a means of diagnosing HC.

It has also been shown that mutations in the non-coding regions of the β-myosin heavy chain gene and the contiguous α-myosin heavy chain gene are not a major cause of HC.[8] This was done by taking all the familes in whom RNase protection of the proband's cardiac β-myosin heavy chain genes had revealed no abnormality and testing these for linkage to the CMH-1 locus. In every informative kindred linkage to the cardiac myosin genes was excluded. These data independently confirm the sensitivity and specificity of RNase protection assays in screening for β-MHC mutations. No other screening method has been objectively assessed in this context.

The molecular mechanism by which myosin mutations cause HC is not clear. Simple structural observations do not suggest clustering of mutations within active sites of the myosin molecule although the mutations do appear to be confined to the head or head/rod junction regions.[5] More rigorous definition of specific functional domains in the light of the recently described three-dimensional crystallographic structure of myosin may be more informative.[9]

Functional studies suggest that some mutant myosins may exhibit reduced ATPase activity. This has been associated with other abnormalities of actomyosin motility and myofibrillar assembly in various *in vitro* systems.[10,11,12] Detailed dissection of the molecular mechanisms by which hypertrophy arises may have to await the generation, by homologous recombination or other techniques, of mouse and larger animal models of cardiac myosin disease. The continued clinical investigation of the effects of myosin mutations and their genetic and environmental modifiers will complement the insights gained from basic science.

The identification of myosin mutations in FHC led to the hypothesis that the syndrome might be a collection of specific inherited diseases whose common denominator was a reduction in myocardial contractile function. In this model the apparently pathognomonic features of HC would therefore be the result of the strength, duration and timing of the hypertrophic stimulus rather than the activation of a discrete hypemophic pathway.

Genetic heterogeneity

Solomon *et at* first documented kindreds with typical FHC whose disease did not map to the CMH- 1 locus on chromosome 14.[13] The extent of the genetic heterogeneity in FHC has since become obvious. The abundance of readily typed and highly informative short tandem repeat polymorphisms dispersed throughout the genome has recently enabled genetic linkage analysis to be undertaken in smaller families. There are now four other loci known; on chromosome 1 (CMH2), chromosome 15 (CMH-3), chromosome 11 (CMH-4) and chromosome 7 (CMH-5/WPW).[14,15,16,17] Several groups also have evidence of at least one further locus, as yet undefined. The relative incidence of disease caused by mutations in the various genes is unclear at this stage but none of the new loci appears to be so common as CMH- 1. It is possible that mutations in many other genes may cause HC.

While novel polymorphic markers have enabled the mapping of smaller kindreds, the lack of informative meioses within such kindreds has prevented the use of extensive physical cloning approaches to identify the disease-causing genes at new loci. Geneticists have therefore taken a candidate gene approach. Using the CMH- 1 locus as a model, investigators have mapped and screened several sarcomeric contractile proteins for mutations at the CMH-2 and CMH-3 loci. This approach has led to the identification of mutations in the cardiac troponin T gene at the CMH-2 locus and in the α-tropomyosin gene at the CMH-3 locus *(Table 21.2)*.

"Sarcomeric" protein gene mutations cause FHC

α-Tropomyosin

The initial candidate gene at the CMH-3 locus, the α-cardiac actin gene, was rapidly excluded using a published polymorphism. Schleef *et al* subsequently mapped the mouse α-tropomyosin gene to mouse chromosome 9, to a genetic interval homologous or syntenic with the region of interest on human chromosome 15.[18] This finding made the α-tropomyosin (αTPM) gene an important candidate for FHC at this locus.

The human α-tropomyosin gene was cloned and an informative short tandem repeat polymorphism isolated from this clone. Using this polymorphism it was possible to demonstrate that there were no definitive recombinants between human α-tropomyosin and disease in the two whose disease mapped to the CMH3 locus. Subsequent sequencing of all of the exons of the αTPM gene expressed in striated muscle revealed mutations in exon 5 in affected individuals from both these families.[19]

Affected individuals from one family were heterozygous for an A->G transition at nucleotide 595 (original human cDNA). This changes codon 180 from GAG to GGG and results in the replacement of α-glutamic acid residue with α-glycine residue in the final protein. In the second family a mutation was also discovered in exon 5; a G->A transition this time at nucleotide 579. The final result in this case would be the substitution of an asparagine for an aspartic acid.

As with the β-cardiac myosin heavy chain gene the evidence supporting these nucleotide substitutions as the causative mutations in these families is threefold. These changes were confirmed by independent means and were not present in over 200 normal chromosomes. The mutated residues are highly conserved in tropomyosin molecules through several phyla and both lie within an active troponin T binding domain. The observation of a *de novo* mutation in the α-tropomyosin gene is the most substantive evidence that these mutations are indeed causing disease.

Cardiac Troponin T

The discovery of mutations in the troponin T binding domain of the α-TPM gene implicated the cardiac troponin T gene as a possible candidate gene at the other FHC loci. The cardiac troponin T gene had not been mapped previously. Using primers from the 3' untranslated region of the published human sequence it was possible to screen by PCR a panel of somatic cell hybrids containing only individual human chromosomes. This demonstrated that the human cardiac troponin T gene was on chromosome 1 making it a strong candidate for the disease gene at the CMH 2 locus.

Early in the course of screening the cardiac troponin T gene a T->C polymorphism was discovered in the gene. This nucleotide substitution does not change the amino acid sense of the mRNA but did allow the gene to be mapped with respect to disease in CMH-2 kindreds. Linkage analysis found no recombinants with disease in the original CMH 2 kindred.

RNAse protection detected mutations in the PCR amplified troponin T cDNAs from affected individuals in three kindreds which were known to map to the CMH-2 locus. The most obvious was an apparent splicing mutation which resulted in the omission of exon 15 of the coding sequence from the mature messenger RNA. This was seen as a shorter cDNA on PCR amplification. The actual mutation which caused this splicing error was a G->A transition in the exon 15 splice donor sequence. Two missense mutations were found in the other two kindreds studied; a G->A transition at nucleotide 287 in one family and T->A transversion at nucleotide 248 in the second.[19] In each case the nucleotide changes fulfilled the previously described criteria for disease-causing mutations.

Table 21.2 *MUTATIONS LEADING TO HC*

Locus	Map location	Mutated gene	Mutations described
CMH-1	Ch14ql	β-cardiac myosin	>30
CMH-2	Ch1q32	Cardiac troponin T	7
CMH-3	Ch15q3	α-Tropomyosin	3
CMH-4	Ch11pl-ql	MYBP-C	>20
CMH-5*	Ch7q3	Unknown	N/A

Cardiac myosin binding protein-C

The assignment of the cardiac myosin binding protein C gene to chromosome 11 lp11.2 led to its proposal as a candidate gene at the CMH-4 locus. Its exact function is unclear but cardiac MYBP-C is arrayed transversely in the sarcomere A-bands and binds both myosin and titin. Mutations were found in the splice donor site of exon M in one family and in the splice acceptor site at nucleotide 1960 in another family.[20,21] These mutations would both be predicted to result in the skipping of an exon and the generation of a premature stop codon which would disrupt the C-terminal, myosin-binding domain of the mature peptide. A third mutation, an 18 base pair duplication in exon P, might also disrupt this domain suggesting a common mechanism for lesions in this gene.[20]

A disease model for FHC

Four of the genes which cause the syndrome of familial HC encode sarcomeric proteins. This suggests that some aspect of sarcomere function may be disrupted in familial HC and that this acts on a final common pathway inducing the phenotype of myocardial hypertrophy with myocyte and myofibrillar disarray.[3,19] Many questions remain however. The extent of ventricular hypertrophy is unrelated to either clinical symptoms or to the risk of sudden death. It may be that these components of the phenotype are the result of parallel pathophysiological pathways and hypertrophy is only a marker for other processes. There is some evidence that the extent or distribution of hypertrophy resulting from mutations at different loci may differ suggesting a heterogeneity in the process at a regional or even cellular level.[2,14,15] The biological complexity may be partly modelled in the flight muscles of *Drosophila* where sarcomeric protein gene mutations affecting contractility also impinge on muscle cell differentiation and viability.[22] The generation of mouse models of HC may help to dissect these disease mechanisms.

The recent data also point the way for the choice of candidate genes at other loci. It is conceivable that many genes involved in cardiac sarcomeric function can cause FHC. The identification of other genetic loci and the characterization of the disease genes at these loci will also test the validity of the sarcomeric model. HC also occurs in association with other phenotypes where sarcomeric genes may not be such obvious candidates

FHC with Wolff-Parkinson-White syndrome

Hypertrophic cardiomyopathy has been known to be associated with the Wolff-Parkinson-White (WPW) syndrome within specific families since it was described, although the exact nature of the relationship was unclear. These families are distinctive in several ways. For example, when WPW was present with HC there appeared to be a higher than expected incidence of complete heart block. Post-mortem data from members of such kindreds suggested that myocardial fibrosis was a more prominent histopathological feature than in other HC cases.

Recently genetic linkage studies in a kindred in which HC cosegregated with the Wolff-Parkinson-White syndrome confirmed that these diverse phenotypes were the result of a single autosomal dominant trait. The gene defect in this disease maps to a novel locus on chromosome 7q3.[17] The relationship of the pathology in this family to HC in general and to 'isolated' ventricular preexcitation is uncertain. It remains to be seen whether mutations in another sarcomeric contractile protein gene cause this syndrome.

FHC with Friedreich's ataxia

Hypertrophic cardiomyopathy is a major feature of the autosomal recessive spinocerebellar degeneration known as Friedreich's ataxia. Approximately 50% of the mortality associated with this disease is attributed to heart failure. The pathological picture is comparable to that of FHC with WPW in that there is increased wall thickness without chamber dilatation in most cases but histologically fibrosis dominates. The gene for Freidreich's ataxia has recently been cloned and found to be a novel gene of unknown function with a possible N-terminal signal peptide.[23]

These last two conditions highlight the imminent reclassification of the cardiomyopathies based on molecular analysis rather than the relatively low resolution of gross ventricular morphology.

Modifying loci

While environmental factors are undoubtedly important, a significant proportion of the variation in expressivity of HC is probably the result of modifying genetic loci. A particular modifier allele may segregate within nuclear families and may even be genetically linked to the disease gene. Testing candidate loci for association with a component of the phenotype is an attractive method to identify such modifiers but is fraught with technical problems. Some preliminary association studies have been performed but the inclusion of several members from each kindred complicates interpretation of the results.[24] Rigorous application of more robust genetic approaches will be required to study genetic modifiers.

Clinical implications

Diagnosis

Hypertrophic cardiomyopathy is almost always an autosomal dominant trait. The 12 lead ECG is more sensitive than echocardiography and is highly specific in the context of an affected family in which 50% of the offspring of affected individuals are at risk. Individual generations may be skipped however, and it is important to document an extended family history.

The role of screening asymptomatic family members is uncertain at present as no clear therapeutic rationale for affected individuals is available. Ideally probands and their families should be referred to centers where screening, genotyping, risk stratification and therapeutic protocols are being evaluated in a formal controlled manner.

Prognosis

There is no apparent relationship between the clinical abnormalities in HC and the cardiovascular risk. Is it possible to relate specific mutations to subsequent risk of cardiovascular morbidity or mortality? Watkins *et al* demonstrated that different mutations in the cardiac β-myosin heavy chain gene were associated with disparate mortality risks.[25] Other groups have observed low death rates in association with the particular mutations which were "malignant" in this study.[26] The apparent discrepancies are possibly due to other genetic and environmental factors affecting the expression of the phenotype within kindreds. Ideally mortality risk should be calculated from the longitudinal observation of large numbers of unrelated individuals with each particular mutation. Multicenter studies will enable such data to be gathered. Similar questions must be asked about variations in the phenotype at the various loci. Until the completion of such prospective studies, the best prognostic index is a careful family history. This may be misleading in the small minority of cases where the mutation has only recently arisen.[7]

Therapy

There is little objective evidence of any prognostic benefit from any current interventions. However, the treatment algorthims being used in the management of HC are derived from studies of genetically heterogeneous populations. The study of genetically homogeneous cohorts of HC patients may change our therapeutic approach dramatically. It will be particularly important to study cohorts of children with defined mutations as they progress through the somatic growth spurt which is associated with the highest risk of sudden death and the development of ventricular hyperetrophy. What is it about this dynamic period which is so critical to these features of the phenotype?

Mutation screening

Screening for mutations in FHC is presently the subject of much discussion. Only 2/3 of FHC is explained by mutations in the four known genes. There is a high rate of new mutations so that entire coding sequences must be screened for each new family. If there are sufficient family members to test for linkage to one of the known loci then the screening could be limited to the disease gene at that particular locus. Currently the benefits of mutation screening are not well defined. Until many of these issues are addressed mutation screening will only be carried out in the context of research studies.

Significant insights into the pathophysiology of hypertrophy and sudden death have already been achieved through the application of molecular genetics to kindreds with HC, a relatively rare disease. The generation of true animal models will enable the pathophysiology of these processes to be understood at a fundamental level. The advance of molecular genetic techniques will also see these insights applied to more complex polygenic traits such as the ventricular hypertrophic response in conditions as diverse as hypertension and valve disease.

REFERENCES

1. McKenna WJ and Watkins H. Hypertrophic cardiomyopathy In: Scriver CR, Beaudet AL, Sly WS and Valle D Eds. The Metabolic and Molecular Bases of Inherited Disease, 7th edn., 1995.

2. Jarcho J A et al. Mapping a gene for familial hypetrophic cardiomyopathy to chromosome 14q 1. N Engl J Med 1989: 321:1372.

3. Geisterfer-Lowrance A, et al. A molecular basis for familial hypeertrophic cardiomyopathy: A β cardiac myosin heavy chain gene missense mutation. Cell 1990: 62: 999.

4. Watkins H, et al. Sporadic hypertrophic cardiomyopathy due to de novo myosin mutations. J Clin Invest 1992:90:1666.

5. Watkins H, Seidman JG, Seidman CE. Familial hypertrophic cardiomyopathy: a genetic model of cardiac hypertrophy. Human Molecular Genetics 1995: 4:1721.

6. Watkins H, et al. Independent origin of identical β cardiac myosin heavy chain mutations in hypertrophic cardiomyopathy. Am J Hum Genet 1996: 53:1180.

7. Dausse E, et al. Familial hypertrophic cardiomyopathy. Microsatellite haplotyping and identification of a hot spot for mutations in the beta-myosin heavy chain gene. J Clin Invest 1994: 92:2807.

8. MacRae CA, et al. An evaluation of Rnase protection assays for the detection of β cardiac myosin heavy chain gene mutations. Circulation 1994: 89:33.

9. Rayment I, et al. Structural interpretation of the mutations in beta-cardiac myosin that have implicated in familial hypertrophic cardiomyopathy. Proc Natl Acad Sci 1995: 92:3864.

10. Cuda G, et al. Skeletal muscle expression and abnormal funaction of beta-myosin in hypertrophic cardiomyopathy. J Clin Invest 1993: 91:2861.

11. Straceski AS, et al. Functional analysis of myosin missense mutations in familial hypertrophic cardiomyopathy. Proc Nat Acad Sci 1992: 91:589.

12. Lankford EB. Abnormal contractile properties of muscle fibres expressing beta-myosin heavy chain mutations in patients with hypertrophic cardiomyopathy. J Clin Invest 1995: 95:1409.

13. Solomon SD, et al. Familial hypertorphic cardiomyopathy ia a genetically heterogeneous disease. J Clin Invest 1990: 86:993.

14. Watkins HC, et al. A disease locus for familial hypertrophic cardiomyopathy maps to chromosome 1q3. Nature Genetics 1993: 3:33.

15. Theirfelder L, et al. A familial hypetrophic cardiomyopathy locus maps to chromosome 15q2 Proc Nat Acad Sci 1993: 90:6270.

16. Carrier L, et al. Mapping of a novel gene for familial hypertrophic cardiomyopathy to chromosome 11. Nature Genet 1993: 4:311.

17. MacRae CA, et al. Familial hypertrophic cardiomyopathy with Wolff-Parkinson-White syndrome maps to a locus on chromosome 7q3. Clin Invest 1995: 96:1216.

18. Scleef M, et al. Chromosomal location and genomic cloning of the mouse α-tropomyosin gene Tpm-1. Genomics 1993: 17:519.

19. Theirfelder L, et al. α-Tropomyosin mutations and cardiac troponin T mutations cause familial hypertrophic cardiomyopathy. Cell 1994: 77:1.

20. Watkins HC, et al. Mutations in the cardiac myosin binding protein-C gene on chromosome 11 cause familial hypertrophic cardiomyopathy. Nature Genetics 1995: 11:434.

21. Bonne G, et al. Cardiac myosin binding protein-C gene splice acceptor site mutation is associated with familial hypertrophic cardiomyopathy. Nature Genetics 1995: 11:438.

22. Fyrberg E, et al. Drosophila melanogaster troponin-T mutations engender three distinct syndromes of myofibrillar abnormalities. J Mol Biol 1990: 216:657.

23. Campuzano V, et al. Freidreich's ataxia: autosomal recessive disease caused by an intronic GAA triplet repeat expansion. Science 1993: 271: 1423.

24. Marian Aj, et al. Angiotensin converting enzyme polymorhism in hypertrophic cardiomyopathy and sudden death. Lancet 1993: 342:1085.

25. Watkins HC, et al. Distribution and prognostic significance of myosin missense mutations in familial hypertrophic cardiomyopathy. N Engl J Med 1993: 326:1108.

26. Fananapazir L, Epstein ND. Genotype phenotype correlations in hypertrophic cardiomyopathy. Circulation 1994: 89:22.

22 GENE THERAPY FOR CARDIOVASCULAR DISEASES

David W.M. Muller

The full potential of genetic therapies for the management of cardiovascular diseases has only recently become apparent. Although most diseases of the heart and vascular tree were for many years assumed to be acquired and multifactorial in origin, rapid and dramatic progress in molecular biology over the past decade has permitted identification of genetic defects responsible for a vast array of cardiovascular disease processes. Techniques such as chromosomal mapping by linkage analysis[1,2] have allowed large populations to be screened for single gene defects. One or more mutations of single genes have been shown to be responsible for familial hypertrophic cardiomyopathy[3], some dilated cardiomyopathies[4], Marfan's syndrome[5], torsade de pointes[6], some inherited thrombotic disorders[7], and supravalvular aortic stenosis.[8]

In addition to these clinical studies of family traits, experimental approaches, including overexpression of normal genes by gene transfer[9-14], and overexpression or deletion of genes using transgenic models and genetic knockouts[15-20], have allowed the selective investigation of the functional importance of individual genes and of their protein products in such processes as intimal hyperplasia[9-11], angiogenesis[11,12], systemic hypertension[13-15], atherogenesis[16-18], vascular thrombosis[19], and the myocardial response to acute ischemia.[20] Although many of these processes are clearly multifactorial in origin, identification of a genetic rather than an acquired basis for the disease process in some patients offers the potential firstly, for treatment by gene replacement for processes characterized by the absence of a specific, essential protein or by the presence of a mutant, dysfunctional protein, and secondly, by gene inhibition using antisense oligonucleotides. Local expression of other proteins with stimulatory or inhibitory activity may also provide a novel therapy for acquired disorders whose pathogenesis is multifactorial.

Somatic gene therapy

Of the several approaches to molecular therapeutics, the method with the most immediate clinical application is direct gene therapy. Although originally conceived as a means of curing inherited genetic diseases by replacing mutant genes in germ cells, the term is most frequently applied to the introduction of foreign DNA into somatic cells. The introduced DNA achieves its therapeutic effect by encoding the production of a protein that has local, regional or systemic effects depending on whether it is retained within the treated cell or is actively secreted into the extracellular space. Several methods have been examined as means of introducing DNA into somatic cells *(Table 22.1)*. These include the use of viral vectors (in particular, adenoviruses, adeno-associated viruses, and retroviruses), viral conjugate vectors (adenovirus-augmented receptor-mediated vectors and hemagglutinating virus of Japan (HVJ) liposomes), and nonviral vectors (cationic liposomes, direct injection, synthetic polymers, and physical methods such as electroporation).[21] Viral vectors allow the uptake of foreign DNA through their interaction with specific membrane receptors. Replication-defective adenoviruses appear to be most efficient in transfecting mammalian cells (including non-prolifer-

Table 22.1   VECTORS CURRENTLY IN USE IN CLINICAL TRIALS APPROVED BY THE RECOMBINANT DNA ADVISORY COMMITTEE (RAC) OF THE NATIONAL INSTITUTES OF HEALTH.

Vector	Number of Clinical Trials	Advantages	Disadvantages
Viral			
Retrovirus	76	Intermediate efficiency Easy to make	Small DNA capacity Random DNA integration Dividing cells only Replication risk
Adenovirus	15	Efficient DNA transfer Nondividing cells Possibly targetable	Immunogenic Replication risk Short duration
Adeno-associated virus	1	Nonimmunogenic	Small capacity Difficult to make
Herpesvirus	0	Nonimmunogenic Targets CNS	Risks unclear Difficult to make
Nonviral			
Liposomes	12	No replication risk Nonimmunogenic	Low efficiency
Naked or particle mediated DNA	3	No replication risk Nonimmunogenic	Low targetability Low efficiency

Adapted from Reference 116 with permission.

ating cells), but are associated with the shortest duration of expression of the foreign gene. DNA introduced using adenoviral vectors remains episomal, and is not integrated into the host cell nucleus. This may reduce the potential for insertional mutagenesis and malignant transformation, but is associated with a shorter duration of gene expression. In addition, since prior adenoviral infection is almost universal in the adult population, the use of these vectors carries the potential risk of inducing an immunological response to the introduced gene and its vector, and to cells expressing the foreign protein. Some of these potential side effects may be avoided using modifications of the adenoviral backbone to prevent expression of immunogenic viral proteins[22], or by using adenovirus conjugates. The latter combine an inactivated adenovirus with a receptor ligand, such as transferrin, to facilitate the passage of the DNA into the cell through the interaction of transferrin with its membrane receptor and to minimize lysosomal degradation of the foreign DNA.[23]

In contrast to adenoviral gene transfer, retrovirus-mediated gene transfer is associated with minimal risk of immunogenicity and a long duration of expression. However, it is also associated with a theoretical potential for mutagenesis because of random insertion of the DNA into the host cell genome, and with a relatively low efficiency of transfection of non-proliferating cells. HVJ liposome conjugates may offer a relatively efficient and safe alternative to retroviruses.[14] Liposomal gene transfer, in which the foreign DNA is coated with a cationic layer of lipid that binds to the target cell membrane, is also a safe alternative with a modest efficiency and intermediate duration of gene expression.

Evaluation of molecular therapies for focal vascular diseases has progressed rapidly from the initial demonstration of the feasibility of ex vivo gene transfer to endothelial cells[24], to in vivo direct gene transfer of marker genes[25], evaluation of the function of individual growth factors when overexpressed in the vascular wall[9-12], and the identification of potential therapies for the inhibition of restenosis[26,27], atherosclerosis[28,29], and for promoting angiogenesis.[12] The principal aim of this chapter is to review the progress made in the application of gene transfer technology to the study and treatment of myocardial diseases and systemic disorders that may promote disease in cardiovascular tissues.

Myocardial gene transfer

Multiple studies have now reported the feasibility of gene transfer to both neonatal cardiac myocytes in cell culture, and to cardiac muscle in vivo. The importance of exogenous DNA transfer to the intact myocardium stems not only from its potential value as a therapeutic strategy but also from its value in improving the understanding of cardiac myocyte gene regulation. Cardiac myocytes possess several unique features that hinder traditional approaches to the study of cell differentiation and regulation. Since permanent cardiac myocyte cell lines are not readily available, the study of cardiac phenotype regulation has relied on the use of fetal and neonatal cardiac myocytes in cell culture.[30-34] However, significant differences in gene expression between neonatal and adult myocardial cells have been reported. These include differences in expression of contractile protein isoforms, atrial natriuretic factor, and various transcription factors.[35] In vivo gene transfer studies are also limited.

Although potentially limited by the fact that adult mammalian myocytes are incapable of proliferation and regeneration[36], gene transfer has been explored in adult myocardium. The potential for direct injection of DNA into the rat myocardium was demonstrated by Lin and colleagues[37] after Wolff and colleagues[38] reported the somewhat surprising finding that murine skeletal myocytes took up and expressed plasmid DNA for a period of at least 2 months after direct injection in vivo. Subsequent studies of concurrent cardiac and skeletal muscle gene transfer[39] suggested that, in fact, the level of gene expression was considerably higher after cardiac gene transfer than after injection of comparable doses of DNA in skeletal muscle. In spite of this, however, the levels of gene expression after direct injection of unescorted, plasmid DNA have remained very low in all animal species examined including rats[37,39-41], dogs[42], rabbits[43], and swine.[43] In general, expression of the introduced DNA has been confined to the myocardium immediately adjacent to the needle tracks [40,41] and estimates of the number of myocytes expressing the introduced gene have been as low as 60 to 100 cells per injection.[40]

Considerably more efficient gene transfer to cardiac myocytes has been achieved using replication-deficient adenoviral vectors. Some studies have indicated transfection rates approaching 100% in vitro.[43-46] As noted above, adenoviruses have several advantages over other gene transfer vector systems. Adenoviral particles are relatively stable and can be purified and concentrated to high titers (10^{12}pfu/ml). In cells that express the appropriate viral receptor and uptake pathway, adenovirus-mediated gene transfer does not require host cell proliferation for efficient genomic expression and may therefore be well suited to DNA transfer into terminally differentiated, non-dividing cardiac myocytes. Relatively large foreign genes (up to 6- to 8-kb size) can be accommodated in the adenoviral genome, increasing the opportunities for producing a variety of therapeutic genes. These vectors also allow the transgene to be under the control of tissue-specific promoter elements[47,48], as well as a variety of viral and mammalian constitutive promoter elements[50], thereby restricting the sites of expression of the foreign gene. Finally, although high titers of adenovirus may be cytolytic, modest titers appear to have no adverse effect on cell survival or morphology in cardiac myocyte cell cultures.[45]

Adenovirus-mediated myocardial gene transfer has been described in a variety of animal model systems using direct injection[46,50,51], catheter infusion delivery systems[52], and intravenous injection[53] in mice[53], rats[46,50], rabbits[52] and pigs.[51] Direct intramyocardial injection of adenoviruses carrying reporter genes achieved levels of gene expression several orders of magnitude higher than after direct injection of plasmid DNA.[46,50,51] In a porcine model[51], gene expression was detected in up to 75% of cardiac myocytes within 5mm of the injection site needle track. There was no evidence of spread beyond the injection site, and little expression by cells other than myocytes. In adult rabbits[52], intracoronary infusion resulted in gene expression both within the coronary arterial wall and in the surrounding myocardium. The proportion of cardiac myocytes expressing the transgene in the area of distribution of the injected coronary artery was estimated to be 32%, considerably higher than previous estimates of the proportion of cells transfected after direct injection of plasmid DNA.[37,39-43] After intravenous injection of 10^9 pfu of virus, murine cardiac myocyte transfection was relatively uniform with an estimated efficiency of 0.2%.[53] In these animals, gene expression was also noted in multiple other organs including the lung, liver, intestine and skeletal muscle.

One major limiting factor in each of the studies of adenoviral gene transfer into adult ventricular myocardium has been a relatively short duration of gene expression. Gene expression tends to peak within the first 1-2 weeks, and then declines rapidly in adults. Prolonged gene expression for as long as 12 months has been reported after gene transfer to neonatal mouse cardiac and skeletal muscle.[53] Ongoing studies examining modifications of the adenoviral genome[22] and the role of immunosuppression[40,54] may also allow persistence of adenovirus-mediated gene expression in the myocardium. One further potential limitation of adenoviral gene transfer to the myocardium has been the local inflammatory response observed at the site of gene expression in some studies.[50,51] Although this may not be unique to adenoviral vectors (it has also been observed after direct injection of plasmid DNA[39,43], the inflammatory response may be responsible for the early loss of gene expression.[51,54] Whether it has any other long-term deleterious consequences remains to be determined.

A third, novel approach to myocardial gene transfer is the engraftment of fetal myocytes or embryonic stem cells. This has been described for both skeletal muscle[55-57] and cardiac muscle cell transplants.[58] In the latter study[58], fetal cardiomyocytes isolated from transgenic mice carrying a fusion gene of the α-cardiac myosin heavy chain promoter with a β-galactosidase reporter were delivered directly into the left ventricular myocardium of syngeneic, nontransgenic hosts. Grafted cells, identified by their expression of the β-galactosidase enzyme, were observed up to 2 months after implantation aligned in circumferential arrays parallel to the host myocardium. Electron microscopy studies demonstrated the presence of intercalated disks between the host and graft cells suggesting the formation of a functional syncytium and the possibility of electrical and mechanical coupling between grafted and host cardiac myocytes.[58] Although it is unlikely that sufficient numbers of myocytes could be transplanted to contribute substantially to the overall contractile function of the ventricular myocardium, local elaboration of therapeutic proteins from the engrafted cells may become a valuable strategy for the treatment of a variety of myopathic processes.

Therapeutic potential of myocardial gene transfer

In addition to providing a means of studying cardiac gene regulation and growth in vivo[39], myocardial gene transfer may provide a unique therapeutic strategy for patient management by introducing genes encoding proteins that are absent or defective due to an inherited genetic defect, or by bestowing regenerative capacity or augmented contractile function on the diseased and failing myocardium *(Table 22.2)*.

a) Inherited disorders. The mutations responsible for several cardiac diseases have now been characterized.[3-6,8] Among the best studied of these are familial hypertrophic cardiomyopathy (FHC) and Duchenne muscular dystrophy. Familial hypertrophic cardiomyopathy is a clinically and genetically heterogeneous disease transmitted as an autosomal dominant trait with variable penetrance, and characterized histologically by myocyte hypertrophy and fiber disarray. The disease arises from a variety of missense mutations of the β-myosin heavy chain (β-MHC), localized most frequently in exons coding for the head and head rod regions of the protein on chromosome 14q11-q12.[3,59] β-MHC is the predominant isozyme of the contractile protein in the ventricular myocardium of adult mammals, and is also present in skeletal muscle.[60] Although mutations of the gene are also expressed in skeletal muscle and other tissues[61], tissue dysfunction appears to be confined to the left ventricular myocardium. Gene transfer of the β-MHC gene has not yet been well studied. However, the rapid advances in the field of myocardial gene transfer may eventually provide a molecular therapeutic approach for this condition. In addition to direct myocardial gene transfer, other approaches such as the selective inhibition of expression of the mutant allele and promotion of transcription of the normal allele may also prove to be possible.[62]

A second inherited condition that may be amenable to treatment by gene replacement or augmentation is Duchenne muscular dystrophy. This lethal, X-linked disease is caused by the absence of dystrophin, a 472K protein encoded by a 14 kilobase transcript.[63] The protein has structural homology to the spectrin family of cytoskeletal proteins, and is expressed at the inner surface of the plasma membrane of skeletal and cardiac muscle.[64] The clinical syndrome is characterized by myonecrosis, fibrosis and fatty infiltration, resulting in a severe skeletal and cardiac

Table 22.2 POTENTIAL MYOCARDIAL GENE THERAPIES.

Disease Gene	
1. Inherited diseases	
• Hypertrophic cardiomyopathy	β-MHC
• Duchenne muscular dystrophy	dystrophin
2. Acquired diseases	
• Heart failure	β-adrenergic receptor
	β-adrenergic receptor kinase (β-ARK) inhibitor
	Angiogenic factors e.g. VEGF, FGF
	Vasodilators e.g. kallikrein

Abbreviations: β-MHC=β-myosin heavy chain; FGF=fibroblast growth factor; VEGF=vascular endothelial growth factor.

myopathy with conduction disturbance. Research into the molecular mechanisms of the disease and potential therapies has been aided by the availability of an appropriate model, the mdx mouse.[65] Several approaches to correcting the defect have been explored in this model.[55,66,67] In a study by Partridge and colleagues[55], muscle precursor cells from normal neonatal mice were grafted into the hind limb muscles of mdx (dystrophin-deficient) mice to determine whether dystrophin synthesis could be induced in the mdx muscle fibers. The normal donor cells were shown to fuse with host cells. Dystrophin of normal size was identified in the normal sarcolemmal location in a substantial proportion of mdx fibers, an observation thought to reflect de novo synthesis by the diseased fibers, rather than passive carriage of the protein from donor cells. Thus, although no functional correlate of the successful transplant was performed, the biochemical defect appeared to have been at least partially corrected. Similar approaches have been attempted to correct other murine muscular dystrophies[68] and inherited phosphorylase kinase deficiency.[69]

Gene transfer approaches to correcting the myopathy associated with dystrophin deficiency have also been described.[66,67] Ragot and colleagues[66] used adenovirus-mediated gene transfer to introduce a 6.3 kilobase pair human dystrophin cDNA into skeletal muscles of mdx mice. As noted above, native dystrophin is encoded by a 14 kilobase transcript which is too large to be incorporated into the adenoviral genome. The 6.3 kilobase cDNA used in this study encodes a "minidystrophin" which was identified in a patient with mild clinical features of Becker muscular dystrophy. This is an inherited muscular dystrophy in which dystrophin is present but is quantitatively or qualitatively abnormal. Transfer of the minidystrophin cDNA into skeletal myocytes and in vivo gene expression was confirmed with sarcolemmal dystrophin immunostaining being detectable in 5-50% of fibers for up to 3 months.[66] This level of expression contrasts with the relatively poor efficiency of expression (approximately 1%) after direct in vivo injection of plasmid DNA encoding human dystrophin or minidystrophin.[67]

Data from a double-blind clinical trial of myoblast transfer for Duchenne muscular dystrophy have now been reported.[68] In 12 patients, myoblasts obtained from genotypically normal male relatives were injected unilaterally into one biceps muscle; the contralateral biceps muscle served as a sham-injected control. Patients were also randomized to receive cyclosporine or placebo to determine the effects of immune suppression on efficacy of the treatment. Intramuscular injections of myoblasts were performed monthly for 6 months and muscle strength was determined monthly for 12 months. Donor-derived dystrophin expression ranged from 0% to 10% of biopsied muscle cell fibers. However, no difference in muscle strength was apparent between the treated and control sides in any patient at any time in the total population or in the cyclosporine treated group. Therefore, although myoblast fusion was documented in some patients, this was insufficient to achieve a recognizable clinical effect.

b) Acquired disorders. In contrast to skeletal muscle, in which satellite cell proliferation and differentiation may regenerate injured muscle, myofiber loss in the

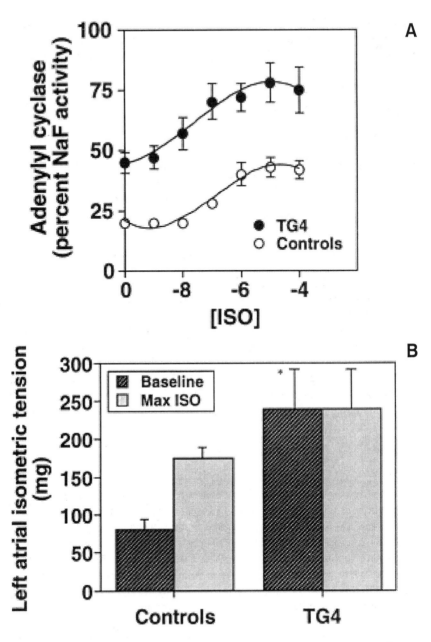

Figure 22.1 Myocardial function in transgenic mice (TG4) overexpressing the β_2-adrenergic receptor. When compared with control animals, transgenic animals had a greater myocardial adenylyl cyclase activity (panel A), baseline isometric tension (panel B), and basal left ventricular dP/dt_{max} (panel C). Baseline levels were comparable to control values after maximal isoproterenol stimulation. * p<0.05 vs control (panel A); *p<0.005, †p<0.05 vs control (panel C). Reproduced from Ref 79 with permission.

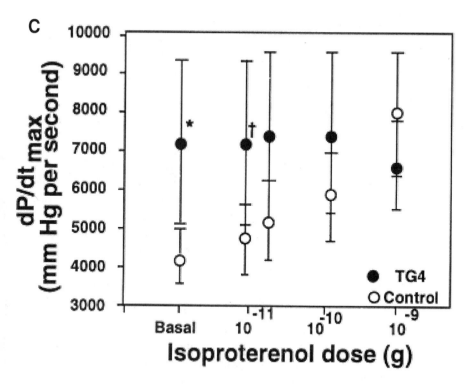

C

mammalian heart is irreversible due to the absence of a regenerative stem cell system and permanent cessation of the cardiac myocyte cell cycle in the early postnatal period.[71,72] Attempts have been made using transgenic mice and cardiac specific promoters to stimulate cardiac hyperplasia using c-myc[73] or SV-40 T antigen oncogenes.[74] However, unless regulation of oncogene expression can be reliably achieved, use of these mitogens will not be suitable as treatments for acquired myocardial disease because of the inherent risks of malignant cell growth and cardiac arrhythmias.[74]

In contrast to the risks inherent in the uncontrolled expression of oncogenes, overexpression of myocardial b-adrenergic receptors may be well tolerated and may permit the augmentation of cardiac function in patients with heart failure. In congestive cardiac failure, myocardial exposure to chronically elevated catecholamine levels results in down-regulation of the β_1-adrenergic receptor population at the myocyte cell surface, thereby decreasing myocardial sensitivity to inotropic stimuli.[75] This down-regulation or desensitization appears to result from phosphorylation of the activated receptors by specific G protein-coupled receptor kinases.[76] Thus, manipulation of the expression of myocardial β-receptors or of the β-receptor kinases offers a potentially novel mechanism of treating myocardial failure.

Several studies have examined this possibility. In one study, transgenic mice overexpressing myocardial β_1-adrenergic receptors did not exhibit a significant increase in myocardial contractility.[77] In contrast, overexpression of β_2-adrenergic receptors, which do not appear to undergo significant down-regulation and which couple more efficiently to adenylyl cyclase than do β_1-adrenergic receptors, was associated with a markedly elevated basal rate of cyclic AMP formation, an increased basal heart rate, a three-fold greater isometric tension development in isolated atria, and a 70% increase in left ventricular dp/dt_{max} when compared with control tissue *(Figure 22.1)*.[78] At baseline, left atrial isometric tension and left ventricular dP/dt_{max} in the transgenic animals were comparable to those at maximal inotropic stimulation in the control animals, but did not increase further after the administration of isoproterenol *(Figs 22.1B-C)*. It was hypothesized that the apparent maximal stimulation of adenylyl cyclase activity in the absence of agonist binding was the result of direct stimulation associated with an extreme increase in density of β_2 receptors.

Increased myocardial contractility was also observed in transgenic mice expressing a β-adrenergic receptor kinase (βARK) inhibitor which prevents phosphorylation and desensitization of activated β-receptors.[79] Baseline left ventricular dP/dt_{max} and left ventricular systolic pressure were significantly higher, and increased to a greater extent during isoproterenol stimulation, than in control animals *(Figs 22.2A-B)*. These studies suggest that it may be possible to augment the contractile function of the failing myocardium of adult patients with ischemic or non-ischemic cardiomyopathies by introducing one or more exogenous genes. It should be noted, however, that these studies were performed in animals with normal myocardial systolic function. Augmented function of diseased cardiac muscle, in which post-receptor dysfunction may also be present, has not yet been demonstrated. Additional approaches to the management of dilated cardiomyopathies might include the use of vasodilator genes such as kallikrein to reduce myocardial work, and overexpression of genes that promote myocardial angiogenesis (such as vascular endothelial growth factor (VEGF) or fibroblast growth factor (FGF) in patients with end-stage ischemic cardiomyopathies.

Gene transfer for systemic cardiovascular disorders

Familial hypercholesterolemia

Familial hypercholesterolemia is an autosomal dominant disorder caused by dysfunction or absence of the low density lipoprotein (LDL) receptor. Dysfunction of the receptor at the hepatocyte membrane surface results in impaired binding, uptake and degradation of circulating LDL and thus, to hypercholesterolemia and premature atherosclerosis.[80] The molecular basis for the disease is a mutation of the LDL receptor gene. Several genetic abnormalities have been described including deletions, insertions, missense and nonsense mutations.[81,82] Heterozygotes, who inherit one abnormal LDL gene, constitute approximately 5% of all patients with acute myocardial infarction before the age of 45 years and have a prevalence in the general population of 1 in 500. The clinical course of patients with homozygous

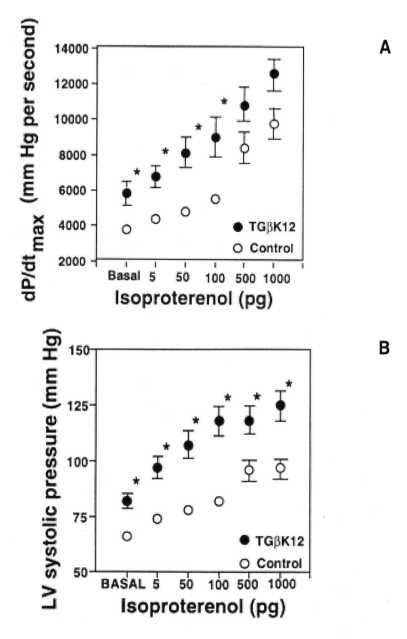

Figure 22.2 Myocardial function in transgenic mice (TGβK12) overexpressing the β-adrenergic receptor kinase (βARK) inhibitor. Left ventricular dP/dt_{max} (panel A) and left ventricular pressure (panel B) were higher at baseline and rose to a greater extent after isoproterenol stimulation than in normal control animals. Reproduced from Ref 79 with permission.

familial hypercholesterolemia depends on their level of LDL receptor expression. Patients with <2% receptor activity (receptor-negative) often develop manifestations of severe coronary artery disease including sudden death during their first decade of life.[82] The atherosclerotic process typically involves the coronary ostia and may also cause aortic valvular or supravalvular thickening and stenosis. Receptor defective patients (>2% receptor activity) have less severe hypercholesterolemia and the onset of symptomatic coronary disease in their second or third decade of life. Untreated, the majority of receptor defective patients die from coronary artery disease before the age of 30 years.

The therapeutic options available for the management of familial hypercholesterolemia are extremely limited. Lipid lowering agents such as bile acid resins and HMG CoA reductase inhibitors typically achieve minimal lowering of serum cholesterol levels in these patients. Substantial metabolic improvement has been achieved by orthotopic liver transplantation.[83] The success of hepatic transplantation, and the dramatic difference in survival between receptor defective and receptor negative patients, led Wilson and colleagues to examine the potential for hepatocellular transfer of the LDL receptor gene as a means of achieving a partial correction of the metabolic defect in familial hypercholesterolemia without the hazards inherent in organ transplantation. In a series of experimental studies, these investigators demonstrated successful engraftment of autologous hepatocytes that were genetically modified ex vivo using a recombinant retrovirus. [84-87] Initial studies were performed in Watanabe heritable hyperlipidemic (WHHL) rabbits, a strain genetically deficient in LDL receptors in which animals homozygous for the condition develop severe hypercholesterolemia, extensive atherosclerosis and premature death. Gene transfer was accomplished by partial hepatectomy, isolation and culture of individual hepatocytes, retrovirus-mediated transfection, and return of the transfected, autologous cells to the liver by infusion into the portal vein.[84] Stable engraftment and partial metabolic correction were evident for the six month duration of the study.[84] Longer term studies in dogs and baboons demonstrated expression of the transgene for up to 18 months after gene therapy.[85,86]

Based on these experimental studies, hepatic gene transfer was performed in a pilot study of 5 patients using the same ex vivo gene transfer approach *(Figure 22.3)*.[87,88] Transgene expression was evident in hepatic tissue obtained by liver biopsy in all patients 4 months after gene transfer. A significant reduction in serum LDL cholesterol was achieved in 3 of the 5 patients with a corresponding increase in LDL catabolism.[88] The first patient treated[87] realized a 20% reduction in serum cholesterol which has now been stable for more than 3 years (*Figure 22.4*). Importantly, although expression of a 'foreign' protein at the hepatocyte cell surface may theoretically have resulted in a rejection response, histological and biochemical studies showed no evidence of hepatitis in any of the 5 treated patients.[88] Thus, a strategy of ex vivo gene transfer to autologous hepatocytes was shown to be safe and to have a variable efficiency and clinical effect. Current efforts to improve the therapeutic efficacy of this treatment include the use of adenoviral constructs for in vivo gene transfer[89-91], and the use of modified adenoviruses[22] or adenoviral conjugates[23] to

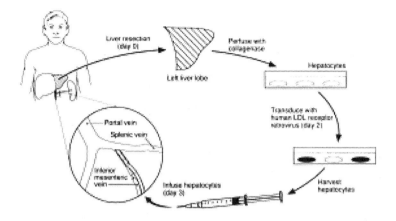

Figure 22.3 Clinical protocol for ex vivo *hepatic gene transfer for familial hypercholesterolemia. Reprinted from Reference 87 with permission.*

further improve the efficiency of transfection or the duration of gene expression. It is expected that these and other modifications will ultimately obviate the need for hepatic resection and ex vivo gene transfer.

Other potential gene therapy strategies described for the management of hypercholesterolemia include overexpression of apolipoprotein A-1 (apo A-1) as a means of augmenting circulating high-density lipoprotein (HDL) cholesterol levels.[92-93] Epidemiological studies suggest an inverse relationship between the levels of circulating HDL cholesterol and the incidence and severity of atherosclerosis.[94-95] Experimental studies have also indicated a protective effect of homologous HDL infusion in hypercholesterolemic rabbits.[96] HDL appears to exert this effect by mobilizing cholesterol from peripheral tissues and promoting its transport to the liver. A critical determinant of the level of circulating HDL appears to be the rate of production of apo A1, its principal protein constituent. Genetically determined deficiencies and excesses of apo A-1 have been described. Individuals with deficiencies of apo A1 and HDL are predisposed to premature coronary artery disease[96] whereas those with increased apo A1 and HDL cholesterol (hyperalphalipoproteinemia) have a relative resistance to atherosclerosis.[98] Consistent with these observations are studies indicating that transgenic mice that express the human apo A-1 gene have increased HDL levels and resistance to the effects of an atherogenic diet.[99]

Importantly, overexpression of apo A1 may also confer resistance to the accelerated atherosclerosis that results from genetic disorders other than hypoalphalipoproteinemia. Apolipoprotein E (apoE)-deficient mice, for example, develop severe hypercholesterolemia, xanthomata, and rapidly progressive atherosclerosis. In a study

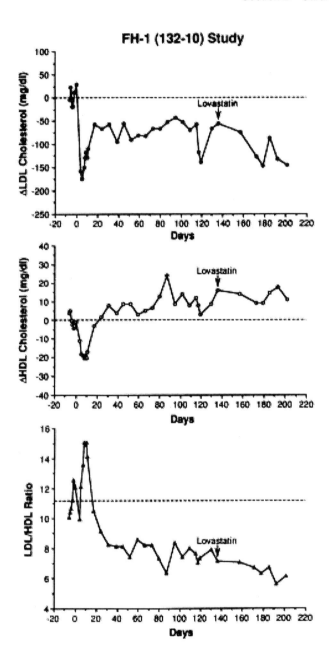

Figure 22.4 Lipid profiles in the first patient with familial hypercholesterolemia treated by ex vivo LDL receptor gene transfer. Adapted from Reference 87 with permission.

reported by Paszty and colleagues[93], inbred strains of apo E knockout mice that also express the human apo A1 transgene were shown to have a 2-3-fold greater HDL level than control animals, and a 6-fold decrease in susceptibility to atherosclerosis when compared with apo E knockout mice without the apo A1 transgene, despite a similar degree of elevation of the serum cholesterol. These observations suggest that overexpression of apo A1 in individuals predisposed to atherosclerosis may be a valuable therapeutic strategy, even in patients with a polygenic etiology for their disease. The feasibility of a gene therapy approach has been reported in one study[92] in which adenovirus-mediated transfer of the human apo A1 gene into normal mice resulted in a transient increase in circulating HDL levels by up to 35% of the baseline levels.

Together, the above studies suggest that there may be several potential gene therapy strategies for inhibiting lipid deposition in the arterial wall in patients genetically predisposed to atherosclerosis. In addition to these systemic approaches, strategies for inhibiting focal lipid accumulation have also been explored. Aorto-coronary saphenous vein grafting, for example, is characterized by early inflammatory cell infiltration and intimal thickening[100-101] with a propensity for early thrombotic occlusion and accelerated atherosclerosis. Transfer of the genes encoding proteins that inhibit thrombus formation, monocyte binding or cell proliferation, performed at the time of vein harvesting and implantation has been suggested as a means of prolonging graft patency[102-103]. In contrast to strategies that aim to correct a genetic disorder, in which sustained expression for many years may be required to slow the atherosclerotic process, it is possible that short-term inhibition of neointimal hyperplasia may render the vein segment relatively resistant to lipid uptake and intimal thickening. Mann and colleagues[29], for example, used an antisense approach to inhibit two cell cycle regulatory proteins, proliferating cell nuclear antigen (PCNA) and cell division cycle 2 (cdc2) kinase, to promote vascular medial hypertrophy rather than intimal hyperplasia in a rabbit jugular vein model of vascular grafting. The medial hypertrophy, or "arterialization", that occurred in vein segments treated with antisense oligonucleotides to PCNA and cdc2 kinase appeared to protect the grafts from macrophage infiltration and lipid uptake over the 10 weeks study period. Thus, a therapy with a relatively short duration of activity may have a long-term impact on graft patency.

Systemic hypertension

Essential hypertension represents a major risk factor for morbidity and mortality from cardiovascular causes.[102] The pathogenesis of this condition is likely to be the interaction between one or more genetic determinants and several environmental stimuli.[103] Genetic manipulations have recently provided the opportunity not only for elucidating the role of individual factors in the pathogenesis of the disease, but also for providing novel therapeutic strategies. Transgenic models of hypertension have produced variable results. Rats expressing the mouse Ren-2 gene have been reported to develop fulminant hypertension[15], but mice expressing the human renin gene were normotensive.[104] Overexpression of the human renin gene in rats by gene transfer using hemagglutinating virus of Japan (HVJ)-liposomes resulted in a significant elevation of the systemic blood pressure in proportion to the level of circulating human renin and angiotensin II.[105] The elevated blood pressure was successfully treated by administration of a specific human renin inhibitor, suggesting that the hypertensive response was due to cleavage of the expressed human renin by rat angiotensinogen.

Gene transfer has also been used to examine the effects of mediators of hypertension on vascular and myocardial hypertrophy. Morishita and colleagues[14] transfected rat carotid arteries with the human angiotensin converting enzyme (ACE) gene to determine the local effects of the angiotensin system independent of the effects of this system on the systemic blood pressure. An increase in vascular ACE activity was documented and was associated with a parallel increase in indices of medial smooth muscle cell proliferation and wall thickness in the absence of an elevation in systemic blood pressure.

These and other studies suggest that a gene therapy approach might also be effective in the treatment of hypertension. Human tissue kallikrein is one potentially therapeutic gene.[106-107] Tissue kallikreins are serine proteases that act on kininogen substrates to form the vasodilator bradykinin. Intravenous injection of the DNA for human tissue kallikrein into spontaneously hypertensive rats resulted in a substantial lowering of the blood pressure for at least 6 weeks.[106] Expression of the transgene was detected in the heart, lung and kidney. Similar results were achieved by intramuscular injection.[107] Thus, if prolonged expression of kallikrein can be achieved in vivo, this may become a useful strategy for the management of essential hypertension.

Pulmonary vascular disorders

The biology of the pulmonary vasculature is complex and distinct from that of the systemic circulation. Management of pulmonary vascular diseases, both primary and secondary, is one of the most difficult and often least satisfying clinical challenges faced by cardiovascular specialists. Extensive experimental studies have, to date, not identified consistently effective pharmacological therapies, but have identified a number of potential targets for therapies based on gene manipulation. Endothelin-1, elastase, platelet-derived growth factor, transforming growth factor, and insulin-like growth factor have been implicated in the genesis of pulmonary hypertension.[108-113] Local expression of genes encoding vasodilators or inhibitors of vascular smooth muscle cell proliferation may therefore provide effective therapies for this otherwise difficult to treat condition. With this in mind, several investigators have examined the possibility of introducing DNA into the pulmonary circulation.[114-115] In one study[114], adenovirus-mediated and liposomal transfer of the human alkaline phosphatase gene demonstrated uptake and expression in the endothelium of pulmonary arteries, veins, capillaries and in the adjacent pulmonary interstitium, but not in large bronchi, for periods up to 2 weeks after introduction. Importantly, there was no evidence of an inflammatory response within the lung parenchyma or in tissues remote from the site of introduction. Whether this approach can be used to reduce pulmonary vascular pressure, particularly once irreversible structural arterial changes have occurred, remains to be determined.

Challenges for clinical application of gene therapy

Like any new technology, it is highly likely that the clinical application of gene therapy will be met with frustration, doubt, and questions about the viability of this approach.[116] Already, more than 100 clinical trials are underway to examine the efficacy of gene therapy in a variety of single gene defects, AIDS, cancer and arterial disease. Reports from the earliest of these trials have been disappointing [68,88,117], predominantly because of the low efficiency of gene transfer and the short duration of gene expression. Clearly, conditions requiring lifelong gene expression in a large number of cells will require major advances in viral biology or in the development of non-viral vectors. On the other hand, disease processes characterized by the need for short-term gene expression, or in which a very low level of gene expression can have a profound biological effect, may be well suited to management by gene transfer in the near future. However, even for these conditions, numerous issues still need to be addressed (Table 22.3). These include the need for minimally invasive access to appropriate organ tissues using effective catheter delivery systems; the requirement for cell targeting and specificity of gene uptake and expression, for example by receptor-mediated DNA transfer [118] and through the use of cell-specific

Table 22.3   CHALLENGES FOR CLINICAL APPLICABILITY OF
             CARDIOVASCULAR GENE THERAPY.

- Efficiency of gene transfer
- Stability of gene expression
- Need for cell specific gene expression
- Local catheter delivery systems
- Immunogenicity of foreign gene or vector
- Risk of mutagenesis from random integration
- Need for intracellular regulation
- Limitations on size of transgene
- Cost-effectiveness

promoters, to allow intravenous gene delivery; the need for in vivo regulation of the transgene [119]; the need to overcome constraints on the size of the gene that can be delivered; and the need to rationalize the risk- and cost-benefits of this technically demanding therapeutic approach.

A large body of experimental data now gives credence to the enormous potential of gene therapy as a therapeutic tool. In spite of the limitations apparent from the early clinical trials, it is highly likely that this technology will continue to develop at a feverish pace and ultimately, will prove to be a valuable adjunctive therapy for a variety of inherited and acquired cardiovascular diseases.

REFERENCES

1. Hetjmancik JF, Roberts R. Molecular gentics and application of linkage analysis. In Roberts R (ed). Molecular Basis of Cardiology. Cambridge, Blackwell Scientific Publications. 1993: 355.

2. Weissenbach J, et al. A second generation linkage map of the human genome. Nature 1992: 39: 794.

3. Jarcho JA, et al. Mapping a gene for familial hypertrophic cardiomyopathy to chromosome 14q1. N Engl J Med 1989: 321: 1372.

4. Kass S, et al. A gene defect that causes conduction system disease and dilated cardiomyopathy maps to chromosome 1p1 - 1q1. Nature Genet 1994: 7: 546.

5. Lee B, et al. Linkage of Marfan syndrome and a phenotypically related disorder to two different fibrillin genes. Nature. 1991: 352: 330.

6. Keating M, et al. Linkage of a cardiac arrythmia, the long QT syndrome and the Harvey ras-1 gene. Science 1991: 252: 704.

7. Bertina RM, et al. Mutation in blood coagulation factor V associated with resistance to activated protein C. Nature 1994: 369: 64.

8. Ewart AK, et al. A human vascular disorder, supravalvular aortic stenosis, maps to chromosome 7. Proc Natl Acad Sci USA. 1993: 90: 3226.

9. Nabel EG, et al. Recombinant platelet-derived growth factor B gene expression in porcine arteries induces intimal hyperplasia in vivo. J Clin Invest 1993: 91: 1822.

10. Nabel EG, et al. Direct transfer of transforming growth factor β1 gene into arteries stimulates fibrocellular hyperplasia. Proc Natl Acad Sci USA 1993: 90: 10759.

11. Nabel EG, et al. Recombinant fibroplast growth factor-1 promotes intimal hyperplasia and angiogenesis in vivo. Nature 1993: 362: 844.

12. Takeshita S, et al. In vivo evidence of enhanced angiogenesis following direct arterial gene transfer of the plasmid encoding vascular endothelial growth factor. Circulation 1993: 88: I-476.

13. Morishita R, et al. Autocrine and paracrine effects of atrial natriuretic peptide gene transfer on vascular smooth muscle and endothelial cellular growth. J Clin Invest 1994: 94: 824.

14. Morishita R, et al. Evidence for direct local effect of angiotensin in vascular hypertrophy : in vivo gene transfer of angiotensin converting enzyme. J Clin Invest 1994: 94: 978.

15. Mullins JJ, Peters J, Ganten D. Fulminant hypertension in transgenic rats harbouring the mouse Ren-2 gene. Nature 1990: 344: 541.

16. Lawn RM, et al. Atherogenesis in transgenic mice expressing human apolipoprotein (a). Nature 1992: 360: 670.

17. Purcell-Huynh DA, et al. Transgenic mice expressing high levels of human apolipoprotein B develop severe atherosclerotic lesions in response to a high fat diet. J Clin Invest 1995: 95: 2246.

18. Wilson JM, et al. Hepatocyte-directed gene transfer in vivo leads to transient improvement of hypercholesterolemia in low density lipoprotein receptor-deficient rabbits. J Biol Chem 1992: 267: 963.

19. Carmeliet P, et al. Physiological consequences of loss of plasminogen activator gene function in mice. Nature 1994: 368: 419.

20. Marber MS, et al. Overexpression of the rat inductible 70-kD heat stress protein in a transgenic mouse increases the resistance of the heart to ischemic injury. J Clin Invest 1995: 95: 1446.

21. Mulligan RC. The basic science of gene therapy. Science 1993: 260: 926.

22. Engelhardt JF, et al. Ablation of E2A in recombinant adenoviruses improves transgene persistence and decreases inflammatory response in mouse liver. Proc Natl Acad Sci USA. 1994: 91: 6196.

23. Wagner E, et al. Coupling of adenovirus to transferrin-polylysine/DNA complexes greatly enhances receptor-mediated gene delivery and expression of transfected genes. Proc Natl Acad Sci USA 1992: 89: 6099.

24. Nabel EG, et al. Recombinant gene expression in vivo within endothelial cells of the arterial wall. Science 1989: 244: 1342.

25. Nabel EG, Plautz G, Nabel GJ. Site-specific gene expression in vivo by direct gene transfer into the arterial wall. Science 1990: 249: 1285.

26. Ohno T, et al. Gene therapy for vascular smooth muscle cell proliferation after arterial injury. Science 1994: 265: 781.

27. Von der Leyen HE, et al. Gene therapy inhibiting neointimal vascular lesion: *In vivo* transfer of endothelial cell nitric oxide synthase gene. Proc Natl Acad Sci USA 1995: 92: 1137.

28. Chen S-J, Wilson JM, Muller DWM. Adenovirus-mediated gene transfer of soluble vascular cell adhesion molecule to porcine interposition vein grafts. Circulation 1994: 89: 1922.

29. Mann MJ, et al. Genetic engineering of vein grafts resistant to atherosclerosis. Proc Natl Acad Sci USA 1995: 92: 4502.

30. Parker TG, et al. Differential regulation of skeletal α-actin transcription in cardiac muscle by two fibroblast growth factors. Proc Natl Acad Sci USA. 1990: 87: 7066.

31. Tsika RW, et al. Thyroid hormone regulates expression of a transfected human alpha-myosin heavy-chain fusion gene in fetal rat heart cells. Proc Natl Acad Sci USA 1990: 87: 379.

32. Thompson WR, Nadal-Ginard B, Mahdavi V. A MyoD1-independent muscle-specific enhancer controls the expression of the beta-myosin heavy chain gene in skeletal and cardiac muscle cells. J Biol Chem 1991: 266: 22678.

33. Kariya KL, Karns LR, Simpson PC. Expression of a constitutively activated mutant of the beta-isozyme of protein kinase-C in cardiac myocytes stimulates the promoter of the beta-myosin heavy chain isogene. J Biol Chem 1991: 266: 10023.

34. Kovacic-Milivojevic B, Gardner DG. Divergent regulation of the human atrial natriuretic peptide gene by c-jun and c-fos. Mol Cell Biol 1991: 266: 10023.

35. Zimmeramann KA, et al. Differential expression of myc family genes during murine development. Nature 1986: 319: 780.

36. Korecky B, Rakusan K. Normal and hypertrophic growth of the rat heart : changes in cell dimensions and numbers. Am J Physiol 1978: 234: H123.

37. Lin H, et al. Expression of recombinant genes in myocardium in vivo after direct injection of DNA. Circulation 1990: 82: 2217.

38. Wolf JA, et al. Direct gene transfer into mouse muscle in vivo. Science 1990: 247: 1465.

39. Kitsis RN, et al. Hormonal modulation of a gene injected into rat heart in vivo. Proc Natl Acad Sci USA 1991: 88: 4138.

40. Acsadi G, et al. Direct gene transfer and expression into rat heart in vivo. New Biol 1991: 3 : 71.

41. Buttrick PM, et al. Behaviour of genes directly injected into the rat heart in vivo. Circ Res 1992: 70: 193.

42. Von Harsdorf R, et al. Gene injection into canine myocardium as a useful model for studying gene expression in the heart of large mammals. Circ Res 1993: 72: 688.

43. Gal D, et al. Direct myocardial transfection in two animal models : evaluation of parameters affecting gene expression and percutaneous gene delivery. Lab Invest 1993: 68: 18.

44. Sen A, et al. Terminally differentiated neonatal rat myocardial cell proliferate and maintain specific differentiated functions following expressio of SV40 large T antigen. J Biol Chem 1988: 263: 19132.

45. Kirshenbaum LA, et al. Highly efficient gene transfer into adult ventricular myocytes by recombinant adenovirus. J Clin Invest 1993: 92: 381.

46. Kass-Eisler A, et al. Quantitative determination of adenovirus-mediated gene delivery to rat cardiac myocytes in vitro and in vivo. Proc Natl Acad Sci USA 1993: 90: 11498.

47. Friedman JM, et al. Cellular promoters incorporated into adenovirus genome : cell specificity of albumin and immunoglobin expression. Mol Cell Biol 1986: 6: 3791.

48. Babiss LE, Friedman JM, Darnell JE Jr. Cellular promoters incorporated into the adenoviral genome : effects of viral regulatory elements on transcription rates and cell specificity of albumin and b-globin promoters. Mol Cell Biol 1986: 6: 3798.

49. Mittal SK, et al. Monitoring foreign gene expression by a human adenovirus-based vector using the firefly luciferase gene as a reporter. Virus Res 1993: 28: 67.

50. Guzman RJ, et al. Efficient gene transfer into myocardium by direct injection of adenovirus vectors. Circ Res 1993: 73: 1202.

51. French BA, et al. Direct in vivo gene transfer into porcine myocardium using replication-deficient adenoviral vectors. Circulation 1994: 90: 2414.

52. Barr E, et al. Efficient catheter-mediated gene transfer into the heart using replication-defective adenovirus. Gene Ther 1994: 1: 51.

53. Stratford-Perricaudet LD, et al. Widespread long-term gene transfer to mouse skeletal muscles and heart. J Clin Invest 1992: 90: 626.

54. Yang Y, et al. Cellular immunity to viral antigens limits E1-deleted adenoviruses for gene therapy. Proc Natl Acad Sci USA 1994: 91: 4407.

55. Partridge TA, et al. Conversion of mdx myofibres from dystrophin-negative to -positive by injection of normal myoblasts. Nature 1989: 337: 176.

56. Salminen A, et al. Implantation of recombinant rat myocytes into adult skeletal muscle : a potential gene therapy. Hum Gene Ther 1991: 2: 15.

57. Koh GY, et al. Differentiation and long-term survival of C2C12 myoblast grafts in heart. J Clin Invest 1993: 92: 1548.

58. Soonpaa MH, et al. Formation of nascent intercalated disks between grafted fetal cardiomyocytes and host myocardium. Science 1994: 264: 98.

59. Dausse E, et al. Familial hypertrophic cardiomyopathy : microsatellite haplotyping and identification of a hot spot for mutations in the β-myosin heavy chain gene. J Clin Invest 1993: 2807.

60. Sartorelli V, et al. Muscle specific gene expression : a comparison of cardiac and skeletal muscle transcription strategies. Circ Res 1993: 72: 925.

61. Yu Q-T, et al. Hypertrophic cardiomyopathy mutation is expressed in messenger RNA of skeletal as well as cardiac muscle. Circulation 1993: 406.

62. Roberts R. Molecular genetics : therapy or terror ? Circulation 1994: 89: 499.

63. Koenig M, et al. Complete coning of the Duchenne muscular dystrophy (DMD) cDNA and preliminary genomic organization of the DMD gene in normal and affected individuals. Cell 1987: 50: 509.

64. Koenig M, Kunkel LM. Detailed analysis of the repeat domain of dystrophin reveals four potential hinge segments that may confer flexibility. J Biol Chem 1990: 265: 4560.

65. Bulfield G, et al. X chromosome - linked muscular dystrophy (mdx) in the mouse. Proc Natl Acad Sci USA 1984: 81: 1189.

66. Ragot T, et al. Efficient adenovirus-mediated transfer of a human minidystrophin gene to skeletal muscle of mdx mice. Nature 1993: 361: 647.

67. Acsadi G, et al. Human dystrophin expression in mdx mice after intramuscular injection of DNA constructs. Nature 1991: 52: 815.

68. Mendell JR, et al. Myoblast transfer in the treatment of Duchenne's muscular dystrophy. N Engl J Med 1995: 333: 832.

69. Law PK, Goodwin TG, Wang MG. Normal myoblast injections provide genetic treatment for murine dystrophy. Muscle Nerve 1988: 11: 525.

70. Morgan JE, et al. Partial correction of an inherited biochemical defect of skeletal muscle by grafts of normal muscle precursor cells. J Neurol Sci 1988: 86: 137.

71. Rumyantsev PP. Interrelations of the proliferation and differentiation processes during cardiac myogenesis and regeneration. Int Rev Cytol 1977: 51: 186.

72. Jackson T, et al. The *c-myc* proto-oncogene regulates cardiac development in transgenic mice. Mol Cell Biol 1990: 10: 3709.

73. Swain JL, Stewart TA, Leder P. Parental legacy determines methylation and expression of an autosomal transgene : a molecular mechanism for parental imprinting. Cell 1987: 50: 719.

74. Field LJ. Atrial natriuretic factor-SV40 T antigen transgene produce tumors and cardiac arrhythmias in mice. Science 1988: 239: 1029.

75. Bristow MR, et al. Decreased catecholamine sensitivity and beta-adrenergic-receptor density in failing human hearts. N Engl J Med 1982: 307: 205.

76. Lohse MJ, et al. Inhibition of β-adrenergic receptor kinase prevents rapid homologous desensitization of β2-adrenergic receptors. Proc Natl Acad Sci USA 1989: 86: 3011.

77. Bertin B, et al. Specific atrial overexpression of G protein coupled human beta 1 adrenoreceptors ib transgenic mice. Cardiovasc Res 1993: 27: 1606.

78. Milano CA, et al. Enhanced myocardial function in transgenic mice overexpressing the β2-adrenergic receptor. Science 1994: 264: 582.

79. Koch WJ, et al. Cardiac function in mice overexpressing the β-adrenergic receptor kinase or the βARK inhibitor. Science 1995: 268: 1350.

80. Brown MS, Goldstein JL. A receptor-mediated pathway for cholesterol homeostasis. Science 1986: 232: 34.

81. Russel DW, Esser V, Hobbs HH. Molecular basis of familial hypercholesterolemia. Arteriosclerosis 1989: 9 (suppl 1): 8.

82. Goldstein JL, Brown MS. Familial hypercholesterolemia. In : Scriver CR, Beaudet AL, Sly WS, Valle D, eds. *The Metabolic Basis of Inherited Disease*. New York, McGraw-Hill, 1991, 201.

83. Bilheimer DW, et al. Liver transplantation to provide low density lipoprotein receptors and lower plasma cholesterol in a child with homozygous familial hypercholesterolemia. N Engl J Med 1984: 311: 1658.

84. Chowdhury JR, et al. Long-term improvement of hypercholesterolemia after ex vivo gene therapy in LDLR deficient rabbits. Science 1991: 254: 1802.

85. Grossman M, Raper SE, Wilson JM. Transplantation of genetically modified hepatocytes in non-human primates. Hum Gene Ther 1992: 3: 501.

86. Grossman M, Wilson JM, Raper SE. A novel approach for introducing genetically modified hepatocytes into the portal circulation. J Lab Clin Med 1993: 121: 472.

87. Grossman M, et al. Successful ex vivo gene therapy to liver in a patient with familial hypercholesterolaemia. Nature Genetics 1994: 6: 335.

88. Grossman M, et al. A pilot study of ex vivo gene therapy for homozygous familial hypercholesterolemia. Nature Med 1995: 1: 1148.

89. Ishibashi S, et al. Hypercholesterolemia in low density lipoprotein receptor knockout mice and its reversal by adenovirus-mediated gene delivery. J Clin Invest 1993: 92: 883.

90. Kozarsky KF, et al. In vivo correction of low density lipoprotein receptor deficiency in the Watanabe heritable hyperlipidemic rabbit with recombinant adenoviruses. J Biol Chem 1994: 269: 13695.

91. Li J, Fang RC, et al. In vivo gene therapy for hyperlipidemia : phenotypic correction in Watanabe rabbits by hepatic delivery of the rabbit LDL receptor gene. J Clin Invest 1995: 95: 768.

92. Kopfler WP, et al. Adenovirus-mediated transfer of a gene encoding human apolipoprotein A-1 into normal mice increases circulating high-density lipoprotein cholesterol. Circulation 1994: 90: 1319.

93. Paszty C, et al. Apolipoprotein A1 transgene corrects apolipoprotein E deficiency-induced atherosklerosis in ice. J Clin Invest 1994: 94: 899.

94. Miller NE. Associations of high-density lipoprotein subclasses and apolipoproteins with ischemic heart disease and coronary atherosclerosis. Am Heart J 1987: 113: 589.

95. Gordon DJ, et al. High density lipoprotein cholesterol and cardiovascular disease : four prospective American studies. Circulation 1989: 79: 8.

96. Badimon JJ, Badimon L, Fuster V. Regression of atherosclerotic lesions by high-density lipoprotein plasma fraction in the cholesterol fed rabbit. J Clin Invest 1990: 85: 1234.

97. Orvados JM, et al. Apolipoprotein A-1 gene polymorphism associated with premature coronary artery disease and familial hypoalphalipoproteinemia. N Engl J Med 1986: 314: 671.

98. Glueck CJ, et al. Longevity syndromes : familial hypobeta and familial hyperalpha lipoproteinemia. J Lab Clin Med 1976: 88: 941.

99. Rubin EM, et al. Inhibition of early atherogenesis in transgenic mice by human apolipoprotein A-1. Nature 1991: 353: 265.

100. Lie JT, Lawrie GM, Morris GC. Aortocoronary bypass saphenous vein graft atherosclerosis. Am J Cardiol 1977: 40: 906.

101. Kroncke GM, et al. Five-year changes in coronary arteries of medical and surgical patients of the Veterans Administration randomized study of bypass surgery. Circulation 1988: 78: 144.

102. MacMahon S, et al. Blood pressure, stroke and coronary heart disease : part 1, prolonged differences in blood pressure : prospective observational studies corrected for regression dilution bias. Lancet 1990: 335: 765.

103. Caulfield M, et al. Linage of the angiotensinogen gene to essential hypertension. N Engl J Med 1994: 330: 1629.

104. Fukamizu A, et al. Tissue-specific expression of the human renin gene in transgenic mice. Biochem Biophys Res Commun 1991: 165: 826.

105. Tomita N, et al. Hypertensive rats produced by in vivo introduction of the human renin gene. Circ Res 1993: 73: 898.

106. Wang C, Chao L, Chao J. Direct gene delivery of human tissue kallikrein reduces blood pressure in spontaneously hypertensive rats. J Clin Invest 1995: 95: 1710.

107. Xiong W, Chao J, Chao L. Muscle delivery of human kallikrein gene reduces blood pressure in hypertensive rats. Hypertension 195: 25: 715.

108. Stelzner TJ, et al. Increased lung endothelin-1 production in rats with idiopathic pulmonary hypertension. Am J Physiol 1992: 262: L614.

109. Giaid A, et al. Expression of endothelium -1 in the lungs of patients with pulmonary hypertension. N Engl J Med 1993: 1732.

110. Maruyama K, et al. Chronic hypoxic pulmonary hypertension in rats and increased elastolytic activity. Am J Physiol 1991: 261: H1716.

111. Katayose D, et al. Increased expression of PDGF A- and B-chain genes in rat lungs with hypoxic pulmonary hypertension. Am J Physiol 1993: 264: L100.

112. Botney MD, et al. Transforming growth factor -beta is decreased in remodeling hypertensive bovine arteries. J Clin Invest 1992: 89: 1629.

113. Perkett EA, et al. Insulin-like growth factor-1 and pulmonary hypertension induced by continous air embolization in sheep. Am J Respir Cell Mol Biol 1992: 6:82.

114. Muller DWM, et al. Percutaneous pulmonary vascular gene transfer and in vivo gene expression. Circ Res 1994: 75: 1039.

115. Schatner SK, et al. In vivo adenovirus-mediated gene transfer via the pulmonary artery of rats. Circ Res 1995: 76: 701.

116. Marshall E. Gene therapy's growing pains. Science 1995: 269: 1050.

117. Knowles MR, et al. A controlled study of adenoviral-vector-mediated gene transfer in the nasal epithelium of patients with cystic fibrosis. N Engl J Med 1995: 333: 823-31.

118. Wu GY, et al. Recetor - mediated gene delivery in vivo : partial correction of genetic analbuminemia in Nagase rats. J Biol Chem 1991: 266: 14338.

119. Kitsis RN, et al. Hormonal modulation of a gene injected into rat heart in vivo. Proc Natl Acad Sci USA 1991: 88: 4138.

Section E

NONINVASIVE CARDIOLOGY

23 NUCLEAR IMAGING TECHNIQUES

Diwakar Jain, Barry L. Zaret

Nuclear imaging techniques play an important role in the non-invasive evaluation of patients with established or suspected coronary artery disease.[1] A number of different radiopharmaceuticals and scintigraphic imaging techniques are available for obtaining important diagnostic and prognostic information about myocardial perfusion, cardiac function and myocardial necrosis in patients with cardiovascular disorders. This article briefly describes various cardiac nuclear imaging techniques, their applications in clinical practice and the recent developments in this field.

Myocardial perfusion imaging

The basic pathology in coronary artery disease is the luminal narrowing of coronary arteries due to the deposition of atheromatous material in its walls. This is a very complex and slowly evolving process, perhaps over several decades. Symptoms occur relatively late in the course of disease and appear only after significant narrowing of coronary arteries has already occurred. Coronary arterial narrowing interferes with myocardial perfusion downstream. With partial luminal narrowing, myocardial perfusion may be normal at rest, but fails to increase appropriately during conditions of increased demand such as during physical exertion or vasodilation. This is the basis of myocardial perfusion imaging with physical or pharmacological stress in clinical practice.

Radiotracers

Exercise myocardial perfusion imaging with Thallium-201 (^{201}Tl) is the most widely used technique for the detection of coronary artery disease.[2-4] The patient is stressed on a treadmill or bicycle with continuous electrocardiographic and blood pressure monitoring and 2-3 mCi of ^{201}Tl is injected intravenously at peak exercise. [201]Tl is rapidly extracted from the blood pool by the myocardium, skeletal muscle and several organs within next few minutes. Approximately 2%-4% of the injected dose of ^{201}Tl goes to the myocardium. Myocardial uptake is proportional to the blood flow. Cardiac imaging is started soon after the exercise. Myocardial segments perfused by narrowed coronary arteries or with scar due to prior myocardial infarction show diminished tracer uptake on these images. [201]Tl shows a continuous redistribution after the initial tissue extraction. Stress images are followed by redistribution images 2.5-4 hour later to detect reversibility in the segments with stress related perfusion abnormality. Perfusion abnormality due to ischemia reverses on redistribution images whereas that due to scar remains unchanged. Sometimes scar and ischemia coexist in the same segments in patients with prior myocardial infarction. This is characterized by partial reversibility of the perfusion abnormality. Stress ^{201}Tl imaging has a sensitivity of nearly 85-92% and a specificity of 90% or above for the detection of coronary artery disease.[1,5] In a significant proportion of defects due to ischemia ^{201}Tl redistribution may be incomplete.[6] Thus the standard stress-redistribution Tl-201 imaging may underestimate the true extent of myocardial viability. A number of different strategies have been proposed for overcoming this limitation.[7] A second injection of ^{201}Tl at rest, either on the same day or on a separate day, appears to be the most satisfactory way of overcoming this limitation in selected cases.[6-9]

Although, ^{201}Tl has been in clinical use for nearly 2 decades, it has several limitations. It has long physical half life (approximately 3 days) which limits the dose which can be used safely without causing undue radiation exposure to the patients. Furthermore, ^{201}Tl emits low energy photons (69-83 KeV) which can be easily attenuated by the thoracic wall and the soft tissue lying anterior to the heart. The attenuation can be particularly troublesome in obese patients and in women. This has lead to the development of a number of technetium-99m (^{99m}Tc) labeled myocardial perfusion agents. [99m]Tc has a shorter half life (approximately 6 hours) and emits slightly higher energy photons (140 KeV). These agents can be used in much higher dose and provide better quality images. Two agents: Sestamibi (Cardiolite, Du Pont Merck Inc.) Teboroxime (Cardiotech, Squibb Inc.) and Tetrofosmin (Myoview, Amersham Healhtcare Inc.) have been approved and are available for routine clinical use.[10,11] Sestamibi and tetrofosmin show little, if any, redistribution after its initial cardiac uptake. Therefore, 2 separate injections are required for stress and rest imaging. Teboroxime shows very rapid washout after initial myocardial uptake. This is an important drawback and therefore it is rarely used in clinical practice these days. Another new ^{99m}Tc labeled agents: Tetrofosmin (Myoview, Amersham Healthcare Inc.) and Q-12 (Furifosmin, Mallinckrodt Inc.) is undergoing advanced clinical studies.[12-14] Tetrofosmin and Q-12 have some advantage over sestamibi because of lower liver uptake and better target to background ratio. Q-12 has not yet been approved for routine clinical use (Table 23.1). Figure 23.1a and 23.1b shows ^{201}Tl and ^{99m}Tc-tetrofosmin images of a patient with atypical chest pain. There

Table 23.1   DIFFERENT AGENTS FOR MYOCARDIAL PERFUSION IMAGING
AND THEIR SALIENT FEATURES.

Agent	Physical 1/2 Life	Myocardial Redistribution	Retention	Main Route of Excretion
Tl-201	72 hrs	Good	Yes	Renal
99mTc-sestamibi	6 hrs	Good	Minimal	Hepatobiliary
99mTc-Teboroxime	6 hrs	Poor	Yes	Hepatobiliary
99mTc-Tetrofosmin	6 hrs	Good	Probably none	Hepatobiliary
99mTc-Furifosmin	6 hrs	Good	Unknown	Hepatobiliary

is significant soft tissue attenuation on Tl-201 images which can interfere with image interpretation, but there is no soft tissue attenuation on ^{99m}Tc-tetrofosmin images.

Another advantage of ^{99m}Tc labeled agents is that first pass imaging can also be carried out during injection of radiotracer during stress and rest.[15] This can provide additional information about left and right ventricular function. Thus it is possible to obtain information about myocardial perfusion and cardiac function with a single test.

Instrumentation

Imaging can be carried out using a planar camera or a tomographic camera (SPECT imaging). With planar camera, imaging is carried out in 3 different views: anterior, left anterior oblique and left lateral (Figures 23.1, 23.2). Whereas tomographic camera acquires a series of images (32-64 images) in a 180-360° orbit around the heart. These images are processed in a manner similar to that for CT images so that left ventricular myocardium is displayed in a series of slices of varying thickness (Figure 23.3). Planar imaging equipment is simpler and less expansive than tomographic imaging equipment. Tomographic imaging particularly with ^{99m}Tc labeled agents allows better anatomic delineation of the perfusion abnormalities. Both techniques have comparable sensitivity for the detection of coronary artery disease, but tomography allows a better angiographic correlation. However, tomographic imaging is prone to a number of artifacts as a result of patient motion during imaging, and attenuation by various extracardiac structures. A meticulous effort is required to prevent false interpretation of the images due to these artifacts. A number of image processing techniques are under development for the prevention of artifacts during tomographic imaging. The tomographic images can be gated with ECG (gated SPECT) for the simultaneous assessment of myocardial perfusion and function.

Types of stress

Treadmill exercise is the preferred method of stress testing. Information about total exercise capacity; changes in heart rate and blood pressure; adverse symptoms such

Thallium

Stress   Redist.

Breast markers

Stress   Redist.

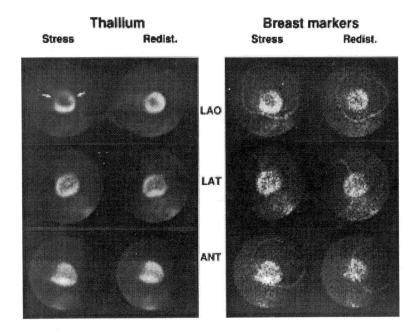

LAO

LAT

ANT

Tc-99m-tetrofosmin

Stress (8.5mCi)   Rest (23mCi)
30 min PI   60 min PI

Breast markers

Stress   Rest

LAO

LAT

ANT

as chest pain and undue fatigue; and electrocardiographic changes such as ST segment depression and arrhythmias are important clinically. In patients who are unable to perform any kind of exercise due to severe peripheral vascular disease, musculoskeletal disorders or pulmonary disease, pharmacological agents can be used for myocardial perfusion imaging. Dipyridamole (Persantine) is the most widely used agent for this purpose.[16-18] Following intravenous administration, this causes marked coronary vasodilatation and can increase myocardial blood flow 2-4 times the resting flow. However, blood flow increase is blunted in the myocardial segments perfused by narrowed coronary arteries. This produces flow heterogeneity and results in apparent perfusion abnormalities on the perfusion images.

Dipyridamole imaging is used routinely for identifying patients at high risk for adverse cardiac events following surgery for peripheral vascular disease.[17,18] Cardiac related causes account for a large proportion of morbidity and mortality following peripheral vascular surgery. Figure 23.2 shows an abnormal dipyridamole ^{201}Tl images of a patient with severe coronary artery disease and impaired left ventricular function. Intravenous adenosine can also be used in place of dipyridamole.[19] At a cellular level, dipyridamole acts by inhibiting the intracellular uptake of adenosine. Thus adenosine is more directly acting than dipyridamole and has more predictable effect on the coronary blood flow. Adenosine has an extremely short half life and its side effects are transient. Theophylline derivatives including caffeine act as antagonists of dipyridamole and adenosine at the cellular level and should be stopped prior to performing dipyridamole or adenosine stress ^{201}Tl imaging. Recently, intravenous dobutamine has been used for stress imaging.[20] This acts by increasing the heart rate and myocardial oxygen demand. This can be used in patients where dipyridamole or adenosine are contraindicated such as in patients with severe bronchopulmonary disease or congestive heart failure or in those where theophylline can not be stopped. Another analog of dobutamine, arbutamine is undergoing clinical studies.[21] Table 23.2 lists various pharmacological agents for myocardial perfusion imaging and their important characteristics.

Clinical applications of myocardial perfusion imaging

Detection of coronary artery disease. Myocardial perfusion imaging is useful for establishing the diagnosis of coronary artery disease in patients presenting with chest pain or in those with a high clinical suspicion of coronary artery disease because of the presence of one or more risk factors for coronary artery disease. This

---

Figure 23.1 (a). Stress-redistribution ^{201}Tl images and breast markers of a female patient with long standing hypertension and atypical chest pain. (b). Stress and rest ^{99m}Tc-tetrofosmin (Myoview) images and corresponding breast markers of the same patient. Standard 3 view planar images are displayed. Note significant soft-tissue attenuation on Tl-201 images (arrows) which can interfere with image interpretation. There is no attenuation with ^{99m}Tc-tetrofosmin. LAO= Left Anterior Oblique view; LAT= Lateral view; ANT= Anterior view.

Dipyridamole Thallium
Stress   Redist.

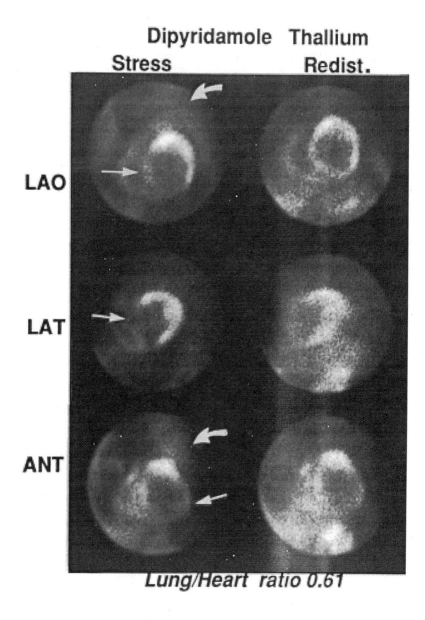

Lung/Heart ratio 0.61

Figure 23.2 Dipyridamole stress ^{201}Tl and redistribution images in 3 standard planar views of a patient with peripheral vascular disease. Note dilated left ventricle with a large partially reversible perfusion abnormality involving the anterior wall, septum and apex (straight arrows). In addition there is increased lung ^{201}Tl uptake (curved arrows). Lung to heart ratio was 0.69 (normal is <0.50).

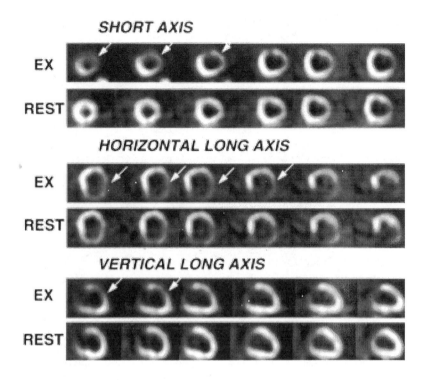

Figure 23.3 Exercise and rest tomographic images with ^{99m}Tc-sestamibi of a patient with anterior and lateral wall ischemia (arrows). The images are displayed in standard short axis, horizontal and vertical long axis.

is an important non-invasive test for identifying patients who should be considered for further invasive studies. Addition of myocardial perfusion imaging to exercise ECG increases the sensitivity as well as specificity of the test for the detection of coronary artery disease.[22] The sensitivity and specificity of exercise ECG alone are 50-60% and 60% respectively for the detection of coronary artery disease, whereas myocardial perfusion imaging has a sensitivity of 85-90% and specificity of 90% for the detection of coronary artery disease. Myocardial perfusion imaging has particular advantage over exercise ECG in patients with left ventricular hypertrophy, LBBB and other abnormalities interfering with proper interpretation of ST segment changes on exercise.

Risk stratification of patients with CAD. Information about the severity, location and extent of myocardial ischemia is useful for risk stratification of patients with known coronary artery disease. Large area of perfusion abnormality or multiple areas of perfusion abnormality identify patients at high risk for cardiovascular events on follow up. Increased lung ^{201}Tl uptake and transient left ventricular dilatation on stress images are also indicative of severe coronary artery disease and are predictive

Table 23.2   DIFFERENT AGENTS FOR PHARMACOLOGICAL STRESS
PERFUSION IMAGING

Agent	Mode of Action	Effect on HR	Effect on SBP	Effect on Double product
Dipyridamole	Coronary vasodilation	slight increase	Decrease	minimal change
Adenosine	Coronary vasodilation	slight increase	Decrease	minimal change
Dobutamine	Increased myocardial oxygen demand	Increase	increase or no change	increase
Arbutamine	Increased myocardial oxygen demand	Increase	increase or no change	increase

of poor prognosis in patients with known coronary artery disease.[23-25] Normal myocardial perfusion imaging is associated with an excellent long term prognosis and a very low incidence of cardiac events on follow up even in the presence of angiographically documented coronary artery disease.[26,27]

Post myocardial infarction evaluation. Submaximum stress ^{201}Tl imaging is an established technique for risk stratification of patients with uncomplicated myocardial infarction prior to hospital discharge.[28,29] Patients with fixed defects have low incidence of adverse cardiac events whereas those with reversible defects have higher incidence of adverse cardiac events. This test can be used to identify patients with recent myocardial infarction who can benefit from cardiac cathetrization and revascularization. With the routine use of thrombolysis in patients with acute myocardial infarction, a substantial reduction in in-hospital mortality as well as 1 year mortality has been achieved.[30] Whether routine predischarge submaximum stress ^{201}Tl in these patients is still useful for risk stratification similar to that in the prethrombolytic era is not clear. However, at this stage the use of predischarge stress ^{201}Tl imaging is still recommended.

Detection of acute myocardial infarction. Resting myocardial perfusion imaging can be used for early detection of acute myocardial infarction in patients presenting with chest pain in the absence of typical electrocardiographic changes of evolving myocardial infarction.[31] Serial myocardial perfusion imaging at rest has been used for studying the efficacy of thrombolytic agents in reducing myocardial infarct size.[32,33]

Risk stratification prior to non-cardiac surgery. Adverse cardiac events are important cause of morbidity and mortality following non-cardiac surgery.[34] Appropriate use of nuclear imaging techniques can significantly lower this complication. The frequency of occurrence of adverse cardiac events in the perioperative period depends upon a number of factors: the prevalence of coronary artery disease in the patient population and the nature and severity of hemodynamic stress during the perioperative period. Patients with a high prevalence of coronary artery disease either symptomatic or occult are particularly vulnerable to cardiac events. Prolonged vascular surgery involving cross-clamping of the aorta, major shifts between intra-vascular and extravascular fluid compartments and hypotension impose significant stress on the cardiovascular system and can result in arrythmias, pulmonary edema or myocardial infarction in the perioperative period in patients with coronary artery disease. Patients with peripheral vascular disease have a high prevalence of coronary artery disease and are at a high risk of perioperative cardiac events. Even after peripheral vascular surgery, these patients continue to have very high morbidity and mortality due to cardiac events.[35] A number of studies have established the role of dipyridamole ^{201}Tl imaging for identifying patients at high risk for preoperative cardiac events.[17,18,36] Dipyridamole ^{201}Tl imaging is particularly suitable for this patient population because of their inability to do exercise. Abnormalities on dipyridamole ^{201}Tl are not only predictive of perioperative morbidity and mortality but also of long term mortality and morbidity.[37,38]

Assessment of left ventricular function

Left ventricular function can be assessed by first pass imaging or equilibrium radionuclide angiocardiography.

First pass imaging

First pass imaging is done by dynamic imaging of the passage of radioactivity from the superior vena cava to right heart, lungs and then to left heart after injecting a bolus of radiotracer into the peripheral arm. Right and left ventricular ejection fraction can be calculated from these data. An important advantage of the newer ^{99m}Tc labeled myocardial perfusion imaging agents is that dynamic first pass imaging can be carried out during the injection of these agents. Thus information about perfusion and function can be obtained from the same injection of radiopharmaceutical.[15]

Equilibrium radionuclide angiocardiography

Equilibrium radionuclide angiocardiography (ERNA) is performed by labeling the blood pool with ^{99m}Tc-pertechnetate. The ECG gated images of the heart are acquired in three standard views (anterior, left anterior oblique and left lateral) to assess the left ventricular wall motion and to calculate left ejection fraction. Left ventricular ejection fraction (LVEF) is the most widely used index of left ventricular function. In patients with coronary artery disease, left ventricular ejection fraction is an important determinant of long term prognosis.[39,40]

Determination of left ventricular ejection fraction also has important therapeutic implications in patients with coronary artery disease. Progressive spontaneous deterioration of LVEF occurs in patients with moderately impaired LVEF (EF<40%) due to ventricular remodeling. This process can be arrested by appropriate use of angiotensin converting enzyme inhibitors.[41]

Serial LVEF monitoring is also useful for the prevention of congestive heart failure in patients receiving doxorubicin therapy. Congestive heart failure is an important complication of doxorubicin therapy. However, with use of appropriate guidelines, it is possible to reduce the incidence of congestive heart failure from 20% to 2-3%.[42,43]

Exercise ERNA. ERNA can also be carried out during exercise. Initially this was used for the detection of coronary artery disease. However, with the wide spread use of myocardial perfusion imaging, exercise radionuclide angiocardiography is rarely used these days for the detection of coronary artery disease. Exercise radionuclide angiocardiography has also been used for the risk stratification of patients with known coronary artery disease. A significant drop in left ventricular ejection fraction with exercise is indicative of poor prognosis despite a preserved left ventricular ejection fraction at baseline.[44]

Left ventricular volumes and pressure volume relations

From the equilibrium radionuclide angiocardiography absolute left ventricular end-diastolic, end-systolic and stroke volumes can also be measured.[45] By knowing the heart rate and blood pressure it is also possible to measure the cardiac output and peripheral vascular resistance. Thus a comprehensive assessment of hemodynamic status can be obtained using this test. Recently, exercise radionuclide angiocardiography has been used in conjunction with another non-invasive device for indirect measurement of ascending aortic pressure, to study the pressure-volume based indices of left ventricular contractility.[46] This appears to be a promising technique for studying intrinsic left ventricular contractility and left ventricular contractile reserve.[47]

Ambulatory left ventricular function monitoring

A combination of the principle of equilibrium radionuclide angiocardiography with Holter monitoring has resulted in a device for the continuous ambulatory monitoring of left ventricular function over several hours.[48] After blood pool labeling with ^{99m}Tc-pertechnetate, a miniature radiation detector is positioned on the chest which monitors and records the left ventricular blood pool activity on a modified Holter monitor. This technique has been used for studying the effects of interventions such as mental stress on left ventricular function and for detecting spontaneous changes in left ventricular function in patients with coronary artery disease.[49] *Figure 23.4* shows the left ventricular function and heart rate, relative end-diastolic and end-systolic volume trends at baseline, with mental stress and with exercise in a patient with chronic stable coronary artery disease. This patient shows a significant fall in LVEF with two different forms of mental stress which was not accompanied by any symptoms or ST segment depression. A recent study indicates that mental stress induced left ventricular dysfunction is predictive of adverse cardiac events in patients with chronic stable angina.[50] *Figure 23.5* shows the incidence of adverse cardiac events over one year in coronary artery disease patients with and without mental

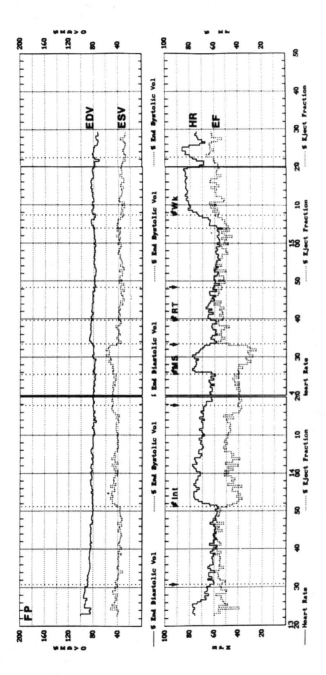

Figure 23.4 Continuous data trend over 2.5 hours of left ventricular ejection fraction (EF), heart rate (HR)) (lower panel) and relative end-diastolic (EDV) and end-systolic volumes (ESV) (upper panel) of a patient with chronic stable angina. The EF and HR are normal at baseline. After a period of stabilization patient underwent psychological interview (Int). This was accompanied by a slight increase in HR, a significant fall in EF and increase in ESV. Mental arithmetic (MS), another form of mental stress produced similar changes. In contrast, computer choice reaction time (RT), a non-stressful task produced no change in EF or HR. Walking (Wk) resulted in marked increase in HR but no change in EF.

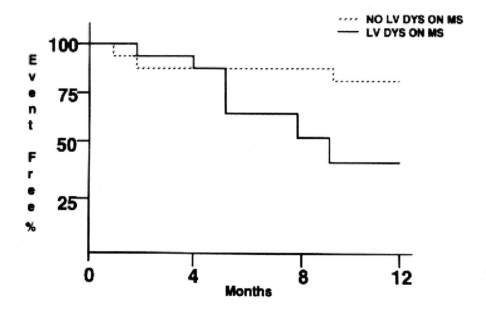

Figure 23.5 Cardiac event free survival rate in 2 groups of patients with chronic stable angina. One group of patient had left ventricular dysfunction in response to mental stress (MS) and the other group had no left ventricular dysfunction in response to mental stress. A significantly greater proportion of patients with mental stress induced left ventricular dysfunction developed cardiac events over 1 year. (Reproduced with permission[50]).

stress induced left ventricular dysfunction. Spontaneous episodes of left ventricular dysfunction can be detected by ambulatory left ventricular function monitoring in patients with non-Q wave myocardial infarction, unstable angina and Q-wave myocardial infarction treated with thrombolytic agents.[51] Preliminary studies have shown, that, in patients with acute myocardial infarction treated with thrombolytic agents, episodes of spontaneous left ventricular dysfunction are predictive of poor prognosis.[52] However, this observation needs to be verified in larger patient population.[33]

Myocardial necrosis imaging

[99m]Tc-pyrophosphate was used for imaging acute myocardial necrosis in 70s and 80s. However due to several technical drawbacks this is only rarely used these days. Recently, indium-111 (^{111}In) labeled Fab fraction of antibody against cardiac myosin (^{111}In-antimyosin) (Centocor Inc.) has been used for imaging necrotic myocardium. This agent is highly selective for necrotic myocardium.[53] This has high sensitivity and specificity for diagnosing acute myocardial infarction. ^{111}In-antimyosin imaging can be used for confirming the diagnosis of acute myocardial infarction in patients with atypical clinical presentation or in those where electrocardiographic

changes are absent or unreliable for diagnosing of acute myocardial infarction.[54] This agent is also useful for diagnosing acute myocarditis, and for detection of cardiac rejection in recipients of heart transplantation.[55,56] ^{111}In-antimyosin imaging has also been used for evaluating the cardiotoxicity of antineoplastic agents such as doxorubicin.[43,57]

Positron emission tomography

Positron emission tomography involves the use of positron emitting isotopes (^{11}C, ^{18}F, ^{13}N, ^{15}O). Positrons disintegrate into two gamma rays released at 180° and can be detected by an array of detectors placed around the patient. These tracers are of relatively short half life and require an on-site cyclotron for production. A detailed description of these agents is beyond the scope of this article. These isotopes can be incorporated into a number of metabolic substrates such as deoxyglucose, fatty acids and acetate and are useful for studying the metabolic activity of myocardium.[58]

New radiotracers

A number of new radiotracers are in various stages of clinical development. Monoclonal antibodies to platelet glycoprotein IIb/IIIa and fibrin labeled with indium-111 or ^{99m}Tc have been used for thrombus imaging.[59] Metaiodobenzylguanidine (MIBG) labeled with iodine-123 has been used for imaging cardiac sympathetic neuronal activity.[60] ^{123}I-labeled fatty acids such as iodophenylpentadecanoic acid (IPPA) and 15-(p-iodophenyl)3R, S-methylpentadecanoic acid (BMIPP) have been used for studying regional myocardial fatty acid metabolism. This is useful in studying the extent of myocardial viability.[61]

Conclusion

Radionuclide imaging techniques have greatly enhanced our understanding of cardiovascular physiology and pathology. These techniques play a crucial role in the proper evaluation of patients with definite or suspected coronary artery disease and for optimal utilization of various therapeutic options.

REFERENCES

1. Zaret BL, Wackers F J Th. Nuclear cardiology (Two Parts). New Engl J Med 1993: 329:775.

2. Ritchie JL, et al. Myocardial imaging with Thallium-201 : a multicenter study in patients with angina pectoris or acute myocardial infarction. Am J Cardiol, 1978: 42: 345.

3. Strauss HW, et al. Thallium-201 for myocardial imaging. Relation of thallium-201 to regional myocardial perfusion. Circulation, 1975: 51:641.

4. Kaul S, et al. Determination of the quantitative thallium imaging variables that oprimize detection of coronary artery disease. Am Coll Cardiol, 1986: 7:527.

5. Wackers F J Th, et al. Quantitative planar thallium-stress scintigraphy: a critical evaluation of the method. Sem Nucl Med 1985: 15:46.

6. Jain D, Zaret BL. Nuclear Imaging Techniques for the Assessment of Myocardial Viability. Cardiology Clinics 1995: 13:43.

7. Wackers FJTh. The maze of myocardial perfusion imaging protocols in 1994. J Nucl Cardiol 1994: 1:180.

8. Dilsizian V, et al. Enhanced detection of ischemic but viable myocardium by the reijection of thallium after stress-redistribution imaging. N Engl J Med 1990: 323: 141.

9. Kayden DS, et al. Thallium-201 for assessment of myocardial viability : quantitative comparison of 24-hour redistribution imaging with imaging after reinjection at rest. J Am Coll Cardiol 18: 1480.

10. Wackers F J Th, et al. Technetium-99m Hexakis 2-Methoxyisobutyl Isonitrile : Human biodistribution, dosimetry, safety and preliminary comaprison to thallium-201 for myocardial perfusion imaging. J Nucl Med 1989: 30:301.

11. Hendel RC, et al. Diagnostic value of new myocardial perfusion agent. Teboroxime (SQ 30217), utilizing a rapid planar imaging protocol : preliminary results. J Am Coll Cardiol 1990:161:855.

12. Jain D, et al. Biokinetics of 99mTc-Tetrofosmin : Myocardial Perfusion Imaging Agent: Implications for a One Day Imaging Protocol. J Nucl Med 1993: 34:1254.

13. Zaret BL, et al. Myocardial perfusion imaging with technetium-99m tetrofosmin: Comparison to thallium-201 imaging and coronary angiography in a phase III multicenter trial. Circulation 91: 313.

14. Rossetti C, et al. Q 12 : A new 99mTc myocardial perfusion agent with optimized imaging properties : Evaluation in humans. J Nucl Med 1991: 32: 1007.

15. Iskandrian AS, et al. Use of technetium-99m isonitrile in assessing left ventricular perfusion and function at rest and during exercise in coronary artery disease and comparison with coronary angiography and exercise thallium-201 SPECT imaging. Am J Cardiol 1989: 64: 270.

16. Shaw L, et al. Prognostic value of dipyridamole thallium-201 imaging in elderly patients. J Am Coll Cardiol 1992: 1390.

17. Eagle KA, et al. Dipyridamole-thallium scanning in patients undergoing vascular surgery : oprimizing preoperative evaluation of cardiac risk. JAMA 1987: 257: 2185.

18. Boucher CA, et al. Determination of cardiac risk by dipyridamole-thallium imaging before peripheral vascular surgery. N Engl J Med 1985: 312: 389.

19. Nishimura S, et al. Equivalence between adenosine and exercise thallium-201 myocardial tomography : a multicenter, prospective, crossover trial. J Am Coll Cardiol 1992: 20: 265.

20. Pennell DJ, et al. Dobutamine thallium myocardial perfusion tomography. J Am Coll Cardiol 1991: 18: 1471.

21. Hammond HK, McKirnan MD. Effects of dobutamine and arbutamine on regional myocardial function in a porcine model of myocardial ischemia. J Am Coll Cardiol 1994: 23:475.

22. Beller GA, Gibson RS. Sensitivity, specificity and prognostic significance of noninvasive testing for occult or known coronary disease. Prog Cardiovasc Dis 1987: 24: 241.

23. Boucher CA, et al. Increased lung uptake of thallium-201 during exercise myocardial imaging : Clinical, hemodynamic and angiographic implications in patients with coronary artery disease. Am J Cardiol, 1980: 46: 189.

24. Jain D, et al. Lung thallium uptake on rest, stress and redistribution cardiac imaging : State-of-the-art-review. Am Jour Card Img 1990: 4:303.

25. Gill JB, et al. Prognostic importance of thallium uptake by the lungs during exercise in coronary artery disease. N Engl J Med, 1987: 317: 1485.

26. Wackers FJT, et al. Prognostic significance of normal quantitative planar thallium-201 stress scintigraphy in patients with chest pain. J Am Coll Cardiol 1985: 6: 27.

27. Wahl JM, et al. Prognostic implications of normal exercise Tl-201 images. Arch Intern Med 1985: 145: 253.

28. Gibson RS, et al. Prediction of cardiac events after uncomplicated myocardial infarction : a prospective study comparing predischarge exercise thallium-201 scintigraphy and coronary angiography. Circulation 1983: 68: 321.

29. Brown KA, et al. Usefulness of residual ischemic myocardium within prior infarct zone for identifying patients at high risk late after acute myocardial infarction. Am J Cardiol 60: 15.

30. Haber HL, et al. Exercise thallium-201 scintigraphy after thrombolytic therapy with or without angioplasty for acute myocardial infarction. Am J Cardiol 1993: 71: 1257.

31. Wackers FJTh, et al. Potential value of Thallium-201 scintigraphy as a means of selecting patients for the coronary care unit. Br Heart Jour 1979: 41: 111.

32. Wackers F J Th, et al. Serial quantitative planar technetium-99m isonitrile imaging in acute myocardial infarction :Efficacy for noninvasive assessment of thrombolytic therapy. J Am Coll Cardiol 1989: 14: 861.

33. Jain D, et al. Radionuclide imaging techniques in the thrombolytic era : In Becker R Ed: the modern era of Coroanry Thrombolysis, pub Kluver Academic Publishers, Norwell MA, first edition 1994.

34. Jain D, et al. Diagnosing perioperative myocardial infarction in noncardiac surgery. International Anesthesiology Clinics 1992: 30: 199.

35. Farkouh ME, et al. Influence of coronary heart disease on morbidity and mortality after lower extremity revascularization surgery : A population-based study in Olmstead county. Minessota . J Am Coll Cardiol 1994: 24: 1290.

36. Leppo JA. Preoperative cardiac risk assessment for noncardiac surgery. Am J Cardiol 1995: 75: 42D.

37. Hendel RC, et al. Prediction of late cardiac events of dipyridamole thallium-201 imaging in patients undergoing elective vascular surgery. Am J Cardiol 1992: 70: 1243.

38. Fleisher LA, et al. Preoperative dipyridamole thallium imaging and Holter monitoring as a predictor of perioperative cardiac events and long term outcome. Anesthesiology 1995:25:122.

39. Lee KL, et al. Prognostic value of radionuclide angiography in medically treated pateints with coronary artery disease : a comparison with clinical and cathetrization variables. Circulation 1990 : 82: 1705.

40. Cohn JN. The vasodilator heart failure trial (V-HeFT). Mechanistic data from the cooperative studies : introduction. circulation 87 (suppl): VI 1.

41. The SOLVD Investigators. Effects of enalapril on mortality and the development of heart failure in asymptomatic patients with reduced left ventricular ejection fractions. N Engl J Med 1992: 327: 685.

42. Schwartz RG, et al. Congestive heart failure and left ventricular dysfunction complicating doxorubicin therapy : Seven-year experience using serial radionuclide angiocardiography. Am J Med 1987: 82: 1109.

43. Jain D, Zaret BL. Antimyosin cardiac imaging : Will it play a role in the detection of doxorubicin cardiotoxicity ? J Nucl Med 1990 :1970.

44. Bonow RP, et al. Exercise-induced ischemia in mildy symptomatic patients with coronary artery disease and preserved left ventricular function: identification of subgroups at risk of death during mediacl therapy. N Engl J Med 1984: 311: 1339.

45. Massardo T, et al. Left ventricular volume calculation using a count-based ratio method applied to multigated radionuclide angiography. J Nucl Med 1990: 31: 450.

46. Marmor A, et al. Left ventricular peak power during exercise : A noninvasive approach for assessment of contractile reserve. J Nucl Med 1993: 34: 1877.

47. Marmor A, et al. Beyond ejection fraction. J Nucl Cardiol 1: 477.

48. Zaret BL, Jain D. Continuous monitoring of left ventricular function with miniaturized nonimaging detectors. In Zaret Bl,.Beller CA Ed : Nuclear Cardiology : State of the art and future directions, pub. Mosby Year Book, St. Louis, 1993 p 137.

49. Burg MM, et al. Role of behavioral and psychological factors in mental stress induced silent left ventricular dysnfunction in coronary artery disease. J Am Coll Cardiol 1993: 22: 440.

50. Jain D, et al. Prognostic significance of mental stress induced left ventricular dysfunction in patients with coronary artery disease. Am J Cardiol July 1995: 76: 31.

51. Jain D, et al. Transient silent left ventricular dysfunction in non-Q wave myocardial infarction and unstable angina. J Nucl Med 1991, 32 Suppl 938.

52. Kayden DS, et al. Silent left ventricular dysfunction during routine activity after thrombolytic therapy for acute myocardial infarction. J Am Coll Cardiol 1990: 15: 1500.

53. Jain D, et al. Indium-111 Antimyosin images compared with Triphenyl Tetrazolium Chloride Staining in a patient 6 days after myocardial infarction. J Nucl Med 1990:31:231.

54. Jain D, et al. Immunoscintigraphy for detecting acute myocardial infarction without electrocardiographic changes. Br Med J 1990: 300, 151.

55. Dec GW, et al. Antimyosin antibody cardiac imaging : its role in the diagnosis of myocarditis. J Am Coll Cardiol 1990: 16:97.

56. Jain D, Zaret BL. Antimyosin cardiac imaging in acute myocarditis. J Am Coll Cardiol 1990: 16: 105.

57. Estorch M, et al. ^{111}In-antimyosin scintigraphy after doxorubicin therapy in patients with advanced breast cancer. J Nucl Med 1990: 31: 1965.

58. Schelbert HR. Positron emission tomography as a biochemical probe for human myocardial ischemia. In Zaret BL, Kaufman L, Dunn R, Berson A eds. Frontiers of cardiac imaging. New York : Raven Press 53.

59. Straton JR, Ritchie JL. 111In-platelet imaging of left ventricular thrombi : predictive value for systemic emboli. Circulation 1990:1182.

60. Schofer J, et al. Iodine-123 metaiodobenzylguanidine scintigraphy : A noninvasive method to demonstrate myocardial adrenergic nervous system integrity in patients with idiopathic dilated cardiomyopathy. J Am Coll Cardiol 1988: 12:1252.

61. Matsunari I, et al. Kinetics of iodine-123-BMIPP in patients with prior myocardial infarction: assessment with dynamic rest and stress images compared with stress thallium-201 SPECT. J Nucl Med 1994: 35: 1279.

24 ECHOCARDIOGRAPHY IN THE EVALUATION OF CORONARY ARTERY DISEASE

Rebecca T. Hahn, Richard B. Devereux

Multiple facets of coronary artery disease can be evaluated by a number of currently available echocardiographic techniques with new technologies holding the promise of direct noninvasive evaluation of distal coronary arteries in the future. Assessment of regional left ventricular wall motion abnormalities and global function, and the detection of complications of acute myocardial infarction are well established uses of echocardiography. With the growing use of stress echocardiography, the diagnosis of significant coronary artery stenosis as well as risk stratification of patients with or without coronary artery disease have become additional uses of echocardiography. The evaluation of myocardial viability, coronary flow reserve and collateral circulation are areas of ongoing research and may soon become accepted uses for this versatile technique.

Acute myocardial infarction

The extent of regional left and/or right ventricular systolic dysfunction is related to the severity and duration of the reduction of coronary blood flow. Upon coronary artery occlusion, myocardial necrosis progresses from the subendocardium to the epicardium[1] with approximately 60% of the myocardium at risk undergoing necrosis after 3 hours of total occlusion. Following 6 hours of total occlusion, 70-80% of the myocardium at risk necroses. Echocardiographic wall motion abnormalities are very sensitive early marker for ischemia or infarction.[2-4] These wall motion abnormalities are characterized by a reduced amplitude and rate of endocardial excursion, and reduction and delay in wall thickening. The sensitivity of echocardiographic wall motion abnormalities for coronary occlusions, however, varies with the amount of myocardium involved, the extent of transmural involvement and the method used to describe the wall motion abnormality.

Canine studies have shown that the larger the acute infarct, the higher the sensitivity of echocardiography to detect wall motion abnormalties.[5,6] In general, there has been excellent correlation between quantitative estimates of circumferential infarct size by echocardiography, scintigraphy and histology.[7-9] The presence and degree of wall motion abnormalities visualized by echocardiography also varies depending on the extent of transmural involvement.[7] Dog studies have shown that wall thickening decreases by approximately 50% when the transmural extent of infarction is < 20% whereas wall thinning occurs when the transmural extent involves >20% of the wall thickness.[10] Consequently, many nontransmural infarcts can be visualized by echocardiography.[11] However, only one-third of patients presenting with a nontransmural infarct exhibit akinesis or dyskinesis, half of the patients exhibit some wall motion abnormality and the remaining patients have no detectable wall motion abnormality by echocardiography. In contrast, in approximately two-thirds of patients presenting with a transmural infarct the infarcted segments are akinetic or dyskinetic with severe hypokinesis seen in the remaining one-third of patients.

Regional myocardial function can be assessed semi-quantitatively (visually) or quantitatively. The two echocardiographic descriptors of regional ventricular function are endocardial excursion and wall thickening. Although the accuracy of visual assessments of both endocardial excursion and wall thickening clearly depend upon the echocardiographer's experience, the correlation between visual and quantitative measures depends on the severity of wall motion abnormality: agreement is high for regions of dyssynergy but more disparate for regions of hypokinesis. Many algorithms have been developed to assist in the assessment of regional wall motion abnormalities, including automatic border detection algorithms and, more recently, color kinesis. The latter is an algorithm in which time-related spatial charges in wall motion are color-coded to enable the physician to quickly semiquantitate wall motion abnormalities. Both automatic border detection and color kinesis are highly dependent on the skill of the examining sonographer, , and as such, can introduce further error into semiquanititative readings. Wall motion assessment remains one of the most difficult tasks of even the most experienced reader.

Complications of acute myocardial infarction

Left ventricular failure

Severe systolic dysfunction: As described above, echocarcardiography is an ideal tool for the noninvasive evaluation of regional and global left ventricular systolic function in the setting of actue ischemia or infarction. In addition, altered systolic function can be detected by echocardiography in myocardial segments adjacent to the ischemic-infarcted region (nonischemic border regions), possibly due to increased wall stress in these regions. After reperfusion of ischemic myocardium, a delay in functional recovery can occur. This delay, termed "stunning", can vary from minutes to days and can be followed over time noninvasively by echocardiography.

Although echocardiography may be helpful in the management and risk assessment of hemodynamically stable patients with myocardial infarction, it may be most useful in the differentiation among causes of cardiogenic shock in acute myocardial infarction. Cardiogenic shock is characterized by organ hypoperfusion and systemic hypotension secondary to cardiac dysfunction. The etiologies of cardiogenic shock in patients with coronary artery disease include not only severe, extensive left ventricular infarction, but also severe right ventricular infarction, papillary muscle infarction and ventricular septal rupture. Echocardiography is frequently the test of choice in the differentiating among these etiologies of cardiogenic shock.

Echocardiographic assessment of functional infarct size and remote asynergy also have prognostic importance. In one study, all patients with infarct areas involving less than 35% of the left ventricular surface area survived; in contrast, 59% of patients with infarcts >35% of the left ventricular surface area were nonsurvivors.[12] Two other studies showed that a high echocardiographic wall motion score was 85-89% sensitive and 82-83% specific for predicting cardiac complications including pump failure, malignant arrhythmias and death.[13,14] Remote asynergy are wall motion abnormalities outside the electrocardiographic infarct region. Its presence predicts an increased incidence of death, cardiogenic shock, high Killip classification and reinfarction.[15]

Diastolic dysfunction: Multiple studies have shown alterations in the transmitral diastolic flow velocity profiles in the setting of acute ischemia or infarct [16,17]. Although these changes are thought to reflect alterations in both relaxation and ventricular compliance, the results have been variable and unreliable, probably secondary to the multitude of factors that influence transmitral flow, including: preload, afterload, left atrial function, right ventricular function and pericardial constraint. To date, there is no reliable echocardiographic index for separating changes in relaxation-phase and atrial filling phase left ventricular diastolic function from effects of altered filling pressures.

Mitral regurgitation

Mild to moderate mitral regurgitation is common following acute myocardial infarction[18] and is secondary to ischemia or infarction of the papillary muscle or myocardium underlying the papillary muscle. The anterolateral papillary muscle has a dual blood supply from the left anterior descending and circumflex coronary arteries. The posteromedial papillary muscle typically is perfused by only the posterior descending coronary artery and therefore is most frequently dysfunctional. Echocardiography with Doppler evaluation is useful in identifying this complication. On two-dimensional images, leaflets fail to close below the annular plane, within the left ventricle and appear "tethered". Color and pulsed Doppler allow quantitative assesment of mitral regurgitation[19,20] with a close correlation to invasive methods. Patients will usually tolerate mild to moderate degrees of mitral regurgitation without significant hemodynamic compromise; however, patients with severe mitral regurgitation may develop signs and symptoms of low forward cardiac output and pulmonary congestion.

In patients with severe mitral regurgitation, it is essential to rule out a flail mitral valve secondary to acute papillary muscle rupture. Although this entity occurs in only 1% of myocardial infarctions, it accounts for 5% of infarct-related deaths.[21,22] Patients present with florid pulmonary edema and a low-output state. Transthoracic echocardiography reveals typically a flail mitral leaflet with a mass of tissue representing the ruptured papillary muscle head that prolapses into the left atrium in systole. Transesophageal echocardiography (TEE) may be required to confirm the diagnosis and degree of mitral regurgitation given the improved resolution and optimal position of the TEE probe behind the left atrium *(Figure 24.1)*. Once the diagnosis is made and the patients are medically stable, early surgical correction has been shown to slightly improve survival compared to conservative management.[23]

Myocardial infarct expansion and aneurysms

Infarct expansion occurs early following myocardial infarction[24] and can be visualized as infarct wall thinning and regional dilatation on transthoracic echocardiogram. Expansion occurs in 12-29% of patients[25] and is the precursor to aneurysm formation. Patients with evidence for expansion and aneurysm formation have a significant increase in 1 year mortality (61%) compared to patients without expansion (9%).[26]

True aneurysms are the result of infarct expansion and thinning of the expanded wall. Pathologically, the aneurysm contains all layers of the ventricular wall but can fibrose and calcify with time. They are defined echocardiographically *(Figure 24.2)* as a distortion in left ventricular shape in systole and diastole, with a wide neck (typically as wide as the body of the aneurysm).[27] There is typically a distinct demarcation between the functionally normal portion of the left ventricular wall and the aneurysm, which may or may not be dyskinetic. The majority of aneurysms involve the cardiac apex and thrombi are seen echocardiographically in up to one-third.[28]

Pseudoaneurysms

False aneurysms result from rupture of the left ventricular free wall and containment of blood by adherent parietal pericardium. The pseudoaneurysm thus is composed of pericardial tissue without myocardial cells. Echocardiographically *(Figure 24.3)* the neck (site of myocardial rupture) is narrow and less than 40% of the diameter of the aneurysm.[29-31] Pseudoaneurysms have a high incidence of early and late rupture.[32]

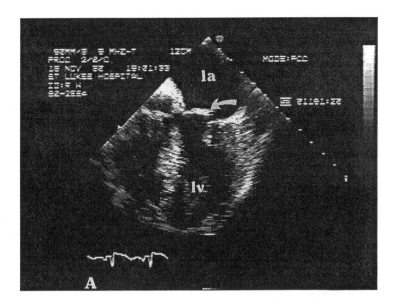

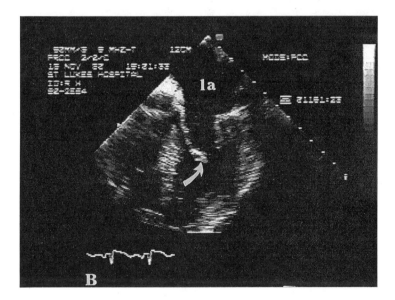

Figure 24.1 *Transesophageal echocardiogram in a patient following an acute myocardial infarction with acute mitral regurgitation secondary to a partially ruptured papillary muscle head. A: Flail anterior mitral valve leaflet in systole. B: Ruptured head of the posteromedial papillary muscle head* (pm) *seen in diastole.* lv, *left ventricle;* la, *left atrium.*

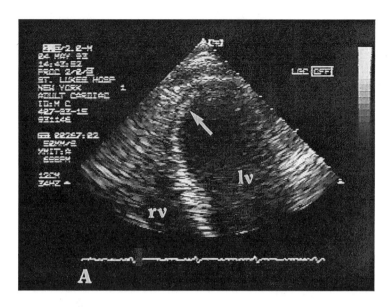

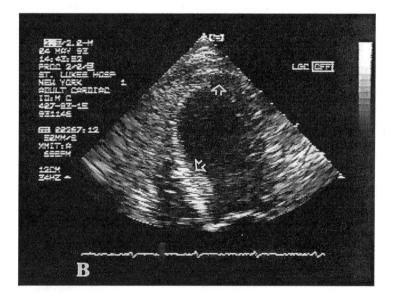

Figure 24.2 Four chamber view of the left and right ventricles in a patient with a history of an anterior wall myocardial infarction and a large apical aneurysm. A: Diastolic frame showing a thin-walled, dilated apex. B: Systolic frame showing persistent distortion of the apex bordered by normal myocardium. lv, left ventricle; rv, right ventricle.

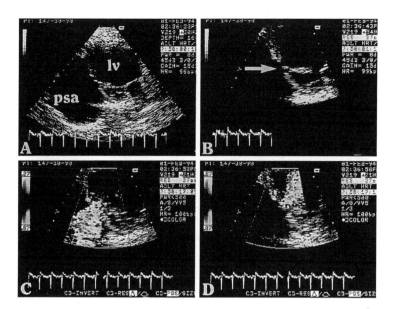

Figure 24.3 A: Parasternal long-axis view (low-window) in a patient with a history of an inferior wall myocardial infarction with a pseudoaneurysm. Marked thinning of the posterior wall with a large localized posterior pericardial effusion. B: Close-up of the posterior wall with clear regions of echo-dropout consistent with myocardial rupture. C: Color Doppler in systole revealing flow into the pericardial space through a narrow-necked break in the myocardium, consistent with a pseudoaneurysm. D. Color Doppler in diastole revealing flow from the pseudoaneurysm into the left ventricle. lv, left ventricle; psa=pseudoaneurysm.

Ventricular septal rupture

Another potentially catastrophic complication of myocardial infarction, ventricular septal rupture occurs in 0.5%-2% of patients but accounts for 1-5% of all infarct-related deaths.[33] It occurs with equal frequency in anterior, inferior or posterior infarctions and usually occurs between 2 to 7 days of initial infarction. Septal rupture is unrelated to hypertension, angina, congestive heart failure or the use of thrombolytics.[34,35] Two-dimensional echocardiography with Doppler is the test of choice for diagnosis of ventricular septal rupture.[36,37] Identification of a ventricular septal rupture includes: direct visualization of the defect or defects, usually in regions of extensive myocardial dysfunction; negative contrast in the right ventricle on intravenous injection of agitated saline contrast; and Doppler identification of high velocity left to right flow across the ventricular septum *(Figure 24.4)*. In addition, assessment of overall left and right ventricular function, as well as Doppler estimation of right ventricular systolic pressure and of the pulmonic systemic flow

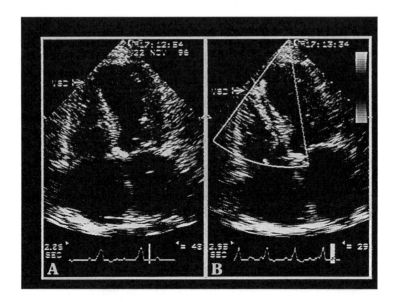

Figure 24.4 Apical four-chamber views of a patient with a history of an acute anterior wall myocardial infarction one week ago and a ventricular septal defect. A: Four-chamber view with markedly thin apical septum with a region of echo-dropout consistent with a ventricular septal defect. B: Color Doppler revealing turbulent flow from the left ventricle into the right ventricle across a ventricular septal defect.

ratio can be made. Surgical intervention has improved mortality over conservative therapy.[38]

Post-infarction pericarditis

Early episterno-pericarditis. This form of post-infarction pericarditis typically occurs within the first 24-96 hours following infarction and is typically a result of localized pericaridal inflammation overlying a transmural infarction. Its incidence may be decreasing in the era of thrombolytic therapy.[39] Patients may be asymptomatic or complain of chest pain (usually nonpericarditic). In the setting of persistent ST segment elevation on ECG, echocardiography can be helpful in differentiating this entity from recurrent ischemia/infarct or aneurysm formation.

Delayed pericarditis. The incidence of delayed pericarditis or "Dressler's Syndrome" may also be decreasing in the era of thrombolytic therapy.[40] Typically this post-myocardial infarction syndrome occurs one week to several months after initial myocardial infarction. Typical percarditic chest pain and a pericardial friction rub are uniformly present however pericardial effusions on echocardiogram may not be seen.

Pericarditis associated with cardiac rupture. The incidence of cardiac rupture following myocardial infarction is approximately 3%, however, it accounts for 10-

20% of deaths in this population.[41,42] Rupture typically occurs within the first week following infarction with one third occuring within the first 24 hours. Predisposing factors include advanced age, female sex, antecedent hypertension and first infarction without prior history of coronary artery disease. Time to thrombolytic therapy may influence the risk of cardiac infarct.[43] Premortem diagnosis is rare since rapid onset of tamponade ensues. However, in those patients with subacute rupture, echocardiographic criteria are very sensitive and specific in diagnosing ventricular wall rupture.[44] Classic echocardiographic signs include the presence of pericardial fluid; diastolic inversion of the right ventricular free wall and right atrial invagination in the setting of a pericardial effusion; and the presence of intrapericardial echoes of high acoustic density. Additional echocardiographic signs of tamponade include respiratory variability in right and left ventricular filling, and plethora of the inferior vena cava with Doppler signs including marked respiratory variability of transvalvular, superior vena cava and hepatic vein flow.[45]

Right ventricular infarction

Right ventricular (RV) involvement is recognized in nearly half of all inferior myocardial infarctions, and in up to 13% of anterior myocardial infarctions.[46,47] There are four subgroups of RV infarcts: Type I in which <50% of the RV inferior wall is involved, Type II in which the whole inferior RV wall is infarcted; Type III in which part of the RV free wall or anterior wall is infarcted and Type IV in which there is infarction of both inferior and anterior RV walls.[48] In Types III and IV, low output state and cardiogenic shock are more common. Two dimensional echocardiography is both sensitive and specific for hemodynamically important RV infarction.[49] Classic echocardiographic findings include: dilatation of the RV, RV asynergy, and abnormal interventricular septal motion.[50] In addition, patients who manifest bowing of the interatrial septum into the left atrium indicative of high right atrial pressures have more hypotension, more heart block and higher mortality.[51]

Left ventricular thrombus

Up to 60% of acute myocardial infarctions may by complicated by the development of left ventricular mural thrombus[52,53]. Echocardiographic detection of mural thrombi early following myocardial infarction carries negative prognostic implications.[54,55] Thrombi are recognized echocardiographically as echo-producing masses in regions of akinesis to dyskinesis, which overlie the true endocardium and distort the intracavitary contour (Figure 24.5). Although typically speckled appearing, regions of echodensity can be seen in more organized thrombi. Prospective studies have shown that the following characteristics of the thrombus increase the risk of embolization: mobility, protrusion into the LV cavity; and location adjacent to zones of hyperkinesis.[56-58]

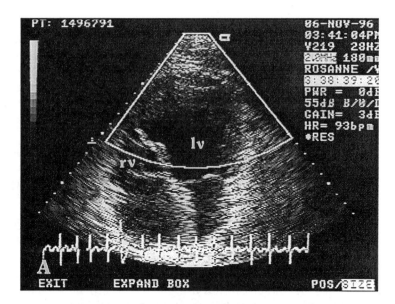

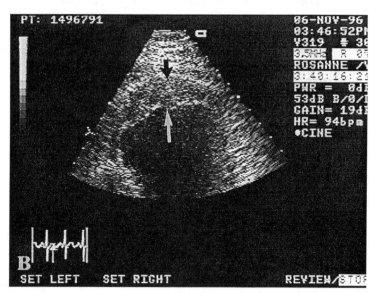

Figure 24.5.   Apical four-chamber view of a patient with a large apical aneurysm, who presented with a transient neurologic event. A: Apical aneurysm with tissue-density echoes in the apex. B: Close-up of the apex with tissue density echoes overlying a thin-walled aneurysm (endocardium marked by) consistent with a mural thrombus.

Stress echocardiography

Exercise echocardiography

The presence of stress-induced wall motion abnormality is an early and sensitive marker of ischemia[59] which may persist longer than ischemic electrocardiographic changes, thus making the addition of echocardiography to routine exercise testing ideal for evaluating both regional and global ischemic ventricular function. The addition of echocardiography to routine exercise testing, has significantly increased the diagnostic yield of stress tests and has been recognized "as a valid, clinically useful and accepted procedure".[60] Because of its availability, safety and low cost, exercise echocardiography has become a commonly used noninvasive test to evaluate coronary artery disease.

A variety of exercise methods have been used in combination with echocardiography.[61] Although early studies used supine bicycle exercise, upright bicycle ergometry is more commonly used. Most studies have shown that the peak values for heart rate during upright cycle ergometry are similar to treadmill exercise. However VO_2 max is 5-10% lower and systolic blood pressure is somewhat higher, probably due to the more limited muscle mass utilized and the gradual contribution of isometric hand grip required to stabilize the torso. The advantage of bicycle ergometry is that continuous echocardiographic imaging can be performed, allowing the assessment of an ischemic threshold as well as detecting areas of asynergy which may disappear rapidly following exercise. Imaging during exercise however can be limited, particularly in the upright position.

Studies have shown that wall motion abnormalities persist for at least two minutes after treadmill exercise, making treadmill exercise ideal for combining with post-exericise echocardiographic imaging. The advantages of this type of protocol are the attainment of maximal workload with treadmill exercise and the ease of imaging (in the left lateral decubitus position). However, to minimize false negative results, on-axis images must be obtained rapidly after of end-exercise, thus making exercise echocardiographic testing an operator/reader dependent test requiring a high level of expertise. The common use of digital image acquisition, which allows for side-by-side comparisons of rest and exercise "cine loops" of systolic and early diastolic images in comparable views, has facilitated the clinical use and interpretation of exercise echocardiography by minimizing artifact due to respiration and tachycardia. Video-tape evaluation is, however, equally accurate but requires greater expertise. Studies are usually interpreted qualitatively with quanititative assessment of ejection fraction reserved for patients who develop global dysfunction, ie: with severe three vessel or left main coronary artery disease. Standard images obtained include: 1) parasternal long axis view, 2) parasternal short axis view, 3) apical four-chamber view and 4) apical two-chamber view. The normal response to exercise is an increase in contractility in all segments with an increase in global left ventricular function and a reduction in left ventricular systolic volume. In addition to two-dimensional imaging, Doppler echocardiography may be useful in the assessment of valvular heart disease or in detecting mitral regurgitation induced by exercise in patients with unexplained dyspnea.

Suggested indications for treadmill stress echocardiography include the following:

a. Abnormal resting ECG (LVH with strain, LBBB, pacemaker)

b. Conditions commonly associated with positive stress ECG responses despite normal larger coronary arteries (hypertrophic cardiomyopathy, LVH, MVP, resting ST segment abnormalities, women, medications (digitalis or type Ia antiarrythmics),

c. Secondary testing in the setting of a positive exercise ECG without symptoms and low clinical index for coronary artery disease (CAD),

d. Evaluation of the following in patients with known CAD:

   -effect of therapy and ischemic threshold

   -extent of myocardium at risk

   -ischemia with underlying preexistent wall motion abnormalities

   -preoperative risk assessment

   -post-myocardial infarction risk assessment

   -suspected angina equivalent,

e. Assessment of left ventricular fucntion during exercise in the presence of: chronic regurgitant valvular lesions, dyspnea on exertion and hypertrophic cardiomyopathy.

f. Assessment of other valvular lesions: mitral stenosis (to assess transvalvular gradients and pulmonary artery pressures with exercise) and aortic stenosis (clinical relevance uncertain).

The overall accuracy of exercise echocardiography is summarized in *Table 24.1* [62-70]. The overall sensivitity ranges from 74-97% with an overall specificty of 64-88%. As with all imaging modalities, the sensivity of exercise echocardiography is highest in patients with multivessel disease (89-100%) and lowest in patients with patients with single vessel disease (60-92%) and those with no prior myocardial infarction (78-91%).

Factors influencing the accuracy of stress echocardiography are shown in *Table 24.2*. They include physiologic factors such as the severity or extent of the CAD, the workload achieved, the presence of nonischemic cardiomyopathy. Technical factors, particularly time to image and imaging plane become primary factors affecting overall accuracy. Finally, there are interpretive factors which may vary depending on the experience of the reader.

Studies comparing exercise echocardiography with thallium 201 scintigraphy [64,66,69-71] are shown in *Table 24.3*. These studies have shown similar sensitivities with overall higher specificity for exercise echocardiography. The lower specificity of Thallium 201 imaging may be accentuated in certain subgroups of patients, particulary women. On the other hand, Thallium 201 imaging detected more "ischemia" compared to echocadiography, in segments with baseline regional dysfunction.

Table 24.1 ACCURACY OF EXERCISE ECHOCARDIOGRAPHY FOR
DIAGNOSING CORONARY ARTERY DISEASE

| Author | Technique | n | Sensitivity % | | | | Specificity % |
			Overall	SVD	MVD	No MI	
Armstrong[62]	Treadmill	123	88	81	93	78	86
Crouse[63]	Treadmill	228	97	92	100	–	64
Pozzoli[64]	Upright Bic	75	71	60	94	–	96
Marwick[65]	Treadmill	150	84	77	93	80	86
Quinones[66]	Treadmill	112	74	58	90	–	88
Hecht[67]	Supine Bic	180	93	84	100	91	86
Ryan[68]	Upright Bic	309	91	86	95	83	78

Assessment of both regional and global effects of revascularization[72], as well as assessment of restenosis following coronary artery bypass grafting[73,74], have been studied using exercise echocardiography. In the latter two studies, the sensitivity in detecting graft stenosis was 94-98% with a specificity of 83-92%.

In patients who present following myocardial infarction, Ryan et al[75] showed a higher sensitivity for exercise echocardiography in predicting future cardiac events when compared to routine treadmill testing (80% vs 55%). Jaarsma et al[76] also showed a high sensitivity and specificity for detecting multivessel disease in the presence of remote asynergy predictive of future cardiac events. Specificity is also higher (95% vs 65%). In patients who present with chest pain, a negative exercise echocardiogram predicted a very low cardiac event rate (0.85-3% per year).[77,78] However, most comparisons between stress echocardiography and stress electrocardiography have failed to take advantage of recent advances in the latter methodology.[79-80]

Pharmacologic stress echocardiography

In patients who cannot achieve an adequate level of exercise or patients in whom myocardial viability is in question, pharmacologic stress testing may be useful. The three most commonly used agents are dipyridamole, adenosine and dobutamine. Dipyridamole is a vasodilator which acts primarily by inhibiting adenosine re-uptake into endothelial and blood cells, thus increasing local adenosine levels. Adenosine is an endogenously produced vasodilator substance with acts through receptors on smooth muscle cells as well as endothelial cells causing vascular smooth muscle cell relaxation, and consequent vasodilatation. Its half-life is <10 seconds. Dobutamine is a synthetic catecholamine that acts on 1, 1, and 2 receptors. At low dose, its primary effect is to increase myocardial contractility whereas at high doses, a

Table 24.2   FACTORS AFFECTING ACCURACY OF STRESS ECHO CARDIOGRAPHY

Physiologic	Technical	Interpretive
Severity of and extent of CAD	Adequacy of Images	Criteria for normality/ischemia
Workload achieved: Blood pressure and heart rate response	R wave triggering/acquisition	Particular knowledge/recognition of: Heterogeneity of normal contraction Variations of basal inferior wall/septal contraction translation (after CAG)
Dose of pharmacologic agent	Tomographic planes: Foreshortening Comparability of tomographic planes	Effect of LBBB, LVH
Cardiomyopathy	Time to imaging (after treadmill) Technical limitations	

LBBB, left bundle branch block; *LVH*, left ventricular hypertrophy; *CAD*, coronary artery disease; *CAB*: Coronary artery bypass grafting. .

(From Nagueh SF and Zoghbi WA. Stress echocardiography for the assessment of myocardial ischemia and viability. Curr Prob Cardiol 1996; 21:445-520. Reproduced with permission.)

Table 24.3   ASSESSMENT OF CAD COMPARISON OF EXERCISE ECHO AND
             EXERCISE THALLIUM 201 SCINTIGRAPHY

Study	N	Echo Sensitivity (%) (	Echo Specificity %)	Thallium Sensitivity (%)	Thallium Specificity (%)
Maurer and Nanda[69]	48	86	92	74	92
Pozzoli et al.[64]	75	71	96	84	88
Galanti et al.[70]	53	93	96	100	92
Quinones[66]	112	74	88	76	81
Hecht et al.[71]	71	90	80	92	65

(From Nagueh SF and Zighbi WA. Stress echocardiography for the assessment of myocardial ischemia and viability. Curr Prob Cardiol 1996;21:445-520. Reprinted with permission.)

chronotropic effect is seen. Recent reviews[81-82] discuss the protocols, side effects, indications and contraindications for each agent. Overall sensitivities for dipyridamole are 52-92% (on average 70%), with a specificity of >90%. Overall sensitivities for adenosine are 40-91% with a specificity of >90%. Overall sensitivities for dobutamine are 68-96% with specificities of 60-100%. Arbutamine is a newer synthetic catecholamine that acts primarily on 1 and 2 receptors which yields similar degrees of inotropic and chronotropic stimulation. Although initial studies with Arbutamine stress echocardiography show a slight improvement in sensitivity compared with exercise echocardiography[82-84], further evaluation is necessary, particularly in view of the fact that this agent is only available for use with a proprietary infusion system.

Imaging planes and wall motion scoring for pharmacologic stress studies are the same as with exercise echocardiography; however, with continuous infusion of dobutamine, imaging can easily be performed at incremental doses thus allowing the assessment of ischemic threshold. Myocardial viability can be documented when hypokinetic or akinetic segments improve their function in response to low-dose dobutamine infusion.

The suggested indications for pharmacologic stress echocardiography include the following:

a. Inability to exercise because of claudication, neurologic deficits, rheumatologic or orthopedic conditions, chronic lung disease or other debilitating conditions.

b. Need for simultaneous evaluation of ischemia and myocardial viability.

c. Evaluation of viable myocardium in patients with left ventricular dysfunction.

d. Risk stratification prior to noncardiac surgical procedures.

e. Inability to achieve target heart rate during exercise because of medical therapy with -blockers and calcium channel blockers, which can be circumvented by dipyridamole or adenosine.

f. Risk stratification after myocardial infarction.

g. Assessment of wall motion or restenosis following revascularization proce-dures.

h. Assessment of left ventricular and valvular function during pharmacologic stress in the setting of chronic or ischemic valvular lesions, dyspnea on exertion and hypertrophic cardiomyopathy.

Prognostic information

a. In patients presenting with suspected coronary artery disease, dipyridamole stress echocardiography successfully stratifies groups at high and low risk for future car-diac events.[85-86] In addition, its negative predictive value was higher than exercise echocardiography.[86] A new wall motion abnormality on dobutamine stress echocar-diography was also highly predictive of cardiac death, myocardial infarction and revascularization procedure[87] in such patients.

b. In patients presenting following an acute myocardial infarction, two studies confirm the significant prognostic power of dipyridamole echocardiography[88-89] with a positive predictive value of 52%, a negative predictive value of 83% and a relative risk for cardiac death with a positive test of 4.4. Preliminary data on the use of dobutamine stress echocardiography in similar patients shows that death and inf-arction were 1.9-2.7 times more likely in patients with positive tests.[90-91]

c. In patients presenting with chronic stable coronary artery disease and a low risk of new cardiac events, dipyridamole echocardiography was effective in prog-nostic stratification; a positive response at low dose identified patients with a high incidence of hard events (sensitivity 50%, specificity 96%).[92] Panza et al.[93] indirect-ly correlated results of dobutamine stress echocardiography with prognosis in pa-tients with chronic coronary artery disease. They studied 104 patients with trans-esophageal echocardiography and assessed the ischemic threshold by measuring the amount of dobutamine infused at the first onset of wall motion disturbance. The ischemic threshold correlated with two variables which are associated with progno-sis: angiographically determined severity of coronary disease as well as mean fall in ejection fraction by radionuclide angiography .

d. In patients presenting with severe peripheral vascular disease, multiple stud-ies show the utility of dobutamine stress echocardiography in the preoperative as-sessment of cardiac risk.[94-95] Poldermans et al.[95] studied 302 patients presenting for major vascular surgery and found that dobutamine stress echocardiography identi-fied a high and intermediate risk group based on ischemic threshold. Although the positive predictive value was only 38%, the negative predictive value was 100%, indicating that the test was especially successful in identifying patients at very low risk.

e. Assessment of revascularization: Multiple small studies have documented the utility of dipyridamole[96-97] and dobutamine[98-100] stress echocardiography in the assessment of revascularization as well as restenosis following either coronary angioplasty or coronary artery bypass grafting. Although only 24 patients were studied, Kao et al.[99] showed that dobutamine stress echocardiographic ischemic responses accurately predicted which patients would improve following angioplasty. Likewise, the suggestion of hibernating myocardium on dobutamine stress echocardigraphy was also highly predictive of wall motion improvement. In 18 patients undergoing coronary artery bypass grafting, Perrone-Filardi et al.[100] showed that dobutamine stress echocardiography accurately identified hibernating myocardium which functionally improved following surgery.

Myocardial viability

In patients with resting wall motion abnormalities, viable myocardium may exist in two situations: myocardial stunning or myocardial hibernation. Stunning occurs when myocardial dysfunction persists following transient coronary occlusion (with restored coronary blood flow). Hibernating myocardium exists in the setting of severe coronary stenosis with reduction in contractility, a teleologic adaptation to preserve cardiac energy.

Early catheterization studies[100-101] suggested that -adrenergic stimulation of dysfunctional but viable myocardial segments could result in enhanced contractility. Recent studies of dobutamine stress echocardiography following acute myocardial infarction (presumed stunned myocardium) have confirmed a high sensitivity and specificity for the identification of viable myocardium. As early as 1990, Pierard et al[102] studied 17 patients following acute myocardial infarction and showed a 78% concordance between assessment of viability and functional recovery by dobutamine echocardiography, and evidence of metabolic activity by positron emission tomography. Duchak et al[103] compared low dose dobutamine with resting thallium-201 SPECT imaging for predicting recovery of ventricular dysfunction in 65 patients after acute myocardial infarction. The study confirmed similar sensitivity and better specificity for low dose dobutamine (81 and 75% respectively), when compared with thallium imaging (73% and 35% respectively). Watada et al[104] studied 21 patients following acute myocardial infarction and found an 83% sensitivity and 86% specificity for detecting improvement in wall motion after subsequent reperfusion (by percutaneous angioplasty) using intermediate dose (10 µg/kg/min) dobutamine. Salustri et al[105] studied 57 patients following acute myocardial infarction (27 received thrombolytics) and found the low dose dobutamine predicted wall motion recovery with a sensitivity of 87% and a specificity of 93%. Slightly lower sensitivity and specificity (79% and 68% respectively) were found in a similar patient population studied by Previtali et al.[106] Overall sensitivity in six studies of dobutamine echocardiography[103-108] range from 66-86% while specificity ranges from 68-94%.

A number of studies[109-113] have evaluated the accuracy of dobutamine stress echocardiography in determining myocardial viability in patients with known coronary disease and chronic left ventricular dysfunction (presumed hibernating myocardium). Dobutamine stress echocardiography was performed prior to revascularization procedures and at set time points following revascularization. Overall sensitivity for dobutamine stress echocardiography ranged between 74-92% with specificities of 73-93%. Afridi et al[113] noted four possible wall motion responses to incremental doses of dobutamine: a biphasic response with improvement in wall motion at low dose and worsening at high dose; sustained improvement in wall motion; sustained worsening in wall motion; and no change in wall motion. The highest sensitivity and specificity for predicting functional recovery was found in segments that exhibited either a biphasic response or progressive worsening (74% and 73% respectively).

New echocardiographic techniques

Contrast echocardiography

Intravascular contrast agents have recently been developed for both intracoronary injection and intravenous injection. These agents are microbubbles (<10 microns) typically formed by sonication of various agents such as Renograffin® or albumin. Injected directly into the coronary arteries, contrast is useful in the following situations: assessing blood flow and anatomic or functional areas at risk[114]; assessing collateral blood flow[115]; assessing the adequacy of myocardial perfusion intraoperatively[116]; and assessing coronary blood flow reserve using contrast with papaverine or dipyridamole.[117-118] Sonicated albumin and newer agents have now been intravenously used to enhance left-heart visualization after injection, which may expand the role of contrast echocardiography in the detection of coronary artery disease.[119-120]

Doppler tissue imaging

This new technique uses pulsed wave Doppler to interrogate high amplitude, low frequency signals that arise from myocardial tissue. The velocity of tissue movement is calculated and encoded for display in a variety of color maps. Color intensity or hue phasically varies with the magnitude and direction of velocity or acceleration of motion i.e.: motion toward the transducer is represented in red, and motion away from the transducer is represented in blue and velocities in excess of the Nyquist limit are represented in yellow-green. This technique may become most useful in the rapid qualitative and quantitative assessment of wall motion abnormalities during stress echocardiography.[121-123]

Transesophageal echocardiography and coronary flow reserve

Many studies have documented imaging of the proximal coronary arteries with transesophageal echocardiography (TEE). Yoshida et al[122] also showed that TEE is both sensitive and specific in detecting significant left main artery stenosis. Proximal left anterior artery (LAD) imaging and Doppler is also feasible allowing for monitoring of coronary blood flow during pharmacologic interventions (i.e., dipyridamole, adenosine, or dobutamine). Thus, the response of coronary flow to maximal coronary dilatation or coronary flow reserve, can be assessed noninvasively.[125-127] Current application of this technique is limited but deserves further evaluation.

Acknowledgment: We would like to thank Virginia Burns for her assistance in preparation of this manuscript.

REFERENCES

1. Reimer KA, et al. The wave front phenomenon of ischemic cell death: I. Myocardial infarct size vs duration of coronary occlusion in dogs. Circulation 1977: 56: 786.

2. Kisslo JJ, et al. A comparison of real-time, two-dimensional echocardiography and cineangiography in detecting left ventricular asynergy. Circulation 1977:55:134.

3. Heger JJ, et al. Crosss-sectional echocardiography in acute myocardial infarction: detection and localization of regional left ventricular asynergy. Circulation 1979:60:531-8.

4. Horowitz RS, et al. Immediate diagnosis of acute myocardial infarction by two-dimensional echocardiography. Circulation 1982:65:323.

5. Weyman AE, et al. Correlation between extent of abnormal regional wall motion and myocardial infarct size in chronically infarcted dogs. Circulation 1977: 56 (Suppl. 2):72.

6. Pandian NG, et al. Myocardial infarct size threshold for two-dimensional echocardiographic detection: sensitivity of systolic wall thickening and endocardial motion abnormalities in small versus large infarction. Am J Cardiol 1985: 55: 551.

7. Weiss JL, et al. Two-dimensional echocardiographic recognition of myocardial injury in man: comparison with post-mortem studies. Circulation 1981:63:401.

8. Meltzer RS, et al. Two-dimensional echocardiographic quantification of infarct size alteration by pharmacologic agents.Am J Cardiol 1979:44:257.

9. Wyatt HL, et al. Experimental evaluation of the extent of myocardial dyssynergy and infarct size by two-dimensional echocardiography. Circulation 1981:63:607.

10. Lieberman AN, et al. Two-dimensional echocardiography and infarct size: relationship of regional wall motion and thickening to the extent of myocardial infarction in the dog. Circulation 1981:63:739-46.

11. Loh IK, et al. Early diagnosis of nontransmural myocardial infarction by two-dimensional echocardiography. Am J Cardiol 1982: 104: 963.

12. Rogers EW, et al. Predicting survival after myocardial infarction by cross-sectional echo. Circulation 1978:58(Suppl 2): II-233.

13. Horowitz RS et al. Immediate detection of early high risk patients with acute myocardial infarction using two-dimensional echocardiographic evaluation of left ventricular regional wall motion abnormalities. Am Heart J 1982: 103:814.

14. Nishimura RA, et al. Role of two-dimensional echocardiography in the prediction of in-hospital complications after acute myocardial infarction. J am Coll Cardiol 1984: 4: 1080.

15. Gibson RS, et al. Value of early two-dimensional echocardiography in patients with acute myocardial infarction. Am J Cardiol 1982: 49:1110.

16. Labovitz AJ, et al. Evaluation of left ventricular systolic and diastolic dysfunction during transient myocardial ischemia reduced by angioplasty. J Am Coll Cardiol 1987:10:748.

17. Johannessen KA, Cerqueria MD, Stratton JR: Influence of myocardial infarction size on radionuclide and Doppler echocardiographic measurements of diastolic function. Am J Cardiol 1990: 65:692.

18. Heikkila J. Mitral incompetence complicating acute myocardial infarction. Br. Heart J 1967: 29:162.

19. Helmcke F, et al. Color Doppler assessment of mitral regurgitation with orthogonal planes. Circulation 1987: 75:175.

20. Miyatake K, et al. Semiquantitative grading of severity of mitral regurgitation by real-time two-dimensional Doppler flow imaging technique. J Am Coll Cardiol 1986: 7: 82.

21. Nishimura RA, et al. Papillary muscle rupture complicating acute myocardial infarction: analysis of 17 patients. Am J Cardiol 1983: 51:373.

22. Wei JY, Hutchins GM, Bulkley BH: Papillary muscle rupture in fatal acute myocardial infarction. Ann Intern Med 1979: 90:149.

23. Shah PK, Swan HJC. Complications of acute myocardial infarction, in Chatterjee K, Parmley WW (eds): Cardiology. Philadelphia, Lippincott-Gower, 1991, p 7.179.

24. Erlebacher JA, et al. Early dilatation of the infarcted segment in acute transmural myocardial infarction: Role of acute left ventricular enlargement. J Am Coll Cardiol 1984: 4:201.

25. Picard MH, et al. Natural history of left ventricular size and function after acute myocardial infarction: assessment and prediction by echocardiographic endocardial surface mapping. Circulation 1990: 82: 484.

26. Meizlish JL, et al. Functional left ventricular aneurysm formation after acute anterior transmural myocarial infarction: Incidence and natural history and prognostic implications. N Engl J Med 1984: 311: 1001.

27. Weyman AE, et al :Detection of left ventricular aneurysms by cross-sectional echocardiography. Circulation 1976: 54:936.

28. Bauer HR, Daniel JA, Nelson RR: Detection of left ventricular aneurysm in two-dimensional echocardiography. Am J Cardiol 1982: 50:191.

29. Catherwood E, et al. Two-dimensional echocardiogaraphic recognition of left ventricular pseudoaneurysm. Circulation 1980: 62:294.

30. Roelandt JR, et al. Improved diagnosis and characterization of left ventricular pseudoaneurysm by Doppler color flow imaging. J Am Coll Cardiol 1988: 12:807.

31. Stoddard MF, et al. Transesophageal echocardiography in the pseudoaneurysm. Am Heart J 1993: 125:534.

32. Roberts WC, Morrow AG.: Pseudoaneurysm of the left ventricle: an unusual sequela of myocardial infarction and rupture of the heart. Am J Med 1967: 43:639.

33. Fox AC, Glassman E, Isom OW: Surgically remediable complications of myocardial infarction. Prog Cardiovasc Dis 1979: 21:461.

34. Mann JM, Roberts WC: Acquired ventricular septal defect during acute myocardial infarction: Analysis of 38 unoperated necropsy patients without rupture. Am J Cardiol 1988:62:8.

35. Kleiman NS, et al. Mechanisms of early death despite thrombolytic therapy: Experience from the thrombolysis in myocardial infarction Phase II (TIMI II) study. J Am Coll Cardiol 1992:19:1129.

36. Smith G, et al. Ventricular septal rupture diagnosed by simultaneous cross-sectional echocardiography and Doppler ultrasound. Eur Heart J 1985: 6:621.

37. Bhatia SJS, et al. Trans-septal Doppler flow velocity profile in acquired ventricular septal defect in acute myocardial infarction. Am J Cardiol 1987: 60:372.

38. Gray RJ, Sethna D, Matloff JM: The role of cardiac surgery in acute myocardial infarction with mechanical complications. Am Heart J 1983: 106:723.

39. Correale D, et al. Comparison of frequency, diagnostic and prognostic significance of pericardial involvement in acute myocardial infarction treated with and without thrombolytics (GISSI). Am J Cardiol 1993: 71:1377.

40. Gregoratos G. Pericardial involvement in acute myocardial infarction. Cardiol Clin 1990: 8:601.

41. Kouchoukos NT. Surgical treatment of acute complications of acute myocardial infarction. Cardiovasc Clinic 1981:11:141.

42. Rasmussen S, et al. Cardiac rupture in acute myocardial infarction. Acta Med Scand 1979:205:11.

43. Honan MB, et al. Cardiac rupture, mortality and the timing of thrombolytic therapy: a meta-analysis. J Am Coll Cardiol 1990:16:359.

44. Lopez-Sendon J, et al. Diagnosis of subacute ventricular wall rupture after acute myocardial infarction: sensitivity and specificity of clinical, hemodynamic and echocardiographic criteria. J Am Coll Cardiol 1992:19:1145.

45. Appleton CP, Hatle LK, Popp RL: Cardiac tamponade and pericardial effusion: respiratory variation in transvalvular flow velocities studied by Doppler echocardiography. J Am Coll Cardiol 1988:11:1020.

46. Kinch JW, Ryan TJ. Right ventricular infarction. N Engl J Med 1994: 330:1211.

47. Cabin HS, et al. Right ventricular myocardial infarction with anterior wall left ventricular infarction: an autopsy study. Am Heart J 1987:113:16.

48. Isner JM: Right ventricular myocardial infarction. JAMA 1988:259:712.

49. Bellamy GR, et al. Value of two-dimensional echocardiography, electrocardiography, and clinical signs in detecting right venricular infarction. Am Heart J 1986:112:304.

50. Jugdutt BI, et al. Right ventricular infarction: two-dimensional echocardiographic evaluation. Am Heart J 1984: 107:505.

51. Lopez-Sendon J, et al. Inversion of the normal interatrial septum convexity in acute myocardial infarction: incidence, clinical relevance and prognostic significance. J Am Coll Cardiol 1990: 15:801.

52. Yater WM, et al. Comparison of clinical and pathologic aspects of coronary artery disease in men of various age groups: a study of 950 autopsied cases from the Armed Forces Institute of Pathology. Ann Intern Med 1951:34:352.

53. Rao G, et al. Experience with sixty consecutive ventricular aneurysm resections. Circulation 1974: 49, 50(Suppl. 2):149.

54. Spirito P, et al. Prognostic significance and natural history of left ventricular thrombi in paitents with acute anterior myocardial infarction: a two-Dimensional echocardiographic study. Circulation 1985:72:774.

55. Kupper AJ, et al. Left ventricular thrombus incidence and behavior studied by serial two-dimensional echocardiography in acute anterior myocarial infarction: left ventricular wall motion, systemic embolism and oral anticoagulation. J Am Coll Cardiol 1989:13:1514.

56. Visser CA, et al. Embolic potential of left ventricular thrombus after myocardial infarction: a two-dimensional echocardiographic study of 119 patients. J Am Coll Cardiol 1985:5:1276.

57. Jugdutt BI, et al. Prospective two-dimensional echocardiographic evaluation of left ventricular thrombus and embolism after acute myocardial infarction. J Am Coll Cardiol 1989:13:554.

58. Keren A, et al. Natural history of left ventricular thrombi: their appearance and resolution in the posthospitalization period of acute mycardial infarction. J Am Coll Cardiol 1990:15:790.

59. Grover-McKay M, Matsuzaki M, Ross J Jr.: Dissociation between regional myocardial dysfunction and subendocardial ST segment elevation during and after exercise-induced ischemia in dogs. J Am Coll Cardiol 1987:10:1105.

60. American College of Cardiology. Policy statement: stress echocardiography. 1990: Oct 14.

61. Quinones MA. Technical considerations in exercise echocardiography: preference of exercise methodology, imaging approach, and comparison with radionuclide techniques. Coronary Artery Disease 1991: 2: 536.

62. Armstrong WF, O'Donnell JO, Feigenbaum H. Exercise echocardiography: Effect of prior myocardial infarction and extent of coronary disease on accuracy. J Am Coll Cardiol 1987:10: 531.

63. Crouse LJ, et al. Exercise echocardiography as a screening test for coronary artery disease and correlation with coronary arteriography. Am J Cardiol 1991:67:1213.

64. Pozzoli MM, et al. Exercise echocardiography and technetium-99-m MIBI single-photon emission computed tomography in the detection of coronary artery disease. Am J Cardiol 1991: 67: 350.

65. Marwick TH, et al. Accuracy and limitations of exercise echocardiography in a routine clinical setting. J Am Coll Cardiol 1992: 19: 74.

66. Quinones MA, et al. Exercise echocardiography versus thallium-201 single-photon emission computed tomography in the evaluation of coronary artery disease: Analysis of 292 patients. Circulation 1992: 85: 1026.

67. Hecht HS, et al. Digital supine bicylce stress echocardiography: a new technique for evaluating coronary artery disease. J Am Coll Cardiol 1993: 21:950.

68. Ryan T, et al. Detection of coronary artery disease with upright bicycle exercise echocardiography. J Am Soc Echocardiogr 1993:6:186.

69. Maurer G, Nanda NC. Two-dimensional echocardiographic evaluation of exercise-induced left and right ventricular asynergy: correlation with thallium scanning. Am J Cardiol 1981:48:720.

70. Galanti G, et al. Diagnostic accuracy of peak exercise echocardiography in coronary artery disease: comparison with thallium-201 myocardial scintigraphy. Am Heart J 1991:122:1609.

71. Hecht HA, DeBoard L, Shaw R. Supine bicycle stress echocardiography versus tomographic thallium-201 exercise imaging for the detection of coronary artery disease. J Am Soc Echocardiogr 1993: 6:177.

72. Labovitz AJ, et al. The effects of successful PTCA on left ventricular function: assessment by exercise echocardiography. Am Heart J 1989:117:1003.

73. Crouse LJ, et al. Exercise echocardiography after coronary artery bypass grafting. Am J Cardiol 1992:70:572.

74. Sawada SG, et al. Upright bicycle exercise echocardiography after coronary artery bypass graft. Am J Cardiol 1989:64:1123.

75. Ryan T, et al. Risk stratification after acute myocardial infarction by means of exercise two-dimensional echocardiography. Am Heart J 1987:114:1305.

76. Jaarsma W, et al. Usefulness of two-dimensional exercise echocardiography shortly after myocardial infarction. Am J Cardiol 1986:57:86.

77. Sawada SG, et al. Prognostic value of a normal exercise echocardiogram. Am Heart J 1990:120:49.

78. Krivokapich J, et al. Prognostic usefulness of positive or negative exercise stress echocardiography for predicting coronary events in ensuing twelve months. Am J Cardiol 1993:71:646.

79. Okin PM, et al. Electrocardiographic identification of increased left ventricular mass by simple voltage duration products. J A Coll Cardiol 1995:25:417.

80. Okin PM, et al. Prognostic value of heart rate adjustment of exercise ST segment depression in the Multiple Risk Factor Intervention Trial. J Am Coll Cardiol 1996:27:1437.

81. Verani, MS. Pharmacologic stress myocardial perfusion imaging. Curr Prob Cardiol 1993:18:481.

82. Nagueh SF, Zoghbi WA. Stress echocardiography for the assessment of myocardial ischemia and viability. Curr Prob Cardiol 1996:21:445.

83. Dennis CA, et al. Stress testing with closed-loop arbutamine as an alternative to exercise. J Am Coll Cardiol 1995:26:1151.

84. Cohen JL, et al. Arbutamine echocardiography: efficacy and safety of a new pharmacologic stress agent to induce myocardial ischemia and detect coronary artery disease. J Am Coll Cardiol 1995:26:1168.

85. Picano E, et al. Prognostic importance of dipyridamole echocardiography test in coronary artery disease. Circulation 1989:80:450.

86. Severi S, et al. Diagnostic and prognostic value of dipyridamole echocardiography in patients with suspected coronary artery disease: comparison with exercise electrocardiography. Circulation 1994:89:1160.

87. Kamaran M, et al. Prognostic value of dobutamine stress echocardiography in patients referred because of suspected coronary artery disease. Am J Cardiol 1995:76:887.

88. Bolognese L, Rossi L, Sarasso G. Silent versus symptomatic dipyridamole-induced ischemia after myocardial infarction: clinical and prognostic significance. J Am Coll Cardiol 1992: 19:953.

89. Camerieri A, et al. Prognostic value of dipyridamole echocardiography early after myocardial infarction in elderly patients: Echo Persantine Italian Cooperative (EPIC) Study Group. J Am Coll Cardiol 1993:22:1809.

90. Bigi R, et al. The prognostic value of dobutamine-atropine stress echocardiography early after acute myocardial infarction. Circulation 1994:90:I-267.

91. Sonel AF, et al. Assessment of post-infarction prognosis using dobutamine stress echocardiography. Circulation 1994:90:I-453.

92. Coletta C, et al. Prognostic value of high dose dipyridamole echocardiography in patients with chronic coronary artery disease and preserved left ventricular function. J Am Coll Cardiol 1995:26:887.

93. Panza JA, et al. Relation between ischemic threshold measured during dobutamine stress echocardiography and know indices of poor prognosis in patients with coronary artery disease. Circulation 1995:92:2095.

94. Davila-Roman VG, et al. Dobutamine stress echocardiography predicts surgical outcome in patients with an aortic aneurysm and peripheral vascular disease. J Am Coll Cardiol 1993:21:957.

95. Poldermans D, et al. Improved cardiac risk stratification in major vascular surgery with dobutamine-atropine stress echocardiography. J Am Coll Cardiol 1995:26:648.

96. Pirelli S, et al. Comparison of usefulness of high-dose dipyridamole echocardiography and exercise electrocardiography for detection of asymptomatic restenosis after coronary angioplasty. Am J Cardiol 1991:67:1335.

97. Bongo AS, et al. Early assessment of coronary artery bypass graft patency by high-dose dipyridamole echocardiography. Am J Cardiol 1991:67:133.

98. Kao HL, et al. Dobutamine stress echocardiography predicts early wall motion improvement after elective percutaneous transluminal coronary angioplasty. Am J Cardiol 1995:76:652.

99. Perrone-Filardi P, et al. Dobutamine echocardiography predicts improvement of hypoperfused dysfunctional myocardium after revascularization in patients with coronary artery disease. Circulation 1995:91:2556.

100. Horn HR, et al. Augmentation of left ventricular contraction pattern in coronary artery disease by an inotropic catecholamine: the epinephrine ventriculogram. Circulation 1974:49:1063.

101. Popio KA, et al. Postextrasystolic potentiation as a predictor of potential myocardial viability: preoperative analyses compared with studies after coronary bypass surgery. Am J Cardiol 1977:39:944.

102. Pierard LA, et al. Identification of viable myocardium by echocardiography during dobutamine infusion in patients with myocardial infarction after thrombolytic therapy: comparison with positron emission tomography. J Am Coll Cardiol 1990:15:1021.

103. Duchak J, et al. Low dose dobutamine induced infarction zone wall thickening correlates with thallium by delayed SPECT imaging.[abstract] Circulation 1992:86:I-384.

104. Watada H, et al. Dobutamine stress echocardiography predicts reversible dysfunction and quantitates the extent of irreversibly damaged myocardium after reperfusion of anterior myocardial infarction. J Am Coll Cardiol 1994:24:624.

105. Salustri A, et al. Prediction of improvement of ventricular function after first acute myocardial infarction using low-dose dobutamine stress echocardiography. Am J Cardiol 1994:74:853.

106. Previtali M, et al. Dobutamine stress echocardiography for assessment of myocardial viability and ischemia in acute myocardial infarction treated with thrombolysis. Am J Cardiol 1993:72:124G.

107. Barilla F, et al. Low dose dobutamine in patients with acute myocardial infarction identifies

viable but not contractile myocardium and predicts the magnitude of improvement in wall motion abnormalities in response to coronary revascularization. Am Heart J 1991:122:1522.

108. Smart S, et al. Low dose Dobutamine echocardiography detects reversible dysfunction after thrombolytic therapy of acute myocardial infarction. Circulation 1993:88:405.

109. Marzullo P, et al. Value of rest thallium-201/technetium-99m sestimibi scans and dobutamine echocardiography for detecting myocardial viability. Am J Cardiol 1993:71:166.

110. Cigarroa CG, et al. Dobutamine stress echocardiography identifies hibernating myocardium and predicts recovery of left ventricular function after coronary revascularization. Circulation 1993:88:430.

111. La Canna G, et al. Echocardiography during infusion of dobutamine for identification of reversible dysfunction in patients with chronic coronary artery disease. J Am Coll Cardiol 1994:23:617.

112. Charney R, et al. Dobutamine echocardiography and resting-redistribution thallium-201 scintigraphy predicts recovery of hibernating myocardium after coronary revascularization. Am Heart J 1994:128:864.

113. Afridi I, et al. Dobutamine echocardiography in myocardial hibernation: optimal dose and accuracy in predicting recovery of ventricular function after coronary angioplasty. Circulation 1995:91:663.

114. Kaul S, et al. Contrast echocardiography in acute myocardial ischemia: I. In vivo determination of total left ventricular "area at risk". J Am Coll Cardiol 1984:4:1272.

115. Sabia PJ, et al. An association between collateral blood flow and myocardial viability in patients with recent myocardial infarction. N Engl J Med 1992: 372:1825.

116. Matthew TL, et al. Assessment of myocardial perfusion during coronary artery bypass graft operations in humans using myocardial contrast echocardiography. Surgical Forum 1989: 40:248.

117. Keller MW, Glasheen W, Kaul S. Myocardial contrast echocardiography in humans: II. Assessment of coronary blood flow reserve. J Am Coll Cardiol 1988: 12:925.

118. Kaul S, Jayaweera AR. Myocardial contrast echocardiography has the potential for the assessment of coronary microvascular reserve. J Am Coll Cardiol 1993:21:356.

119. Falcone RA, et al. Intravenous albunex during dobutamine stress echocardiography: enhanced localization of left ventricular endocardial borders. Am Heart J 1995:130:254.

120. Villanueva FS, Kaul S. Assessment of myocardial perfusion in coronary artery disease using myocardial contrast echocardiography. Coron Artery Dis 1995:6:18.

121. Sutherland GR, et al. Color Doppler myocardial imaging: a new technique for the assessment of myocardial function. J Am Soc Echocardiogr 1994:7:441.

122. Donovan CL, Armstrong WF, Bach DS. Quantitative Doppler tissue imaging of the left ventricular myocardium: validation in normal subjects. Am Heart J 1995:130:100.

123. Uematsu M, et al. Myocardial velocity gradient as a new indicator of regional left ventricular contraction: detection by two-dimensional tissue Doppler imaging technique. J Am Coll Cardiol 1995:26:217.

124. Yoshida K, et al. Detection of left main coronary artery stenosis by transesophageal color Doppler and two-dimensional echocardiography. Circulation 1990:81:1271.

125. Hutchinson SS, et al. Transesophageal assessment of coronary flow velocity reserve during "regular" and "high" dose dipyridamole stress testing. Am J Cardiol 1966: 77:1164.

126. Radvan J, et al. Coronary flow response to dipyridamole using transesophageal echocardiography correlates with myocardial blood flow measured by PET. J Am Coll Cardiol 1994: 8: 360A.

127. Redberg RF, et al. Adenosine-induced coronary vasodilation during transesophageal Doppler echocardiography. Rapid and safe measurement of coronary flow reserve ratio can predict significant left anterior descending coronary stenosis. Circulation 1995: 92:190.

25 TRANSESOPHAGEAL ECHOCARDIOGRAPHY

Alan S. Katz

Since its introduction, transthoracic echocardiography has been somewhat limited by the structures interposed between the ultrasound transducer on the patient's chest and the heart. Patients with chest deformities (pectus excavatum, barrel chest), small intercostal spaces, obese patients, patients with chronic obstrucive lung disease, patients with breast implants, and patients recovering from chest surgery are known to be difficult to image. In ultrasound, there is a physical trade-off. The higher the frequency of the incident beam, the greater the image resolution but the lower the energy for penetration. Transesophageal echocardiography obtains images using an ultrasound transducer at the distal end of an endoscope. Imaging through the esophagus and stomach requires less energy for tissue penetration. Therefore, higher frequency transducers can be used; typically 5.0 to 7.5 MHz, allowing for higher resolution images.

In 1976, M-mode imaging transesophageal echocardiography was introduced for patients in whom transthoracic imaging was difficult.[1] Two-dimensional imaging[23] and pulsed wave spectral Doppler[4] became feasible in the 1980's. In the late 1980's, color flow Doppler[5,6,7] and continuous wave Doppler[8] imaging were added. The ability to view two orthogonal images (biplane)[9,10,11] was introduced in 1990, soon followed by multiplane[12] imaging. Today transesophageal echocardiography has become a practical clinical modality in the community hospital as well as the academic medical center. In is performed in ambulatory clinics, intensive care units, endoscopy suites, and in the operating room. The volume of transesophageal echocardiograms performed has grown steadily and in most laboratories represents 5% to 9% of all transthoracic examinations. It is not the aim of this chapter to describe the mechanics of transesophageal imaging or to summarize the published literature. I have focused on topics in transesophageal echocardiography that have most evolved in recent years. No doubt there will be important developments introduced after this book goes to press which will futher advance the utility of transesohageal echocardiography.

Safety of transesophageal echocardiography

Transesophageal echocardiography is a combination of two well known techniques: echocardiography and esophageal endoscopy. It should be performed by a cardiologist who has received additional training in endoscopy. In the operating room an anesthesiologist, well trained in echocardiography technique, may replace the cardiologist. In 1992, the American Society of Echocardiography published guidelines for physician training in transesophageal echocardiography.[13]

The technique is semi-invasive but major complications are rare. In 1991, Daniel et al[14] reviewed the experience of 15 European centers, performing transesophageal echocardiography for at least one year. This is to date, the largest tranesophageal echocardiographic study reported. A total of 10,419 transesophageal echocardiography examinations were performed in the participating institutions. Major complications reported were 6 bronchospasms, 2 episodes of hypoxia, 3 non-sustained ventricular tachycardia, 3 transient atrial fibrillation, 1 third degree atrioventricular block, and one severe angina pectoris. One of the patients with bleeding complications died (mortality rate 0.0098%). The autopsy revealed a malignant lung tumor with esophageal infiltration. Kjanderia et al[15] published similar statistics from the Mayo clinic. In a study of 5500 transesophageal echocardiograma the incidence of complications, both major and minor, was 2.8%. Only one death was reported. Thus, though semi-invasive, transesophageal echocardiography is a low risk procedure.

Antibiotic prophylaxis

There has been considerable debate on the necessity of endocarditis prophylaxis for patients undergoing transesophageal echocardiography. The risk of endocarditis is associated with both the incidence of bacteremia and with the presence of cardiac pathology. Patients who undergo transesophageal echocardiography have a high prevalence of valvular heart disease.[16-19] The incidence of bacteremia reported with esophagogastroscopy has been reported to be between 4% and 8%.[20-24] The risk of bacteremia from transesophageal echocardiography appears to be minimal. Chandrasekaran et al[25] reported that all cultures in their series of 85 patients were negative except in two patients with preexisting bacteremia. Melendez et al[26] in a study of 140 patients who underwent transesophageal echocardiography reported that the incidence of positive blood cultures after the procedure was no higher than that of samples taken before the procedure. Only one small series[27] of 24 patients reported an incidence of bacteremia of 17%. The organisms isolated were all mouth flora, and would not be susceptible to the recommended antimicrobial prophylaxis recommended by the American Heart Association. Final reccomendations are pending from the American Heart Association, but at this time antibiotic prophylaxis appears to be warranted only for high risk patients- patients with prosthetic heart valves, devices , poor dentition or a history of endocarditis.

Endocarditis

Transesophageal echocardiography has become an important tool in the diagnosis and management of suspected infective endocarditis *(Figure 25.1)*. It has been shown to be superior to transthoracic echocardiography for the detection of both valvular vegetations[28-31] and perivalvular complications.[32] Sochowski et al, using a monoplane scope, recently demonstrated that a negative transesophageal echocardiography study reduces the likelihood that endocarditis is present. They cautioned that in high risk patients, such as those with prosthetic valves, a repeat examination is warranted. With a multiplane scope, the sensitivity of transesophageal echocardiography for diagnosing endocarditis may be even higher.

There remains controversy over the necessity of transesophageal echocardiography in diagnosing and managing endocarditis. Karalis et al[33] published an interesting paper on the utility of transesophageal echocardiography in aortic valve endocarditis. The authors found that subaortic complications were present in 13 of 24

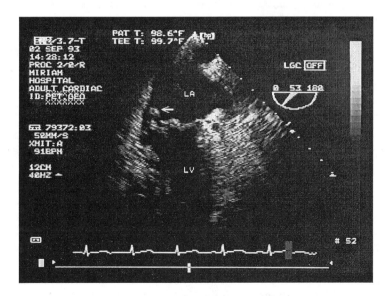

*Figure 25.1 **Endocarditis**. Multiplane transesophageal image 53 from the transverse axis of a patient with endocarditis of the mitral valve. The arrow points to a mass attached to the posterior leaflet. LA-left atrium, LV-left ventricle.*

patients (54%) studied. In many of these cases, the medical and surgical management was altered by the echocardiographic findings.

Atrial fibrillation

The current recommendation for management of atrial fibrillation of greater than two days duration is that patients should receive warfarin therapy for three weeks before cardioversion and four weeks after cardioversion.[34] These recommendations are based largely on a study published by Bjerkelund and Orining in 1969.[35] The authors reported the results of a prospective, controlled study comparing long-term anticoagulant prophylaxis with no anticoagulant prophylaxis in 437 patients undergoing electrical cardioversion for atrial arrhythmias. The incidence of systemic embolization in the group receiving long-term anticoagulant therapy was only 0.8%, whereas the incidence in the group without anticoagulant therapy was 5.3%.

The left atrial appendage has been implicated as the location of thombus formation in serveral studies. Transthoracic echocardiography is limited in its ability to detect left atrial thrombi with sufficient sensitivity. Pollick and Taylor studied 82 patients by transesophageal Doppler echocardiography and observed an association between thrombus formation and increased left atrial appendage size, as well as poor atrial appendage contraction. Spontaneous echo contrast in the left atrium is thought to be a marker of stasis and has been associated with thrombus formation. Pozzoli et al., using pulsed Doppler transesophageal echocardiography, reported a relationship between left atrial appendage dysfunction, spontaneous echo contrast and thrombus formation. Verhorst et al. reported that left atrial appendage forward and reverse peak flow velocities were lower in patients with a recent episode of systemic embolization than in those without a history of thromboembolic events. Garcia-Fernandez et al found that impaired atrial appendage function was associated with the presence of thrombus. These findings were true for both atrial fibrillation and sinus rhythm *(Figure 25.2)*.

One great advantage of transesophageal echocardiography over transthoracic imaging is the ability to image the left atrial appendage. Because of this, several groups suggested that transesophageal echocardiography may be useful in screening patients for thromboembolic complications prior to electrical cardioversion. However, Fatkin et al reported thromboembolic complications occuring after electrical cardioversion in 4 of 65 patients who had had a negative transesophageal echocardiogram. One explanation for these observations is that thrombi which may be large enough to lodge in small cerebral vessels may be too small to be detected by transesophageal echocardiography. An alternative explanation that the authors proposed is that thrombus formation occured after the cardioversion procedure with "atrial stunning". In support of this theory, the authors reported the development of spontaneous echo contrast in several patients post electrical cardioversion.

Certainly, the report of cerebral events in patients with negative transesophageal echocardiograms should make the clinician cautious in proceeding with early

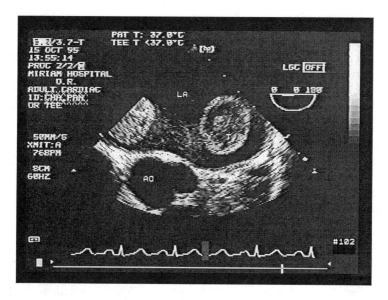

*Figure 25.2 **Left atrial thrombi**. This transesophageal image depicts two masses 2.8 cm in diameter which were proven to be thrombi (T) after surgical excision. This patient had rheumatic mitral stenosis but remained in normal sinus rhythm. LA-left atrium, AO-aortic root.*

cardioversion. Grimmm et al have proposed an algorithm in which transesophageal echocardiography is used in deciding upon anticoagulation. They suggest that all patients should undergo therapeutic anticoagulation at the time of as well as after cardioversion but a negative transesophageal echocardiogram would shorten the time of anticoagulation prior to electrical cardioversion. Manning and colleagues recently studied 230 patients admitted to the hospital for conversion of atrial fibrillation. All patients with no contraindication received anticoagulation with heparin. If no thrombus was visualized by transthoracic or transesophageal echocardiography, the patients underwent pharmacologic or electrical cardioversion. Patients with a positive echocardiographic study received at least three weeks of anticoagulation with warfarin prior to cardioversion. All eligible patients received warfarin for at least three weeks after cardioversion. No thromboembolic events were observed. These results support the concept of shortening the period of anticoagulation prior to cardioversion when transesophageal echocardiographic imaging is negative. Because of the low incidence of thromboembolic events with cardioversion, a large, prospective, randomized trial is necessary to confirm these results. A multicenter trial entitled the Assessment of Cardioversion Using Transesophageal Echocardiography (ACUTE) is currently underway to answer this question.

None of these trials addressed the risk of thromboembolic events with atrial flutter. Bikkina and colleagues recently studied 24 patients admitted to the hospital with atrial flutter with transesophageal echocardiograms. Patients with prior doc-

umented atrial fibrillation, a prosthetic valve or current anticoagulation were excluded from the study. Intra-atrial thrombus was detected in 5 of the 24 patients
(21%) with atrial flutter. This contrasted with 6 thrombi in 184 consequetive control patients studied during the same period of time. Male gender and left ventricular ejection fraction <40% were predictors of left atrial thrombus formation in
patients with atrial flutter.

Aortic dissection

Dissection of the thoracic aorta is a life-threatening emergency and requires prompt
diagnosis and treatment. Patients with DeBakey type I or type II (Stanford type A)
aortic dissection usually require immediate surgery, whereas patients with DeBakey
type III dissection (Stanford type B) can generally be managed medically.

Transesophageal echocardiography has emerged as a powerful tool for diagnosing aortic dissection *(Figure 25.3)*. Simon et al. diagnosed dissection in 32 of 32
patients with transesophageal echo. Erbel et al. found that transesophageal echocardiography missed the diagnosis in 1 of 82 patients. When that patient underwent
aortic valve replacement for severe aortic regurgitation a localized type II dissection was noted. Ballal et al. used transesophageal echocardiography to correctly
diagnose aortic dissection in 33 of 34 patients (sensitivity 97%) Their one false
negative had a localized dissection close to the aortic valve leaflet in a large ascending aortic aneurysm. Nienaber et al. compared transesophageal echocardiography
to magnetic resonace imaging and x-ray computer tomography for diagnosing aortic
dissection They reported similar sensitivities for magnetic resonance imaging (98%),
transesophageal echocardiography (98%) and x-ray computer tomography (94%).
However, the specificity of transesophageal echocardiography (77%) was lower than
magnetic resonance imaging (98%).

Bansal et al. studied the reasons for false negative diagnosis of aortic dissection by transesophageal echocardiograpy and by aortography. In 65 patients studied by both methods, transesophageal echocardiography correctly diagnosed dissection in 63 patients (97%) while aortography diagnosed 50 patients correctly (77%).
The two patients in whom aortic dissection was not recognized by transesophageal
echocardiography had type II dissections localised to the inner margin of the distal
ascending aorta. This region is difficult or impossible to image by transesophageal
echocardiography because of the presence of the air-filled trachea.

Intraoperative transesophageal echocardiography in mitral valve repair

Intraoperative epicardial echocardiography has long been recognized as a useful
tool in patients undergoing mitral valve surgery. Mitral valve repair is preferable to
mitral valve replacement whenever technically possible, because valve repair has
lower short-term morbidity and mortality, stable long-term results, and better left

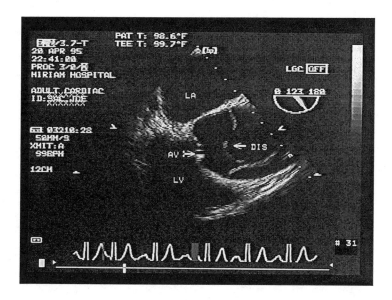

*Figure 25.3 **Aortic dissection**. This is an image of a proximal aortic dissection. The dissection (dis) begins about 2 cm distal to the aortic valve (AV) and continued to the descending aorta. LA-left atrium, LV-left ventricle.*

ventricular function, probably because of the tethering effect of papillary muscles and chordae. However, residual mitral regurgitation after repair remains a problem and intraoperative echocardiography has been shown to be an invaluable aid.

The introduction of transesophageal imaging, made intraoperative imaging more practical since the sterile field is not affected *(Figures 25.4, 25.5)*. Sheikh and colleagues studied 154 consecutive patients undergoing different types of valve surgery to assess the utility of intraoperative transesophageal echocardiography.[36] Prebypass imaging yielded unsuspected findings that either assisted or changed the planned operation in 29 (19%) of the patients. In the subset of patients undergoing mitral valve operations, surgical decisions based on echocardiographic results were made in 26(41%) of 64 cases. Postbypass imaging revealed unsatisfactory operative results that necessitated immediate further surgery in 10 (6%) of the 154 patients. Postbypass imaging also identified patients at risk for an adverse postoperative outcome resulting from valve dysfunction or from reduced left ventricular function. Furthermore, Reichert and colleagues studied 23 patients undergoing mitral valve reconstruction for severe mitral regurgitaion and found that residual mitral regurgitation, as assessed by transesophageal color flow mapping in the operating room, correlated highly with the ultimate mitral regurgitation by contrast cineventriculography.[37]

When assessing mitral regurgitation in the operating room, it is important to remember that regurgitation is particularly sensitive to the afterload state. Careful consideration should be given to the patient's peripheral systolic blood pressure

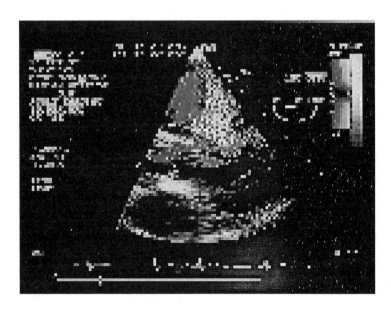

Figure 25.4 **Severe mitral regurgitation.** *This is a color Doppler image of a patient with a flail anterior leflet and severe eccentric mitral regurgitation (MR). LA-left atrium, LV-left ventricle*

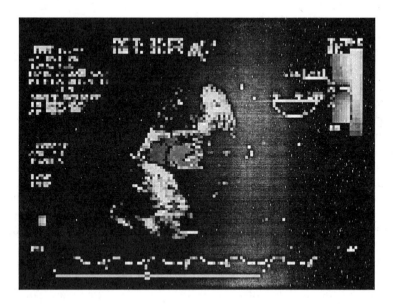

Figure 25.5 **Mitral valve repair.** *This image was taken from the same patient as Figure 4 after successful mitral valve repair. A Cosgrove ring was placed in the mitral position and no residual mitral regurgitation is noted. LA-left atrium LV-left ventricle.*

when evaluating mitral regurgitaion.[38] For this reason, the decision to perform mitral valve surgery in a patient undergoing other cardiac surgery should be made prior to going to the operating room whenever possible. In addition to assessing the extent of mitral regurgitation transesophageal echocardiography is extremely helpful in identifying the mechanical cause for regurgitation. It has been demonstrated to be helpful in assessing the feasibility of repair and the method of reconstruction.[39]

One complication of mitral valve repair is the development of systolic anterior motion of the mitral apparatus. Freeman and and associates reported that severe systolic anterior motion of the mitral apparatus caused significant mitral regurgitation in 13 of 143 patients (9.1%).[40] Importantly, they observed that systolic anterior motion resolved with correction of the postcardiopulmonary bypasss hyperdynamic state typically caused by hypovolemia and intravenous catecholamine infusions. In their study, contrary to previous reports[41,42,43], no patient had left ventricular outflow tract obstruction induced by systolic anterior motion on predischarge transthoracic echocardiogram.

It is important to note that delineation of the mitral reguitant jet is affected by the instrument used, gain settings and available windows. The mitral regurgitant volume and orifice, left ventricular systolic pressure, left atrial pressure and compliances, as well as the mechanism of leaflet malcoaptation, all affect the assessment of mitral regurgitation. Eccentric mitral regurgitant jets, typically seen with mitral prolpase or flail leaflet segments, adhere to the wall of the left atrium because of the Coanda effect, decreasing the apparent size of the regurgitant signal by Doppler color echocardiography.[44] Pulsed wave Doppler echocardiography of the pulmonary venous inflow, with pulmonry venous systolic flow reversal being a highly sensitive finding for severe mitral regurgitation[45], provides complementary information and should be routinely performed.

Conclusion

Transesophageal echocardiography is an essential diagnostic tool for the modern cardiologist. Advances in techniques, image processing, and adjuvant procedures will no doubt make transesophageal imaging increasingly important. Because of space limitations, I have limited my discussion of intraoperative transesophageal echocardiography to mitral valve surgery, but many institutions have found it usesful for intraoperative left ventricular function monitoring. No doubt the development of ultrasonic contrast agents will improve assessment of ventricular function and assessment of myocardial viability. Furthermore, I have not discussed the enormous utility of transesophageal echocardiography in congenital heart disease. Advances in three dimensional reconstruction techniques will increase the utility of transesophageal echocardiography in evaluating complex congenital heart disease. Finally, improved border detection techniques and digital storage and retrieval of echocardiograms will improve the accuracy of transesophageal imaging and make distant review of studies more accessible.

REFERENCES

1. Frazin L, et al. Esophageal echocardiography. Circulation 1976;54:102.

2. Hisanaga K, et al. High speed rotating scanner for transesophageal cross-sectional echocardiography. Am J Cardiol 1980;46:837.

3. Schluter M, et al. Transesophageal cross-sectional echocardiography with a phased array transducer system: technique and initial clinical results. Br Heart J 1982;48:67.

4. Schluter M, et al. Assessment of transesophageal pulsed Doppler echocardiography in the detection of mitral regurgitation. Circulation 1982;66:784.

5. Takamoto S, Omoto R. Visualization of thoracic dissecting aortic aneurysm by transesophageal Doppler color flow mapping. Herz 1987;12:187.

6. De Bruijn NP, Clements FM, Kisslo J. Transesophageal application of color flow imaging. Echocardiography 1987;4:557.

7. Nellessen U, et al. Transesophageael two-dimensional echocardiography and color Doppler flow velocity mapping in the evaluation of cardiac valve prostheses. Circulation 1988;78:848.

8. Weintraub A, et al. CW Doppler in transesophageal echocardiography allows anaylsis of high velocity flows and enhances the utility of transesophageal echo. Circulation 1990;82(suppl III):669.

9. Bansal RC, et al. Biplane transesophageal echocardiography: technique, image orientation, and preliminary experience in 131 patients. J Am Soc Echocardiogr 1990;3:348.

10. Seward JB, et al. Biplanar transesophageal echocardiography: anatomic correlations, image orientation, and clinical applications. Mayo Clin Proc 1990;65:1193.

11. Omoto R, et al. New trend in transesophageal echocardiography: combined use of matrix biplane proble and real-time side-by-side biplane imaging system. Circulation 1990;82(suppl III):667.

12. Eiachskampf FA, Hoffman R, Hanrath P. Experience with a transesophageal echo-transducer allowing full rotation of the viewing plan: the omniplane probe. J Am Coll Cardiol 1991;17:34A.

13. Pearlman AS, et al. Guidelines for physician training in transesophageal echocardiography: Recommendations of the American Society of Echocardiography Committee for Physician Training in Echocardiography. J Am Soc Echocardiogr 1992;5:187.

14. Daniel WG, et al. Safety of transesophageal echocardiography — a multicenter survey of 10,419 examinations. Circulation 1991;83:817.

15. Khandheria BK. The transesophageal echocardiographic examination: Is it safe? Echocardiography 1994;11:55.

16. Seward J, et al. Transesophageal echocardiography: technique, anatomic correlations, implementations, and clinical applications. Mayo Clin Proc 1988;63:649.

17. Currie PJ. Transesophageal echocardiography: new window to the heart. Circulation 1989;80:215.

18. Gussenhoven EJ, et al. Transesophageal two-dimensional echocardiography: its role in solving clinical problems. J Am Coll Cardiol 1986;8:975.

19. Foster E, et al. Streptococcal endocarditis temporally related to transesophageal echocardiography. J Am Soc Echo 1990;3:424.

20. Perucca PJ, Meyer GW. Who should have endocarditis prophylaxis for upper gastrointestinal procedures? Gastrointest Endosc 1985;31:285.

21. Shorvon PJ, Eykyn SJ, Cotton PB. Gastrointestinal instrumentation, bacteremia, and endocartidis. Gut 1983;24:1078.

22. Leitch DG, et al. Bacteremia following endoscopy. Br J Clin Pract 1986;40:341.

23. Norfleet RG, et al. Does bactermia follow upper gastrointestinal endoscopy? Am J Gastroenterol 1981;76:420.

24. Botoman VA, Surawicz CM. Bacteremia with gastrointestinal endoscopic procedures. Gastrointest Endosc 1986;32:342.

25. Chandrasekaran K, et al. Impact of transesophageal color flow Doppler echocardiography in current cardiology practice. Echocardiography 1990;7:114.

26. Melendez LJ, et al. Incidence of bacteremia in transesophageal echocardiography: A prospective study of 140 consecutive patients. JACC 1991;18:1650.

27. Gorge G, et al. Positive blood cultures during transesophageal echocardiography. Am J Cardiol 1990;65:1404.

28. Daniel WG, et al. Conventional and transesophageal echocardiography in the diagnosis of infective endocarditis. Eur Heart J 1987;8 (suppl):287-92.

29. Erbel R, et al. Improved diagnostic value of echocardiography in patients with infective endocarditis by transesophageal approach: a prospective study. Eur Heart J 1988;9:43.

30. Mugge A, et al. Echocardiography in infective endocarditis: reassessment of prognostic implications of vegetation size determined by the transthoracic and the transesophageal approach. J Am Coll Cardiol 1989;14:631.

31. Shively BK, et al. Diagnostic value of transesophageal compared with transthoracic echocardiography in infective endocarditis. J Am Coll Cardiol 1991;18:391.

32. Daniel WG, et al. Improvement in the diagnosis of abscesses associated with endocarditis by transesophageal echocardiography. N Engl J Med 1991;324:795.

33. Karalis DG, et al. Transesophageal echocardiographic recognition of subaortic complications in aortic valve endocarditis. Clinical and surgical implications. Circulation 1992;86:353.

34. Laupacis A, et al. Antithrombotic therapy in atrial fibrillation. Third ACCP Conference on Antithrombotic Therapy. Chest 1992;102 Suppl:426S.

35. Bjerkelund CJ, Orning OM. The efficacy of anticoagulant therapy in preventing embolism related to DC electrical conversion of atrial fibrillation. Am J Cardiol 1969;23:208.

36. Shrestha MK, et al. Two dimensional echo diagnosis of left atrial appendage thrombus in rheumatic heart disease. A clinicopathologic study. Circulation 1983;67:341.

37. Jordan RA, Scheifey CH, Edwards JE. Mural thrombus and arterial embolism in mitral stenosis: a clinicopathologic study of fifty one cases. Circulation 1951;3:363.

38. Schweizer P, et al. Detection of left atrial thrombi by echocardiography. Br Heart J 1981;45:148.

39. Bansal RC, et al. Detection of left atrial thrombi by two-dimensional echocardiograpy and surgical correlation in 148 patients with mitral valve disease. Am J Cardiol 1989;64:243.

40. Pollick, C, Taylor D. Assessment of left atrial appendage function by transesophageal echocardiography, Implications for the development of thrombus. Circulation 1991;84:223.

41. Iliceto S, et al. Dynamic intracavitary left atrial echoes in mitral stenosis. am J Cardiol 1985;55:603.

42. Daniel W, et al. Left atrial spontaneous echo contrast in mitral valve disease: an indicatior for increased thromboembolic risk. J Am Coll Cardiol 1988;11:1204.

43. Erbel R, et al. Detection of spontaneous echocardiographic contrast within the left atrium b transesophageal echocardiography: spontaneous echocardiographic contrast. Clin Cardiol 1986;9:245.

44. Black IW, et al. Left atrial spontaneous echoc contrast: a clinical and echocardiographic analysis. J Am Coll Cardiol 1991;18:398.

45. Pozzoli M, et al. Left atrial apendage dysfunction: a cause of thrombosis? Evidence by transesophageal echocardiography-Doppler studies. J AM Soc Echocardiography 1991;4:435.

46. Verhorst P, et al. Left atrial appendage flow velocity assessment using transesophageal echocardiography in nonrheumatic atrial fibrillation and systemic embolism. Am J Cardiol 1993;71:192.

47. Garcia-Fernandez MA, et al. Left atrial appendage doppler flow patterns: implications of thrombus formation. Am Heart J 1992;124:955.

48. Orsinelli DA, Pearson AC. Usefulness of transesophageal echocardiography to screen for left atrial thrombus before elective cardioversion for atrial fibrillation. Am J Cardiol 1993;72:1337.

49. Manning WJ, et al. Cardioversion from atrial fibrillation without prolonged anticoagulation with use of transesohpageal echocardiography to exclude the presence of atrial thrombi. N Engl J Med 1993;328:750.

50. Fatkin D, et al. Transesophageal echocardiography before and during direct current cardioversion of atrial fibrillation: evidence for "atrial stunning" as a mechanism of thromboemblic complications. J Am Coll Cardiol 1994;23:307.

51. Grimm AG, et al, Should all patients undergo transesophageal echocardiograpy before electrical cardioversion of atrial fibrillation? J Am Coll Cardiol 1994;23:533.

52. Manning WJ, et al. Transesophageal echocardiographically facilitated early cardioversion from atrial fibrillation using short-term anticoagulation: Final results of a prospective 4.5 year study. J Am Coll cardiol 1995;25:1354.

53. Bikkina M, et al. Prevalence of intraatrial thrombus in patients with atrial flutter. Am J Cardiol 1995;76:186.

54. Debakey ME, et al. Surgical management of dissecting aneurysms of the aorta. J Thoracic Cardiovasc Surg 1965;49:130.

55. Simon P, et al. Transesophageal echocardiography in the emergency surgical management of patients with aortic dissection. J Thorac Cardiovasc Surg 1992;103:1113.

56. Erbel R, et al. Echocardiography in the diagnosis of aortic dissection. Lancet 1989;1:457.

57. Ballal RS, et al. Usefulness of transesophageal echocardiography in assessment of aortic dissection. Circulation 1991;84:1903.

58. Nienaber CA, et al. The diagnosis of thoracic aortic dissection by noninvasive imaging procedures. N Engl J Med 1993;328:1.

59. Bansal RC, et al. Frequency and explanation of false negative diagnosis of aortic dissection by aortography and transesophageal echocardiograpy. J Am Coll Cardiol 1995;25:1393.

60. Johnson ML, et al. Usefulness of echocardiography in patients undergoing mitral valve surgery. J Thorac Cardiovas Surg 1972;64:922.

61. Goldman ME, et al. Intraoperative echocardiography for the evaluation of valvular regurgitation: experience in 263 patients. Circulation 1986;74:143.

62. Maurer G, et al. Intraoperative Doppler color flow mapping for assessment of valve repair for mitral regurgitaion. Am J Cardiol 1987;60:333.

63. Yacoub M, et al. Surgical treatment of mitral regurgitation caused by floppy vlves: repair versus replacement. Circulation 1981;64:210.

64. Carpentier. cardiac valve surgerey-the "French correction." J Thorac Cardiovasc Surg 1983;86:323.

65. Bonchek LI, et al. Left ventricular performance after mitral valve reconstruction for mitral regurgitation. J Thorac Cardiovasc Surg 1984;88:122.

66. Stewart W, et al. Intraoperative Doppler color flow mapping for decision-making in valve repair for mitral regurgitation: Thechnique and results in 100 patients. Circulation 1990;81:556.

67. Sheikh KH, et al. The utility of transesophageal echocardiography and Doppler color flow imaging in patients undergoing cardiac valve surgery. J Am Coll Cardiol 1990;15:363.

68. Reichert SL, et al. Intraoperative transesophageal color-coded Doppler echocardiography for evalvuation of residual regurgitation after mitral valve repair. J Thorac cardiovas Surg 1990;100:756.

69. Maurer G, et al. Intraoperative Dopper Color flow mapping for assessment of valve repair for mitral regurgitaion. Am J Cardiol 1987;60:333.

70. Pieper EP, et al. Additional value of biplane transesophageal echocardiography in assessing the genesis of mitral regurgitation and the feasibility of valve repair. Am J Cardiol 1995;75:489.

71. Freeman WK, et al. Intraoperative evaluation of mitral valve regurgitation and repair by transesophageal echocardiography: incidence and significance of systolic anterior motion. J Am Coll Cardiol 1992;20:599.

72. Galler M, et al. Long-term follow-up after mitral valve reconstruction: incidence of postoperative left ventricular outflow obstruction. Circulation 1986:74(suppl I):I-99.

73. Schiavone WA, et al. Long-term follow-up of patients with left ventricular outflow tract obstruction after Carpentier ring mitral valvuloplasty. Circulation 1988;78(suppl I):I60.

74. Mihaileanu s, et al. Left ventricular outflow obstruction after mitral valve repair (Carpentier's technique). Circulation 1988;78(suppl I):I-78.

75. Cape EG, et al. Adjacent solid boundaries alter the size of regurgitant jets on Doppler color flow maps. J Am Coll Cardiol 1991;17:1094.

76. Klein AL, et al. Transesophageal echocardiography of pulmonary venous flow: a new marker of mitral regurgitaton severity. J Am Coll Cardiol 1991;18:518.

26 DUPLEX VASCULAR ULTRASONOGRAPHY

Aris Antoniou, Lampros Vlahos

Cardiovascular disease is the leading cause of death in the United States. For example in 1987 46% of the estimated 2.127.000 deaths recorded in the USA, 976,706 deaths were attributable to diseases of the heart and blood vessels.[1,2] Most of these deaths can be attributed to atherosclerosis. Stroke remains the third most common and leading cause of death in the western world and the major cause od disability in adults. Approximately 750,000 Europeans will each year experience a stroke which may lead to death or disability disease. Atherosclerosis in the carotid arteries is responsible for up to 25 - 50% of strokes.[3,4]

The pathogenesis of atherosclerosis is not completely understood as the processes involved are complicated and multifactorial. The modified response-to-injury hypothesis of atherosclerosis development was originally proposed in 1976 by Ross and Glomset[5], who hypothesized that the arteriosclerotic lesions were the result to factors released from platelets that had adhered to sites of hypercholesterolemia - induced endothelial denundation. The original hypothesis has undergone several revisions since then.[6,7]

An overview of how an atherosclerotic plaque is formed is given by the response to injury hypothesis. The vessel lumen is covered by a monolayer of endothelial cells which are joined tightly together to form a semipermeable barrier that limits the eflux of large low-density lipoprotein molecules to enter the subendothelial spaces.[8]

The endothelial cells play an important role by inhibiting the platelet aggregation first by the negative surface charge of the endothelium and mainly by the release of the platelet inhibitors prostacyclin (PGI_2) and endothelium - derived relaxing factor or nitric oxide (EDRF - NO) which also relax the smooth muscle of the media and increase the lumen diameter of the vessel. Thrombolysis is also promoted by secretion of tissue plasminogen activator (tPA). When injury of the endothelium happens the loss of tight junctions increases penetration of large molecules into subendothelial space and the function of endothelial cells is impaired. Reduction of the PG2, EDRF - NO, and tPA secretions promotes platelet aggregation and vasoconstriction. The smooth muscle of the media is proliferated by increased secretion of platelet - derived growth factor and endothelin - 1. Leucocytes and T-lymphocytes are recruited to sites of injury - by the damaged endothelial cells which secret monocyte chemoattractant protein - 1 (MCP-1). Endothelial cell damage is promoted by a lot of factors such as aging, hypertension, hyperlipidemias, diabetes, smoking etc which affect one or more functions of the endothelial cells, for example EDRF - NO (nitric acid) secretion is diminished by aging, smoking and hypercholesterolemie, diabetes and hypertension.[9-11]

When primary endothelial cell damage happens the cycle of plaque formation begins. Fatty streak formation is the earliest atherosclerotic lesion noted in the vicinity of arterial branches where irregular hemodynamic phenomena happen. Fatty streaks are relatively flat intimal lesions consisting of macrophages and smooth muscle which contain droplets of lipids.[12] Fatty streaks most commonly progress into fibrotic lesion and rarely regress.[13] Fibrotic lesions are characterized by a fibrotic cap composed of smooth muscle cells recruited from both the subendothelium and the media.[2,12,14]

As the disease progresses the fibrotic plaque may rupture and intraplaque hemorrhage and subsequent thrombus is formed.[15] Other hypotheses on plaque formation like the monoklonal hypothesis[16] and the immunology hypothesis[17] have been described based on x-linked chromosome studies and T-lymphocytes of the fibrotic cap activation.

Questions arise on the implications of radiology in the diagnosis of the disease, quantification of the stenosis and qualification of the process. The fourth dimension of radiology, time and disease, should always appreciated as traditionally radiographs or sonograms represent a frozen image of a dynamic process at an instant time and based on diagnostic criteria, reflect the morbid anatomy (pathology) findings.[18]

Atherosclerosis is a dynamic process that evolves over time provoked by a number of factors affecting the progress of the disease and also the changes of morphology and composition of the lesions.

Various invasive and non-invasive techniques have been developed and have been used to characterize the atherosclerotic lesions and quantify the vessel narrowing. Among them angiography, conventional and recently digital, is useful in distinguishing between simple and complex plaques if the lesions are viewed at the appropriate angle. It has been shown however on clinical and animal studies that angiography tends to understimate the degree of arteriosclerosis and this is mainly due to the compensatory arterial lumen enlargement as the disease progress and the lumen reduction is not apparent until the area occupied by the plaque reaches a 40% of the area are encircled by the internal elastic lamina.[19,20]

High resolution ultrasound (duplex scanning and color flow doppler imaging C.F.D.I.) has become the first line of investigation in the diagnosis of arterial and venous disease and is extensively used to determine the degree of stenosis and plaque morphology. Recent studies have indicated that the morphology of plaque is of significant importance[21-25] as some types are accompanied by a high risk of cerebral infarction.

In a recent study presented at North Amer Chapter of ISCVS, June 1995 computed assisted plaque morphology study, it was shown that the incidence of CT infarction was increased with echolucent plaques from 10,5% to 66%.[26]

B-mode or gray scale images provide information of the vessel wall anatomy. High-resolution ultrasound images reflect the normal anatomy of the carotid artery wall by demonstrating the adventitia and intima as these layers define the outer and inner margins of the artery. A thin line at the site of the intima does not represent the actual thickness of the structure as it is only a reflection. Between the parallel lines of the adventitia and the intima an echopoor area represents the media. Thickening or undulation of the intimal reflection represents plaque formation. Certain arteries e.g. the carotids, coronary, distal aorta and iliofemosal have a high prevalence of plaque formation. At the carotid bifurcation plaque formation is more pronounced at the outer wall of the common carotid artery and the outer lateral wall of the proximal segment of the internal carotid *(Figure 26.1)*. Studies have shown that oscillations in flow direction occur at the lateral wall in the region of flow separation, the wall shear stress is low and blood flow remains undirectional throughout the cardiac cycle.[27,28] Thus results in a longer exposure of the endothelial cells to atherogenic substances circulating in the blood[29] and is termed "increased particle residence time". Thereafter the formation of the plaque follows the "response-to-injury hypothesis *(Figure 26.2)*.

Plaque vary in composition and some are soft (echolucent) and friable and others sclerotic and heavily calcified (echogenic). The appearance of plaque is not uniform and contain in different percentages clusters of cholesterol, fibrous tissue and calcium. B-mode classification of plaque according to their characteristics :

TYPE I : Uniformely echolucent. A tiny thin echogenic cap at the margin of the plaque may be visible. In our institution we call this type of plaques "Ghost plaque" as sometimes are not visible on gray. Scale image and only the increased Doppler signal or the disturbed C.F.D.I. suggests their presence.

TYPE II : Predominantly echolucent with <50% echogenic areas which represent the fibrous tissue *(Figure 26.3)*.

TYPE III : Predominantly echogenic with <50% echolucent areas *(Figure 26.4)*.

TYPE IV : Uniformly echogenic *(Figure 26.5)*

TYPE V : Plaque that cannot be classified due to heavy calcification.

Gray - scale sonograms in traverse and longitudinal plane with or without C.F.D.I. are necessary to evaluate the carotid lumen, to estimate the luminal reduction, the plaque extension as well as the characterisation of the plaque content and its surface assessment (smooth - irregular - ulcerated). In addition vertebral arteries are always evaluated for reverse blood flow *(Figure 26.6)*

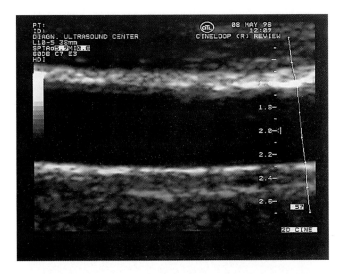

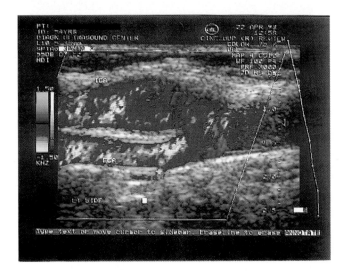

Figure 26.1 Normal bifurcation of the common carotid.

Doppler spectal analysis at site of maximum stenosis demonstarted on Gray Scale or C.F.D.I. is necessary to quantify the hemodynamic changes and grade the stenosis in mild - moderate - severe or occluded. The Duplex criteria for grading internal carotid artery (ICA) stenosis *(Table 26.l)* using the STRANDNESS criteria (D, D+), ratio of peak systolic velocity of ICA to end - diastolic velocity of common carotid artery (CCA), end-diastolic velocity of CCA.

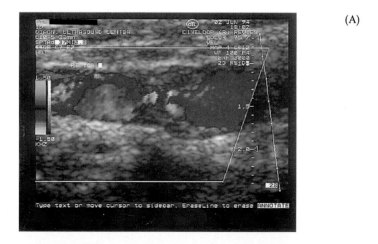

(A)

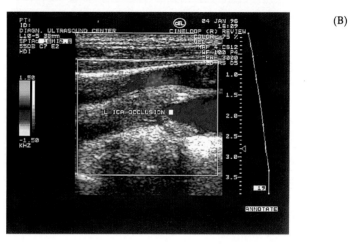

(B)

*Figure 26.2 Concentric plaque type II-III at the right ICA (A). Concetric plaque at the
origin of left ICA causing complete occlusion (B).*

Duplex criteria for grading carotid stenosis

Condition that may affect the velocity criteria is arrhythmia, hypertension, aortic
valve insufficiency, severe proximal CCA stenosis, occlusion or severe distal ICA
stenosis, contralateral ICA or CCA severe stenosis or occlusion. Anatomic variations such as kinking and coiling of the carotid artery and other pathology such as
aneurysm, dissection, A-V malformation or carotid body tumor.

C.F.D.I. has proved especially useful in the cases of "pseudo-occlusion" a term
describing very severe stenoses. The identification of a minimal flow by CFDI suggests a string - like remaining lumen thus affecting the desicion making for endarterectomy.[30]

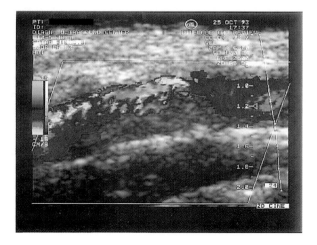

Figure 26.3 Soft-tissue eccentric plaque type II at the origin and proximal part of ICA, causing severe stenosis.

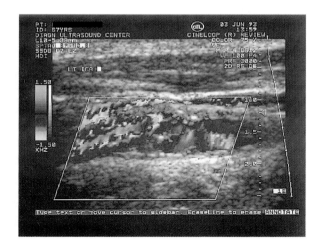

Figure 26.4 Ulcerated atheromatous plaque type III at the proximal part of ICA causing severe stenosis.

Peripheral arterial sonography

Color flow Doppler Imaging (C.F.D.I.) has emerged as a useful tool in the diagnosis of peripheral arterial disease, in the last decade. C.F.D.I. provides mapping and description of focal stenosis or occlusions, documentation of the site and extension

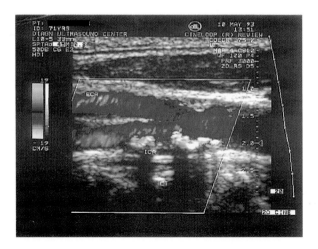

Figure 26.5 Multiple calcified plaques at the ICA origin (TYPE IV).

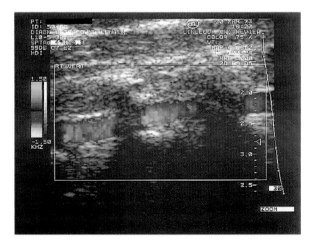

Figure 26.6 *Reversed flow in the vertebral artery due to severe stenosis of the innominate artery.*

of plaques, lumen diameter reduction and flow disturbances, that effectively could be treated by non-surgical interventional angiographic techniques and non invasively monitor the effects of such procedures [31,32].

Diagnostic difficulties arise in 1) patients with diffuse arterial wall calcification e.g. diabetics, 2) in the presence of multiple tandem lesions in which the hemody-

Table 26.I DUPLEX CRITERIA FOR GRADING ICA STENOSIS

STENOSIS(%)	PSV	EDV	PSV_{ICA} / PSV_{CCA}
0-29	<100	<40	
30-49	110<PSV<130	<40	
50-59	>130	<40	<3,2
60-69	>130	40<EDV<110	3,2/<PSV<4 ratio
70-79	>210	110<EDV<140	>/4
80-95	>210	>140	>/4
96-99		STRING FLOW	
OCCLUSION		ABSENCE OF FLOW	

PSV=peak systolic velocity, EDV=end-diastolic velocity

namic significance of more distal lesions may be difficult to assess, 3) focal lesions in the adductor canal (HUNTER'S canal) region.

The most common sites of involvement in arteriosclerosis in the lower extremity is the superficial femoral artery at the lower third in the HUNTER's canal which produces minimal to moderate claudication because of collaterals developed through the profunda femoris, the second most common site being the arto-iliac segment which often produces serious claudication and for reasons poorly understood involvement of this region is more common in the non-diabetic patient. Standard sonographic examination of the lower extremity includes the evaluation of abdominal aorta and iliac arteries - with special interest at the aortic bifurcation. Thus the patient is examined in the supine and lateral decubitus positions slightly oblique. In this position in the majority of patients both common iliac arteries are visualised and waveforms demonstrating the typical triphasic spectrum is elicited from each vessel.

The external iliac artery becomes the femoral artery as it passes deep to the inguinal ligament. Common femoral artery is a 6 - 8 mm diam. vessel and the patient is examined in supine position with the leg slightly adducted and externally rotated. As bifurcations show a predilection for the development of arteriosclerotic plaques special attention should be paid at the origin of superficial and deep femoral arteries. The superficial femoral artery, a 4-6 mm diam. vessel is traced down to the Hunter's canal (adductor canal), a difficult site to be evaluated as the artery crosses posteriorly towards the popliteal fossa. The popliteal artery (Figure 26.7-26.8) is examined in decubitus or prone position with the knee slightly flexed and has a triphasic waveform. Posterior tibial and peroneal arteries are also examined but as they have rich intercommunicating collaterals which provide adequate blood flow to the foot all three arteries should be involved to give rise to clinical manifestations. Diabetic patients have a greater prevalence of involvement of these vessels than non-diabetic patients.

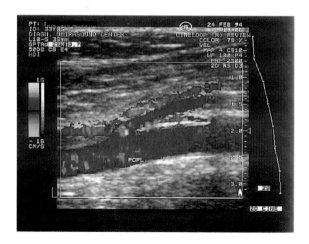

Figure 26.7 Normal popliteal artery bifurcation

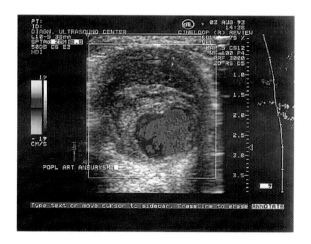

Figure 26.8 Popliteal artery aneurysm

Quantification of peripheral vascular disease relies in a complex study using the C.F.D.I. mapping of the diseased arteries and at the site of maximum stenosis depict the pulsed - Doppler waveform C.F.D.I. alone can depict a stenosis that is seen as a narrowing of the color flow lumen.[33] Sites of significant narrowing of the peripheral arteries will cause focal color Doppler flow abnormalities in which aliasing and flow reversal will appear. Doppler waveform changes at the site of maximum lumen stenosis and proximal arterial segments are taken. Minimal lumen reduction (0 - 19% reduction) consists of mild spectral broadening while the triphasic waveform is preserved. Moderate narrowing (20 - 49% narrowing) is characterized

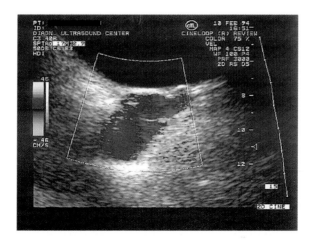

Figure 26.9 Right internal iliac pseudo-aneurysm in a patient operated for pelvic tumor (ovarian cancer)

by spectral broadening, the reverse flow component is preserved but the peak velocity at the site of narrowing increases up to double that in the proximal segment. In severe stenosis, which is surgically significant, there is an increase of peak systolic velocity of >2 m/sec, loss of the reverse flow component thus producing a high-velocity monophasic waveform with continous diastolic flow. Duplex sonography compared to arteriography has a sensitivity of 82% and specificity of 92% in identifying lesions with more than 50% stenosis.[34]

Occlusion is suspected whenever flow signals are not detected either on C.F.D.I. or Doppler, while they are easily detected in the adjacent deep vein portion. C.F.D.I. has been also used as an easy non-invasive method to evaluate post - angioplasty or post - angioplasty complications such as the development of a pseudoaneurysm[35] (Figure 26.9).

Conclusion

C.F.D.I. has emerge as a useful non-invasive tool in the diagnosis of arterial disease and better understanding the natural history of plaque formation. The obvious advantages of C.F.D.I. such as cost and time effectiveness, diagnostic accuracy and high resolution in the characterization of plaque morphology and texture may supplant angiography and for the time being M.R. angiography as the primary imaging modality in arterial disease.

REFERENCES

1. American Heart Association, 1990. Heart and Stroke facts. Dallas: American Heart Association; 1990.

2. P. Macke Consigny: Pathogenesis of Atherosclerosis. Am J Roentgenol 1995; 164:553-558.

3. Harrison MJG: Pathogenesis. In Warlow C, Morris P.J. (eds). Transient Ischemic Attacks p.p. 21-46. Marcel Delkker Inc. New York, 1982.

4. Bogonsslavsky J, et al: Cardiac and arterial lesions in transient ischemic attacks. Arch Neurol. 1986; 43:223-228.

5. Ross R, Glomset J.A. The pathogenesis of atherosclerosis. N Engl J Med 1976; 295:369-377.

6. Ross R. The pathogenesis of atherosclerosis - an update. N Engl J Med 1986; 314:488-500.

7. Ross R. The pathogenesis of atherosclerosis: a perspective for the 1990s. Nature 1993; 362:801-809.

8. Steinberg D, Witztum J.K. Lipoproteins and the pathogenesis of atherosclerosis. Circulation 1990; 264:3047-3052.

9. Flavahau N.A. Atherosclerosis or lipoprotein-induced endothelial dysfunction. Potential mechanisms underlying reduction in EDRF/nitric oxide activity. Circulation 1992; 85:1927-1938.

10. Zeiher A.M, et al. Endothelium-mediated coronary blood flow modulation in humans: effects of age, atherosclerosis hypercholesterolemia, and hypertension. J. Clin Invest 1993; 92:652-662.

11. Pauza J.A, et al. Role of endothelium-derived nitric oxide in abnormal endothelium-dependent vascular relaxation in patients with essential hypertension. Circulation 1993; 87:1468-1474.

12. Stary HC, et al. A definition of initial, fatty streak, and intermediate lesions of atherosclerosis: a report from the Committee on Vascular Lesions of the Council on Arteriosclerosis. American Heart Association. Arterioscler Thromb 1994; 14:840-856.

13. Blankenhorn DH, Kramsch DM. Reversal of atherosis and sclerosis: the two components of atherosclerosis. Circulation 1989; 79:1-7.

14. Faggiotto A, Ross R. Studies of hypercholesterolemia in the non-human primate. II. Fatty streak conversion to fibrons plaque. Arteriosclerosis 1984; 4:341-356.

15. Fuster V, et al. Atherosclerotic plaque rupture and thrombosis: evolving concepts. Circulation 1990; 82 (suppl II): 11-47-11-59.

16. Benditt E.P, Benditt J.M. Evidence for a monoclonal origin of human atherosclerotic plaques. Proc Natl Acad Sci USA 1973; 70:1753-1756.

17. Hansson G.K, Jonasson L, Seifert P.S, Stemme S. Immune mechanisms in atherosclerosis. Arteriosclerosis 1989; 9:567.

18. Dwyer J.A. Time and Disease: The Fourth Dimension of Radiology. Radiology 1989; 173:17-21.

19. Glascov S, et al. Compensatory enlargement of lumen size and wall morphology in normal subjects and patients with coronary artery disease. N Engl J Med 1987; 316:1371-1375.

20. Zarins CK, et al. Differential enlargement of artery segments in responce to enlarging atherosclerotic plaques. J Vasc Surg 1988; 7:386-394.

21. Langsfield M, Gray-Weale A.C, Lusby R.J. The role of plaque morphology and diameter reduction in the development of new symptoms in asymptomatic carotic disease. J Vasc Surg 1989; 9:548-557.

22. Sterpetti A.V, et al. Ultrasonographic features of carotid plaque and the risk of subsequent neurologic deficits. Surgery 1988; 104:652-660.

23. Belcaro G, et al. Ultrasonic classification of carotid plaques causing less than 60% stenosis according to ultrasound morphology and events. J Cardiovasc Surg 1993; 34:287-294.

24. O'Halloran LW, et al. Natural history of asymptomatic carotid plaque. Am J Surg 1987, 154:659.

25. European carotic plaque study group. Carotid plaque composition relation to ultrasound B-mode imaging and clinical presentation. Eur J Vasc Surg in press.

26. Nikolaides A.N, et al. The value of computer analysis of ultrasonic plaque echolucency in identifying high risk carotid bifurcation lesions. North Am Chapter of ISC VS, 1995. J Vasc Surg in press.

27. Phillips DJ, et al. Flow velocity patterns in the carotic bifurcations of young presumed normal subjects. Ultrasound Med Biol 1983; 9:39-49.

28. Middeton WD, Foley WD, Lawson TL. Flow reversal in normal carotid bifurcatim: Color Doppler flow imaging analysis. Radiology 1988; 167:207-210.

29. Zarius CK, Glagov S, Giddens DP. What do we find in human atherosclerosis that provides insight into the hemodynamic factors in atherogenesis? In Glagov S, Newman WP, Schaffer S.A. eds. Pathobiology of the human atherosclerotic plaque. New York: Springer-Verlag, 1990:317-332.

30. Carroll B.A. Carotid sonography. Radiology 1991; 178:303-313.

31. Taylor LM Jr, Edwards JM, Porter JM. Present status of reversed vein bypass grafting: five year results of a modern series. J Vasc Surg 1990; 11:193-206.

32. Adar R, Critchfield G.C, Eddy DM: A confidence profile analysis of the results of femoropopliteal percutaneous transluminal angioplasty in the treatment of lower-extremity ischemia. J Vasc Surg 1989; 10:57-67.

33. Erickson S.J, et al. Stenosis of the internal carotid artery: assessment using color Doppler imaging compared with angiography. AJR 1989; 152:1299.

34. Kohler TR, et al. Duplex scanning for diagnosis of aortoiliac and femoropopliteal disease: a prospective study. Circulation 1987; 76:1074.

35. Sacks D, et al. Evaluation of the peripheral arteries with duplex US after angioplasty. Radiology 1990; 176:39.

Section F
INTERVENTIONAL CARDIOLOGY

27 TREATMENT OPTIONS FOR CORONARY REVASCULARIZATION

Roxana Mehran, Martin B. Leon

The discovery of the use of balloon angioplasty was accomplished by Dotter in 1963, when he recanalized an occluded right iliac artery by passing a percutaneously introduced catheter retrograde through the occlusion to perform an abdominal aortogram in a patient with renal artery stenosis.[1-5] On September 16th, 1977, the first percutaneous transluminal coronary angioplasty (PTCA) in a human was performed by Gruentzig, in Zurich. Gruentzig et al. followed this first report with the first 50 coronary angioplasties in 1979.[6-10]

At its infancy stage in the early years, the coronary angioplasty equipment was cumbersome and primitive. The balloons were of high profile and made of polyvinyl chloride, which was noncompliant and had a low rupture threshold of 6 atm. In the early 1980's the new guiding catheters were constructed with smaller profiles and improved usability. The indications of percutaneous coronary angioplasty hence expanded from the discrete lesions in one coronary artery in stable patients to more complex lesions in more than one coronary artery in patients with acute coronary syndromes. By 1980, 1000 angioplasties were performed in the USA. This number has now exploded into the current >300,000 annual procedures in the USA alone; a staggering growth.[11]

New device angioplasty

The development of the new devices were based on the premise that balloon angioplasty has limitations in treating a subset of lesions with increased risk of acute complications i.e. elastic recoil, dissections and abrupt closure, usually warranting emergency coronary artery bypass operation which is less optimal than elective coronary artery bypass surgery (CABG). Eccentric, ostial, long and calcified lesions fit in this category.

Several laser angioplasty devices have been investigated since the early 1980's [13-15]. The current excimer laser angioplasty catheter emits pulsed energy in the ultraviolet range and ablates plaque by photochemical rather than thermal mechanisms. This technology has been applied to vein graft lesions with some success.[16] The Amsterdam-Rotterdam (AMRO) trial, however showed no benefit from excimer laser (followed by adjunct PTCA) compared with PTCA alone in treating long diffuse lesions. At 6 month s follow-up the restenosis rate was 52% for the laser group and 41% for the PTCA group (p=0.13).[17]

In 1985, Simpson developed the directional atherectomy (DCA) catheter, reporting successful results in removing plaque.[18-22] The emergence of this new device provided basis for the first randomized trial comparing this technique to balloon angioplasty alone.[23,24] The CAVEAT trial used a conservative approach to plaque removal in an attempt to minimize deep vessel wall injury showed a significantly higher procedural success with DCA vs. PTCA (<50% diameter stenosis, 89% vs. 80%, p<0.001). The technique was associated with higher cost, at least as many acute complications and late adverse outcomes, and a similar restenosis rate. Likewise, the CCAT which compared DCA and PTCA in patients undergoing non-ostial proximal left anterior descending angioplasty, showed slightly improved acute procedu-ral success with DCA (94% vs. 88%, p=0.06), but similar angiographic restenosis rates (46% vs. 43%, p=0.7) and clinical events between the two groups.[25] More recent trials have evaluated evaluate the efficacy of aggressive tissue removal, as "optimal DCA" might improve the restenosis rates over PTCA.[26,27] In this context, the acute results of the BOAT and the OARS trials were positive, favoring aggressive directional atherectomy (see relevant chapter). These trials stress the importance of the specific operator in influencing acute procedural outcomes and subsequent restenosis.

In an effort to treat more diffuse and calcified lesions in the coronary arterial tree, a high speed rotational pulverizing device capped by a diamond-studded conical end (Rotablator) was developed.[28,29] This device preferentially pulverizes hard atheromatous tissue with relative sparing of plaque-free wall. The calcified atheromatous plaque is rendered more susceptible to balloon dilation after ablation with rotational atherectomy. This device is associated with a high procedural success rate (>90%), and low complication rate (<5%). The event free survival (i.e., freedom from death, infarction, CABG, or repeat PTCA) was present in about 70% of patients in one year, according to one report.[30-32] The comparison of this technology to balloon angioplasty based on a prospective randomized trial is currently being evaluated.

Despite the development of these new devices the problem of restenosis still remained and occurred in about 35-50% of patients. Restenosis is a complex array of events which occurs almost immediately after vessel wall injury with platelet aggregation, thrombus formation, elastic recoil, intimal hyperplasia and geometric remodeling.

Stents: the final frontier?

Dotter et al. reported the experimental peripheral arterial placement of stainless steel coils in 1969 and nitinol coils in 1983, with mixed results.[33,34] Sigwart et al., innovators of the spring-loaded self-expanding stainless steel Wallstent (Medinvent SA, Lausanne, Switzerland) reported the first use of coronary stents in human in 1987.[35] The next generation of stents were the balloon expandable stents including the Palmaz-Schatz (Johnson & Johnson Interventional Systems, Warren, N.J.) slotted articulated stainless steel device and the Gianturco-Roubin flexible, stainless steel, coil stent (Flex-Stent, Cook, Inc.).[36-38]

In two large randomized trials in Europe (BENESTENT) and the United States (STRESS), stents were found to reduce restenosis in focal de novo native coronary lesions compared with balloon angioplasty.[39-41] Stents offer arterial scaffolding and therefore eliminate recoil and subsequent remodeling. The acute gain offered by stenting is larger than any other device thus far used, and translates into improved long-term outcome. In STRESS, the initial procedural success (92% vs. 88%, p=0.018), as well as the angiographic restenosis rates (32% vs. 42%) were significantly improved in the stent group. The improved restenosis rates for stents in these two trials were offset by a higher rate of vascular complications and longer hospital stay in the stent group. In 1995, Colombo et al. described the utility of intravascular ultrasound guidance in stent placement and thereby eliminating the need for systemic anticoagulation.[42] The reduced anticoagulation dramatically decreased the acute bleeding complications without increasing the sub-acute thrombosis rate. Recently the BENESTENT II Pilot reported the very low restenosis rate using the heparin coated stent with 0% sub-acute thrombosis rate.[43] New stent designs are being developed in an attempt to further improve the results of stenting. The different geometry and material of the new stents may confer more flexible stents with variable sizes to treat the longer lesions in more tortuous arteries. Whether the positive impact of stents on restenosis will remain dominant in the less favorable subgroup of lesions, i.e.: small vessels or diffuse lesions is not as yet known. Despite the improved restenosis rate s achieved with stents, the restenosis rate remain at 20 to 30%. Restenosis within tubular slotted stents is primarily secondary to neointimal hyperplasia. This has been documented by serial intravascular ultrasound studies and confirmed by histologic evidence.[44-48] In-stent restenosis is now a growing problem. Ways to reduce in-stent restenosis, either by improving stent designs, use of ablative techniques prior to stent implantation(to achieve maximal acute lumen dimensions), and combining stent implantation with antiproliferative pharmacologic agents or radiation therapy may further impact the improved restenosis rates over balloon or other new device angioplasty.[49-52]

The emerging trends in percutaneous revascularization include a more "aggressive" operator behavior. Patients are now higher risk with more complex lesions in more than one coronary artery. In pursuit of the "optimal" angiographic result (lower final % diameter stenosis), adjunct athero-ablative techniques with heavy reliance on stenting as the final common pathway are being used. The use of intravascular ultrasound and adjunct pharmacology (e.g. platelet GPIIb/IIIa inhibitors) have been helpful in guiding device use and reducing the acute complications associated with the procedure.[53,54] As a result angiographic success rates have improved (>95%), the procedures are safer with fewer major complications (1-2%), the patient cohort has expanded with improving results in previously unfavorable lesion subsets. Finally percutaneous revascularization is now more definitive with lower repeat clinical revascularization rates (10-20%).

Revascularization of patients with multivessel disease

Approximately 600,000 patients undergo myocardial revascularization in the USA each year at a current estimated cost that exceeds $13.5 billion dollars. It is therefore essential that we determine the best strategy to treat patients with coronary disease that would be safe, efficacious and cost effective.

Introduced in 1969 by Favaloro and colleagues, CABG has become the most completely studied operation in the history of surgery. This established procedure has proven efficacious in many clinical trials [55-59]. In the 1990s patients undergoing bypass surgery are older, more likely to have depressed ejection fractions, and are more likely to have had a prior myocardial infarction. Cardiac surgeons are performing more re-operations, and more emergent surgeries.

Patients with significant valvular disease or left ventricular aneurysms requiring revascularization are best treated with CABG at the time of valve or aneurysm repair. Currently, CABG is also favored when large amounts of myocardium are supplied by one or more chronically occluded vessels, or in the narrowing of "old" saphenous vein grafts. This is secondary to the fact that percutaneous revascularization may not the best choice for these patients Recently the use of CABG has increased in the elderly with reported survival rate of 87% in octogenarians at three year follow-up.

With the use of improved myocardial protection, the mortality rates for multivessel CABG is 1-2% and the risk of perioperative MI approximately 5%. Re-operations may be performed with a mortality of 2-4%, and risk of MI of 8%. Gross neurologic defects result from embolization of atherosclerotic debris, or from air embolization, and the prevalence is 0.5% in young patients, but 5% in patients older than 70, and 8% in patients over 75. As many as 75% of patients demonstrate neurobehavioral disturbances when tested 8 days postoperatively, but by 3 months only 10-30% of patients exhibit them.[60-62]

The 10 year patency of saphenous vein grafts appears variable, with some reporting only 50% patency. Some authors report 80% patency of SVG to LAD, and 70-75% patency in other vessels.[63-65] The internal mammary artery has become the preferred conduit for direct coronary revascularization, and patency rates of up to 90% at 10 years have been described.[66] Use of bilateral internal mammary artery grafting has become popular, but the risk of sternal wound infection is increased in obese or diabetic patients. When the internal mammary arteries are unavailable, the right gastroepiploic artery, inferior mesenteric artery or the inferior epigastric artery may be used. The long-term patency rates for arterial conduits other than LIMA has not yet been demonstrated.

Trials comparing CABG vs. PTCA

The *Argentine Randomized Trial of Coronary Angioplasty vs. Bypass Surgery in Multi-vessel Disease* (ERACI) released one year results in October 1993.[67] This study was designed to compare freedom from combined cardiac events(angina, myocardial infarction, and death) at one, three, and five year follow-up. Results revealed no differences in survival or myocardial infarction rates, and no significant differences in major in-hospital complications. Functional revascularization was similar in both groups. Patients receiving CABG were more likely to have complete revascularization (88 vs. 51%) and were more frequently free of angina, re-interventions and combined cardiac events (84% vs. 64%, p<0.005).

The *Randomized Interventional Treatment of Angina* (RITA) study, from the United Kingdom, aimed to compare the long-term incidence of death and non-fatal myocardial infarction in patients with single or multivessel disease, in whom complete revascularization is feasible with either treatment.[68] Totally occluded vessels could be included if the surgeon and cardiologist agreed that there was an equal chance of restoring blood flow tot the distal artery by either method. At 2.5 year follow-up, 8.6% of patients undergoing CABG vs. 9.8% of PTCA patients had died or suffered a myocardial infarction (p=NS). The need for subsequent revascularization was less for CABG patients 4.8% vs. 37% (p<0.0001). Patients in the PTCA group did report more angina, but using the use of anti-anginals as a marker is not sufficient, since many centers prescribe these drugs routinely post-PTCA, as well as for hypertension or to improve postinfarction mortality. Only 4.8% of the referred patients were randomized, and although this rate is comparable to that obtained in other studies, many of the angiographically eligible patients were not randomized on non-clinical grounds (i.e., patient refusal).

The *German Angioplasty and Bypass Investigation* (GABI) enrolled patients with multivessel disease and Class II to IV angina according to the Canadian Cardiovascular Society (CCS).[69] Out of 8981 patients screened, 359 patients were enrolled. To be included, complete revascularization had to be necessary and technically feasible in at least two arteries supplying different myocardial territories. Perioperative myocardial infarction occurred more frequently in the CABG group 8.1% vs. 2.3% (p<0.05), whereas procedural mortality was no different (2.5% vs. 1.1%). Freedom form angina at discharge was reached in 74% of CABG patients vs. 71% of PTCA patients (p=NS); and at one year, angina CCS class >III was evident in 7% of both groups. In regard to antianginal use, 22% of the CABG group did not require antianginals as opposed to 12% of the PTCA group. At one year there was no difference in myocardial infarction rates, however, re-interventions were necessary in more PTCA patients (p=0.05). In fact, 44% of the patients in the PTCA group required re-intervention (repeat PTCA in 23%, CABG in 18%, and both in

3%). If only the patients who actually underwent the assigned treatment were included in the analysis, the mortality was 11% in the CABG group and 5% in the PTCA group (p=0.047). In this study only 4% of patients screened were randomized and 80% of the patients were men.

The *Coronary Artery Bypass Revascularization Investigation* (CABRI) is a multicenter randomized trial conducted in Western Europe including 26 centers and 11 countries, that used stress thallium studies and repeat cardiac catheterizations in its comparison of the two procedures.[70] This study has demonstrated no significant differences in the rates of myocardial infarction (2.9% vs. 3.3%) at one year among patients assigned to PTCA or CABG, respectively. The need for repeat vascularization was five times greater in the PTCA group, and when the study's intention to treat analysis was abandoned, the differences became sharper. The strongest predictors of persistent angina at one year were a history of infarction, a high CCS angina class, angina on exercise testing, a low maximum heart rate on exercise, and high total burden of coronary artery disease. Investigators conclude that peripheral vascular disease, cerebral vascular disease, and age are predictors of survival, but choice of intervention does not predict survival or freedom from angina.

The *Emory Angioplasty vs. Surgery Trial* (EAST) used primary endpoints of incidence of death, Q-wave infarction, or large defect on SPECT radionuclide scan [71]. Secondary endpoints included the achievement of complete revascularization, incidence of repeat revascularization, left ventricular function, exercise capacity, need for additional procedures, quality of life, and economic considerations. Data were analyzed by an intention-to-treat analysis. A total of 5118 patients were screened, 842 patients (16.5%) were deemed eligible by angiographic, clinical and operator assessment, but 450 were not randomized secondary to physician refusal (353) and patient refusal. The 392 patients enrolled had multivessel disease and ejection fractions>40%. Follow-up angiograms were performed 3 years after the procedure. Complete revascularization was achieved in 66% of CABG patients vs. 44% of PTCA patients. Overall mortality was 6.2% for CABG vs. 7.1% for PTCA, and Q wave infarction was slightly increased in the CABG group, 19.6% vs. 14.6% for PTCA (p=0.2). Left ventricular ejection fraction was 69% in both groups at the time of follow-up. Incidence of large ischemic defects in SPECT scan were similar in both groups: 5.7% of patients in the CABG group vs. 9.6% in the PTCA group (p=0.17). Of the PTCA patients, 22% eventually underwent CABG and 54% had either repeat PTCA or CABG, while only 1% of CABG patients had repeat CABG and 13% PTCA. Angina was more prevalent in the PTCA group at 3 years: 20% of PTCA patients had CCS class II-IV angina, compared with 12% of the CABG patients.

The *Bypass Angioplasty Revascularization Investigation* (BARI), enrolled 1829 patients with signs of clinically severe angina or objective evidence of ischemia and multivessel disease by angiography.[72] The primary endpoint is death at 5 years. Other major endpoint criteria include myocardial infarction, angina, subsequent revascularization, resource use, quality of life, and measures of left ventricular function and angiographic criteria at five years. At a mean follow-up of 5.4 years there was no statistically significant difference in survival between CABG and PTCA (89% vs. 86%). Although the in-hospital rate of myocardial infarction was higher in the CABG group, the PTCA group had a substantially greater need for additional revascularization procedures, especially in the first year after PTCA. Furthermore, a 15% difference in 5-year survival was demonstrated with CABG over PTCA in a *post hoc* subgroup analysis of the diabetic patients of the BARI trial.

The overall message of all these trials is that when comparing the two strategies in treatment of patients with multivessel disease, there is no difference in the long-term prognosis between the two strategies. However, PTCA is associated with higher need for repeat revascularization.[73] Although these trials were randomized with long-term follow-up, they no longer reflect the current practice of percutaneous coronary interventions or CABG. Currently, 30-50% of percutaneous coronary interventional strategies involve the use of stents. The current advances in coronary artery bypass surgical techniques, including grafting off cardio-pulmonary bypass, have decreased the in-hospital morbidity. In these trials, off-bypass CABG was rarely performed. In addition, there were too few arterial conduits used in patients undergoing CABG. Importantly, the follow-up period for most of the trials is too short (average of <3 years), antedating the window of saphenous vein graft disease vulnerability, a factor which may influence longer-term results. Therefore, one has to evaluate the limitations of each strategy, in order to better understand the optimal revascularization strategy for patients with multivessel disease in the current growing phase of percutaneous and surgical revascularization techniques.

Limitations of percutaneous coronary revascularization

Despite the evolution of the multidevice era, we remain perplexed with the problem of restenosis, which remains the major limitation of percutaneous revascularization (see also relevant chapter). Our efforts to diminish this process had not been successful until the development of endovascular stents. However we are still seeking for perfection, as stents are associated with neointimal proliferation which may result in in-stent restenosis, especially in specific lesion subsets (ostial, calcified, small vessel, diffuse disease). Over the years it has become obvious that there are certain factors which may increase the risk for developing restenosis.[74] These include clinical as well as peri-procedural conditions. The clinical predisposing factors for angiographic restenosis include: unstable angina and insulin dependent diabetes mellitus. Hypertension, end-stage renal failure and vasospastic angina have also been implicated.[75,76] The procedural factors associated with increased restenosis rates were explored in the M-HEART study.[75] The variables which correlated best with restenosis were the initial native coronary artery diameter, lesion length, left anterior descending or saphenous vein graft lesion location, percent diameter stenosis pre and post procedure. The restenosis rate varied from 20% in the "low risk" group to 61% in the "high risk" group. Other studies have implicated the coronary lesion morphology factors highly associated with restenosis, namely complex lesion morphology, intraluminal thrombus, or reduced coronary flow (TIMI-grade). Violaris et al. reported the long-term luminal renarrowing after PTCA of total occlusions by quantitative coronary angiography. A significantly higher angiographic restenosis rate at 6 months was observed in patients with total coronary occlusions as compared to those with coronary stenoses (45% vs. 34. %, p<0.001).[77] The fundamental theory of Kuntz and Baim that the acute lumen gain at the time of intervention is the major determinant of greater lumen gain at 6 months has held true in the randomized trials.[78,79] In CAVEAT, the final minimal lumen diameter after the procedure was the single most important determinant of subsequent lumen caliber. This concept continues to hold true with many other randomized trials.

Lesion location. The left anterior descending artery (LAD) lesion location may be an important predictor of restenosis after percutaneous revascularization. In the CAVEAT population, although the subgroup of patients with proximal LAD lesions had a lower angiographic restenosis if treated with DCA, the rate was 51% in the DCA group compared with 63% in the angioplasty group (p=0.04). The restenosis rate for other lesion locations (non-LAD) was 48% in the DCA group compared with 50% in the PTCA group, both significantly lower than the LAD restenosis rates. This trial along with other randomized trials established an association between LAD location and high rate of restenosis. In the STRESS trial, when LAD lesion location was compared to non-LAD lesion location, at the time of intervention, the vessels in the LAD group were smaller (2.850.40 vs. 3.090.48,P<0.0001), with less acute gain (1.370.49 vs. 1.570.53, p<0.0001), which translated into a smaller minimal lumen diameter (1.460.60 vs. 1.760.61, p<0.0001), and a higher diameter stenosis (48.8519.03 vs. 42.9018.73, p0.001) at follow-up. The target lesion revascularization rate of patients with LAD lesions was 19% vs. 11% in the non-LAD location. In the PTCA group, the lesions in the LAD location had a restenosis rate of 62% compared to 32% in the non-LAD location. These data support that LAD lesion location is associated with higher restenosis rate and increased incidence of target lesion revascularization if treated percutaneously.

In-stent restenosis. It is important to note that since STRESS and BENESTENT, the technique of coronary stenting has changed. This has reflected the lower vascular complications and restenosis rates in lesion subsets included in these studies. However, with the current increased use of stents in "non-STRESS or BENESTENT" lesions, the rate of in-stent restenosis is higher.[80] In-stent restenosis occurs about 20-30% of lesions treated with stents, and is usually treated with repeat PTCA. The results after repeat treatment of in-stent restenosis are not adequate and the rate of subsequent target lesion revascularization is high especially in diffuse lesions (lesion length >10mm).[81,82] Therefore it is important to identify predictors of diffuse in-stent restenosis, so that other revascularization techniques can be applied to treat these lesions.

Limitations of CABG

Most patients prefer angioplasty to CABG because it is less invasive, has less morbidity, with a lower frequency of major complications. There is accelerated recovery with angioplasty resulting in early return to normal daily activity and work.

One of the more important complications associated with CABG on cardiopulmonary bypass is the neurologic events that occur with this procedure, especially in the elderly.[83] In a retrospective review of complications among cardiac surgery patients, the frequency of altered mental status was reported to be 3.4%, with a 1% reported rate of stroke.[84] Prospective testing has revealed a 24-34% rate of occurrence of permanent neurologic or neuropsychological deterioration after cardiac surgery. Focal neurologic deficits can occur in association with a large air embolism as a result of restarting cardiac pulsation without completely evacuating air in the cardiac chambers. Focal neurologic deficits can also occur in association with local hypoperfusion and microemboli (atherosclerotic debris at the site of aortic clamping or cannulation). Diffuse neurologic and neuropsychological deficits are presumably due to global cerebral hypoperfusion as a result of microemboli.[85,86] In spite of major improvements in CPB over the years, neurologic event still occur. It is for these reasons that recently coronary artery bypass without cardiopulmonary bypass has been implemented , especially in high risk patients. Other limitations of CABG include the longer recovery associated with the usual healing process post sternotomy.

The fate of vein graft conduits. The saphenous vein graft is prone to progressive intimal proliferation. Angiographic studies have shown that a 2 percent per year vein-graft attrition rate from the 1st to the 7th post operative year increases to approximately 5 percent per year form the tenth to the 12th year.[87] It is felt that the gradual increase in the rate of sudden death beginning 3.5 years after saphenous vein bypass grafting is probably due more to vein-graft closure than to progression of native coronary artery disease and it is associated with a decline survival rates and an increase in the rates of reoperation and other cardiac events by 7-10 years after the operation. When disease does occur in vein grafts, percutaneous techniques are associated with higher procedural complications (distal embolization, myocardial infarction), sub-optimal results, and poor long-term outcome.[88,89]

Arterial conduits (internal mammary artery, IMA) on the other hand have patency rates which greatly exceed those of the vein grafts. Several reports have shown patency rates of 85 to 95% up to 10 years after the operation.[90] Long-term follow-up of patients with IMA grafts show that these patients have lower rate of late infarction, lower incidence of angina, and improved survival over those with venous conduits, reflecting the higher patency rate of the IMA graft.[91-94] Importantly, the data on the patency of arterial conduits are based on clinical rather than angiographic follow-up of patients.

The importance of the left anterior descending artery

The LAD is a strategically important artery, and its patency is an major determinant of survival. Autopsy studies of patients who die suddenly with acute myocardial infarction show lesions in the proximal segment of the LAD more frequently than other coronary lesions.[93] There is evidence that anterior wall myocardial infarction is associated with poorer prognosis most likely secondary to the large territory of myocardium supplied by this artery. The 10-year actuarial survival (excluding hospital deaths) for patients who received an internal -mammary artery graft reported by Loop et al. was 87%, as compared with 76% for those who had saphenous vein grafts (p<0.0001).[94] Improved survival with the IMA graft was evident already at 5 years, and the improvement was even greater at 10 years. Although angiographic data are not available to document the patency of the IMA graft, it is clear from the long-term clinical follow-up of these patients and historical controls of PTCA, that the left IMA to the LAD may even be preferable to percutaneous revascularization especially if the lesion in the LAD is calcified, long, ostial or on a bend.

Hybrid revascularization

The optimal revascularization strategy for patients with multivessel disease is yet to be determined. The more favorable surgical techniques should include 1) off-by-pass, 2) use of arterial conduits, 3) minimally invasive. The percutaneous approach should include patients with favorable lesions for stenting as described earlier. The technique of coronary artery bypass surgery without cardiopulmonary bypass has been well established in multiple centers.[95-97] More recently the technique of minimally invasive direct myocardial revascularization has been described.[98] The minimally invasive CABG, performed off-bypass through a limited anterior thoracotomy, offers a left IMA graft to the LAD. Patients can be extubated in the recovery room and ambulate on post-operative day-1 and be discharged to home in 2-3 days.

The combination of minimally invasive CABG of the LAD using IMA, with conventional percutaneous revascularization of non-LAD lesions using endovascular stents may be an option. It seems that the "hybrid revascularization" approach may be a safe and efficacious treatment of patients with multivessel disease. Percutaneous revascularization of the non-LAD vessels should include utilization of stents or ablative techniques, perhaps even intraoperatively or very early post- or pre-operatively, in order to facilitate early discharge to home. This combination may offer the patient "the best of two possible worlds". To further assess feasibility and efficacy of this strategy, multicenter, randomized trials comparing this novel strategy to the conventional CABG are warranted. However prior to that, the patency of IMA graft to LAD with minimally invasive CABG technique must be established and compared to the conventional method of IMA grafting.

REFERENCES

1. Dotter CT. Presented at the 1963 Czech Radiological Congress, June 10, 1963.
2. Dotter CT. Transluminal angioplasty: a long view. Radiology 1980;135:561.
3. Dotter CT, Judkins MP. Transluminal treatment of arteriosclerotic obstruction: description of a new technic and a preliminary report of its application. Circulation 1964;30:654.
4. Dotter CT. Cardiac catheterization and angiographic techniques: the future. Czech Radiologie 1965;19:217.

5. Dotter CT, Judkins MP. Percutaneous transluminal treatment of arteriosclerotic obstruction. Radiol 1965;31:453.

6. Gruentzig A. Die perkutane rekanalisation chronischer arterieller verschlusse (Dotter-Prinzip) mit einem neuen dopplleumigen dilation-skatheter. Fortschr Roentgenstr 1976;124:80.

7. Gruentzig A. Perkutane dilatation von coronarstenosen-beschriebungeines neuen kathetersystems. Klin Wochenschr 1976;54:543.

8. GruentzigA, Turina MI, Schneider JA. Experimental percutaneous dilatation of coronary artery stenosis. Circulation 1976;54.

9. Hurst JW. The first coronary angioplasty as described by Andreas Gruentzig. Am J Cardiol 1986;57:185.

10. Gruentzig A, Senning A, Siegenthaler WE. Nonoperative dilatation of coronary artery stenosis: percuataneous transluminal coronary angioplasty. N Engl J Med 1979;301:61.

11. Mueller RL, Sanborn TA. The history of interventional cardiology:: Cardiac catheterization, angioplasty , and related interventions. Am Heart J 1995;129:146.

12. Livesay JJ, et al. Preliminary report on laser coronary endarterectomy in patients. Circulation 1985;72.

13. Cumberland DC, et al. Percutaneous laser thermal angioplasty: intial clinical restults with a laser probe in total peripheral artery occlustions. Lancet 1986;1:1457.

14. Cumberland DC, et al. Percutaneous laser-assisted coronary angioplasty. Lancet 1986;2:214.

15. Litvack F, et al. Percutaneous excimer laser coronary angioplasty: Results in the first consecutive 3,000 patients. J Am Col Cardiol 1994;23:323.

16. Strauss BH, et al. Early and late quantitative angiographic evaluation of vein graft lesions treated by excimer laser with adjunctive balloon angioplasty. Circulation 1995;92:348.

17. Appleman YEA, et al. Ranomised trial of excimer laser angioplasty versus balloon angioplasty for treatment of obstructive coronary artery disease. Lancet 1996;347:79.

18. Simpson JB, et al. Transluminal atherectomy: a new approach to the treatment of atherosclerotic vascular disease. Circulation 1985;72:146.

19. Simpson JB. How atherectomy began: a personal history. Am J Cardiol 1993;73:3-5E.

20. Simpson JB, et al. Transluminal coronary atherectomy: results in 21 human cadaver vascular segments. Circulation 1986;74:202.

21. Simpson JB, et al. Transluminal atherectomy: initial clinical results in 27 patients. Circulation 1986;74:203.

22. Simpson JB, Robertson GC, Selmon MR. Percutaneous coronary atherectomy. Circulation 1988;78:82.

23. Topol E, et al. A comparison of directional atherectomy with coronary angioplasty in patients with coronary artery disease. N Engl J Med 1993;329:221.

24. Elliott JM, et al. One-year follow-up in the coronary angioplasty versus excisional atherectomy trial (CAVEAT I). Circulation 1995; 91:2158.

25. Adelman A, et al. A comparison of directional atherectomy with balloon angioplasty for lesions of the left anterior descending coronary artery. N Engl J Med 1993;329:228.

26. Baim DS, et al. Acute results of the randomized phase of the balloon versus optimal atherectomy trial (BOAT). Circulation 1995;92(Suppl):I-544.

27. Popma JJ, et al . Early and late quantitative antiographic outcomes in the Optimal Atherectomy Restenosis Study (OARS). J Am Coll Cardiol 1996; Suppl A:291A.

28. Ahnn S, et al. Treatment of focal atheromatous lesions by angioscopically guided high speed rotary atherectomy. J Vasc Surg 1988;7:292.

29. Zacca NM, et al. Treatment of syptomatic peripheral atherosclerotic disease with a rotational atherectomy device. Am J Cardiol 1989; 63:77.

30. Warth D, et al. Rotational atherectomy multicenter registry: acute results, complications and 6-month angiographic follow-up in 709 patients. J Am Coll Cardiol 1994;24:641-648.

31. Ellis S, et al. Relation of clinical presentation, stenosis morphology, and operator technique to the procedural results of rotational atherectomy-facilitated angioplasty. Circulation 1994;89:882.

32. MacIsaac AI, et al. High speed rotational atherectomy: outcome in calcified and noncalcified coronary artery lesions. J Am Coll Cardiol 1995;26:731.

33. Dotter CT. Transluminally placed coil-spring endarterial tube grafts: long-term patency in canine popliteal artery. Invest Radiol 1969, 4:329.

34. Dotter CT, et al. Tranluminal expandable nitinol coil stent grafting: preliminary report. Radiology 1983, 147:259.

35. Sigwart U, et al. Intravascular stents to prevent occlustion and restenosis after transluminal angioplasty. N Engl J Med 1987;316:701.

36. Palmaz JC, et al. Expandable intraluminal graft: a preliminary study. Radiology 1985, 156:73.

37. Palmaz JC, et al. Expandable intraluminal vascular graft: afeasibitlity study. Surgery 1986;99:199.

38. Roubin GS. Early and late results of intracoronary arterial stenting after coronary angioplasty in dogs. Circulation 1987;76:891-897.

39. Serruys PW et al, for the Benestent Study Group. A comparison of balloon-expandable-stent implantation with balloon angioplasty in patients with coronary heart disease. N Engl J Med. 1994;331:489.

40. Schatz RA et al, for the STRESS investigators. Stent REStenosis Study (STRESS): analysis of in-hospital results. Circulation 1993;88(Suppl):594.

41. Fischman DL, et al, for the Stent Restenosis Study Investigators. A randomized comparison of coronary-stent placement and balloon angioplasty in treatment of coronary artery disease. N Engl J Med 1994;331:496.

42. Colombo A, et al. Intracoronary stenting without anticoagulation accomplished with intravascular ultrasound guidance. Circulation 1995;91:1676.

43. Serruys PW and the BENESTENT Study Group. BENESTENT-II pilot study: 6 months follow-up of phase 1, 2, and 3. Circulation 1995;92(Suppl I): I-542.

44. Hoffmann R, et al. Patterns and mechanisms of in-stent restenosis: a serial intravascular ultrasound study. Circulation 1996;94:1247.

45. Dussaillant GR, et al. Small stent size and intimal hyperplasia contribute to restenosis: a volumetric intravascular ultrasound analysis. J Am Coll Cardiol 1995;26:720.

46. Mintz GS, et al. Arterial remodeling after coronary angioplasty: A serial intravascular ultrasound study. Circulation 1996;94:35.

47. Painter JA, et al. Serial intravascular ultrasound studies fail to show evidence of chronic Palmaz-Schatz stent recoil. Am J Cardiol 1995;75:398.

48. Mintz GS, et al. Endovascular stent reduce restinosis by eliminating geometric arterial remodeling: a serial intravascular ultrasound study. J Am Coll Cardiol 1995;25(Suppl A):36A.

49. Leon M, Wong C. Intracoronary stents: A breakthrough technology or just another small step? Circulation 1994;89:1323.

50. Laird JR, et al. Inhibition of neointimal proliferation with low-dose irradiation from a b-emitting stent. Circulation 1996;93:529.

51. Hong MK, et al. Continuous subcutaneous angiopeptim reduces neointimal hyperplasia in a porcine coronary in-stent restenosis model. Circulation, in press.

52. de Scheerder IK, et al. Angiopeptin loaded stents inhibit the neointimal reaction induced by polymer coated stents implanted in porcine coronary arteries. J Am Coll Cardiol 1995; Suppl A:36A.

53. Goldberg SL, et al. Benefit of intracoronary ultrasound in the deployment of Palmaz-Schatz stents. J Am Coll Cariol 1994;24:996.

54. EPIC Investigators. Use of a monoclonal antibody directed against the platelet glycoprotein IIb/IIa recptor in high-risk coronary angioplasty. N Engl J Med 1994;330:956.

55. Hollman Jl. Myocardial Revascularization: coronary angioplasty and bypass surgery indications. Med Clin North Am 1992;76:1083.

56. ACC/AHA guidelines and indications for coronary artery bypass graft surgery. Circulation 1991;83:1125.

57. The Veterans Administration Coronary Artery Bypass Surgery Cooperative Study Group. Eleven year survival in the VA trial of bypass surgery for stable angina. N Engl J Med 1984;311:1333.

58. Eurpean Coronary surgery Study Group. Prospective randomized study of coronary artery bypass surgery in stable angina pectoris. Circulation 1982;65 (Supp I):1167.

59. Coronary Artery Surgery Study Principal Investigators and their associates. Myocardial infarction and mortaligy in the CASS randomized trial. N Eng J Med 1984;310:750.

60. Hise JH, Nipper ML, Schnitker JC. Stroke associated with coronary artery bypass surgery. Am J Neuroradiol 1991;12:811.

61. Shaw PJ, et al. Neurologic and neuropsychological morbidity following major surgery: comparison of coronary artery bypass and peripheral vascular surgery. Stroke 1987;18:700.

62. Smith PLD, et al. Cerebral consequences of cardiopulmonary bypass. Lancet 1986;1:823.

63. Campeau L, et al. Aortocoronary saphenous vein bypass graft changes 5 to 7 years after surgery. Circulation1978, 58(Suppl I): I-170-1755.

64. Compeau L, et al. Patency of saphenous vein bypass grafts at two weeks and at one year in two series of consecutive patients. Circulation 1975;52:369.

65. Compeau L, et al. The relation of risk factors to the development of atherosclerosis in saphenous vein bypass grafts and the progression of disease in the native circulation. A study 10 years after aortocoronary bypass surgery. N Engl J Med 1984;311:1329.

66. Cameron A, Kemp HG, Green GE. Bypass surgery with the internal mammary artery graft: 15 year follow-up. Circulation 1986; 74(Suppl III): III30-36.

67. Rodriquez A, et al. Argentine Randomized Trial of Percutaneous transluminal Coronary Angioplasty vs. Coronary Artery Bypass Surgery in Multivessel Disease. In hospital results and 1 year follow-up. J Am Coll Cardiol 1993;22:1060.

68. RITA Trial Participants. Coronary angioplasty vs. coronary artery bypass surgery: the Randomized InterventionTreatment of Angina trial. Lancet 1993;34:573.

69. Hamm CW, et al. A randomized study of coronary angioplasty compared with bypass srugery in patients with symptomatic multivessel coronary disease. N Engl J Med 1994;331:1037.

70. CABRI Trial Participants. First-year results of the Coronary Angioplasty vs Bypass Revascularisation Investigation. Lancet 1995;346:1179.

71. King S, et al. A randomized trial comparing coronary angioplasty with coronary bypass surgery. N Engl J Med 1994;331:1044.

72. The Bypass Angioplasty Revascularization Investigation (BARI) Investigators. Comparison of coronary bypass surgery with angioplasty in patients with multivessel disease. N Engl J Med 1996;335:217.

73. Pocock SJ, et al. Meta-analysis of randomised trials comparing coronary angioplasty with bypass surgery. Lancet 1995;346:1184.

74. Popma JJ, Topol EJ. Factors influencing restenosis after coronary angioplasty. Am J Med 1990;88:1-16N.

75. Hirshfeld JW, et al. Restenosis after coronary angioplasty: A multivariate statistical model to relate lesion and procedure variables to restenosis. J Am Coll Cardiol 1991;18:647.

76. de Groote P, et al. Local lesion-related factors and restenosis after coronary angioplasty.

Evidence from a quantitative angiographic study in patients with unstable angina undergoing double-vessel angioplasty. Circulation 1995;91:967.

77. Violaris AG, Meldert R, Serruys PW. Long-term luminal renarrowing after successful elective coronary angioplasty of total occlusions. Circulation 1995;91:2140.

78. Kuntz RE, et al. Generalized model of restenosis after conventional balloon angioplasty, stenting and directional atherectomy. J Am Coll Cardiol 1993;21:15.

79. Kuntz RE, Baim DS. Defining coronary restenosis. Newer clinical and angiographic paradigms. Circulation 1993;88:1310.

80. Mehran R, et al. Mechanisms and results of balloon angioplasty for the treatment of In-stent restenosis. Am J Cardiol 1996; 78:618.

81. Yokoi H, et al. Long-term clinical and quantitative angiographic follow-up after the Palmaz-Schatz stent restenosis. J Am Coll Cardiol 1996;27(Suppl A): 224A.

82. Coffee CE, et al. Natural history of cerebral complications of coronary artery bypass graft surtery. Neurology 1983;33:1416.

83. Sotaniemi KA, Mononen H, Hokkanen TE. Long term cerebral outcome after open heart surgery. A five year neuropsychological follow-up study. Stroke 1986;17:410.

84. Aris A, et al. Arterial line filtrationduring cardio-pulmonary bypass. J Thorac Cardiovasc Surg 1986;91:526.

85. Smith PLC, et al. Cerebral consequences of cardiopulmonary bypass. Lancet 1986;1:823.

86. Kirklin JW, Blackstone Eh, Rogers WJ. The plights of the invasive treatment of ischemic heart desease. J Am Coll Cardiol 1985;5:158.

87. Holmes DR Jr, et al. A multicenter, randomized trial of coronary angioplasty versus directional atherectomy for patients with saphenous vein bypass graft lesions. Circulation 1995;91:1996.

88. Douglas JS, et al. Randomized trial of coroanry stent and balloon angioplasty in the treatment of saphenous vein graft stenosis. J Am Coll Cardiol 1996;Suppl A:178A.

89. Barner HB, et al. Late patency of the internal mammary artery as a coronary bypass conduit. Ann Thorac Surg 1982;34:408.

90. Tector AJ, et al. The internal mammary artery graft. Its longevity after coronary bypass. JAMA 1983;246:2181.

91. Grondin CM, et al. Comarison of late changes in internal mammary artery and saphenous vein grafts in two consecutive series of patients 10 years after operation. Circulation 1984;70:Suppl 1: I-208.

92. Schuster EH, Griffith LS, Bukley BH. Preponderance of acute procimal left anterior descending coronary arterial lesions in fatal myocardial infarction. A clinicopathologic study. Am J Cardiol 1981;47:1189.

93. Loop FD, et al. Influence of the internal-mammary artery graft on 10-year survival and other cardiac events N Engl J Med 1986;314:1.

94. Benetti F, et al. Direct myocardial revascularization without extracorporeal circulation. Chest 1991;100:312.

95. Pfister AJ, et al. Coronary artery bypass without cardiopulmonary bypass AnnThora Surg 1992;54:1085.

96. Fannin W, Kakos G, Williams T. Reoperative coronary bypass without coronary pulmonary bypass. Ann Thorac Surg 1993;55:46.

97. Acuff TE, et al. Minimally invasive coronary artery bypass grafting. Ann Thorac Surg 1996;61:135.

28 CORONARY ATHERECTOMY

Samin K. Sharma, Annapoorna S. Kini

Transluminal coronary angioplasty (PTCA) has grown rapidly in the last decade with increasing operator experience and advances in balloon technology. It is estimated that more than 500,000 procedures will be performed in the United States this year. Recent data document a very high procedural success rate of PTCA; upwards of 95%.[1,2] However, there remains three major limitation to the balloon technique: 1) acute closure causing ischemic complications in about 5%[3] 2) lesions unsuitable for intervention in about 45%[4] and 3) restenosis rate of about 50%.[5] There has been a great deal of enthusiasm in developing alternative mechanical means to alter luminal geometry in order to decrease restenosis and intense research efforts are being focused on pharmacological means of preventing smooth muscle hyperplasia; the histologic etiology of restenosis.[6] Secondary goals driving the development of new devices have been to reduce the incidence of acute complications and extend the applicability of percutaneous interventional technique to lesions that previously were considered unsuitable.

Directional coronary atherectomy

The first new interventional device to receive FDA approval for clinical use in 1990, is directional coronary atherectomy (DCA) developed by John B. Simpson at Sequoia Hospital in California. The Simpson Coronary Atherocath physically removes atherosclerotic plaque from the coronary artery, leaving smooth cut surfaces devoid of intimal flaps and dissections which is in sharp contrast to the mechanism of balloon angioplasty.

Description of the device and the procedure

Atherectomy equipment consists of a large guiding catheter (9.5 to 11 French), the Simpson Coronary Atherocath (SCA), the motor drive unit (MDU), a rotating hemostatic valve (RHV) and a low pressure indeflator device. The guiding catheters are available in various sizes and shapes to accommodate all usual and unusual coronary artery and vein graft takeoffs. The SCA catheter is comprised of a housing with a cutter inside it and a nosecone at the distal end. The distal end of SCA has a halo radio-opaque gold plated 17 mm rigid stainless steel metal housing mounted on a torque cable shaft. Spanning the length of the housing is a support balloon made of either compliant Surlyn material (SCA-1) or polyethylene terephthalate (PET) material (SCA-EX or GTO). The housing has a window, creating a 'cutting chamber', across which the cutter blade travels. The cutter spins at 2000 rpm and is advanced through the cutting chamber manually over a conventional 0.014 inch guide wire. The cutting chamber is contiguous with the nosecone made of either stainless steel braid covered with Surlyn (SCA-1) or polyurathane spring coil (EX & GTO) and serves as a collection chamber for the shaved atheromatous material. The balloon mounted opposite the window serves to stabilize the device and prolapses the atheroma into the cutting chamber. At the proximal end of the SCA catheter there is a rotater (which allows for directional rotation of the housing) and a proximal adapter with two side ports, one for saline flushing of the central lumen and other for balloon inflation/deflation. The MDU, which rotates the cutter, attaches in a press fit fashion to the proximal end adapter and has a lumen for guide wire passage. The SCA devices are now available in several sizes and configurations (Table 28.1). Device size 5 or 6 are used for vessel 2.5 or 3.0 mm diameter while 7 or 7G are used for vessels 3.0-3.7 or > 3.7mm respectively.

Patients are treated in similar fashion to those undergoing standard PTCA (aspirin, sedation, heparin), with few differences. Pre-treatment with a calcium blockers is recommended. Intravenous Heparin is administered to maintain an activated coagulation time (ACT) of 350-400 sec. A coaxial position of the guiding catheter with reference to the ostium of the coronary artery is particularly important during DCA. A 0.014 inch guide wire, preferably extra support, is positioned across the

Table 28.1   TYPES OF SIMPSON CORONARY ATHEROCATH.

Type	Housing Length (mm)	Window Size (mm)	Balloon Material	Sizes (F)	Nose Cone
SCA-1	17	10	Surlyn	5,6,7,7G	Stiff notched transition
SCA-EX	17	9	PET	5,6,7G	Polyurethane spring coil
SCA-EX SC	9	5	PET	5,6,7	Polyurethane spring coil
SCA-GTO	17	9	PET	5,6,7	Polyurethane spring coil

PET = Polyethlene terephthalate.

lesion and SCA catheter is advanced out of the guide and into the coronary artery. A combination of gentle pushing and corkscrew rotation of the device is used to cross the lesion. Predilatation with a small diameter balloon may be required in some cases. The window is then rotated in the desired direction, balloon is then inflated, the MDU turned on and the cutter is slowly advanced manually across the cutting chamber thus shearing off a segment of atheroma. The atheromatous material is rolled and stored in the nosecone untill the device is removed *(FIG 28.1)*. This sequence is repeated with the housing window facing different quadrants of the arterial wall until an adequate angiographic result is obtained with the initial cuts directing towards the bulkiest portion of the plaque followed by circumferential cuts. The nosecone usually can hold the contents of ten to twelve cuts. Postdilatation by an appropriate size balloon is usually recommended to attain larger lumen with smooth angiographic borders. After successful completion of the procedure, heparin is generally discontinued and arterial sheath is pulled after 4-5 hours.

Mechanism of action

While it is conceptually appealing to physical remove plaque from an artery it is important to recognize that this is not the only means by which DCA improves luminal diameter. In addition to tissue removal, two other possible mechanism may contribute to increase luminal diameter and volume [7]. First inflation of the support balloon may be particularly important, as once the internal elastic lamina has been

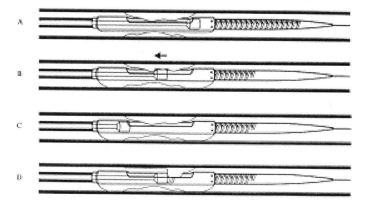

Figure 28.1 (A) The Simpson Coronary AtheroCath is advanced over a 0.014-inch guidewire and cross the lesion. The housing is rotated until the window is directed toward the angiographic evidence of disease. (B) The balloon is inflated and the advancement control lever is retracted until the cutter is located within the proximal portion of the housing. (C) The balloon is inflated to the desired pressure to position the lesion in the window and hold the housing securely within the vessel. (D) The attached motor drive unit is activated and the cutter is advanced through the lesion. The cutter is then fully advanced, and the excised atheroma extracted.

broken by the atherectomy cuts, the radial compliance of the vessel increases and subsequent cuts with balloon inflations will further dilate the base of the atherectomy cuts. This has been termed "facilitated angioplasty". Secondly, there is the 'Dotter' effect produced by mechanical dilatation due to passage of a high profile device across the lesion. Some operators[8] attempt to obtain the largest possible post-procedural luminal diameter (initial gain) with the hypothesis that subsequent intimal hyperplasia may cause a partial decrease in the luminal diameter (late loss) without resulting in a clinically and/or angiographically significant restenosis. In this "Bigger is Better" hypothesis, the resultant higher net gain (initial gain - late loss) is due to the larger initial gain and translates into the observed lower restenosis with DCA. This is in contrast to the findings of Umans and Serruys[9] that the higher initial gain achieved by DCA is offset by a greater late loss resulting in no significant difference in follow-up luminal diameter when compared to TCA of matched lesions.

Histopathological Findings. Directional coronary atherectomy provides an unique opportunity to study human atherosclerotic plaque. A mean of 11.6 ± 6 specimens with an average weight of 18.5 mg (range 5.8-45.1) are derived from each lesion.[10] Tissue samples from primary lesions include atherosclerotic plaque in about 95%, media in about 50%, and adventitia in about 25% specimens. Fibro-intimal proliferation, a hallmark of restenosis, is present in 97% of restenotic lesions and also in about 33% of primary lesions. Although presence of deep wall components (media and adventitia) is not uncommon in atherectomy specimens obtained from successful procedures, but in cases with coronary perforation, the incidence of retrieval of deep wall component is very high and is seen on multiple specimens.[11] The relation of retrieval of deep wall components to subsequent fibromuscular hyperplasia was an issue of great controversy after the results of Garratt et al[12] demonstrating the higher restenosis with deep tissue resection in vein graft and restenotic lesions but not in the primary lesions. A subsequent report by Kuntz et al[13] in a larger series of DCA lesions failed to establish the above hypothesis and found no relation of deep wall resection with restenosis in any coronary lesion subsets. Coronary thrombus is also frequently (about 40%) detected in atherectomy specimens especially in patients with acute coronary syndromes (post-MI and unstable angina with ECG changes) and complex angiographic lesions.[14-16] These unique observations underscores the key role of coronary thrombus in the pathophysiology and clinical manifestations of acute coronary syndromes.

Results and clinical trials

The early and late acute success of the DCA can be summarized by various single and multiple center results and from the results of various randomized trials.

Earlier multicenter results. Ellis et. al. analyzed the results of DCA of 400 lesions in 378 patients from 1988 to 1990 in terms of correlates of lesion success and ischemic complications.[17] There was an overall procedural success rate of 87.8% with major ischemic complications of death, infarction (MI) or emergency bypass surgery (CABG) occurring in 6.3% of patients: death 1.0%, MI 1.8% and emergency

CABG 5.5%. Operator experience was an important factor in reducing the rate of ischemic complications as patients who underwent DCA early in the experience had a 10% rate of major ischemic complications while those done later had a 4.6% complication rate. Other factors that predicted complications were bend lesions and a primary rather than restenotic lesion. Lesion success was predicted by the presence of a complex lesion, presumably containing a small thrombus and by a restenotic lesion. Negative correlates of lesion success were proximal tortuosity, lesion angulation, eccentricity and calcification. It is important to note that these data reflect the relatively early experience with DCA and results have improved over time with increased operator experience and refinements in technology.

Popma et al studied the factors predisposing to abrupt vessel closure following DCA in 1140 lesions in 1020 patients at 14 clinical centers.[18] Abrupt vessel closure occurred in 43 lesions (4.2%) mostly occurring in the catheterization laboratory (79%). Univariate predictors of abrupt closure were de novo lesions (p<0.001), lesions in right coronary artery (p=0.001) and diffuse lesions (p=0.04). Also there was a trend towards lower acute closure in vein graft lesions compared to native lesions (1.6% vs. 4.4%; p=0.08). Subsequent balloon angioplasty was attempted in 32 of 41 cases with abrupt closure and was successful in about half of the cases particularly when the etiology was thrombotic or indeterminate rather than coronary dissection. A total of 25 patients underwent emergency bypass surgery and three patients died; 2 after abrupt closure and one after attempted salvage angioplasty. Therefore abrupt vessel closure is relatively infrequent after DCA.

Hinohara et al[19] reported the long term results of 332 lesions treated by DCA from 1986 to 1989. The mean post procedure residual stenosis was 11.6 ± 19.2% and 71% of patients were left with <20% residual stenosis. Restenosis (defined as >50% stenosis at follow-up angiography obtained in 82% of cases) was observed in 42% with an overall restenosis rate of 37% for native coronary arteries. The predictors of restenosis were hypertension, longer lesion (≥10mm), noncalcified lesion, smaller vessel diameter (<3mm) and use of a smaller (6F) device. In a subgroup analysis of primary lesions for vessels ≥ 3mm, restenosis rates were 12% for lesions treated with 7F device. Fishman[20] reported similar long-term results of 225 lesions in 190 patients treated by DCA at Beth Israel Hospital from 1988 to 1991. Procedural success was 91% for DCA alone and 98% for post-DCA adjunctive balloon angioplasty. Follow-up angiography was obtained in 77% of patients at a mean of 179 ± 57 days. The overall restenosis (>50% diam. stenosis) rate was 32%. Predictors of a lower restenosis rate were serum cholesterol <200 mg/dl (18%), recent MI (16%) and a post-DCA MLD of ≤ 3 mm (24%).

Saphenous vein grafts (SVG), which are generally large in size seems to be the ideal targets for DCA. Conventional balloon angioplasty is has a very high restenosis rate upto 70% in this setting and DCA by improving the post-procedure lumen diameter could reduce the restenosis rates. Available data are conflicting in this regard. Hinohara et al[19] reported an overall 63% angiographic restenosis rate in 64 SVG lesions; 53% in primary lesions, 58% in lesions treated with one prior angioplasty and 82% for lesions treated with ≥2 prior angioplasties. Less restenosis was observed in focal (< 5mm) lesions (46%) and in lesions with a post-DCA lumen diameter of ≥3mm (52%). On the contrary Fishman et al[20] reported an overall angiographic restenosis rate of only 28% in 35 SVG lesions in their study.

CAVEAT. In the Coronary Angioplasty Versus Excisional Atherectomy Trial (CAVEAT) 1012 patients with de novo focal lesion in native coronary arteries were randomized to DCA (512) or TCA (500) and a higher procedural success rates was observed for DCA as compared to PTCA (88.6% versus 80.3%; p=0.001)[21]. The incidence of abrupt vessel closure was 7% in the DCA group vs. 3% in the PTCA group (p=0.02). When a composite acute clinical endpoints consisting of death, MI, coronary bypass surgery or acute closure were analyzed, PTCA patients were significantly less likely to develop one of these endpoints (6% versus 11% in the DCA group; p=0.001). There were no deaths in the DCA group compared to two deaths in the PTCA group[19]. The angiographic restenosis rate (defined as ≥50% stenosis) at six month follow-up of 90% of the eligible patients was slightly lower for DCA compared to PTCA (50% vs 57%; p=0.06). In the proximal LAD artery subgroup, DCA resulted in significantly less restenosis compared to PTCA (51% versus 63%; p=0.04). While the angiographic results favored DCA, when patients were analyzed at six months using a composite clinical endpoints of death, MI, coronary bypass surgery, and repeat percutaneous intervention, there was no significant difference; 60% of patients in the DCA group were event free at 6 months compared to 63% of patients in the PTCA group. A regression analysis of the determinants of six-month MLD revealed that the final post-procedure MLD was the single most important determinant of subsequent lumen caliber (p<0.001) with other important determinants being vessel size before intervention, presence of diabetes mellitus and lesion location in the proximal LAD artery. Possible explanations for unfavorable results after DCA in the CAVEAT trial include the small vessel size (2.9mm) and post-DCA residual stenosis (29%). Of note, in a subgroup analysis of the CAVEAT data, a post-DCA residual stenosis of <20% resulted in a restenosis rate of 31%, which is consistent with the previously published data [22,23]. These observations appear to substantiate the "Bigger is Better" hypothesis. One year follow-up of CAVEAT I trial patients revealed higher death rate in the DCA group as compared to the PTCA group (11 in DCA vs. 3 in PTCA; p=0.035). Univariate predictors of death included age, abrupt closure, periprocedural enzyme elevation and peripheral vascular complications. By multivariate analysis, DCA was the only variable predictive of combined end point of death or MI.[22] Also at one year follow-up cumulative rates of MI were higher in the DCA group compared to PTCA group (8.9% vs. 4.4%; p=0.005)

CCAT. The Canadian Coronary Atherectomy Trial (CCAT), which randomized 274 de-novo lesions of the proximal one-third of left anterior descending (LAD) coronary artery to DCA versus PTCA, demonstrated high procedural success rates for both techniques (94% for DCA and 88% for PTCA; p=0.06) but angiographic success (<50% diameter stenosis) was significantly higher in DCA group versus PTCA (98% vs. 91%; p=0.01) [23]. While there were no significant differences in rates of acute complications between the two techniques, there was a trend towards a higher incidence of emergent bypass surgery in the PTCA group (4.4% vs. 1.4% in the DCA group; p=0.17). These observations, in sharp contrast to the results of CAVE-AT trial, are very intriguing and are perhaps related to the experience of the operators in two trials. In the CCAT trial[21] 6 months angiographic follow-up data of 257 eligible patients revealed no significant differences in restenosis (>50% stenosis) between two treatment groups (DCA 46% vs. PTCA 43%; p=0.71). A stepwise logistic regression analysis revealed only unstable angina as the predictor of restenosis. In this trial of vessels ≥3 mm in diameter, though DCA resulted in a higher post-procedural MLD (2.34 mm vs. 2.10 mm; p<0.0001) and lower post-procedure residual stenosis (25% vs. 33%; p<0.001) than PTCA, there was a significantly greater late loss in the DCA group (0.79 ± 0.61mm vs. 0.47 ± 0.64mm; p<0.001) resulting in similar net gains (0.66 ± 0.65mm for DCA vs. 0.68 ± 0.70mm for PTCA; p=0.81) between the two techniques, and therefore no observed difference in restenosis. Also in CCAT trial there was no difference in mortality between DCA and PTCA at one year.

CAVEAT II . In the CAVEAT II trial 305 patients with de novo vein graft lesions were randomized to DCA (n=149) or PTCA (n=156).[24] Angiographic success was greater with DCA (89% vs. 79%; p=0.02). Major complications of death, Q-wave MI or emergent CABG were similar in the two groups but distal embolization (13.4% vs. 5.1%; p=0.01) and non-Q wave MI (16.1% vs. 9.6%; p=0.09) were higher in the DCA group. At 6 months of follow-up, restenosis rates were similar (45.6% for DCA vs. 50.5% for PTCA; p=0.5) with a trend towards decreased target-vessel revascularization in the DCA group (18.6% vs. 26.2%; p=0.09).

BOAT. By analyzing the results of the CAVEAT and CCAT trials, it became apparent that post procedure MLD after DCA in these trials was higher than reported by various high volume centers and perhaps resulted in higher acute complications and lack of difference in restenosis rates (compared to PTCA). The balloon versus optimal atherectomy (BOAT) trial was formulated on the basis that optimal DCA, if done correctly, can decrease the post procedure stenosis to <15% with a major complications of <4% and this may translate into lower restenosis. A total of 989 patients with de novo focal lesion in native coronary artery of > 3.0mm were randomized to DCA (497) or PTCA (492) with a higher DCA lesion success (98.8% vs. 96.5% for PTCA; p<0.05) and procedural success (93% vs. 86.7% for PTCA; p=0.005) and similar major complication rates (2.8% for DCA and 3.3% for PTCA; p=NS).[25] DCA patients had a higher incidence of CPK-MB elevation >3X normal (14% vs. 5%; p=0.001) in the setting of otherwise uncomplicated procedure. DCA also achieved higher post-procedure MLD (2.82mm vs. 2.33mm; p=0.001) and lower % residual stenosis (15% vs. 28%; p=0.001). Eight month follow-up angiographic data in 80% of the eligible patients revealed a lower restenosis rate (>50% diam stenosis) in the DCA group (32% vs. 40% in PTCA; p=0.02) but no difference in the target site revascularization rate (15.3% vs. 18.35 for PTCA; p=0.23). One year cumulative mortality was 0.6% in DCA group and 1.6% in the PTCA group (p=NS). Therefore BOAT trial seems to have answered various concerns raised by earlier trials and established that DCA done correctly may decrease the angiographic restenosis without increasing acute or long term mortality.

OARS. In the optimal atherectomy restenosis study (OARS) 200 patient at 4 centers assessed the impact of IVUS guided optimal atherectomy on acute and late clinical and angiographic outcomes.[26] Overall procedural success rate was 97.5% and major complications occurred in 2.5% without any in-hospital death. Angiographic restenosis occurred in 29% with a target vessel revascularization rate of 19%. There was no excess mortality on 1 year follow-up.

Indications and limitations

Directional coronary atherectomy is presently indicated for discrete lesions in large vessels (>3mm size), complex lesions, bifurcation lesions and ostial lesions. The use of DCA has declined significantly since the wide spread use of intracoronary stents. Even then ostial and bifurcation lesion poses special problems for stenting and in DCA has a definite niche in these lesion subsets. DCA can also be used as a bail out device to remove small intimal flaps in selected cases. Recently there has been a great enthusiasm about use of DCA for in-stent restenosis in the large vessels (>3.75mm). Other indications for which DCA has shown to be effective are total occlusions, lesions with small thrombus and during recent myocardial infarctions (Table 28.2).

Significant peripheral vascular disease may limit the introduction of a 10 French DCA guiding catheter into the femoral artery. Similarly, the presence of mild left main disease, is a limitation to the DCA because of bulky nature of the device causing ischemia during the procedure.

Tortuous coronary arteries or severely angulated segments proximal to the target lesion may restrict the applicability of the procedure because of the relative stiffness and inflexibility of the SCA device. The ShortCutter and GTO devices have significantly improved the crossing and tracking profile of the current DCA devices.

Table 28.2   INDICATIONS FOR DIRECTIONAL ATHERECTOMY.

Definite
- Noncalcified ostial lesion
- Bifurcation lesion
- Branch point lesions
- Complex,eccentric focal lesion in large vessel (>3mm)

Possible
- Bailout for small dissection post TCA
- Total occlusion - acute or chronic
- Lesion with small thrombus
- In-stent restenosis in large vessels (>3.25mm)

Heavy lesion or vessel calcification remains a major limitation to DCA both because of greatly increased difficulty in crossing the lesion and an inability of the cutter to shave off the calcified plaque. In addition, there appears to be a greater risk of coronary perforation in this setting.

The in-hospital costs of the DCA procedure are greater than associated with PTCA, predominantly due to the higher cost of the atherectomy system.[21] However, the hospital stay is not prolonged, and a cost effectiveness analysis shows that compared to PTCA and coronary stenting, DCA may be the most cost effective procedure.[27] Most of the trials have shown that use of DCA is associated with a higher incidence of CPK and CPK-MB elevation and long term outcome in this setting with otherwise successful procedure is not well known.

In conclusion, DCA is the first of many new interventional techniques approved for treating coronary artery disease and represents an important addition to our current armamentarium. Presently, DCA is a safe and efficacious means of treating discrete coronary lesions in large vessels and lesions in which conventional balloon angioplasty or stent may be associated with suboptimal results. The clinical indications for DCA will continue to expand particularly with recent results of BOAT and OARS trials and future technological advances like larger devices for vessel >5 mm in diameter, long window devices for segmental lesions, small profile devices compatible with 8 or 9 Fr. guides (Bantom catheter), device with ultrasound crystal on the cutter (GDCA) and devices with an enhanced capability to cut calcified plaques. Directional coronary atherectomy also provides the ability to study human coronary atheroma, and thus may add greatly to the body of knowledge about coronary artery disease and restenosis.

Rotational coronary atherectomy

Percutaneous Transluminal Coronary Rotational Atherectomy (PTCRA), also known as Rotablation, was invented by David Auth, PhD, in 1982. The objective of PTCRA is to create a smoother lumen in the arteries with atheromatous plaques when compared with PTCA. This is achieved by a rotating abrasive burr which causes the formation of microparticulate debris (usually 5 - 10 microns), small enough to be cleared by the distal vasculature and taken up by the reticuloendothelial system. This atheromatous debris is also responsible for many of the pathophysiological changes seen during PTCRA. PTCRA works on the novel concepts of differential cutting and orthogonal displacement of friction.

Physical principles

Differential cutting. Differential cutting is the main principle by which Rotablator works and implies that the elastic materials are deflected away from the surface whereas the inelastic materials get pulverized by the abrasive burr. Thus, this effect allows the normal (elastic) coronary arterial wall to be deflected away from the surface of the burr, while calcified, fibrous or fatty atheromatous plaques (inelastic) are ablated by the rotating burr.

Orthogonal displacement of friction. This principle of orthogonal displacement of friction, permits the easy passage of the burr through tortuous and diseased segments of the coronary arterial tree. Friction occurs when the sliding surfaces are in contact, but is minimized by a sliding motion perpendicular or orthogonal to the contact surface. At rotational speeds greater than 60,000 rpm the longitudinal frictional is virtually eliminated and the movement of the burr is unimpeded.

Description of the device and the procedure

The Rotablator system (Boston Scientific) consists of a reusable console that controls the rotational speed of an olive shaped, nickel-plated, brass, abrasive burr which has on its leading edge a coating of 20-30 μm diamond chips embedded into the metal. The burr (8 sizes, diameter 1.25-2.50 mm) is welded to the flexible drive shaft tracking along a flexible guidewire. The drive shaft is enclosed in a 4.3 F flexible Teflon sheath, which protects arterial wall from potential rotating drive shaft and serves as a conduit for saline flush solution which cools and irrigates the system. The speed of the burr rotation is regulated by a compressed-air or nitrogen driven turbine, which is controlled by the console and activated by a foot pedal; rotational speed is monitored by a fiberoptic tachometer. A 0.009-inch stainless steel 310 cm long guide wire is used, and has a floppy 2.2 cm (RotaWire floppy) or a stiff 2.8 cm (RotaWire Extra Support) distal platinum spring with 0.014 inch radiopaque tip. During rotational atherectomy the lesion is initially crossed by guide wire so that the platinum tip of the wire is distal to the lesion. The burr/drive shaft is then advanced over the guidewire until it lies just proximal to the stenosis. Thereafter, rotation is initiated, and using a control knob on the top of the advancer, the rotating burr (160,000-180,000 rpm, depending on burr size) is slowly advanced through the lesion.

The procedural approach to PTCRA is similar, in many respects, to PTCA. All patients receive aspirin 325 mg daily and calcium channel blockers. Heparin is administered to keep the activated clotting time 300 sec. The "Rota Flush" solution, containing heparin, nitroglycerin and verapamil, is continuously infused through the Teflon sheath. Vasopressors such as dopamine and phenylephrine should be readily available to treat hypotension. During and shortly after PTCRA, moderate to severe chest discomfort is common and analgesics such as morphine should be liberally used. Glycoprotein IIb/IIIa inhibitors, such as abciximab (ReoPro), should be used in long and calcified lesions which are especially prone to slow flow. Temporary pacemaker is routinely inserted during PTCRA of the right, circumflex or ostial left anterior descending coronary lesions. Right heart pressures should be monitored in patients requiring long ablations. In cases of severe ventricular dysfunction and large area of myocardial jeopardy, a prophylactic intra-aortic balloon pump should be used.[38]

Rotablator technique. Depending on size of the burr, an 8-10 F sheath is inserted into the femoral artery under local anesthesia.

Guidewire. The positioning of the guidewire is critical in determining the cutting vector and thus the outcome of the procedure. Tangential placement of the wire may result in directing the burr into the vessel wall and thus increase the risk of perforation or dissection.

Burr selection. Burr selection depends on various factors including atherosclerotic plaque, vessel architecture, distal flow and left ventricular function. The aim is to achieve a final burr to artery ratio of 0.7-0.8 with a step-burr approach.

Ablation Technique. Under fluoroscopy the steering guidewire is advanced through the narrowing and directed into the distal part of the coronary artery The burr is introduced into the guiding catheter and advanced along the guidewire, placed just before the stenosis and rotation is started. A 'pecking' technique is usually used wherein the burr is advanced into the lesion momentarily and then brought back for a second and then readvanced. Also, ablative runs should be short, not exceeding 30 sec. The frequency should be maintained at an optimal level (dependent on the burr size) and a >5,000 rpm drop should not be allowed as this increases the risk of vessel trauma and ischemic complications caused by frictional heat and formation of large particles. In cases of persistent chest pain, ECG changes or hypotension, the intervals between runs should be increased (even to several minutes) until these parameters start to normalize. A manual autoflush technique is also employed between ablations: blood is aspirated from the guiding catheter and forcefully injected with additional saline back into the vessel.

Adjunctive Therapy. If PTCRA is used as primary therapy, it can be combined with DCA, stent, or routine PTCA. After PTCRA, routine PTCA is often used with an oversized balloon at 1 atm, to decrease haziness and improve angiographic appearance.

Complications and special issues

Slow flow-No reflow. Slow flow is defined as the delayed clearance of contrast material (TIMI flow 1-2) and no reflow (TIMI flow 0) as cessation of distal flow of contrast material in the absence of angiographic dissection or spasm. There are many factors that contribute to the development of slow flow: large plaque burden, microparticulate aggregation, platelet activation, microvascular spasm, hypotension due to a compromised myocardium and neurohumoral reflex. Studies have shown that 77% of the particles generated were less than 5 microns and 88% were less than 12 m.[39] The best way to avoid slow flow is to prevent it by short burr runs and a gradual, incremental step burr approach and maintenance of adequate systemic blood pressure and coronary perfusion.

Vasospasm. High speed rotating burr is prone to cause vasospasm by direct contact to the vessel wall or heat generation. Its occurrence has been greatly minimized by the routine use of rota flush and intracoronary vasodilators. In refractory cases, low pressure balloon inflation may be necessary to relieve the vasospasm.

Hypotension and ventricular dysfunction. Transient hypotension during ablation occurs commonly due to compromised myocardial contraction in the subtended vessel. Vasopressors such as phenylephrine and dopamine should be liberally used to prevent hypotension (intravenous or intracoronary). In baseline severe ventricular dysfunction or hypotension, an intaaortic balloon pump should be used "prophylactically".

CPK Release. Capillary "plugging" due to atheromatous debris causes myocardial injury and necrosis especially in the setting of slow flow and no flow and can occur in up to 25% of cases. Use of abciximab has been shown to decrease the release of CPK after rotablator (see below) and points to the role of platelets in this process. Studies have shown no change in ventricular function in patients with CPK release after otherwise successful PTCRA.

Perforation. Coronary perforation caused by the device, though rare (0.5%), usually occurs in angulated lesions (>90°). It can be avoided by careful burr selection and avoiding wire bias situation.

Dissection and acute closure. Minor coronary dissection occurs in 10% of cases after PTCRA, usually in angulated lesions and large burr-to-artery ratio. Acute closure is infrequent after PTCRA and represents occult dissection or underdone ablation. These can be avoided by maximal plaque debulking using the step burr approach.

Indications and results

Rotational atherectomy has been shown to be superior to balloon angioplasty in specific coronary lesion subsets *(Table 28.3)*. The PTCRA has undergone evolution with change in technique, equipment and better understanding of the procedure. The indications, safety, and comparison of PTCRA to other revascularization techniques have been presented or are currently tested in several trials.

US Multicenter Registry A multicenter registry of patients treated with rotational atherectomy at 22 sites was maintained from 1988-1993. Analysis of 3,717 lesions in 2,976 patients revealed a procedural success rate (residual stenosis <50% with at least a 20% reduction in diameter stenosis, uncomplicated by death, CABG, or Q-wave MI) of 95%.[40] Other complications included nonQ-wave MI (CK>2.5 x normal), 6.1%; dissection, 13%[41] perforation 0.6%[42] slow flow 7.6%[43] and groin complications 2.2%.[44] The restenosis rate was 39%.

European Experience. Results from 3 European centers using PTCRA in 129 patients repotrted primary success of 86%: by PTCRA alone in 57% and with PTCRA and adjunctive PTCA in 29%. Acute occlusion occurred in 10 patients (7.7%). Recanalization was achieved by PTCA in 7: urgent CABG in 2, Q-wave and non-Q-wave myocardial infarction occurred in 3 and 7 patients, respectively. No deaths occurred. An overall angiographic restenosis rate was 38%.

ERBAC Trial. A randomized trial comparing **E**xcimer **L**aser vs. **R**otablator vs. **B**alloon **A**ngioplasty **C**omparison trial for AHA/ACC type B2/C lesions revealed lower

Table 28.3   INDICATIONS FOR ROTATIONAL ATHERECTOMY.

Definite indications	1. Long diffuse lesions
	2. Calcified lesions
	3. Bifurcation lesions
	4. Ostial lesion
Possible indications	1. Total occlusion
	2. In stent restenosis
	3. Complex calcified lesion
	4. Distal SVG anastomotic lesion
	5. Dart type lesions (>10 mm mildly, calcified lesion in < 3 mm vessel)
Contraindications	1. Thrombus containing lesion
	2. SVG lesions

acute complication of infarction, emergent bypass or death after PTCRA compared to Laser or PTCA (2.3 % vs. 6.2% vs. 4.8% respectively; p=0.04). Angiographic restenosis and target lesion revascularization rates were not different.[45] Restenosis was 1.86 times more likely in long lesions and 2.54 times more likely in noncalcified lesions; restenosis rates were lowest (6.3%) for short calcified lesions and highest (37.2%) for calcified lesions >20 mm in length.

STRATAS. The Study to Determine Rotablator System and Transluminal Angioplasty Strategy tested two methods of using the Rotablator: the *aggressive strategy,* with maximum debulking (0.8-0.9 burr-to-artery ratio) followed by no or low pressure adjunctive PTCA (<1 atm) and the *conventional strategy,* with moderate debulking (0.75 burr-to-artery ratio) followed by standard adjunctive PTCA (>3 atm). The results revealed lower acute major complications with the aggressive vs. the conventional strategy (1.9% vs 5.2%, p<0.02). The long term results showed similar target lesion revascularization rates amongst the two strategies.

DART. The Dilation vs Ablation Revascularization Trial is a randomized trial comparing PTCRA with or without adjunctive low pressure PTCA (< 1 atm) to conventional PTCA in AHA/ACC type A or B lesions, in vessels <3 mm diameter . The primary endpoint is clinical and angiographic restenosis in 500 patients, and substudies of intravascular ultrasound, cost effectiveness, and quality of life will also be include. The trial has been completed and the results are awaited.

CARAT. The Coronary Angioplasty and Rotablator Atherectomy Trial is a prospective multicenter randomized trial which compares the results of Rotablator using small burr (final burr-to-artery ratio <0.7) vs. larger burrs (final burr-to- artery ratio >0.7). The primary end point is restenosis and secondary endpoints include target vessel revascularization and cost.

"RotaStent". PTCRA prior to stenting (RotaStent) represents a true device synergy in that rotational atherectomy by debulking the calcified atheroma increases the lesion compliance allowing adequate stent expansion and maximal luminal dimensions. Mintz et al, using intravascular ultrasound, demonstrated that PTCRA followed by stent resulted in a larger luminal gain (7.3 mm vs. 5.1 mm) and a smaller residual stenosis (12% vs. 27%) when compared with PTCRA followed by adjunctive PTCA.[46] A prospective, multicenter randomized trial comparing stent alone vs RotaStent is being designed (SPORT trial).

"Rota ReoPro". In a prospective, non randomized trial with 200 patients use of ReoPro with PTCRA decreased absolute CK rise by 48%, the incidence of any abnormal CK rise by 50%, and the occurrence of non-Q wave MIs by 67%.[47] The randomized trial is being formulated to investigate this further.

TWISTER *The Trial of Within Stent Treatment of Endoluminal Restenosis.* addresses a demanding challenge to the interventional cardiologist. A registry of PTCRA for in-stent restenosis has demonstrated >99% procedural success and a recurrent restenosis rate of 35%. This is lower than recurrent restenosis rate reported for PTCA treatment of in-stent restenosis. The TWISTER trial, with a total of 500 patients, will have a 3 arm randomization: PTCA alone vs. PTCRA with or without low pressure PTCA vs. PTCRA and adjunctive PTCA.

In conclusion, PTCRA has found a definite niche in specific coronary lesion subsets and is a useful tool in the interventional armamentarium. The technique is still evolving and the device is being improved upon to enhance the procedural results. RotaStent device synergy is exciting and holds great promise to decrease the restenosis.

REFERENCES

1. Topol EJ, et al. Analysis of coronary angioplasty practice in the United States with an insurance claim database. Circulation 1993:87:1489.

2. Detre K, et al. Percutaneous transluminal coronary angioplasty in 1985-1986 and 1977-1981. N Engl J Med 1988:318:265.

3. Lincoff AM, et al. Abrupt vessel closure complicating coronary angioplasty: Clinical, angiographic and therapeutic profile. J Am Coll Cardiol 1992:19: 926.

4. Forrester JS, Eiger N, Litvack F. Interventioanl cardiology: The decade ahead. Circulation 1991:84:942.

5. Nobuyoshi M, et al. Restenosis after successful percutaneous transluminal angioplasty: Serial angiographic follow-up of 299 patients. J Am Coll Cardiol 1988:12:616.

6. Popma JJ, Califf RM, Topol EJ. Clinical Trials of restenosis after coronary angioplasty. Circulation 1991:84:1426.

7. Penny WF, et al. Insights into the mechanism of luminal improvement after directional coronary atherectomy. Am J Cardiol 1991:67:435.

8. Kuntz RE, et al. The importance of acute luminal diameter in determining restenosis after coronary atherectomy or stenting. Circulation 1992:86:1827.

9. Umans VA, et al. Restenosis after directional atherectomy and balloon angioplasty: Comparative analysis based on matched lesions. J Am Coll Cardiol 1993:21:1382.

10. Safian RD, et al. Coronary atherectomy clinical angiographic and histological findings and observations regarding potential mechanisms. Circulation 1990:82:69.

11. Johnson D, et al. Acute complications of directional coronary atherectomy are related to the morphology of excised stenoses. J Am Coll Cardiol 1992:19:76A.

12. Garratt KN, et al. Restenosis after directional coronary atherectomy: Differences between primary atheromatous and restenosis lesions and influence of subintimal tissue resection. J Am Coll Cardiol 1990:16:1665.

13. Kuntz RE, Hinohara T, Safian RD. Restenosis after directional coronary atherectomy: Effects of luminal diameter and deep wall excision. Circulation 1992:86:1394-99.

14. Isner JM, et al, for the CAVEAT Investigators. Coronary thrombus: Clinical features and angiographic diagnosis in 370 patients studied by directional atherectomy. Circulation 1992:86:2583.

15. Christou GP, et al. Histopathological correlation of coronary arteriographic lesion morphology using directed atherectomy derived specimens: frequent thrombus in complex lesions. J Am Coll Cardiol 1992:19:375A.

16. Sharma SK, et al. Lipid rich plaques with thrombus are common in unstable rest angina: Observations from artherectomy tissue analysis. J Am Coll Cardiol 1995 25:281A.

17. Ellis SG, et al. Relation of stenosis morphology and clinical presentation to the procedural results of directional coronary atherectomy. Circulation 1991:84:644.

18. Popma JJ, et al. Abrupt vessel closure after directional coronary atherectomy. J Am Coll Cardiol 1992: 19:1372.

19. Hinohara T, et al. Restenosis after directional coronary atherectomy. J Am Coll Cardiol 1992: 20:623.

20. Fishman RF, et al. Long-term results of directional coronary atherectomy: Predictors of restenosis. J Am Coll Cardiol 1992:20:1101.

21. Topol EJ, et al, for the CAVEAT study group: A comparison of directional atherectomy with coronary angioplasty in patients with coronary artery disease. N Engl J Med 1993:329:221.

22. Elliot JM, et al. One-year follow-up in the coronary angioplasty versus excisional atherectomy trial (CAVEAT I). Circulation 1995:91:2158.

23. Adelman AG, et al. A comparison of directional atherectomy with balloon angioplasty for lesions of the left anterior descending coronary artery. N Engl J Med 1993:329:228.

24. Holmes DR, et al. The CAVEAT-II investigators. A multicenter, randomized trial of coronary angioplasty versus directional atherectomy for patients with saphenous vein bypass graft lesions. Circulation 1995:91:1966.

25. Baim DS, et al. The BOAT investigators. Final results in the balloon vs optimal atherectomy trial (BOAT): 6 month angiography and 1 year clinical follow-up. Circulation1996:94:I-436.

26. Simonton CA, et al. Acute and late clinical and angiographic results of directional atherectomy in the optimal atherectomy restenosis study. Circulation 1995:95:I-544.

27. Cohen DJ, et al. Cost-effectiveness of directional atherectomy, stenting and conventional angioplasty in single-vessel disease: A decision-analytic model. J Am Coll Cardiol 1993:21:227A.

28. O'Murchu B, et al. Role of IABP Counterpulsation in High Risk Atherectomy. J Am Coll Cardiol 1995: 26:1270.

29. Prevosti LG, et al. Particulate debris from rotational atherectomy: size, distribution and physiologic effect. Circulation 1988: 78: II-83.

30. MacIsaac A, et al. Angiographic predictors of outcome of coronary rotational atherectomy from the completed multicenter registry. J Am Coll Cardiol 1994: 23: 353.

31. Brown DL, Buchbinder M. Incidence, predictors and consequences of coronary dissection following high speed rotational atherectomy. Am J Cardiol 1996: 78: 1416.

32. Cohen B, et al. Coronary perforation during rotational ablation: Angiographic determinants and clinical outcomes. J Am Coll Cardiol 1994: 23: 354.

33. Ellis SG, et al. Relation of clinical presentation, stenosis morphology, and operator technique to the procedural results of rotational atherectomy and rotational atherectomy-facilitated angioplasty. Circulation 1994: 89: 882.

34. Warth DC, et al. Rotational atherectomy multicenter registry: Acute results, complications and 6-month angiographic follow-up in 709 patients. J Am Coll Cardiol 1994: 24: 641.

35. Vandormael M, et al. Comparison of excimer laser, rotablator and balloon angioplasty for the treatment of complex lesions: ERBAC study final results. J Am Coll Cardiol. 1994: 23: 57A.

36. Mintz GS, et al. Rotational atherectomy followed by adjunct stents: the preferred therapy for calcified large vessels. Circulation 1995: 92 9(Suppl I): I-329.

37. Braden GA, et al. Abciximab decreases both the incidence and magnitude of creatine kinase elevation during rotational atherectomy J Am Coll Cardiol 1997: 29: 499A.

38. O'Murchu B, et al. Role of IABP Counterpulsation in High Risk Atherectomy. J Am Coll Cardiol 1995: 26:1270.

39. Prevosti LG, et al. Particulate debris from rotational atherectomy: size, distribution and physiologic effect. Circulation 1988: 78: II-83.

40. MacIsaac A, et al. Angiographic predictors of outcome of coronary rotational atherectomy from the completed multicenter registry. J Am Coll Cardiol 1994: 23: 353.

41. Brown DL, Buchbinder M. Incidence, predictors and consequences of coronary dissection following high speed rotational atherectomy. Am J Cardiol 1996: 78: 1416.

42. Cohen B, et al. Coronary perforation during rotational ablation: Angiographic determinants and clinical outcomes. J Am Coll Cardiol 1994: 23: 354.

43. Ellis SG, et al. Relation of clinical presentation, stenosis morphology, and operator technique to the procedural results of rotational atherectomy and rotational atherectomy-facilitated angioplasty. Circulation 1994: 89: 882.

44. Warth DC, et al. Rotational atherectomy multicenter registry: Acute results, complications and 6-month angiographic follow-up in 709 patients. J Am Coll Cardiol 1994: 24: 641.

45. Vandormael M, et al. Comparison of excimer laser, rotablator and balloon angioplasty for the treatment of complex lesions: ERBAC study final results. J Am Coll Cardiol. 1994: 23 : 57A.

46. Mintz GS, et al. Rotational atherectomy followed by adjunct stents: the preferred therapy for calcified large vessels. Circulation 1995: 92 (Suppl I): I-329.

47. Braden GA. Abciximab decreases both the incidence and magnitude of creatine kinase elevation during rotational atherectomy. J Am Coll Cardiol 1997: 29: 499A.

29 EXCIMER LASER ANGIOPLASTY

Henry H. Ting, Farris K. Timimi, John A. Bittl

Although balloon angioplasty has been a significant advance in the treatment of patients with coronary artery disease, this treatment is limited by a significant incidence of restenosis that averages about 50% in most recent reports.[1,2,3] Restenosis after balloon angioplasty is associated with the healing response of vascular tissue to injury and involves platelet deposition, inflammatory cell infiltration, smooth muscle cell proliferation, and extracellular matrix formation.[4] Because the mechanism of vessel dilatation in balloon angioplasty involves significant vessel injury with intimal fissuring, limited penetration into the subintimal space, and occasionally deep dissection into the media, it was hoped that interventional methods causing less vascular injury would decrease the likelihood of restenosis.

Excimer laser angioplasty was first developed in 1988 with the hope that it would precisely remove atherosclerotic plaque and thus reduce the risk of restenosis. After five years of intense clinical investigation, excimer laser angioplasty has evolved in many ways. Through several refinements in procedural technique, patient selection, and operator experience, the procedure is now targeted for lesions that are difficult to treat with other methods. The ultimate value of excimer laser angioplasty, however, depends in part on its ability to maintain long-term vessel patency. The purpose of this paper is to review the current indications for excimer laser angioplasty and emphasize the long-term success rates.

The clinical era of laser angioplasty began in 1984 with continuous-wave systems and bare optical fibers.[5-6] After reports of vessel perforation,[7] thermal probe angioplasty was developed[8] but this was complicated by reduced success, thermal injury, perforation, and restenosis.[9] Limited success was also achieved with the hybrid laser-thermal probe system,[10] balloon-centering argon laser," and laser-balloon angioplasty.[12]

Excimer laser angioplasty emerged in 1988 as an appealing technique to ablate atherosclerotic plaque with minimal thermal injury to the vessel wall. Excimer laser systems were developed to operate over a guide wire, thus ensuring better co-axial alignment and a lower risk of vessel perforation than earlier laser systems. The use of pulsed energy delivery, usually at a frequency of 25 Hz with interpulse delays of approximately 40 ms, allowed for adequate tissue cooling between laser pulses. Tissue ablation with excimer laser angioplasty appeared to result from a combination of photochemical dissociation, photoacoustic effects, and a localized thermal effect.[13,14,15] Dose response curves suggested a linear relationship between the depth of tissue ablation and the number of pulses utilized.[16]

Clinical results

Excimer laser coronary angioplasty has been shown to have favorable acute success rates in preliminary reports.[17,18] In a recent report,[17] excimer laser coronary angioplasty was used to treat 858 stenoses in 764 patients (mean age 61 years, 75% male). Clinical success was achieved in 86% of patients, as defined by residual stenosis <50% and no major complications during hospitalization. Major complications during hospitalization occurred in 7.6% of patients, including death in 0.7%, acute Q wave or non Q wave myocardial infarction in 3.6%, and bypass surgery in 4.1%. Relative risk analysis and comparison with historical controls showed that patients with saphenous vein graft lesions, aorto-ostial lesions, and total occlusions had acceptable success rates and low complication rates. The results of reports for saphenous vein graft lesions, aorto-ostial lesions, and total occlusions are reviewed here.

Saphenous vein graft lesions

Excimer laser coronary angioplasty has been reported in several studies as a potentially useful intervention for patients with saphenous vein graft lesions.[17,18,19,20] The most recent analysis included a total of 495 patients (mean age 63, 77% male) who underwent treatment with excimer laser angioplasty for 545 saphenous vein graft stenoses.[21] The mean age of the saphenous vein grafts was 8 years. Clinical success was achieved in 92% of patients as indicated by residual stenosis <50% and no major complications during hospitalization. Major complications during hospitalization occurred in 6.1% of patients, including death in 1%, acute Q wave or non Q wave myocardial infarction in 4.6%, and bypass surgery in 0.6%. Relative risk analysis demonstrated that excimer laser coronary angioplasty had the most favorable outcome, in terms of highest success rates and lowest complication rates, in discrete lesions located in the ostium of all vein grafts and in the body of smaller (<3mm) vein grafts (Figure 29.1). After controlling for lesion morphology and graft dimension, vein graft age had no effect on the success or complication rates of excimer laser angioplasty.

In comparison, studies of balloon angioplasty for saphenous vein graft lesions

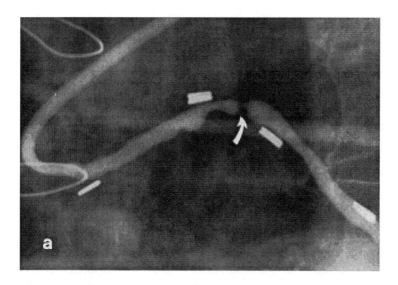

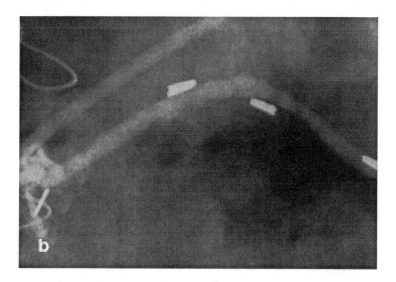

Figure 29.1 Saphenous vein graft lesion. A 61 year-old man developed unstable angina, associated with a complex 80% stenosis in the saphenous vein graft to the first obtuse marginal branch (a, arrow). The lesion was successfully treated with the sequential perfusion strategy of excimer laser angioplasty and directional atherectomy without complication, leaving a 10% residual stenosis (b).

have reported success rates ranging from 80-85%.[22,23,24,25] Complication rates for balloon angioplasty of vein grafts were higher for grafts >3 years of age (4% death rate, 13% risk of embolization and myocardial infarction, and 4% risk for bypass surgery) than those for younger grafts.[25] The overall restenosis rate for vein graft lesions treated by balloon angioplasty was 82%.[25]

Aorto-ostial lesions

Excimer laser coronary angioplasty has also been used to treat patients with aorto-ostial stenoses[17,18,26]. In the most recent analysis, 200 patients (mean age 65, 53% male) underwent excimer laser angioplasty for 209 aorto-ostial stenoses.[26] The distribution of stenoses sites included left main coronary artery in 12%, right coronary artery in 59%, and saphenous vein graft in 28%. Clinical success was achieved in 90%, as defined by residual stenosis <50% and no major complications during hospitalization. A major complication during hospitalization occurred in 10.2% of patients, including acute Q wave or non Q wave myocardial infarction in 6.8% and bypass surgery in 3.4%. There were no deaths reported. Right coronary artery and saphenous vein graft ostial lesions *(Figure 29.2)* had the most favorable outcomes and left main coronary artery ostial lesions had the least favorable outcomes.

In comparison, the largest series of balloon angioplasty for treatment of aorto-ostial lesions reported a lower acute success rate of 79%.[27] Complications included a 5.7% rate of myocardial infarction and a 9.4% rate of acute dissection or vessel closure requiring emergent bypass surgery. There were no deaths reported. Six month follow-up of balloon angioplasty of aorto-ostial stenoses revealed an angiographic restenosis rate of 37%.

Total occlusions

The results with excimer laser angioplasty in treating chronic total occlusions have been reported with excimer laser coronary angioplasty in two recent published studies.[17,28] In a preliminary report of 127 total occlusions that could be crossed with a guidewire, the clinical success rate of excimer laser coronary angioplasty was 84%.[17] Major complications during hospitalization occurred in 2.4% of patients, including death in 0.8%, myocardial infarction in 0.8%, and bypass surgery in 0.8%. In a more recent analysis, a total of 162 patients (mean age 59, 83% male) underwent excimer laser coronary angioplasty for 172 total occlusions.[28] Clinical success was achieved in 90% of patients with total occlusions that could be crossed with a guidewire. Major complications during hospitalization occurred in 3.7% of patients, including death in 0.6%, myocardial infarction in 1.9%, and bypass surgery in 1.2%.

Complications

One of the most serious complications of laser angioplasty is vessel perforation. A

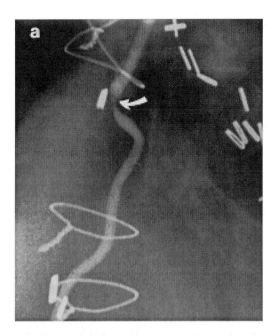

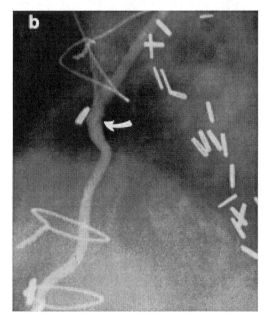

Figure 29.2 *Aorto-ostial lesion. This 45 year-old women developed increasing angina four months after coronary artery bypass surgery associated with subtotal occlusion of the ostium of the graft (a, arrow). The lesion was successfully treated with excimer laser angioplasty and adjunctive angioplasty, leaving no residual stenosis (b, arrow).*

recent series of 764 patients with 858 stenoses treated with excimer laser angioplasty had an incidence of vessel perforation of 3% (23 patients), of which 1% (9 patients) had major complications, including tamponade, myocardial infarction, or need for bypass surgery.[29] No patient with a vessel perforation expired during hospitalization. Multivariable analysis demonstrated that lesions at an increased risk for perforation were lesions at bifurcations, in diabetic patients, and in female patients. Long lesions (>10 mm) and saphenous vein graft lesions were not at increased risk. Vessel perforation was noted in 8.3% of lesions in which the difference between the diameter of the catheter and that of the target vessel was less than 0.5 mm; however, vessel perforation was noted in only 1.5% of lesions in which the difference between the diameter of the catheter and that of the target vessel was greater than 1 mm. Therefore, the risk of vessel perforation may be decreased by using laser catheters more than 1 mm smaller than the diameter of the target vessel.

Another important predictor of clinical success and acute complications is the presence of intracoronary filling defects by angiography prior to laser angioplasty. In a recent series of 142 patients who underwent laser angioplasty, clinical success was achieved in 58% of patients with angiographic evidence of an intracoronary filling defects, as compared with a clinical success rate of 95% in patients without angiographic evidence of intracoronary thrombus. Angiographic demonstration of an intracoronary thrombus was found to be the single most important predictor of acute vessel complications including embolization and acute myocardial infarction.[30]

Lesion eccentricity, as measured by the eccentricity index, is defined by the percent deviation of the midline axis of the stenosis lumen from the midline axis of the vessel lumen, and was found to be an important predictor of acute vessel complications.[31] Eccentric stenoses might be amenable to therapy with eccentric monorail catheters, whose eccentric array of fibers may provide better control and outcome than laser catheters with a concentric array of fibers.

Restenosis

Restenosis is the major drawback of all interventional devices. In a series of 764 patients treated with excimer laser angioplasty, the overall restenosis rate at six month follow-up was 46%, based on the combined angiographic and noninvasive follow-up testing.[17] For saphenous vein grafts, the angiographic restenosis rate was 55% at six month follow-up, with a 44% compliance rate.[32] This restenosis rate may be an overestimate, because symptomatic patients are more likely to comply with the request for six month angiographic follow-up than asymptomatic patients. Restenosis rates, which varied among differing lesion morphologies and graft dimensions, were highest in lesions longer than 10 mm located in saphenous vein grafts smaller than 3 mm. For aorto-ostial lesions, six month angiographic follow-up, which was obtained in 51% of eligible patients, showed a restenosis rate of 39%.[26] The restenosis rate was highest in left main coronary artery lesions (64% restenosis rate) and lowest in right coronary artery and vein graft lesions (35% restenosis rate in

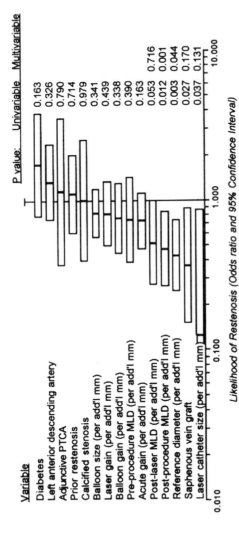

Figure 29.3 Predictors of restenosis. Odds ratios are provided to estimate the probability that a given variable increases or decreases the likelihood of restenosis, as compared with all other lesions without the variable. For polychotomous or continuous variables, such as lesion length or reference diameter of the vessel, the odds ratio refers to the added or reduced risk of one additional mm in lesion length or vessel size. The 95% confidence intervals reflect the statistical reliability of the odds ratios. P values are obtained from univariable and multivariable logistic regression analyses of restenosis, as defined dichotomously as the presence of ≥50.0% stenosis on follow-up angiography. (Reproduced with permission from Journal of American College of Cardiology[21]).

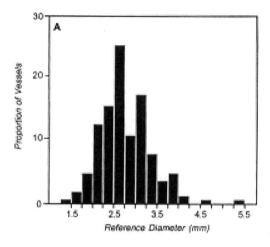

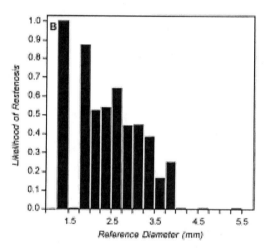

Figure 29.4 Distribution of vessel diameters and restenosis. The distribution of reference diameters containing lesions for excimer laser-facilitated angioplasty ranged from 1.50 to 5.35 mm and approximated a Gaussian function (A). Restenosis was more likely to be observed in vessels with small reference diameters (B). (Reproduced with permission from Journal of American College of Cardiology[21]).

both). Restenosis was less likely when the residual diameter stenosis was <35% after treatment with excimer laser angioplasty. For total occlusions, the overall restenosis rate at six month follow-up was 46%, as assessed with a combination of angiographic and noninvasive testing.[17]

Several studies have demonstrated that the likelihood of restenosis after coronary intervention is inversely related to the lumen diameter achieved at the time of the procedure.[33] A quantitative analysis of luminal narrowing after excimer laser angioplasty has revealed that the overall restenosis rate is 50%.[21] The size of the vessels treated with excimer laser angioplasty ranged from 1.3 to 5.5 mm and followed a normal distribution. The likelihood of restenosis was greatest in smaller vessels *(Figure 29.3)*. Of all predictors of restenosis after excimer laser angioplasty, the strongest factors included the diameter of the target vessel and the immediate post-procedure lumen diameter *(Figure 29.4)*.

Thus, excimer angioplasty produced the lowest restenosis rates in largest native coronary vessels and bypass grafts in which the largest post-procedure minimal lumen diameters can be obtained. With the typical use of excimer laser facilitated angioplasty in smaller diffusely diseased vessels poorly suited for directional atherectomy or coronary stenting, limitations on the size of the posttreatment lumen imposed by the reference vessel size have been reflected by an apparently higher incidence of restenosis than that seen with other new devices. But, this analysis has revealed that smaller vessels are at greater risk of restenosis than larger vessel. The goal of excimer laser angioplasty thus remains to safely achieve the largest lumen possible by combining laser treatment and adjunctive balloon angioplasty, directional atherectomy, or stenting.

Future directions

Excimer laser coronary angioplasty is the most extensively studied laser revascularization technique. Although excimer laser coronary angioplasty is a promising intervention for saphenous vein grafts, aorto-ostial lesions, and total occlusions, these lesions comprise only 10-15% of all lesions treated with conventional balloon angioplasty. Increased acceptance of laser angioplasty awaits a rigorous comparison between excimer laser coronary angioplasty and conventional balloon angioplasty.

A multicenter, randomized trial is planned to evaluate the safety and efficacy of excimer laser coronary angioplasty as compared to that of conventional balloon angioplasty. Patients with saphenous vein bypass graft stenoses in grafts ≤3.0 mm in diameter, aorto-ostial lesions, and total occlusions will be randomized to undergo treatment with percutaneous balloon angioplasty or excimer laser angioplasty. This study has the potential to define in a rigorous, randomized fashion the clinical efficacy and safety of excimer laser coronary angioplasty and expand the general acceptance of this promising interventional tool.

REFERENCES

1. Nobuyoshi M, et al. Restenosis after successful percutaneous transluminal coronary angioplasty : Serial angiographic follow-up of 229 patients. J Am Coll Cardiol 1988: 12: 616.

2. Adelman AG, et al. A comparison of coronary atherectomy with coronary angioplasty for lesions of the proximal left anterior descending coronary artery. N Engl J Med 1993: 329: 228.

3. Topol EJ, et al. A comparison of balloon angioplasty with directional atherectomy in patients with coronary artery disease. N Engl J Med 1993: 329 : 221.

4. Forrester JS, et al. A paradigm for restenosis based on cell biology : clues for the development of new preventive therapies. J Am Coll Cardiol 1991: 17: 758.

5. Geschwind H, Boussignac G, Teisseire B. Percutaneous transluminal laser angioplasty in man. Lancet 1984: 2 : 844.

6. Ginsburg R, et al. Salvage of an ischemic limb by laser angioplasty: Description of a new technique. Clin. Cardiol. 1984: 54.

7. Ginsburg R, et al. Percutaneous transluminal laser angioplasty for treatment of peripheral vascular disease : clinical experience in 16 patients. Radiology 1985: 156 : 619.

8. Cumberland DC, et al. Percutaneous laser thermal angioplasty : initial clinical results with a laser probe in total peripheral artery occlusions. Lancet 1986: 1 : 457.

9. Tobis JM, et al. Laser-assisted versus mechanical recanalization of femoral arterial occlusions. Am J Cardiol 1991: 68: 1079.

10. Belli AM, et al. Total peripheral artery occlusions : Conventional versus laser thermal recanalization with a hybrid probe in percutaneous angioplasty : Results of a randomized trial. Radiology 1991: 181 : 57.

11. Foschi A, et al. Laser angioplasty of totally occluded coronary arteries and vein grafts: preliminary report on a current trial. Am J Cardiol 1989: 9F.

12. Reis GJ, et al. Laser balloon angioplasty : clinical, angiographic and histologic results. J Am Coll Cardiol 1991: 18: 193.

13. van Leeuwen TG, et al. Origin of arteriaal wall dissections induced by pulsed excimer and mid-infrared laser ablation in the pig. J Am Coll Cardiol 1992: 19: 1610.

14. van Leeuwen TG, et al. Intraluminal vapor bubble induced by excimer laser causes microsecond arterial dilation and invagination leading to extensive wall damage in the rabbit. Circulation 1993: 87 : 1258.

15. Clarke R, et al. Gas chromatography light microscopic correlation of excimer laser photoablation of cardiovascular tissues : evidence for a thermal mechanism. Circulation Res 1987: 60 : 429.

16. Litvack F, et al. The excimer laser : From basic science to clinical application. In : Vogel JHK, King SB III, ed. Interventional cardiology: Future directions. St. Louis : C.V. Mosby Co: 1989 : 170.

17. Bittl JA, et al. Clinical success, complications and restenosis rates with excimer laser coronary angioplasty. Am J Cardiol 1992 : 70: 1533.

18. Litvack F, et al. Percutaneous excimer laser coronary angioplasty : Results in the first consecutive 3,000 patients. J Am Coll Cardiol 1994: 23 : 323.

19. Bittl JA, Sanborn TA. Excimer laser-facilitated coronary angioplasty : relative risk analysis of acute and follow-up results in 200 patients. Circulation 1992: 86: 71.

20. Cook SL, et al. Percutaneous excimer laser coronary angioplasty of lesions not ideal for balloon angioplasty. Circulation 1991: 84: 632.

21. Bittl JA, et al. Predictors of luminal narrowing after excimer laser coronary angioplasty. J Am Coll Cardiol 1994: 23: 1314.

22. Liu MW, et al. Angiographic predictors of a rise in serum creatine kinase (distal embolization) after balloon angioplasty of saphenous vein coronary artery bypass grafts. Am J Cardiol 1993: 72: 514.

23. De Feyter PJ, et al. Balloon angioplasty for the treatment of lesions in sapherous vein bypass grafts. J Am Coll Cardiol 1993: 21: 1539.

24. Douglas JS Jr. Percutaneous intervention in patients with prior coronary bypass surgery (Update 8). In : Topol EJ, ed. Textbook of Interventional Cardiology. Philadelphia : Saunders: 1993 : 119.

25. Platko WP, et al. Percutaneous transluminal angioplasty of sapherous vein graft stenosis : long-term follow-up. J Am Coll Cardiol 1989: 14: 1654.

26. Eigler N, et al. Excimer laser coronary angioplasty of aorto-ostial stenoses : Results of the Excimer Laser Coronary Angioplasty (ELCA) Registry in the first 200 patients. Circulation 1993: 88: 2049.

27. Topol Ej, et al. Multicenter study of percutaneous transluminal angioplasty for right coronary artery ostial stenosis. J Am Coll Cardiol 1987: 9 : 1214.

28. Holmes DR Jr, et al. Chronic total obstruction and short term outcome : The excimer laser angioplasty registry experience. Mayo Clin Proc 1993: 68: 5.

29. Bittl JA, et al. Coronary artery perforation during excimer laser coronary angioplaty. 1993: 21 : 1158.

30. Estella P, et al. Excimer laser-assisted angioplasty for lesions containing thrombus. J Am Coll Cardiol 1993: 21: 1550.

31. Ghazzal ZMB, et al. Morphological predictors of acute complications after percutaneous excimer laser coronary angioplasty. Results of a comprehensive angiographic analysis : Importance of the eccentricity index. Circulation 1992: 86: 820.

32. Bittl JA, et al. Predictors of outcome of percutaneous excimer laser coronary angioplasty of saphenous vein graft lesions. Am J Cardiol 1994: 74: 144.

33. Kuntz RE, et al. A generalized model of restenosis following conventional balloon angioplasty, stening and directional atherectomy. J Am Coll Cardiol 1993: 21: 15.

30 NOVEL INTERVENTIONAL TECHNIQUES FOR ACUTE CORONARY SYNDROMES

David R. Holmes Jr.,Robert S. Schwartz

The introduction of percutaneous transluminal coronary angioplasty (PTCA) in 1977 has revolutionized modern cardiology.[1] It not only has offered an alternative means for treating patients with acute coronary syndromes but also stimulated interest in the pathophysiology of these syndromes. Percutaneous revascularization procedures have become the treatment of choice for patients with single vessel disease requiring revascularization and similarly provide an excellent option for selected patients with multivessel coronary artery disease.[2-6] The annual number of dilatation procedures now exceeds the number of coronary bypass surgical procedures.

Although widely used, PTCA has a number of important limitations including acute or threatened closure, inability to achieve complete revascularization in many patients (usually related to the presence of a chronic total occlusion), restenosis, and inadequate initial results with selected lesion characteristics including coronary arterial thrombus-containing lesions. These limitations have stimulated the development of several new groups of interventional devices aimed at improving the initial outcome, decreasing restenosis in the longer-term, or devices able to be used as bailout to treat acute complications. These devices include atherectomy catheters for lesion ablation, lasers, and intravascular stents. Many of these new devices remain investigational, although an increasing number have received F.D.A. approval including directional coronary atherectomy, rotational atherectomy, transluminal extraction catheters, Excimer laser coronary angioplasty, and two different stents. These devices have all been studied and are used with varying frequency in broad subsets of patients requiring revascularization. It must be remembered that all of these new devices also have their own limitations and complication patterns. Some of these are no different than with conventional PTCA while some are unique, such as coronary perforation.

Although initially described in patients with stable angina, because of improved operator experience and technical advancements, percutaneous procedures have been applied with increasing frequency in patients with acute ischemic syndromes. These acute ischemic syndromes include unstable angina, acute myocardial infarction, and postinfarction angina. The pathophysiology of these syndromes has been explored in depth both in animal models and in humans using a variety of techniques such as intravascular ultrasound. In addition, the response of some of these syndromes to specific treatment, for example, acute myocardial infarction and thrombolytic therapy, has provided additional knowledge about the underlying mechanisms.

The pathophysiology of these syndromes includes an active atherosclerotic plaque that becomes unstable either because of plaque rupture or hemorrhage with subsequent exposure of plaque and arterial wall elements to circulating blood.[7,8] This is also associated with endothelial dysfunction and often inappropriate vasoconstriction. Intraluminal thrombus and platelet deposition occur. This may result in vessel occlusion or subtotal stenosis with eventual resolution. In general, acute myocardial infarction is the result of total occlusion with predominant red cell thrombus with some platelet admixture, while unstable angina is the result of a subtotal stenosis often with predominant platelet cell thrombus.

This underlying pathophysiology is responsible for acute ischemic syndromes as well as some of the complications of interventional therapy. The results of this therapy have in general been excellent, although associated with slightly higher mortality, increased potential for acute closure, and a definite increase in restenosis rates compared to treatment of patients with stable angina. Intraluminal filling defects likely representative of coronary arterial thrombus have been a risk factor for dilatation, and in early series were associated with a marked increase in acute closure. In the first small series from 1985, 73% of patients with intracoronary thrombus had acute or threatened closure compared to only 9% of patients without coronary thrombus.[9] Subsequent series have also documented an increased risk in this setting, although the results have improved.[10,11] In a recent series from the Mayo Clinic, the role of thrombus as an independent predictor of angioplasty failure was assessed over time.[12] For this analysis, all patients undergoing angioplasty of a single coronary arterial lesion from 1984 through 1991 were analyzed. Three time periods were analyzed—1984 through 1986, 1987 through 1989, and 1989 through 1991. Of 2,699 patients undergoing initial angioplasty during that time, 1,121 (42%) had angiographic evidence of thrombus. Multivariate analysis documented that thrombus remained an independent predictor of angioplasty failure and that the magnitude of this adverse effect had not changed over the three time periods assessed in this study.

For these reasons, despite the fact that PTCA often gives excellent results, new approaches to the patient with acute ischemic syndromes are being investigated. Some of these new approaches involve the use of new devices while some involve combined drugs and devices to optimize the results. Not all devices are suitable for thrombus-containing lesions.

Directional atherectomy

Directional atherectomy was the first alternative to conventional PTCA which was approved for use. By its design, shape and size, it is ideally suited for short lesions, < 10 to 12 mm, in large vessels which are nontortuous and noncalcified. Both of these latter conditions are associated with decreased success rates with this device. In addition, lesion eccentricity, bulky lesions or lesions containing a focal ulceration are favorable for directional atherectomy because of its ability to selectively remove tissue. These lesion characteristics are relatively common in patients with unstable angina. Directional atherectomy has been used in this setting. Early single and multicenter experience prior to F.D.A. approval identified that angiographically complex, probable thrombus-containing lesions, were associated with an excellent outcome. In our experience, the presence of intraluminal thrombus prior to atherectomy was not associated with decreased success rates compared with what has been documented with conventional PTCA. There was, however, an increased incidence of prolonged angina (p = 0.046) and coronary artery embolization (p = 0.003). In the CAVEAT trial of 1,012 patients, in whom de novo native coronary arterial lesions were randomized to either PTCA or directional coronary atherectomy, approximately 70% of patients had unstable angina defined as postinfarction angina, accelerating angina or rest angina with or without electrocardiographic changes [13]. In this study, the initial success rate assessed by quantitative coronary angiography was 89% versus 80% for conventional dilatation. In this trial, there was no overall difference in restenosis rate between the two therapies, although for the proximal left anterior descending subset, there was a decreased restenosis with directional atherectomy of 50% versus 59%. Directional coronary atherectomy has also been widely used in the treatment of discrete vein graft disease, which may also have associated thrombus. As was true in CAVEAT-1, CAVEAT-2 (which randomized patients with de novo vein graft disease to either directional coronary atherectomy or PTCA)[14], directional coronary atherectomy resulted in improved initial success rates and improved residual stenosis but with an increase in non-Q-wave myocardial infarction and distal embolization. In this trial, as was true with CAVEAT-1, the large majority of patients had unstable angina (89%).

At the current time, directional coronary atherectomy plays an important role in treatment of selected lesions which may be seen in acute ischemic syndromes including thrombus-containing lesions. In these subsets of patients, directional coronary atherectomy can be used to optimize the initial angiographic result, although the restenosis rates are not substantially improved and increased distal embolization rates have been seen. More complete lesion removal may improve the long-term results.

TEC (Transluminal extraction catheter)

TEC has also been approved by the F.D.A. This has the potential advantage of removing thrombus from lesions. It has usually been used in very high risk patients with vein graft disease, again which often contain thrombus and degenerating atheroma. In the initial NACI registry, 240 lesions were attempted with TEC atherectomy.[15] In this experience, adjunctive PTCA was used in 88.8% of the lesions. The initial success rate with the device was 47.5% but after adjunctive dilatation, rose to 80.4%. It must be remembered that these lesions were probably at marked increased risk for complications; 63.8% involved vein graft disease, 41.1% had thrombus, and 17.8% were ulcerated. TEC is currently being evaluated in the treatment of acute myocardial infarction, although as yet the number of patients treated is low.

At the present time, TEC is a useful therapy for patients with diffuse vein graft disease often containing thrombus or lesions in large nonangulated coronary arterial segments with a large thrombus burden.[16] Again, as was true with directional coronary atherectomy, restenosis rates remain increased in these patients and are not improved relative to conventional PTCA.

Rotablator

Rotational atherectomy is now approved and widely used. The principle behind this device is differential ablation of fibrous or calcified plaque compared to the more normal arterial wall. In the presence of a significant amount of intracoronary thrombus or vein graft disease, this device should not be used. In patients with unstable angina and with fibrous or calcified lesions, it remains an excellent treatment option compared to PTCA. Initial experience with the ERBAC trial of patients who could have either laser, PTCA or rotational atherectomy, the latter was associated with significantly improved initial success rates; restenosis rates, however, were somewhat increased with rotational atherectomy.

Lasers

Three laser systems have been approved — two Excimer systems and one Holmium YAG system. The Excimer laser system has been used relatively widely. It consists of a 308 nM XeCL pulsed excimer laser which is magnetically switched with a pulse duration of $\geq$ 200 nsec. Its optimal role involved treatment of longer diffuse lesions which are only mildly calcified. Severe calcification is usually not well treated by these systems. Thrombus-containing lesions accounted for 7.8% and 9.2% of these lesions treated by Excimer laser coronary angioplasty in the initial NACI registry.[17] The device success rates in this experience were again only approximately 45% because of the small fiber size used, but with adjunctive dilatation, the final lesion success rate was approximately 85%. In the most recent AIS multicenter registry experience, thrombus was still associated with decreased success rates compared to other lesion subtypes.[18] In patients with longer diffuse disease with mild calcification or chronic total occlusion, it remains a very reasonable option irrespective of whether the patient has unstable angina or not.

The Holmium YAG laser system operates in the mid infrared spectrum with a wavelength of 2.10 _M. This is avidly absorbed by fresh thrombus. In a multicenter investigation, thrombotic lesions were successfully treated by this device.[19-21] It has been used in the setting of acute myocardial infarction with the laser being advanced to the point of thrombotic occlusion and then very slowly advanced until there was restoration of flow.[19] As with other laser systems, adjunctive PTCA is then required. Whether in the setting of acute myocardial infarction laser offers benefit over conventional PTCA is unknown. Given the excellent success rates with PTCA in this setting, trials comparing Holmium YAG laser to PTCA will require very large numbers of patients to document improved results.

Laser thrombolysis has also been studied.[22-24] The heterogeneous nature of arterial thrombus is related to variation in age, thrombus and composition. These may significantly affect optical properties. Oxyhemoglobin has strong absorption in the ultraviolet waveband from 400-600 nM. Light absorption increases significantly with lasers emitting between 1,000 and 3,000 nM. This data has formed the rationale for laser thrombolysis. Recently pulsed-dye lasers have been tested with pulsing at 1-2 μsec intervals. The catheter is a fluid-core light guide. Conventional radiographic contrast is an excellent optical transmission medium; it also allows for continuous visualization of the coronary vascular bed. During lasing, contrast is flushed down the lasing catheter. Based on preclinical studies which were favorable, a pilot study in patients with acute myocardial infarction who failed thrombolysis or who had a contraindication to thrombolysis has been initiated with favorable early results.[24]

Stents

Stents have been approved for treatment of acute closure and prevention of restenosis.[25-29] A number of other stents are being evaluated. No stent yet has a primary indication in unstable angina or acute ischemic syndromes. They are, however, be used in this setting.

There is an increasing amount of information on the use of stents for acute or threatened closure which has documented a reduction in need for emergency CABG and a decrease in frequency of development of Q-wave myocardial infarction. [25,26,29] Acute or threatened closure may be increased in the setting of dilatation for acute ischemic syndromes and the underlying complex lesions with associated thrombus. Stents in this setting may be associated with increased potential for subacute closure. Subacute stent thrombosis has been reported in 8-20% of series of bailout stenting. Factors associated with subacute closure includes inflow or outflow obstruction, residual untreated dissection, persistent thrombus, inadequate anticoagulation, poor stent expansion and stent diameter < 3.0 mm. The importance of these risk factors was assessed in the Cook stent multicenter registry of patients enrolled from August 1991 to March 1993.[30] Three specific risk factors for stent thrombosis were assessed: 1) stent diameter < 3.0 mm; 2) residual filling defects; and 3) residual dissection. In a group of 1,183 patients, if none of these risk factors were present, the incidence of thrombosis was 5%; if one was present, the incidence increased to 10% and if two or three were present, the incidence of subacute thrombosis was 26% (p = 0.00001).

Stents can be used to treat acute or subacute closure in patients with acute ischemic syndromes and thrombus. If thrombus is seen angiographically, consideration should be given to local delivery of thrombolytic therapy such as urokinase. This can be achieved using one of several types of side hole infusion catheters. These are much better than end hole perfusion catheters because they can be used to bathe the entire stented length of artery. The catheters are positioned using a guidewire across the stented segment. Urokinase, 250,000 to 500,000 units, can be delivered while the patient is in the laboratory over 30-45 minutes. At the end of this time, if thrombus is no longer present and flow is excellent (TIMI-3), the infusion may be terminated. If residual thrombus remains, the patient can be returned to the CCU with a constant infusion of urokinase down the infusion catheter at 50,000 U/hr for several more hours. If this latter option is used, there are several approaches: 1) the guiding catheter can be withdrawn to the descending thoracic aorta and then flushed intermittently with heparin; or 2) the guide catheter can remain in the ostium of the vein graft or the coronary artery. In this latter case, care must be taken to avoid catheter damping. While the guide catheter is in place, it is usually infused with urokinase, also with 50,000 U/hr. At the end of urokinase infusion, angiography is repeated to document arterial patency. Antiplatelet agents should also be given during this time. Following stent implantation in the setting of acute ischemic syndromes, anticoagulation must be maintained with heparin, aspirin, dipyridamole and coumadin.

Recently, ticlopidine has been used in patients undergoing stent implantation. In a series of 238 patients with placement of stents in 244 arterial segments, ticlopidine was administered beginning three days prior to the procedure.[31] During the procedure, intravenous heparin was started and maintained for 20 hours. Following implantation, patients were kept on subcutaneous heparin for one week and ticlopidine for three to six months. Only nine patients on this regimen (3.8%) had subsequent thrombosis by seven days. The use of this regimen obviates the need for long-term anticoagulation and may broaden the utility of this approach.

There is also interest in a variety of coatings on metallic stents to prevent both acute or subacute closure and restenosis. BENESTENT II, a randomized European trial of stenting for native coronary arterial lesions, is evaluating a heparin coated stent.

New devices

Given that the pathophysiology of acute ischemic syndromes is coronary arterial thrombus, there has been an interest in developing devices for thrombus removal. Thrombus removal would have the advantage of treating the obstructing lesion; in addition, it could facilitate gaining more information about the pathophysiology of syndromes. In the case of failed thrombolytic therapy, the thrombus may be mainly platelet and not red cell. Knowledge of these details may facilitate development of new approaches.

Thrombectomy *(Figure 30.1)* has been reported.[32] With this technique, a 5 French catheter is inserted through a conventional 8 French guiding catheter. This 5 French catheter is advanced to the occluded coronary segment. With continued suction, the thrombus can be removed. If the occlusion is proximal or even ostial, the guiding catheter itself may be used to aspirate the thrombus. This technique was attempted in eight patients, seven of whom had an acute or recent infarction. The eighth had chronic angina two months following myocardial infarction with a persistent coronary occlusion. Aspiration thrombectomy removed thrombus and by itself restored flow in four of eight patients. In a single patient with an acute occlusion, reperfusion following thrombectomy alone improved the ongoing ischemia although a critical subtotal stenosis remained. Following attempted thrombectomy, successful PTCA was carried out in seven of eight patients. This technique, while not widely employed, can be helpful in selected patients. In addition, it allows analysis of the material removed which can facilitate clinical investigation into the mechanism of persistent coronary occlusion.

A second approach is the continued development of devices capable of local drug delivery. At the present time, two devices are currently available; several others are in varying stages of development.

The Dispatch™ catheter *(Figure 30.2)* is a perfusion balloon which can be used for local delivery. This unique device has three lumens, one for infusion of drug, one which allows for blood perfusion, and one for "balloon" inflation. The balloon is a helical coil and sealing membrane which is inflated against the vessel wall. Because of the design, this balloon cannot be used for dilatation alone as it has only about 2 atm dilating force when the coils are inflated to 6 atm. Flow rates of 50-70% of normal flow can be maintained during drug infusion. Local thrombolytic therapy has been most widely used and may be effective in treating coronary arterial thrombus. Because this flow allows for maintenance of substantial flow, it can be left inflated for a long duration, optimizing the amount of drug delivered. Substantial investigation will be required to identify the optimal delivery pressure and flow rates.

Another approach currently available involves the use of hydrogel-coated balloons.[33,34] A variety of agents can be absorbed into the hydrogel. During inflation of the balloon, the polymer comes in contact with the arterial surface. Compression of the hydrogel drives the agent into the vessel wall with hydrostatic pressure. Intra-

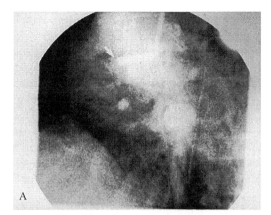

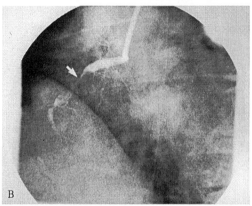

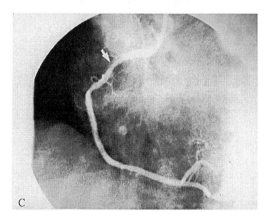

Figure 30.1 A: Left anterior oblique projection of the right coronary artery documenting a proximal occlusion. B: Thrombectomy and removal of thrombus restores patency. C: PTCA after thrombectomy leads in excellent result[32].

mural delivery of drug has been documented for heparin and horseradish peroxidase as a marker. Urokinase has also been tested; in vitro and in vivo pharmacokinetics documented transfer of urokinase from the balloons to the arterial wall and a reduction in platelet deposition at the site of deposition. In a pilot series of 15 patients[35], local site delivery of urokinase using this balloon resulted in improved coronary flow or improvement in the angiographic appearance with less thrombus in all patients. A system such as this has several potential advantages including the fact that lower total drug dose can be used while higher local site concentrations can be achieved. In addition, the mechanical effect of balloon dilatation may expose more thrombus surface to the urokinase. There are at least some disadvantages, however; the total drug delivered is limited, the delivery may be nonuniform unless the balloon is completely apposed to the vessel wall, and no perfusion capacity exists so that the duration of inflation may be relatively short. Finally, the duration of action is also probably quite short. Irrespective of these deficiencies, the system is currently available and can be successfully used to treat refractory thrombus formation.

Other catheter designs are being tested. One is a rheolytic thrombectomy catheter which uses high-velocity jets of saline solution to lyse and remove thrombus [36]. The saline solution is delivered in a jet from an exhaust port at the end of the catheter. This jet of saline at 10,000-15,0000 psi entrains the clot and fragments, and drives them into the high velocity region for dissolution and removal by a Bernoulli effect *(Figure 30.3)*. This catheter has been tested in vitro and in in vivo animal models with promising initial results. Another approach involves a Venturi catheter driven by a power injector.

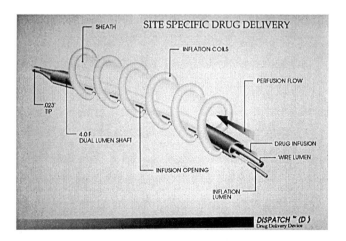

Figure 30.2 Schematic diagram of the Dispatch[TM] catheter. This is a triple lumen catheter; with ballon inflation, the central lumen allows blood perfusion. The membrane and the infusion openings allow local drug delivery, e.g. urokinase. With permission from Sci Med Life Systems, Im., Maple Crore, Minnesota.

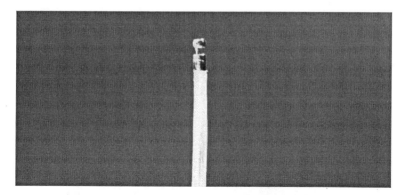

Figure 30.3 Diagram of the rheolytic thrombectomy catheter which uses streamliness of saline to disolve and remove thrombus. With permission from Possis Medical, Mineapolis, Minessota.

Other catheters rely on ultrasound for clot disruption.[37-39] Several different designs are being tested. This approach has been found to be very effective in ablating clots in vitro and in vivo. One ultrasound ablation system has been tested in patients.[39] It consists of a 115 V electrical generator, a piezoelectric transducer and a probe. This sytem, which operates at a frequency of 19.5 KHz, has been found to be relatively atraumatic to the normal arterial wall; it rapidly disrupts at least peripheral arterial thromboses, increases arterial distensibility of calcified lesions, and causes arterial vasodilatation. It has been tested in an initial series of 50 peripheral arterial lesions in 45 patients. In this series, 86% of occluded segments were recanalized. The mean reduction in stenosis after ultrasound ablation was 39%. Prototype ultrasound probes have also been used in the coronary arteries.[40] In this series, patients were treated for a mean of 493 seconds with ultrasonic ablation with resultant improvement in 17 of 19 lesions treated. The role that these catheters will play will depend upon their ability to be delivered into the coronary vascular bed with minimal trauma to the vessel wall. Their role will also depend upon the continued development of improved antiplatelet and antithrombotic strategies which will determine the magnitude of the resistant coronary thrombus problem. At present, these devices could be used in the setting of failed thrombolysis for acute myocardial infarction, a large amount of thrombus in a native coronary artery which would make dilatation problematic, or perhaps most importantly, in degenerating vein grafts with a large thrombus burden. The question is whether these devices offer significant improvement over PTCA alone.

Other catheter designs are being tested. An iontophoretic catheter capable of delivering charged molecules using a low current has been developed.[41,42] In a carotid arterial model, Hirudin could be delivered over a high concentration gradient. This approach also does not currently permit dilatation but can deliver a large amount of drug locally *(Figure 30.4)*.

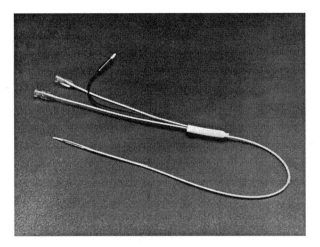

Figure 30.4 Iontophoretic catheter which can be used for local delivery of ions with the support of low voltage. With permission from Cortrak, Mineapolis, Minnesota.

In addition to mechanical devices, conventional adjunctive medications have been used to optimize results. The TAUSA trial (Thrombolysis and Angioplasty in Unstable Angina) assessed the role of intracoronary urokinase during angioplasty for unstable angina. Four hundred sixty-nine patients were studied in two phases using two dosing regimens. All patients received aspirin and heparin. Contrary to what may have been predicted, acute closure was increased in patients treated with urokinase versus placebo (10.2% vs 4.3%, p < .02). The adverse in hospital clinical endpoints of ischemia, infarction or emergency CABG were also increased with urokinase (12.9% vs 6.3%, p < .02) [43]. The mechanism for this adverse effect is unclear but may be related to intramural hemorrhage in the arterial segment dilated, failure of thrombolytic therapy to affect the platelet rich thrombi often seen in unstable angina, or a procoagulant effect. Any of these mechanisms are possible but may be operative to a different extent in individual patients.

In addition to conventional medications and mechanical devices, several new groups of medications will be widely used for treating patients with acute ischemic syndromes. Recently, a randomized trial of a platelet glycoprotein IIb/IIIa receptor blocker has been reported [44,45]. Two thousand ninety-nine patients undergoing high risk angioplasty or directional coronary atherectomy were randomly assigned treatment. Patients were defined as high risk by the following criteria: 1) acute evolving myocardial infarction within 12 hours of onset of symptoms; 2) early postinfarction angina or unstable angina; or 3) high risk lesions. The primary endpoint was a composite of death, nonfatal infarction, unplanned surgical revascularization or repeat percutaneous procedure, unplanned implantation of a coronary stent or refractory ischemia requiring intraaortic balloon pump. In the 696 patients in the placebo limb who were treated with aspirin and heparin, 12.8% of patients had one or more of the outcomes in the primary endpoint compared to only 8.3% of 708 patients treated with bolus and infusion of the drug. There was no difference in mortality but the incidence of nonfatal infarction and repeat PTCA was markedly decreased in the patients receiving the IIb/IIIa receptor blocker. As might have been predicted, the incidence of bleeding was substantially higher. Major bleeding was seen in 7% of the placebo group compared to 14% of the patients treated with bolus and infusion.

Antithrombins and other novel anticoagulant regimens are being evaluated [46-49]. Hirudin has been tested and found to be associated with improved clinical outcome in patients with acute infarction. In TIMI-5, 246 patients with ST segment elevation acute myocardial infarction were treated with either rtPA plus heparin or rtPA plus hirudin. Patients treated with hirudin showed a trend toward improved outcome [48]. This is being tested in the larger TIMI-9 and GUSTO IIb trials. Hirudin is also being studied in dilatation patients in the Helvetica trial from Europe. Other antithrombins include Hirulog, Hirugen and Argatroban.

Although these new therapeutic agents will be useful adjuncts, bleeding will be a significant consideration, particularly vascular access bleeding. Cerebrovascular accident is also of concern. In an initial run-in phase of GUSTO 2 and TIMI-9, there was an excess of mortality from hemorrhagic stroke [50,51]. This required downward titration of both heparin and the Hirudin. More widespread use of effective vascular sealants should make the use of these newer agents safer.

Summary

Treatment of acute ischemic syndromes accounts for a large part of the modern practice of cardiology. The central role of an unstable plaque and coronary arterial thrombus has been increasingly recognized. Treatment of these syndromes requires consideration of this pathophysiology. The continued development of improved devices will allow safer, more effective procedures, particularly when combined with newer, more specific drugs. In contrast to the past experience where the clinical course of these patients was characterized by recurrent ischemia, this will likely be changed to a scenario where recurrent ischemia is less but access site bleeding is greater. Local drug and development of vascular access closure devices will further improve the outcome in these patients.

REFERENCES

1. Gruentzig AR, Senning A, Sieganthaler WE. Nonoperative dilatation of coronary artery stenosis: Percutaneous transluminal coronary angioplasty. N Engl J Med 1979:301:61.

2. Holmes DR, Vlietstra RE. Balloon angioplasty in acute and chronic coronary artery disease. JAMA 1989:261:2109.

3. Detre K, et al. Percutaneous transluminal coronary'angioplasty in 1985-1986 and 1977-1981. N Engl J Med 1988:318:267.

4. Landau C, Lange RA, Hillis LD. Medical Progress: Percutaneous transluminal coronary angioplasty. N Engl J Med 1994:330:981.

5. Detre K, et al. One year follow-up results of the 1985-86 National Heart, Lung, and Blood Institute's Percutaneous Transluminal Coronary Angioplasty Registry. Circulation 1989:80:421.

6. Berger PB, et al. Initial results and long-term outcome of coronary angioplasty in chronic mild angina pectoris. Am J Cardiol 1993:71:1396.

7. Fuster V, et al. The pathogenesis of coronary artery disease and the acute coronary syndromes (Part 1). N Engl J Med 1992:326:242.

8. Fuster V, et al. The pathogenesis of coronary artery disease and the acute coronary syndromes (Part 2). N Engl J Med 1992:326:310.

9. Mabin TA, et al. Intracoronary thrombus: Role in coronary occlusion complicating percutaneous transluminal coronary angioplasty. J Am Coll Cardiol 1985:5:198.

10. Sugrue D, et al. Coronary thrombus as a risk factor for acute vessel occlusion during percutaneous transluminal coronary angioplasty: Improving results. Br Heart J 1986:56:62.

11. Vaitkus P, Herrmann H, Laskey W. Management and immediate outcome of patients with intracoronary thrombus during PTCA. Am Heart J 1992:124:1.

12. Reeder GS, et al. Intracoronary thrombus: Still a risk factor for PTCA failure. Cathet Cardiovasc Diagn in press.

13. Topol EJ, et al. CAVEAT Study Group: A comparison of directional atherectomy with coronary angioplasty in patients with coronary artery disease. N Engl J Med 1993:329:221.

14. Holmes DR Jr, et al. A multicenter, randomized trial of coronary angioplasty versus directional atherectomy for patients with saphenous vein bypass graft lesions. Circulation in press.

15. Baim DS, et al. Evaluating new devices: Acute (in hospital) results from the New Approaches to Coronary Intervention Registry. Circulation 1994:89:471.

16. Safian RD, et al. Clinical and angiographic results of transluminal extraction coronary atherectomy in saphenous vein bypass grafts. Circulation 1994:89:302.

17. Vandormael M, et al. Comparison of excimer lasers, rotational atherectomy and balloon angioplasty for complex disease: The ERBAC study. J Am Coll Cardiol 1994:23. (Special Iss):484A.

18. Holmes DR Jr, Klein LW, Litvack F. Lesion morphology and acute outcome after excimer laser angioplasty: A prospective evaluation. Circulation: in press.

19. Topaz O, et al. Laser facilitated angioplasty and thrombolysis for acute myocardial infarction complicated by prolonged or recurrent chest pain. Cathet Cardiovasc Diagn 1993:28:7.

20. Knopf WD, et al. Multicenter registry report: Holmium laser angioplasty in coronary arteries. Circulation 1992:86(Suppl I):I-511

21. Estella P, et al. Intracoronary thrombus increases the risk of excimer laser coronary angioplasty. Circulation 1992:86(Suppl I):I-654.

22. Gregory KW: Laser thrombolysis. In, *Textbook of Interventional Cardiology*. Topol EJ (ed), Saunders, 1994:982.

23. Gregory KW, et al. Coronary artery laser thrombolysis in acute canine myocardial infarction. Circulation 1989:80:523.

24. Gregory KW, et al. Laser thrombolysis in acute myocardial infarction. J Am Coll Cardiol 1993:21(Suppl A):2898A.

25. Roubin GS, et al. Intracoronary stenting for acute and threatened closure complicating percutaneous transluminal coronary angioplasty. Circulation 1992:85:916.

26. George BS, et al. Multicenter investigation of coronary stenting to treat acute or threatened closure after PTCA: Clinical and angiographic outcomes. J Am Coll Cardiol 1993:22:135.

27. Schatz RA, et al. Clinical experience with the Palmaz-Schatz coronary stent. J Am Coll Cardiol 1991:17(Suppl B):155B.

28. Colombo A, et al. Coronary stenting: Single institutional experience with the initial 100 cases using the Palmaz-Schatz stent. Cathet Cardiovasc Diagn 1992:26:171.

29. Hearn JA, et al. Clinical and angiographic outcomes after coronary stenting for acute or threatened closure after PTCA: Initial results with a balloon expandable stainless steel design. Circulation 1993:88:2086.

30. Liu MW, et al. Risk stratification of stent thrombosis following intracoronary stenting for acute or threatened closure. A Cook stent multicenter registry study. Circulation 1993:88(Suppl A):I-122.

31. Barragan P, Sainsous J, Silvestri M. Ticlopidine and subcutaneous heparin as an alternative regimen following coronary stenting. Cathet Cardiovasc Diagn 1994:32:133.

32. Reeder GS, Lapeyre AC, Edwards WD, Holmes DR. Aspiration thrombectomy for removal of coronary thrombus. Am J Cardiol 1992:70:107.

33. Fram DB, et al. Localized intramural drug delivery during balloon angioplasty using hydrogel-coated balloons and pressure-augmented diffusion. J Am Coll Cardiol 1994:23:1570.

34. Nunes GL, et al. Local delivery of a synthetic antithrombin with a hydrogel-coated angioplasty balloon catheter inhibits platelet-dependent thrombosis. J Am Coll Cardiol 1994:23:1578.

35. Mitchel JF, et al. Inhibition of platelet deposition and lysis of intracoronary thrombus during balloon angioplasty using urokinase-coated hydrogel balloons. J Am Cardiol in press.

36. Drasler WJ, et al. Rheolytic catheter for percutaneous removal of thrombus. Radiology 1992:182:263.

37. Rosenschein U, et al. Ultrasonic angioplasty in totally occluded peripheral arteries. Circulation 1991:83:1976.

38. Steffen W, Siegel RJ. Ultrasound angioplasty: A review. J Interventional Cardiol 1993:6:77.

39. Siegel RJ, et al. Clinical trial of percutaneous peripheral ultrasound angioplasty. J Am Coll Cardiol 1993:22:480.

40. Siegel RJ, et al. Use of therapeutic ultrasound in PTCA. Experimental in vitro studies and initial clinical experience. Circulation 1994:89:1587.

41. Soria I, Hassinger NL, Owen WJ. Local delivery of hirudin into rabbit carotid arteries with an ionotophoretic catheter. Circulation 1993:88:3552A.

42. Fernandez-Ortiz A, et al. A new approach for local intravascular drug delivery: ionotophoretic balloon. Circulation 1994:89:1518.

43. Ambrose JA, et al. Adjunctive thrombolytic therapy during angioplasty for ischemic rest angina. Results of the TAUSA trial. Circulation 1994:90:69.

44. EPIC Investigators. Use of a monoclonal antibody directed against the platelet glycoprotein receptor in high risk coronary angioplasty. N Engl J Med 1994:330:956.

45. Topol EJ, et al. Randomized trial of coronary intervention with antibody against platelet IIb/IIIa integrin for reduction of clinical restenosis. Results at six months. Lancet 1994:343:881.

46. Topol EJ, et al. Use of a direct antithrombin, Hirulog™, in place of heparin during coronary angioplasty. Circulation 1993:87:1622.

47. Lefkovitz J, Topol EJ. Direct thrombin inhibitors in cardiovascular medicine. Circulation in press.

48. Cannon CP, et al. A pilot trial of recombinant desulfatohirudin compared to heparin in conjunction with tissue plasminogen activator and aspirin for acute myocardial infarction. Results of the Thrombolysis in Myocardial Infarction (TIMI) 5 trial. J Am Coll Cardiol 1994:23:993.

49. Topol EJ, et al. Recombinant hirudin for unstable angina pectoris. A multicenter randomized angiographic trial. Circulation 1994:89:1557.

50. Antman EM for the TIMI 9A Investigators. Hirudin in acute myocardial infarction: A safety report from the Thrombolysis and Thrombin Inhibition in Myocardial Infarction (TIMI 9) trial. Circulation in press.

51. Topol EJ for the GUSTO Investigators. A randomized trial of intravenous heparin versus recombinant hirudin for acute coronary syndromes. Circulation in press.

31 INTRACORONARY ULTRASOUND

George Dangas, Paul G. Yock

Selective coronary angiography has been the "gold standard" for the diagnosis and evaluation of coronary artery disease (CAD) since the late 1950's. While angiography provides a detailed map of the spatial distribution of the coronary arterial tree, it has several inherent limitations. Angiographic errors mainly arise from viewing a three-dimensional, often tortuous and/or branching vessel in a planar two-dimensional picture and from the frequent overlap of arterial silhouettes *(Figure 31.1)*. Furthermore, all anatomic information obtained angiographically is limited solely to the coronary lumen and does not describe the pathology of the vessel wall itself. In addition to these theoretical and technical limitations of angiography, a series of studies have provided positive clinical outcomes not accompanied by similar angiographic results, thus leading to a significant debate on whether angiography alone is the most appropriate means of anatomic assessment of coronary syndromes.[1]

In the late 1980's intracoronary ultrasound (ICUS) was introduced as a unique procedure for direct visualization of the coronary vasculature, for tissue characterization of the arterial lesions and for *in vivo* assessment of the pathology of the vessel wall itself.[2] The ICUS catheter contains a high frequency (20-30 MHz) miniaturized ultrasound transducer (<1mm) with an axial resolution of approximately 150 mm. Visualization of each coronary plaque individually and of the whole arterial wall in serial cross-sections can be achieved.[3]

The specific goals for this diagnostic device are multiple. ICUS is unique in visualizing in vivo the vessel wall, providing novel insights in describing plaque composition, arterial remodeling, elastic recoil, restenosis and post-transplant vasculopathy. On that basis, ICUS is the state-of-the-art technique for vascular imaging and assessment of the vessel wall and the atherosclerotic process.[4,5] From a clinical point of view, ICUS may potentially be valuable in pre-intervention device selection

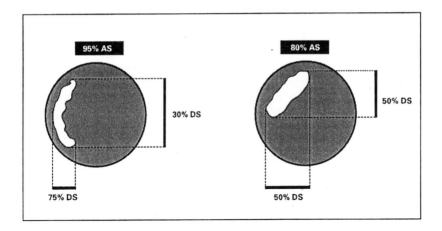

Figure 31.1 Representation of the disadvantage of angiography in accurately assessing lesion severity in casees of eccentric lesions. AS=area stenosis by intravascular ultra-sound, DS=angiographic diameter stennosis.
(Artwork by Ximena Tamvakopoulou, BA).

and for post-intervention assessment of the need for further transcatheter or phar-macologic (e.g. anticoagulation) therapy. Although ICUS appears to have emerged as the "state-of-the-art" technique for intracoronary imaging, the current debate about its clinical utility is underlined by the fact that ICUS cost has just beguun to be reimbursed by the insurance companies.

Tissue characterization

ICUS provides multiple serial cross-sections of the vessel wall. The high frequency of the ultrasound signal allows examination of small structures (<0.2mm) up to a depth of approximately 5mm (image diameter 1cm).[6] The brightness of the reflec-tion is dependent on the angle of the beam to the reflector and the relative stiffness of the neighboring tissue. The overall amount of the imaged substance and the reflectivity of certain molecules such as collagen determine the ultrasonic image within a given location in the vessel wall.[3,4]

Adventitia (the outermost vessel wall layer) is the most echogenic of the nor-mal layers, as it contains large amount of collagen and fibrous tissue. The media is clearly imaged in muscular type arteries (including the coronaries) as a more echolu-cent (gray) ring-layer and the innermost intima-plaque complex is a relatively bright layer. In elastic type arteries (e.g. aorta, carotids) the media is more difficult to distinguish clearly.[7] This distinct three-layered ICUS appearance of the vessel wall is not uniformly present in young adults[8] and depends on the collagen content of the media, the integrity of the internal elastic membrane (IEM) and the intimal thickness[9], frequently accompanied by thinning of the media.[3] This may result in a two-layered rather than a three-layered appearance (the madia is indistinct).

The reliability of ICUS tissue characterization has been validated with comparison to *in vitro* histology in both the presence and absence of atherosclerosis [10,11]. However, even in the era of ICUS imaging, the initial phases of atherosclerosis associated with endothelial dysfunction still precede any detectable anatomic abnormality.[12]

Calcification

Atherosclerotic calcification begins as early as the second decade of life, just following the fatty streaks.[13] However, calcium deposits are greater and more prevalent in elderly patients.[14] The amount of calcium increases with the age of the atherosclerotic plaque, but it is not associated with the degree of angiographic stenosis. Several reports have linked coronary lesion calcification and its potential for plaque rupture. Early stages of calcification have been associated with increased plaque vulnerability, whereas extensive calcium deposits may render the lesion resistant to rupture.[19]

Calcium within the vessel wall may be deep, superficial or both. Fluoroscopy is the usual method for detection of coronary calcification, but it does not accurately localize or quantify the amount of calcium. Since calcium is a powerful reflector of ultrasound, it can be reliably visualized by ICUS. An area of calcification is usually depicted by ICUS as a hyperechoic border with shadowing beyond (obscuring any tissue structures deep to the intimal interface). Often there is also a set of one or more rings or reverberations spaced at regular intervals from the leading border.

ICUS identification of calcium has been validated *in vitro*.[7] The sensitivity of ICUS for detection of dense calcification has been reported as 90% and its specificity as 100% when compared to the "gold standard" pathologic data. However, ICUS was only 64% sensitive, but still highly specific, for overall calcium detection, including small accumulations or scattered microcalcifications (<0.05mm).[16]

ICUS can assess the arc, length, and distribution patterns of coronary artery calcification. Mintz et al. evaluated the pattern of calcium (e.g. amount, location and distribution) in 1155 native coronary lesions.[17] ICUS detected lesion calcium in 73% of lesions (almost as accurate as pathologic samples), which was situated superficially in 48%, deeply in 28% and in both regions in 24%. Angiographic detection of calcium was significantly lower and depended on the configuration, distribution and amount of target lesion and reference segment calcium. The phase I of the GUIDE trial showed similar results.[4] It is generally thought that the clcification has to extend in at least two 90° arcs in the ICUS image in order to be detected fluoroscopically.

The major limitation to the ultrasound assessment of target lesion calcium is the inability of ICUS to identify the thickness of a calcific deposit. Related to this issue is the difficulty for quantification of the calcium content by ICUS. The arc length of calcification is commonly used as an index of the amount of calcium, with the obvious dependence on the distance from the transducer. Longitudinal measurement of calcification with the motorized pullback technique adds some degree of accuracy, but is also limited by the arterial tortuosity, the catheter-calcification angle and the beam thickness.[22]

Fibrotic plaque

Fibrotic plaques constitute the majority of atherosclerotic lesions and contain fibrous tissue, collagen, elastin, proteoglycans and debris. Many of these plaques have calcific elements with characteristic shadowing of the deeper structures. The structured pattern of macromolecules (e.g. collagen) in this tissue does not allow as much "scatter" of the ultrasound beam as in soft plaque. Therefore, the appearance of the tissue is more highly dependent on the relative position of the transducer. The strength of the reflection is sufficient, but there may be "attenuation" of the beam as it penetrates into deeper regions of a fibrous plaque, resulting in a drop-out (darkening) of the image in this area. Thus, deeply situated fibrotic tissue may not be appropriately depicted unless compared with other identified elements in the same depth and intervening tissue using the same gain settings.[3,4]

Lipid-rich plaque

Lipid components of the atherosclerotic plaque are poorly reflected by ultrasound and produce a "non-directive" pattern of backscatter energy, unlike calcium. Therefore, lipid-containing (soft, fibrofatty) plaques are typically echolucent (relatively dark). In *in vitro* study, the sensitivity of 40MHz ICUS in diagnosing lipid-rich plaques was 89% and the specificity was 100%.[19] *In vivo* however, it is much more difficult to identify lipid laden plaque with any reliability. Lipid-rich plaques are more prone to rupture, leading to an acute coronary syndrome and ICUS has confirmed their prevalence in these clinical settings. In a study of unstable angina patients, ICUS found 74% soft plaques and 25% calcific or mixed plaques compared to 41% and 59% respectively in stable angina patients.[20]

Thrombus

Intracoronary thrombosis is the final common pathophysiologic mechanism of the large majority of acute coronary syndromes. Angiographically, thrombus is described as an intraluminal filling defect or a complex lesion and angioscopy is considered the gold standard for evaluating thrombus.[21] Thrombus is generally an intraluminal structure that needs to be distinguished from flowing blood, but it may also become an organized, deeply situated intramural plaque component.

Blood itself is visualized by ICUS as a speckled, low intensity and continuously changing pattern, as the red blood cells can scatter but not directly reflect the sound-beams. Conversely, thrombus appears somewhat brighter than blood and its brightness is related to red blood cells rather than platelets. Thrombus is still very difficult to image reliably with ICUS and in high quality images it may have a characterisitic scintillating or sparkling appearance. In certain cases the geometric configuration of thrombus rather its tissus characteristics may be the clue for the correct ICUS diagnosis. Currently, there is active research in the identification of thrombus involving development of advanced computer software to distinguish subtle differences of videodensitometric data or patterns of the raw radiofrequency signals.[3,4,18]

Imaging of other luminal morphology

Imaging of arterial dissections is an important feature of ICUS, especially in the context of a transcatheter interventions.[3,22] ICUS provides a more complete evaluation of the severity and pattern of the dissection than is available from angiography. ICUS evaluation of dissection includes:

1) accurate estimate of the compromise of the arterial lumen

2) the depth of the dissection (superficial or deep walled)

3) the relation with calcification

4) the position of the catheter with respect to the true or false lumen

ICUS imaging immediately after recanalization of a total occlusion can be useful in identifying the position of the guide wire (true or false lumen).[23]

Quantitative coronary ultrasound (QCU)

Measurement of the vessel size is among the most frequently used and helpful pieces of information gained by ICUS. The ability to accurately resolve lumen and outer plaque borders with good image quality is the first step in accurate sizing of lesions. Measurements may be done on-line or off-line using computer planimetry. Frequently used measurements are (Figure 31.2):

1) Lumen cross-sectional area (LA) and diameter (Ld). Identification of the lumen contour is easily accomplished, especially when the lumen is large enough and the catheter is not encompassed by plaque. When the catheter is partially or completely occlusive, the ability to delineate the lumen is less accurate. Injection of radiographic contrast agent may help outline the lumen with the creation of micro-bubbles.

2) "Vessel" cross-sectional area (VA): area contained within the media-adventitia border (at the level of the internal elastic lamina).

3) Plaque plus media cross-sectional area (plaque burden, PB) is calculated as VA-LA. The ratio PB/VA is the percent plaque burden (%PB).

4) Eccentricity ratio (er). This is the ratio of maximal to minimal total wall thickness. An index of 1.0 indicates a purely concentric plaque distribution.

There are several technical reasons to believe the accuracy of ICUS measurements of the coronary lumen compared to QCA. First, the ICUS pictures provide a clear outline of the lumen, which may be obscure in an angiogram view, even in

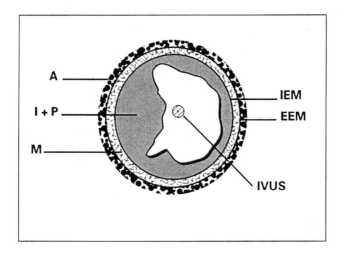

Figure 31.2 *Arterial cross-section as imaged with the intravascular ultrasound catheter (IVUS). Quantitative measuments of the external elastic membrane (EEM), the intima plus plaque area (I+P) and the lumen (L) can be obtained. IEM=internal elastic membrane, M=media.*
(Artwork by Ximena Tamvakopoulou, BA).

orthogonal views, due to overlap and/or forshortening of vessels. In addition, direct planimetry is more reliable than the mathematic area calculation based on the diameter stenosis. The major limitation in the accuracy of the ICUS measurements is non-coaxial positioning of the catheter, resulting in an eliptical distortion of the lumen due to the tilting of the beam plane in relation to a true cross-section.

Eccentric plaques and diffuse disease are the two configurations that highlight the superiority of QCU to quantitative coronary angiography (QCA). The QCU-QCA discrepancy in appropriately assessing lesion eccentricity was described in phase I of the GUIDE trial.[4] QCA and QCU measurements deviate significantly post-angioplasty, probably on the basis of plaque disruption and the development of multiple small channels that can be filled with dye during angiography.[24] However, the main reason for the discrepancy between QCU and QCA results post-intervention was shown to be the occurrence of deep dissection of the vessel wall involving the media.[25]

A motorized pullback system enables the operator to define the exact position of the catheter in reference to a fixed point e.g. the aorto-ostial junction, and to perform axial length measurements which have been validated *in vivo*.[26] The currently available system applies a constant velocity of 0.5 or 1.0 mm/sec (D=TxV; D=distance, T=pullback time and V=catheter velocity). The ability to obtain sequential cross-sections of the vessel wall in a standardized fashion is the first step for the IVUS-guided three-dimensional arterial reconstruction. This goal is already attempted with the support of advanced computer software[27,28] and initial results were presented recently.[29,30] The issue of systolic/diastolic motion artifact can be potentially resolved with EKG-gated pullback.[31]

Another aspect of CAD that has been clarified by ICUS is vessel wall tapering. In an ICUS study of 146 atherosclerotic lesions the phenomenon of lumen tapering was shown to be almost uniform and the cross-sectional narrowing was almost identical pre and post lesion. The latter implied that EEM tapering as well as differential axial plaque distribution may account for the distal tapering of the lumen.[32]

Geometric arterial remodeling

Glagov et al. first described the concept of adaptive enlargement of coronary arteries at the sites of CAD.[33] The proposed mechanism was the preservation of the arterial lumen despite the growth of the atherosclerotic plaque. From the available pathologic data this response of the vessel wall was found inadequate to counterbalance growth of a plaque occupying >40% of the area surrounded by the IEM. This results in the early stages of CAD being underestimated by angiography. In another report by the same group different sites of the coronary tree showed a varying response to plaque growth thereby implying the contribution of additional determinants of arterial remodeling.[34] In fact, intraluminal pressure, vascular injury and differential flow characteristics have been collectively implicated in vascular remodeling[35] and the remodeling process has been suggested to be of significant generalized biologic importance.[36] ICUS has recently provided us with a unique tool in assessing the concept of vascular remodeling at the site of *de novo* and restenotic atherosclerotic lesions as well as the reactivity of the whole vessel wall in physiologic, pathologic and pharmacologic stimuli.[37,38].

The left main coronary artery has been shown by ICUS to be diseased with atherosclerosis much more frequently than with angiography because of the significant degree of compensatory enlargement.[39] In an ICUS study of 80 lesions, the dimension of the EEM was proportional to the plaque area when the stenosis was <30%. Beyond this point the target lumen was decreased relatively to the reference segment in proportion to the plaque area.[40] Other studies have similar results with small differences in the cut-off point for the development of uncompensated lumen narrowing.[38] This model of adaptive vessel enlargement in response to atherosclerosis may apply even to saphenous vein bypass grafts.[41]

A recent pathologic and ICUS study of the femoral arteries systematically assessed the mechanisms of vessel wall response to atherosclerosis.[42] Again, three types of vessel wall remodeling were described: compensatory enlargement, paradoxical shrinkage and neutral response. Paradoxical vessel wall shrinkage occurred in the same arteries which were adaptively enlarged in other sections. The remodeling process was thus found to differ within the same artery and paradoxical shrinkage was shown to contribute significantly to the most severe stenoses.

ICUS has been used for the evaluation of arterial spasm and its relation to atherosclerosis. A diffuse atherosclerotic process was documented in arteries with diffuse spasm, whereas focal spasm was associated with sites of localized atherosclerosis, not necessarily obstructive.[43] In a similar context, another ICUS study evaluated coronary distensibility. This vessel property was found to be compromised in arteries with occult atherosclerosis and their response to vasodilators was diminished if the intima-media complex was thickened.[44] Similarly, the dilation of atherosclerotic arteries in response to nitroglycerin was shown to be primarily due to expansion of the nondiseased part of the vessel wall.[45] Additionally, ICUS has been used for the evaluation of the elastic arterial properties *in vivo* and their dependence on smooth muscle cell relaxation or contraction.[46]

Restenosis

The problem of restenosis following angioplasty remains a puzzling issue in interventional cardiology. Restenotic lesions differ from de novo lesions, but vascular remodeling affects both processes.[47] ICUS provides a tool to evaluate the reaction of the all layers of the vessel wall to angioplasty (PTCA) or other interventional therapy *(Figure 31.3)*. It allows study of the mechanism of lumen enlargement, including plaque redistribution and the development of ruptures and fissures of the plaque surface in response to injury. An optimal initial result is important for restenosis ("bigger is better")[48,49] and quantification of residual plaque burden after the procedure has been shown to correlate with restenosis.[50] The mechanism of very early (within days) lumen loss is currently attributed primarily to elastic recoil. Restenotic arteries have been reported to have significantly greater wall stretch during initial PTCA, suggesting that elastic recoil may be an important factor for restenosis.[51]

The contribution of arterial shrinkage vs. neointimal proliferation to the development of late lumen loss and restenosis is unclear. In one study, restenosis following PTCA was shown to be primarily related to vessel shrinkage, whereas there was relatively more neointimal tissue growth following directional atherectomy (DCA).[52] A sequential ICUS study after PTCA and DCA (SURE trial) was recently reported by a Japanese group.[53] ICUS was performed before and after the procedure, 24h, 1 month, and 6 months after the intervention. The preliminary results showed that the VA increased initially post-PTCA and up to 1 month, but there was a significant late decrease in VA which was associated with restenosis. Shrinkage contributed more to late loss than intimal proliferation, although both mechanisms were operative.

The GUIDE trial is systematically evaluating the problem of restenosis after PTCA and DCA using ICUS. As recently reported in the phase II of this trial, the ICUS determined percent plaque area (%PA) and minimal luminal diameter (MLD) were the most powerful predictors of restenosis; achievement of MLD >1.96mm was associated with decreased restenosis, and residual %PA >64% had a relative risk of 1.7 for late restenosis.[54] On the other hand, the initial results of the European trial PICTURE did not support the utility of ICUS in predicting restenosis.[55] The same issue is also addressed with the INSPIRE trial (post-PTCA).

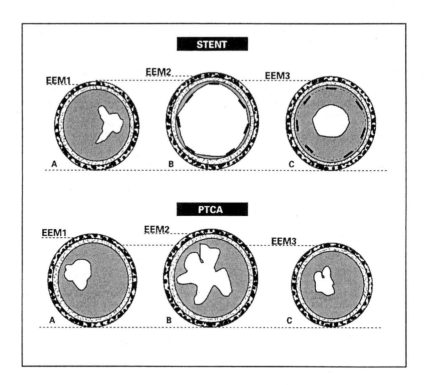

*Figure 31.3 Insights in the pathogenesis of restenosis after balloon angioplasty (PTCA)
and stent. The baseline external elastic membrane (EEM$_1$) expands after stent placement
(EEM$_2$) and does not retract at follow-up (EEM$_3$). After PTCA, the follow-up EEM$_3$
develops shrinkage compared to EEM$_2$. At the same time one may note the importance
of neointimal proliferation for in-stent restenosis. This type of in vivo assessment of the
vascular wall components has been made possible only with the intravascular ultrasound
catheter.*

(Artwork by Ximena Tamvakopoulou, BA).

ICUS in coronary interventions

Mechanisms of lumen gain

ICUS data have provided extensive information on the mechanisms of lumen gain
with the various devices. This information together with the tissue characterization
of the target lesion implicate a potential role for pre-intervention ICUS to optimize
device selection in order to optimize both the short and the long term outcome of
transcatheter therapy.

Arterial stretch is an important mechanism of lumen gain with balloon angioplasty, but there is variable arterial response to balloon injury. Fibrocalcific plaques
do not stretch as much and behave less favorably to PTCA resulting in more dissec-

tions than softer, non-calcific plaques.[22,56] Interestingly, the location of the calcific deposit was directly associated with the origin of the dissection, indicating the importance of locally increased shear stress (next to the non-compressible calcium) during balloon inflation for the development of a dissection. On the other hand, lesions without any plaque disruption have been associated with worse long term outcome, i.e. restenosis.[57] Evidently, the acute lumen gain should be optimal in these cases. The lumen gain from balloon angioplasty is more pronounced at the site of the maximal cross-sectional stenosis, but vascular injury may be more pronounced in the less stenotic areas.[58] A successful angiographic result may still be associated with dissection [25] or extensive vessel wall damage (identifiable with ICUS), which may comrpomise the long term outcome of the procedure. Further increase of the acute gain with ICUS guidance may be beneficial in such cases.[48]

Correlation between the mechanism of balloon dilatation and the preexisting type of arterial remodeling at the lesion site has been attempted.[59] Femoral arteries with paradoxical shrinkage at the lesion siteunderwent stretching with increase in the VA following angioplasty. In comparison, lumen gain in arteries without geometric shrinkage was mostly due to plaque displacement. In these cases, change in VA was positively associated with the magnitude of immediate recoil. The final MLD achieved were similar in both types of arteries.

The mechanism of lumen gain with DCA is a combination of plaque removal with a smaller degree of wall stretch compared to angioplasty. [60,61] The limitation of DCA in successfully extracting calficied plaques (arc>90°) has been elucidated by ICUS studies.[62,63] The final lumen dimensions, the amount of residual plaque, and the weight of tissue retrieved with DCA are related to the size of the arc and the location of the target lesion calcium as determined by ICUS. Additionally, there are potentially deleterious effects of the disruption of the architecture of the vessel wall due to overtly aggressive DCA.[64]

Rotational coronary atherectomy (RCA) utilizes a high speed burr to selectively target inelastic and calcified plaques. Lumen gain after RCA is due to plaque ablation including significant reduction of the arcs of calcium with the production of a smooth cylindrical surface.[65] Adjunctive balloon angioplasty creates vessel expansion without further decrease of the plaque area. Dissections are usually rare and, if present, have limited axial and circumferential extension. It is for these reasons that RCA is the device of choice in heavily calcified lesions particularly when the calcium is near the luminal surface.[66]

Balloon expandable intracoronary stents are currently used broadly.[67,68] They provide a mechanical force ("scaffolding") to keep the artery open. Stents have been shown superior to PTCA and DCA in producing more acute gain especially in concentric plaques.[69] Plaque eccentricity and calcification have been associated with less lumen gain by stenting. As demonstrated with ICUS, stents do not recoil and late restenosis of stented lesions is mostly due to neointimal tissue growth.[70-74] The restenotic process following stent placement appears to be accentuated in areas where the initial post-procedure plaque residual is higher[71] and incases treated with stents with small diameter.[74] Blood flow in any residual space between the stent and the vessel wall is a slow and thus prothrombotic. Optimal stent expansion, as demonstrated with ICUS, can eliminate such an interspace and leads significantly decreased rates of stent thrombosis (see below). At the same time, achievement of a greater lumen diameter with optimal stent expansion is thought to also decrease restenosis and current prospective studies are addressing this issue. Stent expansion can be achieved with the use of an oversized balloon and/or the inflation of a not-oversized balloon at high pressure. Both these techniques constitute a significant vessel wall injury with an unknown long-term impact. ICUS can direct the use of either one of these techniques according to specific information on the proximal and distal vessel diameter and the amount and site of vessel wall calcium.

Pre-intervention use of ICUS

Pre-intervention assessment of the lesion severity by ICUS may be useful in deciding whether treatment of the lesion is necessary. In fact, when Mintz et al. examined the impact of pre-intervention ICUS on changing the therapeutic strategies, the decision to intervene was solely based on ICUS assessment of lesion severity in 13% of the lesions studied. In these patients, MLD obtained by QCU correlated poorly with QCA (r=0.42). A change in the subsequent trancatheter therapy was made in 44% of the total cases; in 50% of angiographically borderline lesions, no intervention was performed. ICUS assessment of target lesion calcification, eccentricity and unusual morphology were the reasons for changing or selecting specific devices.[75]

Although lesions targeted with percutaneous interventions are generally focal, ICUS has showed diffuse atherosclerosis even in "normal" reference segments. This may affect appropriate device sizing. However, there are no definitive prospective data to document a need for device sizing by ICUS. In the CLOUT trial[76] IVUS was used for selective device upsizing based on the VA of the reference segment after an initial "optimal" PTCA. The strategy was safe and yielded a 30% increase in acute lumen gain (attempting to achieve "stent-like" result using ICUS-guided PTCA).

ICUS has a high sensitivity in identifying vessel wall calcification and might have significant input in identifying calcific lesions that would respond unfavorably to PTCA or DCA, but would be optimally treated with RCA. Furthermore, ICUS use may allow the option of a stepwise interventional approach: calcified lesions may be initially treated with RCA and subsequently with DCA or with stenting.

ICUS quantitative measurements add information regarding the target lesion, the reference vessel and lumen tapering. Therapeutic decisions are often related to accurate assessment of lumen dimensions, stenosis severity, and/or the diameter of the "normal" reference segment pre-intervention. The ability to measure lesion length is useful in choosing the balloon length as well as determining the length and number of stents needed to treat the target lesion.[26] Axial lengths also aid in determining the exact location of landmarks like side branches and calcium and their distance to the target lesion. This feature may aid in a more accurate placement of intracoronary stents. In addition, together with the knowledge of the lesion morphology by ICUS, a stepwise strategy of combined transcatheter therapy may be chosen for the patient according to the ICUS findings. The whole issue of the significance of pre-intervention ICUS on device selection and the improvement of the acute and chronic procedural outcome is yet to be prospectively assessed in a randomized trial.

Use of ICUS during intervention

After the determination of the interventional treatment strategy, ICUS can be used to assess the response of the vessel to the treatment in case of complications and to evaluate the need to upsize or change a device. It can provide, for instance, information on the orientation of the DCA cutter in view of the eccentricity of most lesions.

The most common interventional complications are: abrupt vessel closure, dissection, distal embolization, slow-flow/ no-reflow, vasospasm in the treated vessel. ICUS can assist the identification of most of them. Dissections have a characteristic appearance and massive thrombus can be visualized as a substantial increase in plaque mass without a flap and occasionally with a disctinctly abnormal geometric configuration. In case of diffuse arterial spasm ICUS may show a reduction of the caliber of the whole vessel (not only lumen reduction).[3]

Clinical utility of ICUS post-intervention

Optimal lumen gain is the current target of every interventional procedure.[48,49] Angiography is a gross way to identify the procedural outcome. In fact, the higher discrepancy between QCU and QCA has been demonstrated in lumen measurements following an intervention, primarily due to undiagnosed dissections.[24] Therefore, the ICUS guided optimization of the procedural results has gained substantial indirect support. However, it is unknown whether the additional anatomic information provided by ICUS during and after the procedure actually correlates with improved acute and long-term outcome. Therefore, the utility of ICUS post-intervention has been a subject of several current trials.

The optimization of the interventional result with the achievement of maximal luminal gain led to low post-DCA restenosis rate in the OARS trial[77] and the ICUS-guided technique was shown to be safe despite the aggressive plaque excision (post-DCA diameter stenosis 7%). Several reports have also demonstrated the existence of significant residual plaque and/or dissections after PTCA, which were diagnosed by ICUS despite an optimal angiographic result. However, no prospective randomized trial has addressed the issue of the absolute utility of ICUS guidance during intervention.

The utility of ICUS-guided stent implantation has become a widely debated issue. Stent implantation in the large BENESTENT[67] and STRESS[68] trials was followed by prolonged systemic anticoagulation to avoid stent thrombosis. This strategy led to prolonged patient hospitalization, increased bleeding complications and still did not eliminate stent thrombosis. Recently Colombo et al showed that intra-coronary stenting can be performed without subsequent use of coumadin, when deployment is optimized by ICUS guidance.[78] Multiple studies have demonstrated a number of issues related to the conventional stent deployment techniques:[79,80] suboptimal apposition to the vessel wall, under-expansion, asymmetric expansion, unrecognized adjacent lesions, or detection of edge dissections.

The advantage of ICUS-guided stent implantation has been attributed to the diagnosis of these technically suboptimal results. On the other hand, several studies have shown low rates of subacute stent thrombosis ($< 2\%$) with high pressure de-ployment and only angiographic guidance.[69] Therefore, ICUS guidance has a very narrow margin to demonstrate a superior result [81] in respect to subacute stent throm-bosis. However, even with the high pressure stent deployment, 28-34% of the stents are found incompletely expanded by ICUS criteria in the AVID and CRUISE trials; further dilatation yielded larger maximal stent areas (unpublished data). The im-pact of this finding on subacute thrombosis and restenosis is not yet available.The use of strict ICUS criteria for stent expansion with the high pressure balloon tech-nique (target stent diameter $\geq 9mm^2$, or 90% of reference luminal diameter) yielded restenosis rate of 7% in the MUSIC trial (unpublished data). According to these results, the maximal stent area (an ICUS measurement) as an absolute value is imporant for restenosis. The issue of restenosis after high pressure stent deploy-ment with or without ICUS guidance is under investigation.

Given the reports implying the potentially deleterious effect of extremely ag-gressive atherectomy[64] on the long term outcome, similar questions need to be ad-dressed in the context of aggressive stenting with high pressure balloon dilatation .[82] In that setting ICUS might restrict the high pressure technique only to the subopti-mally expanded stents after the regular dilatation. Finally, despite the debate in the field of native coronary stenting, ICUS may offer significant advantage in venous graft stenting.[83]

Conclusion

Several groups have reported on the potential clinical utility of ICUS information. All the previously discussed information provided by ICUS on tissue characteriza-tion of the plaque, the diagnosis of procedural complications, the appropriate sizing of the reference vessel and and devices used as well as the post-procedure evalua-tion of the results can be potentially useful in various stages of a significant number of interventions. The results of ongoing trials on its subjects are expected with great interest. ICUS is not independent from coronary angiography, but complements angiography in such extent, that is considered the "state-of-the-art" technique for intracoronary imaging.

Since ICUS imaging is closely linked to technologic advancements, it will fur-ther evolve in the future. Very high frequency transducers will allow for better image resolution and improved features for tissue characterization. Advanced computer software not only will improve videodensitometry, but it will also help tremendously the concept of the three-dimensional vascular reconstruction. Furthermore, ICUS with forward imaging ability may uncover a totally novel aspect of the pre-intervention lesion evaluation.

REFERENCES

1. Topol EJ, Nissen SE. Our preoccupation with coronary luminology. The dissociation between clinical and angiographic findings in ischemic heart disease. Circulation 1995; 92: 2333.

2. Yock PG, Linker DT, Angelsen BA. Two-dimentional intravascular ultrasound: technical development and initial clinical experience. J Am Soc Echocardiogr 1989; 2: 296.

3. Rosenfield K, Isner JM. Intravascular ultrasound in patients undergoing coronary and peripheral arterial revascularization, in: Topol EJ (ed.) Textbook of Interventional Cardiology, 2nd ed. Saunders (Philadelphia) 1994: 1153.

4. Yock PG, Fitzerald PJ, Sudhir K. Intravascular ultrasound, in: Topol EJ (ed.) Textbook of Interventional Cardiology, 2nd ed. Saunders (Philadelphia) 1994: 1136.

5. Waller BF, Pinkerton CA, Slack JD. Intravascular ultrasound: A histological study of vessels during life. Circulation 1992; 85: 2305.

6. Nissen S, et al. Intravascular ultrasound of the coronary arteries: current applications and future directions. Am J Cardiol 1992;69:18H.

7. Nishimura RA, et al. Intravascular ultrasound imaging: in vitro validation and pathologic correlation. J Am Coll Cardiol 1990; 16: 145.

8. Fitzgerald PJ, et al. Intravascular ultrasound imaging of coronary arteries. is three layers the norm? Circulation 1992; 86: 154.

9. Maheswaran B, et al. Intravascular ultrasound appearance of normal and mildly diseased coronary arteries: correlation with histologic specimens. Am Heart J 1995: 130: 976.

10. Tobis JM, et al. Intravascular ultrasound imaging of human coronary arteries in vivo. Circulation 1991; 83: 913.

11. St. Goar FG, et al. Detection of coronary atherosclerosis in young adult hearts using intravascular ultrasound. Circulation 1992;86:756.

12. Mano T, et al. Endothelial dysfunction in the early stage of atherosclerosis precedes appearance of intimal lesions assessable with intravascular ultrasound. Am Heart J 1996; 131: 231.

13. Stary HC. The sequence of cell and matrix changes in atherosclerotic lesions of coronary arteries in the first forty years of life. Eur Heart J 1990;11(Suppl E):3.

14. Simons DB, et al. Non-invasive definition of anatomic coronary artery disease by ultrafast computed tomographic scanning: a pathologic comparison study. J Am Coll Cardiol 1992; 20: 1118.

15. Richardson RD, Davies MJ, Born GVR. Influence of plaque configuration and stress distribution on fissuring of coronary atherosclerotic plaques. Lancet 1989; 2: 941.

16. Friedrich GJ, Moes NY, Muhlberger VA. Detection of intralesional calcium by intracoronary ultrasound depends on the histologic pattern. Am Heart J 1994; 128: 435.

17. Mintz G, et al. Patterns of calcification in coronary artery disease. a statistical analysis fo intravascular ultrasound and coronary angiography in 1155 lesions. Circulation 1995; 91: 1959.

18. Linker DT. Intravascular imaging, in: Fuster V, Ross R, Topol EJ (eds) Atherosclerosis and Coronary Artery Disease. Lippincott-Raven (Philadelphia) 1996: 1473.

19. DiMario CD, et al. Detection and characterization of vascular lesions by intravascular ultrasound: an in vitro study correlated with histology. J Am Soc Echocadiogr 1992; 5: 135.

20. Hodgson JM, et al. Intracoronary ultrasound imaging: correlation of plaque morphology with angiography, clinical syndrome and procedural results in patients undergoing coronary angioplasty. J Am Coll Cardiol 1993; 21: 35.

21. Mizuno K, et al. Angioscopic evaluation of coronary-artery thrombi in acute coronary syndromes. N Engl J Med 1992; 326: 287.

22. Fitzgerald PJ, Ports TA, Yock PG. Contribution of localized calcium deposits to dissection after angioplasty: An observational study using intravascular ultrasound. Circulation 1992; 86: 64.

23. Kimura B, et al. Subintimal wire position during angioplasty of a chronic total coronary occlusion: detection and subsequent procedural guidance by intravascular ultrasound. Cathet Cardiovasc Diagn 1995; 35: 262.

24. De Scheerder I, et al. Intravascular ultrasound versus angiography for measurement of luminal diameters in normal and diseased coronary arteries. Am Heart J 1994; 127: 243.

25. Nakamura S, et al. an explanation for discrepancy between angiographic and intravascular ultrasound measurements after percutaneous transluminal coronary angioplasty. J Am Coll Cardiol 1995; 25: 633.

26. Fuessl RT, et al. In vivo validation of intravascular ultrasound length measurements using a motorized transducer pullback system. Am J Cardiol ; in press.

27. Evans JL, et al. Accurate three-dimensional reconstruction of intravascular ultrasound data. Circulation 1996; 93: 567.

28. Roelandt J, et al. Three-dimensional reconstruction of intracoronary ultrasound images. Rationale, approaches, problems, and directions. Circulation 1994; 90: 1044.

29. Hodgson JM, Quealy K, Berry J. Volumetric plaque quantification by 3-D intracoronary ultrasound: Validation of accuracy and assessment of in-vivo variability. J Am Coll Cardiol 1996; 27(SupplA): 364A.

30. von Birgelen C, et al. Clinial application of a new computerized method measuring coronary artery dimensions by three-dimentional intracoronary ultrasound: reproducibility in vivo during coronary interventions. Eur Heart J 1995; 16(Suppl): 428.

31. von Birgelen C, et al. Volumatric intracoronary ultrasound: A new maximum confidence approach for the quantitative assessment of progression-regression of atherosclerosis? Atherosclerosis 1995; 118 (Suppl): S103.

32. Javier S, et al. Intravascular ultrasound assessment of the magnitude and mechanism of coronary artery and lumen tapering. Am J Cardiol 1995; 75: 177.

33. Glagov S. et al. Compensatory enlargement of human atherosclerotic coronary arteries. N Engl J Med 1987; 316: 1371.

34. Zarins CK, et al. Differential enlargement of artery segments in response to enlerging atherosclerotic plaques. J Vasc Surg 1988; 7: 386.

35. Gibbons GH, Dzau VJ. The emerging concept of vascular remodeling. N Engl J Med 1994; 330: 1431.

36. Clarkson TB, et al. Remodeling of coronary arteries in human and nonhuman primates. JAMA 1194;271:289.

37. Stiel GM, et al. Impact of compensatory enlargement of atherosclerotic coronary arteries on angiographic asessment of coronary artery disease. Circulation 1989; 80: 1603.

38. Ge J, et al. Coronary artery remodeling in atherosclerotic disease: an intrasvascular ultrasonic study in vivo. Cor Art Dis 1993; 4: 981.

39. Gerber TC, et al. Extent of atherosclerosis and remodeling of the left main coronary artery determined by intravascular ultrasound. Am J Cardiol 1994; 73: 666.

40. Hermiller JB, et al. In vivo validation of compensatory enlargement of atherosclerotic coronary arteries. Am J Cardiol 1993 ;71: 665.

41. Mendelsohn FO, et al. In vivo assessment by intravascular ultrasound of enlargement in saphenous vein bypass grafts. Am J Cardiol 1995; 76:1066.

42. Pasterkamp G, et al. Paradoxical arterial wall shrinkage may contribute to luminal narrowing of human atherosclerotic femoral arteries. Circulation 1995; 91: 1444.

43. Koyama J, et al. Comparison of vessel wall morphologic appearance at sites of focal and diffuse coronary vasospasm by intravascular ultrasound. Am Heart J 1995; 130: 440.

44. Nakatani S, et al. Assessment of coronary artery distensibility by intravascular ultrasound. Circulation 1995; 91: 2904.

45. Yamagishi M, et al. Coronary reactivity to nitroglycerin: intravascular ultrasound evidence for the importance of plaque distribution. J Am Coll Cardiol 1995; 25: 224.

46. Bank AJ, et al. Direct effects of smooth muscle relaxation and contraction on in vivo human brachial artery elastic properties. Circ Res 1995; 77: 1008.

47. Mintz GS, et al. Intravasular ultrasound comparison of restenotic and denovo coronary artery narrowings. Am J Cardiol 1994; 74: 1278.

48. Kuntz RE, et al. Generalized model of restenosis after conveentional balloon angioplasty, stenting and directional atherectomy. J Am Coll Cardiol 1993; 21: 15.

49. Beatt KJ, et al. Restenosis after coronary angioplasty: the paradox of increased lumen diameter and restenosis. J Am Coll Cardiol 1992; 19: 258.

50. Mintz GS, et al. The final percentage cross sectional narrowing (residual plaque burden) is the strongest intravascular ultrasound predictor of angiographic restenosis. J Am Coll Cardiol 1995; 25 (Sp.Iss.): 35A.

51. Rodriguez A, et al. Early decrease in minimal lumen diameter predicts late restenosis. Am J Cardiol 1993; 71: 1391.

52. Di Mario C, et al. Quantitative assessment with intracoronary ultrasound of the mechanisms of restenosis after percutaneous transluminal coronary angioplasty and directional coronary atherectomy. Am J Cardiol 1995; 75: 772.

53. Kimura T, et al. Time course of geometric arterial remodeling after coronary angioplasty: balloon angioplasy vs. directional coronary atherectomy. J Am Coll Cardiol 1996; 27(Suppl-1A): 41A.

54. The GUIDE Trial Investigators. IVUS-determined predictors of restenosis in PTCA and DCA: Final report from the GUICE trial, phase II. J Am Coll Cardiol 1996; 27(SupplA): 156A.

55. Peters RJG on behalf of the PICTURE Study Group. Prediction of angiographic restenosis by intracoronary ultrasound imaging after coronary balloon angioplasty. Eur Heart J 1995; 16(Suppl): 201.

56. Potkin BN, et al. Arterial responses to balloon angioplasty: an intravascular ultrasound study. J Am Coll Cardiol 1992; 20: 942.

57. Honye J, et al. Morphological effects of coronary balloon angioplasty in vivo assessed by intravascular ultrasound imaging. Circulation 1992; 85: 1012.

58. Lugt AV, et al. Comparison of intravascular ultrasonic findings after coronary balloon angioplasty evaluated in vitro with histology. Am J Cardiol 1995; 76: 661.

59. Pasterkamp G, et al. Remodeling of de novo atheroslerotic lesions in femoral arteries: impact on mechanism of balloon angioplasty. J Am Coll Cardiol 1995; 26: 422.

60. Nakamura S, et al. Intracoronary ultrasound imaging before and after directional coronary atherectomy: in vitro and clinical observations. Am Heart J 1995; 129: 841.

61. Umans VA, et al. Angiographic, ultrasonic, and angioscopic assessment of the coronary artery wall and lumen area configuration after directional atherectomy: The mechanism revisited. Am Heart J 1996; 130: 217.

62. Matar FA, et al. Multivariate predictors of intravascular ultrasound end points after directional coronary atherectomy. J Am Coll Cardiol 1995; 25: 318.

63. De Lezo et al. Intracoronary ultrasound assessment of directional coronary atherectomy: Immediate and follow up findings. J Am Coll Cardiol 1993; 21: 298.

64. Dussaillant GR, et al. The "dark side" of overly aggressive multidense atherectomy. J Am Coll Cardiol 1996; 27(Suppl.A): 393A.

65. Mintz GS, et al. Intravascular ultrasound evaluation of the effect of rotational atherectomy in obstructive atherosclerotic coronary artery disease. Circulation 1992; 86: 1383.

66. Kovach JA, et al. Sequential intravascular ultrasound characterization of the mechanisms of rotational atherectomy and adjunct balloon angioplasty. J Am Coll Cardiol 1993; 22; 1024.

67. Serruys PW, et al. A comparison of balloon-expandable stent implantation with balloon angioplasty in patients with coronary artery disease. N Engl J Med 1994; 331: 489.

68. Fischman DL, et al. A randomized comparison of coronary stent placement and balloon angioplasty in the treatment of coronary artery disease. N Engl J Med 1994; 331: 496.

69. Marsico F. De Servi S, Kubica J. Influence of plaque composition on luminal gain after balloon angioplasty, directional atherectomy, and coronary stenting. Am Heart J 1995; 130: 971.

70. Painter JA, et al. Serial intravascular ultrasound studies fail to show evidence of chronic palmaz-schatz stent recoil. Am J Cardiol 1995; 75: 398.

71. Hoffman R, et al. What causes focal restenosis at the margins of Palmaz-Schatz stents? A serial intravascular ultrasound study. J Am Coll Cardiol 1996; 27(SupplA): 321A.

72. Gorge G, et al. Intravascular ultrasound after low and high inflation pressure coronary artery stent implantation. J Am Coll Cardiol 1995; 26: 725.

73. Nakamura S, et al. Intracoronary ultrasound observations during stent implantation. Circulation 1994; 89: 2026.

74. Dussaillant GR, et al. Small stent size and intimal hyperplasia contribute to restenosis: a volumetric intravascular ultrasound analysis. J Am Coll Cardiol 1995; 26: 720.

75. Mintz GS, et al. Impact of preintervention intravascular ultrasound imaging on transcatheter treatment strategies in coronary artery disease. Am J Cardiol 1994; 73: 423.

76. Stone GW, et al. Improved outcome of balloon angioplasty with intracoronary ultrasound guidance-core lab angiographic and ultrasound results from the CLOUT study. J Am Coll Cardiol 1996; 27(SupplA): 155A.

77. Baim DS, et al. Mechanisms of luminal enlargement by optimal atherectomy-ivus insights from the OARS study. J Am Coll Cardiol 1996; 27(Suppl.A): 291A.

78. Colombo A, et al. Intracoronary stenting without anticoagulation accomplished with intravascular ultrasound guidance. Circulation 1995; 91: 1676.

79. Goldberg SL, et al. Benefit of intracoronary ultrasound in the deployment of Palmaz-Schatz stents. J Am Coll Cardiol 1994; 24: 996.

80. Kiemeneij F, Laarman G, Slagboom T. Mode of deployment of coronary Palmaz-Schatz stents after implantation with the stent delivery system: An intravascular ultrasound study. Am Heart J 1995; 129: 638.

81. Hall P, et al. A randomized comparison of combined ticlopidine and aspirin therapy versus aspirin therapy alone after successful intravascular ultrasound-guided stent implantation. Circulation 1996; 93: 215.

82. Allen KM, et al. Is there need for intravascular ultrasound after high-pressure dilatations of Palmaz-Schatz stents? J Am Coll Cardiol 1996;27(Suppl.A):138A.

83. Painter JA, et al. Intravascular ultrasound assessment of "biliary" stent implantation in saphenous vein graft lesions. J Am Coll Cardiol 1994; 23: 484A.

32 RESTENOSIS

George Dangas, Roxana Mehran

More than twenty years since the first performance of percutaneous transluminal coronary angioplasty (PTCA), interventional cardiology has numerous applications and utilizes a wide range of revascularization strategies[1] to treat coronary artery disease (CAD). However, despite the technical advancements of the new techniques, recurrence of the arterial stenoses has persisted. This pathologic process has been referred to as restenosis. It represents a distinct pathophysiologic entity within CAD and its treatment is critical as it will drastically increase the impact of PTCA on the sustained clinical improvement of patients with CAD.

Restenosis represents a significant narrowing of the arterial lumen at the angioplasty site and occurs in 40% of the cases, usually presenting with recurrent chest pain. However, angiographic restenosis may also be totally asymptomatic. The majority of the restenoses develop within the first three months and the lumen narrowing has been shown to be completed by six months.[2-5] Although restenosis can be defined in many ways (i.e., histologic, clinical, angiographic), angiographic restenosis has been considered the gold standard by the interventional cardiologists. A dichotomous definition of an absolute luminal stenosis >50% at the angioplasty site is mostly used. However, a >30% lumen reduction compared to the initial successful result has also been proposed to represent restenosis.[6, 7]

The restenotic process has also been defined as a continuous variable. Atrerial renarowing at the procedure site was serially evaluated and measured arithmetically as the minimal lumen diameter (MLD) by Serruys et al.[6] Restenosis was then defined as any lumen renarrowing that exceeds the mean value by two standard deviations (SD). The "cut-off" number was found to be 0.72mm (with 2.5% false positives) in the studied population. In the same study it was also demonstrated that the amount of lumen renarrowing was directly proportional to the arterial diameter achieved with the initial intervention ("the more you gain, the more you loose"). In contrast to the latter statement the maximal MLD achieved with PTCA has been identified as the most important variable that affects restenosis (see below). This was shown to be irrespective of the specific revascularization technique used ("bigger is better").[7]

Pathogenesis of restenosis

The restenotic process is thought to be an arterial wall response to the direct physical injury which the balloon or other devices create. The complex cascade of numerous subsequent events begins with onset of injury and involves local inflammation, mural thrombosis, neointimal hyperplasia and arterial geometric changes and recoil *(Table 32.1)*.

Early elastic recoil

Balloon dilation causes immediate arterial stretch. Acute lumen loss (up to 50%) has been demostrated following ballon deflation due to elastic recoil. The incidence and extent of early elastic recoil has been investigated with a 24-hour post procedure angiogram. The patient population with an early lumen loss of >10% (and <100%) had 74% incidence of late restenosis[8], whereas restenosis occurred only in 10% of patients with early recoil <10%. This study directly implicated early elastic recoil in the pathogenesis of late restenosis. Furthermore, recent data indicated that the major degree of elastic recoil actually takes place much earlier than 24

Table 32.1 PATHOGENETIC STEPS OF RESTENOSIS

EARLY ELASTIC RECOIL

MURAL THROMBOSIS
Platelet aggregation and thrombosis
Mural thrombus formation
Mural thrombus organization

NEOINTIMAL PROLIFERATION
Smooth muscle cell activation
Vessel wall inflammation
Smooth muscle cell migration
Smooth muscle cell proliferation
Extracellular matrix formation

CHRONIC GEOMETRIC ARTERIAL CHANGES

hours post-PTCA. Angiograms taken serially after successful angioplasties (residual stenosis 17%) showed lumen reduction to 35% one hour post-PTCA and further reduction to 41% 24 hours later. This implies that recoil is for the most part an acute process (81% within the first hour) probably occuring immediately post-procedure.[9] Systematic assessment of elastic recoil may actually be a valid predictor of restenosis. In case it might be assessed reliably even earlier than one hour, its routine evaluation may be feasible in all patients to stratify their risk for restenosis and possibly modify the interventional approach to their coronary lesions. Stenting in cases of increased elastic recoil post-PTCA has been shown to have restenosis rate of 21% in a small study.[10]

Mural thrombosis and neointimal hyperplasia

Initial angiographic success depends on balloon size, inflation pressure and time. These factors contribute to forceful deep arterial injury, subintimal tear, vessel stretch and plaque compression. The endothelium is damaged and denuded from the arterial wall. This allows for immediate apposition of a fibrin layer and subsequent platelet adhesion and aggregation. Arterial injury also exposes to the circulating blood highly thrombiogenic substances of the subendothelium (matrix and collagen). Platelet receptors (integrins) bind to cell adhesion molecules (e.g. fibronectin) and platelet degranulation follows. Damaged and dysfunctional endothelium either contributes or fails to prevent this process. The ultimate step of platelet aggregation process is the binding of the IIb/IIIa integrin to fibrinogen, von Willebrand factor and fibronectin in the surface of the vessel wall. Locally decreased blood low and shear stress augment this process showing the importance of rapid and sustained establishment of high blood flow rates during PTCA for the reduction of future restenosis.[11,12] According to animal models, monocytes and neutrophils are attracted to the area beginning an inflammatory response with the release of cytokines.[13-15]

Platelet degranulation releases locally many hemostatic, vasoconstrictive and mitogenic substances. Thrombin, platelet derived growth factor (PDGF), thromboxanes, serotonin and von Willebrand's factor are some of them and lead to mural thrombus formation.[13] Heparin is inactive against clot-bound and matrix-bound thrombin unlike other direct antithrombins.[16-17] The importance of mural thrombosis in restenosis has therefore developed well justified interest in more effective antithrombotic therapies than heparin alone.

Mural thrombosis promotes neointimal hyperplasia[18] which is the classic histologic hallmark of restenosis.[13] Initially there is smooth muscle cell (SMC) activation by locally induced growth factors (e.g. FGF) and attracted inflammatory cells (macrophages). Fibrosis and organization of the mural thrombus which is now incorporated into the repaired vessel wall are the outcomes of local inflammation. PDGF can expressed by platelets, macrophages and SMC and directly induces SMC migration[19] from the medial to the intimal layer of the arterial wall. This is associated with altered SMC phenotype leading to active proliferation under the action of growth factors (e.g. basic fibroblast growth factor bFGF, insulin-like growth factor

IGF, epidermal growth factor EGF, transforming growth factor TGFb) and cytok-ines.[20-23]

SMC proliferation begins within 24 to 48 hours after the injury and decreases after two to four weeks.[23] Any further luminal narrowing is due to the extracellular matrix produced. The signaling for the termination of the SMC proliferation has not been clarifieed yet, but it may involve accumulation of a critical amount of extracellular matrix in direct contact with the SMC. The collagen and matrix forma-tion are finished by the fourth month after the initial injury, a time course that is in accordance with the angiographic descriptions.

Chronic geometric arterial remodeling

The arterial wall undergoes chronic geometric remodeling in response to injury. Chronic atherosclerosis leads to focal vessel enlargement. This is thought to occur to counterbalance the luminal obstruction by the plaque in order to preserve blood flow.[24-25] In restenotic lesions the initial stretch destructs vasa vasorum which are abundant in the atherosclerotic areas, and possibly leads to local hypoxia of the vessel wall, compression of the medial layer and SMC injury (leading to increased reactive DNA synthesis).[26] Restenotic lesions lead to localized contraction of the artery, which accounts for 66% of the total late lumen narrowing.[27] Three types of lumen progression post-procedure have been described: *late lumen gain* (increased external elastic membrane (EEM) diameter, only mild intimal hyperplasia), *late lumen loss* (minimal change in EEM diameter, significant intimal hyperplasia with still >50% arterial patency) and *restenosis* (decrease in EEM diameter, significant intimal hyperplasia, vessel patency <50%). Remodeling of the vessel wall may be related to local hemodynamic characteristics after PTCA and possibly the destruc-tion of the architecture of the vessel wall.[28]

Predictors of post-PTCA restenosis

The pathogenesis of restenosis could have been better understood if reliable predic-tors of this condition were identified.[29-30] Preprocedural characteristics that increase the incidence of restenosis are unstable angina and diabetes mellitus (especially type I). In unstable angina, culprit lesions showed higher restenosis rate compared to non-culprit.[31] Evaluation of hyperlipidemia as a predictor of restenosis led to contradictory results but high lipoprotein (a) levels were recently reported to corre-late with restenosis.[32] Hypertension, end-stage renal disease and coronary vasos-pasm may also predispose to restenosis, but solid associations have not been made yet. The M-HEART study evaluated 510 patients with 598 lesions and used a sys-tematic approach to identify variables associated with three levels of restenosis in-cidence (low, intermediate, high).[33] The diameter of the native coronary artery, lesion length, lesions in the left anterior descending (LAD) or in saphenous vein graft (SVG) and % diameter stenosis pre and post PTCA were the factors that correlated best with high restenosis rate. There was significant difference in restenosis rates among groups (20% to 61%, with overall restenosis rate 40%). Proximal lesions, bend or bifurcation location, complex lesions in unstable angina patients, intracoronary thrombosis and reduced TIMI flow have high restenosis rate. An extensive recent review [34] showed the restenosis rate (>50% rule) to be 45% for the totally occluded lesions (19% as recurrent total occlusions) and compared to 34% for the subtotal stenoses (5% restenosed as total occlusios). Procedural variables associated with restenosis were the total balloon inflation time and the presence of intracoronary thrombus.

Coronary revascularization techniques

The high incidence of restenosis with balloon angioplasty (40%) has been targeted with the development of newer revascularization devices among other anti-restenotic strategies. However, despite their sophisticated approach to lesions, no significant impact on the post procedure restenosis rate has not been made until recently.

Directional coronary atherectomy (DCA)

Introduced by Simpson in 1986[1], DCA increases the arterial lumen by directly removing (rather than compressing) portions of the atherosclerotic plaque in attempt to minimize vessel wall injury and medial (SMC) damage. Despite better initial angiographic outcome than PTCA , DCA failed to show any difference in the rate of restenosis in two head to head comparison randomized trials (CAVEAT, CCAT).

The CAVEAT I [35] trial (1012 patients) showed a favorable trend but no statistically significant overall restenosis rate between DCA and PTCA (50% vs. 57%). However there was difference in the restenosis rate for the proximal and particularly the non-ostial[36] segment of the LAD (51% DCA, 63% PTCA). The complication rate (death, MI) was increased with DCA and that extended to the one year follow up (11 vs. 3 deaths, 2% vs. 1%).[37]

The CCAT[38] trial (274 patients with proximal LAD lesions) showed similar restenotic rates (46% DCA, 43% PTCA) and complication profile. The CAVEAT II [39] trial (309 patients with SVG lesions) showed no significant difference in restenosis (46% DCA, 51% PTCA) with reduced target vessel reintervention rate for the DCA group (13% vs. 22%). More recent larger trials compared angioplasty with "optimal" atherectomy performed in limited centers to ensure achievement of maximal MLD for all the cases.[40] In the BOAT trial, the DCA technique resulted in greater acute luminal gain and significantly reduced restenosis compared to PTCA (see relevant chapter). The immediate post-procedure MLD achieved in the DCA group was comparable with the post-stent MLD achieved in the STRESS trial (S.K. Sharma, personal communication).

Rotational atherectomy (Rotablator)

This interventional device consists of a sized burr coated with diamond chips rotating at high speed through the stenotic segments of the arterial wall and pulverizing the atherosclerotic plaque into very small particles.[1] The rotablator differentially ablates calcified plaque rather than elastic tissue of the normal wall and usually requires adjunctive angioplasty. The restenosis rate has been recently reported[41] as high as 38% (709 patients, 745 procedures). The rotablator can approach long calcified lesions thought not to be amenable to PTCA, but has not offered any advantage to restenosis rate over any other intervention thus far. Direct head to head comparison of the technique to PTCA is under way (DART).

Transluminal extraction atherectomy (TEC)

The TEC catheter dissects and aspirates parts of the clot and the plaque with subsequent exposure of residual atheroma and organized thrombus to the circulation and usually requires adjunctive PTCA. The restenosis rates for native coronary and SVG lesions (69%) have been disappointingly high.[42,43] This device is currently reserved for thrombus containing lesions with complex anatomy and high procedural risk.

Laser - facilitated PTCA

Laser devices cause tissue ablation and produce acoustic shock waves. They aim in destructing the substrate of restenosis (SMC) while eliminating the occlusive plaque. The Excimer Laser Coronary Angioplasty (ELCA) utilizes 308 nm XeCl pulsed ultraviolet laser with minimal thermal injury to tissue[1] and is able to ablate long, mildly calcified plaques and is followed by balloon dilation to achieve bigger MLD.[44] The overall restenosis rate has been reported 45-50%, but somewhat lower (35%) for SVG lesions.[45] Again, better long term outcome was correlated with better initial result.[46] Direct comparison to PTCA is not available but these results do not imply any improvement in restenosis. Holmium laser is a solid state pulsed mid-infrared (2.1 mm) system otherwise similar to ELCA and has been reported (331 patents, 365 lesions) to have six-month restenosis rate (44%) similar to the other procedures.[47]

Intracoronary stents

Sigwart placed the first intracoronary stent in 1987.[1] Cumulative report by Serruys et al.[48] showed a restenosis rate of 32% (0.72mm MLD reduction) or 14% (>50% stenosis) with identification of early thrombotic occlusion as the most important limitation of the procedure, related to their intrinsic thrombogenicity and to patient selection bias.

The BENESTENT[49] trial (520 patients with chronic stable angina and a single lesion randomized to stent vs. PTCA) showed improved six-month restenosis (>50%

rule) rate (22% vs. 32% to PTCA), decreased need for repeat revascularization (10% vs. 20%) but increased peripheral vascular complications (14% vs. 3%) in the stent group. Similarly, the STRESS [50] trial (410 patients with symptomatic CAD) reported a lower restenosis (>50% rule) rate at six months (32% vs. 42%) and decreased need for repeat revascularizations (10% vs. 15%) with increased bleeding and vascular complications (7% vs. 4%) for the stent group.

In the first study the stent patients were placed on aspirin and dipyridamole for six months and on wartarin (INR 2.5-3.5) for three months. However, in the STRESS trial patients received dipyridamole and warfarin (INR 2-3.5) for one month and aspirin indefinitely. The MLD achieved with stents was larger than in the PTCA group and remained so at the follow up in spite of the greater late loss observed. The immediate post-procedure elastic recoil was reported as 15% for the stent group and 24% for the PTCA group.

Stents provide a new insight in understanding restenosis. They cause some focal medial necrosis at the site of the indentation and mainly offer a geometrical support to keep the arterial lumen enlarged. This has been studied with Intravascular Ultrasound (IVUS) which is used routinely after stent placement for proper expansion and deployment [51,52]. Stents markedly diminish the acute elastic recoil and, as presently reported do not allow geometric arterial remodeling. The stent restenosis seems primarily due to neointimal hyperplasia which appears to be more pronounced in stent cases than other interventions. In addition to mechanical wall support, stents may modify restenosis by providing markedly increased blood flow downstream.[53]

Stent thrombosis is a well described complication and currently vigorous anticoagulation is mandated in most stent centers after stent placement. Colombo et al. however, reported[54] that anticoagulation can be safely avoided with IVUS documented full stent expansion. The regimen used was either aspirin (5 days) and ticlopidine (1 month) or aspirin alone in 359 patients, after initial stent placement with <20% angiographic residual the deployment was optimized with IVUS guidance (good apposition of the stent to the wall, cross sectional area at least equal to the reference vessel, no more than 60% stenosis at the edges). This group reported 94% two-month procedural success, two acute closures (the first day with Q-wave MI), one sub acute and two additional during the months 3-6 with a six-month rate of restenosis 22%, 13% re intervention, 6% CABG, 6% MI, 2% death and 2% stent occlusion over six months. Heparin-coated stents may target successfully both the early thrombosis and the late restenosis. The BENESTENT II evaluates this question, however without direct comparison to conventional stents.[55]

Intracoronary ultrasound (ICUS)

ICUS imaging before and after PTCA has shown that there is more axial plaque redistribution than compression and that failure to cause any dissection leads to early lumen loss by elastic recoil (15% of cases). Spasm associated with eccentric lesions, thrombi and dissections all causes abrupt closure during PTCA and are appreciated better with ICUS than angiography. Lesions with significant plaque burden may be more amenable to ELCA or rotablator as opposed to DCA or PTCA. ICUS can also guide maximal tissue debulking by DCA for optimal result. Mintz et al. reported the residual plaque burden after the intervention to be the most powerful predictor of restenosis.[56] ICUS application for optimal stent deployment especially against eccentric plaques ensures the elimination of any thrombogenic interspace (low flow) between stent and vessel wall and may obviate the need for anticoagulation (see relevant chapter).

Local drug delivery systems

Local drug delivery systems may directly administer selectively to the target lesion pharmacological agents that need higher local concentration which would otherwise be impossible to achieve with systemic administration because of side effects or toxicity.[57,58]

The "balloon over a stent" device facilitates apposition during drug delivery, while the hydrophilic polyacrylic polymer (hydrogel) coated balloon transfer the substances during inflation and wash out to the adventitia in waves.[59] Wolinsky's perforated balloon[60] has 25 mm laser drilled holes, is non-compliant and the infusion pressure delivers the substance to the adventitia, but the fluid jets may cause vascular trauma. In contrast, the microporous balloon has a membrane with thousands of pores (<l mm) and delivers by diffusion avoiding trauma. The iontophoretic porous balloon[61] has the cathode at the catheter and the anode at the skin and showed improved drug delivery than passive diffusion with <10% endothelial denudation and SMC proliferation. The Dispatch catheter has a characteristic helical configuration[62] allowing long infusions at low inflation pressure and is used for the treatment of thrombotic lesions (e.g. for urokinase or heparin administration).

Biodegradable drug-releasing polymer stents have been developed with two pharmacokinetic options: uniform through a monolithic matrix, or controlled by a polymer filter (reservoir type). The drug needs to diffuse widely because the stent actually covers only 5-12% of the arterial area. Obviously there is potential for inflammation and thrombosis locally. Fibrin coated metallic stents, as well as stents covered with genetically modified endothelial cells have been developed.[57,58] The metallic stents can also provide a means for local delivery of any radioactive substance that would aim to abolish local cell proliferation (e.g. ionizing radiation, ί particles). However, one should note that external beam irradiation attempted for decreased restenosis, actually had the opposite effect in the pig model.[63-65]

Detailed evaluation of these new devices is difficult since their failure may be secondary to factors related to the experimental model selected and the technical characteristics of the device itself. Arterial size, possible prior injury, plaque thickness and extent of coronary disease differ in all various experiments. The apposition to the wall may cause damage but also helps eliminate anatomic barriers to drug diffusion. Atherosclerotic plaques appear non-permeable, but in humans the abundant vasa vasorum may facilitate diffusion. The impact on SMC proliferation is important as well as the knowledge of how deep in the wall each drug needs to be delivered . In order for the drug to have an impact on restenosis, some authors have suggested that it is essential to achieve adventitial saturation.[66] Undoubtedly their utility is correlated with the determination of the optimal timing dosage and pharmacodynamics of the specific agents delivered.

Pharmacotherapy for restenosis

Multiple agents have been tried for the reduction of the restenosis rate, targeting all possible mechanisms of its pathogenesis *(Table 32.2)*. So far the majority of the studies has not yielded many successful positive results.

Table 32.2

INTERVENTIONAL APPROACHES TO RESTENOSIS

Stents
"Bigger is better" techniques
Local drug delivery
Coated or biodegradable stents
radioactive stents
hydrogel balloons
Inotophoretic balloons
Dispatch catheter

MEDICAL APPROACHES TO RESTENOSIS

Antiplatlet agents
Antithrombotics
ACE inhibitors
HMG-CoA reductase inhibitors
Fish oils
Antiproliferative agents
Antiserotonin agents
Somatostatin analogs

GENETIC AND MOLECULAR APPROACHES TO RESTENOSIS

Gene therapy
Inhibitors of SMC proliferation
Constitutively active negative regulators
Promoters of SMC inhibition
Factors-targets of pharmacotherapy ("Trojan horse")

Antisense oligonucleotides
Selective (?) inhibition of translation
Genetically engineered cells

Endothelial cells layer on stents (? expression of normal genes)

Conventional agents

Anti-platelet agents. Since the initial event after injury is endothelial denudation and platelet-thrombus formation[13], these agents may be beneficial for prevention of restenosis. However, dipyridamole, ticlopidine and thromboxane-A2 inhibitor studies have been negative. Aspirin therapy showed a trend towards decreased restenosis only in the meta-analysis of all the various trials.[30] Ciprostene is a new prostacyclin analog which has shown some initial positive results.[67,68]

The recent development of a chimeric murine antibody against the human platelet receptor IIb/IIIa integrin by Coller[69] has been a novel approach to antiplatelet therapy. This antibody (c7E3 Fab, or abciximab) was administered to patients undergoing PTCA and showed 80% inhibition of platelet aggregation.[70] In the EPIC[71] trial (2099 patients undergoing high risk PTCA with primary end-point the 30-day major coronary event rate), c7E3 Fab was administered as an intravenous bolus with or without a 12-hour infusion, in addition to standard therapy with aspirin and heparin. This trial showed significant reduction in primary endpoints (13% placebo group, 8% bolus + infusion group), but increased bleeding complications which was attributed to unadjusted, high heparin dosage.[72] Interestingly, the six-month follow up of this cohort showed decreased rates of target vessel revascularization (17% vs. 22%) and major ischemic events (27% vs. 35 %) for the bolus+infusion group compared to placebo.[73] In all comparisons the group treated only with drug bolus had intermediate results. The potential mechanism of this antibody is the "passivation" of the cell surface at the time of the injury and inhibition of fibronectin which may affect neointimal hyperplasia. Other IIb/IIIa inhibitors (MK-383, integrelin) are synthetic peptides against epitopes of the specific platelet receptor. Their evaluation is also under way.

Anti-thrombotic therapy. Since mural thrombus formation is critical for restenosis, such agents may also be useful.[74] Heparin inhibits platelet function and SMC proliferation in addition to thrombin inactivation after it binds to the heparin cofactor antithrombin-III. Heparin did not show any beneficial effect on restenosis in an initial trial[75], possibly because of its inability to bind thrombin situated deeply in the sub-endothelial mural thrombus (important for SMC proliferation as discussed). However, recent report of locally delivered heparin using the Dispatch catheter after PTCA led to the impressively low restenosis rate of 7%.[76] Obviously this finding will be further followed up . Hirudin is considered effective than heparin in the inhibition of mural thrombus. This may be due to its smaller size, and because it functions without a cofactor. However the HELVETICA trial failed to demonstrate a benefit of hirudin on restenosis.[77] Hirulog is a synthetic antithrombin and has been used successfully instead of heparin during PTCA. This drug is currently being evaluated in large trials of PTCA.[78]

Low molecular weight heparin preparations (e.g. enoxaparin) are fragments of the usual heparin with more favorable pharmacokinatic and pharmacodynamic properties (slower clearance and increased activity for factor Xa). Despite positive animal data, these agents did not decrease restenosis in humans, possibly because of the relatively low dose used.[79] Two novel antithrombotic agents have also been tried in preliminary restenosis studies: the synthetic tri-peptide PPACK (with a similar structure to fibrinopeptide A), which has been delivered locally with the hydrogel balloon and inhibited platelet-dependent thrombus in the pig model[80], and a 15-nucleotide (ss-DNA) with a specific direct thrombin inhibitory effect.[81]

Vasodilators. Although adequate support for the use of such agents against restenosis is not available, a trend towards restenosis prevention by routine use of calcium channel blockers is evident in pooled data.[31] Ketanserin is a serotonin receptor antagonist (inhibits vasoconstriction, platelet activation and the mitogenic effect of serotonin on SMC) failed to demonstrate positive clinical or angiographic outcome six months after PTCA.[82]

Lipid-lowering agents. Treatment with an HMG-CoA reductase inhibitor (lovastatin) postPTCA did not achieve any benefit on restenosis despite aggressive LDL-cholesterol lowering achieved.[83] Treatment with w-3 fatty acids was found efficacious in certain small trials and meta-analysis was positive for both clinical and angiographic restenosis.[30,68] Based on these results, larger studies are currently under way. These agents have been shown to inhibited intimal hyperplasia in animal models possibly because of both serum lipid reduction and attenuation of platelet aggregation.

Agents against cell proliferation. Inhibition of cell migration and proliferation has shown some effect in prevention of restenosis. Trapidil, a thromboxane-A$_2$ inhibitor and a PDGF receptor antagonist, was used in the STARC trial.[84] Patients were assigned to 300 mg of trapidil daily or aspirin; therapy was initiated at least three days pre-PTCA for a total of 6 months. This trial showed significant reduction in the restenosis rate with trapidil (26% vs. 44% or 31% vs. 45% according to the restenosis definition applied). The trapidil group had also 58% less episodes of unstable angina and 34% less anginal complaints at 6 months.

Angiopeptin, a somatostatin analog, inhibits both FGF and IGF-1. This agent appears to limit myointimal thickening and restore the vasodilatory response of the vessel wall to acetylcholine. Angiopeptin has been shown to lower the clinical event rate (mainly repeat revascularization) at 12-month follow-up after PTCA, but without affecting angiographic restenosis.[85]

Angiotensin converting enzyme inhibitors have also been investigated for possible restenosis benefit. Initial data in the rat model were promising, but the clinical trials had negative results. However, the dosage used was significantly lower than that needed to produce favorable results in the animal models and drug administration was initiated after PTCA. These agents are now tested for local delivery therapy.[31,67,86,87]

Molecular approaches to restenosis

As the understanding of the pathophysiology of the restenotic process grows, investigators have tried to transform its molecular background. The first practical problem this strategy faces is the way to deliver the genetic material with high specificity and efficiency.[88] Lipofection with cationic liposomes[89], as well as viral vectors can also be used for transfection. Retroviruses lead to DNA integration in the chromosome of the host (insertion), thereby increasing the deleterious potential for mutagenesis. Furthermore, in vivo transfection with retroviruses needs active cell replication and is inhibited by serum and complement. Adenoviral vectors enter the cell via receptor mediated endocytosis but their expression time is limited due to cell death (3 weeks). They also cause local inflammation and bear significant infectious potential on various cell types (brain, liver). Their property to avoid lysosomal degradation, due to their capsid proteins, is unique and has been used in the formation of a transfecting complex: the DNA is bound to an inactivated adenovirus which is coupled to a ligand (e.g. transferrin) and allows the whole complex to be identified by the ligand receptor and enter the cell.[57-58] Indirect gene transfer involves removal and ex vivo genetic engineering of endothelial cells (e.g. for t-PA expression) with subsequent re-implantation of these cells either over a stent or with local delivery systems. The hydrogel balloon or experimental direct peri-adventitial apposition have been used.[90] However, the exact timing of appropriate in vivo activation of these cells is still unclear.

Gene therapy. This includes two approaches according to whether the encoded protein will be retained in the cell, or secreted.[91] In the latter case the desired effect is exerted in more cells than those actually transfected. There are examples of gene therapy strategies against coronary restenosis. Adenoviral vectors have been used in a model of transfection of SMC with the gene encoding HSV-tk, followed by gancyclovir administration.[92] Ganciclovir selectively killed only the HSV-tk expressing cells as well as neighboring cells (paradoxically, or "innocent bystander" effect). An inactivated adenoviral vector was used in a model of insertion of a constitutively active negative regulator (retinoblastoma gene product) which successfully resulted in cell stasis.[93]

Antisense oligonucleotides[94] are short DNA segments which bind the mRNA leading to inhibition of translation. An important limitation is the possibility for non-selective binding of other cellular proteins.[95] Aptamers are short strands of DNA or RNA that can bind specific proteins and successfully inhibit thrombin[81] activity in vitro. Genetically manufactured recombinant fusion proteins consisting of a combination of a potent toxin with a peptide ligand to a cell surface receptor, usually that of a growth factor have also been used ("Trojan horse" strategy). Possible candidates for such toxins are the *Pseudomonas* and the *E.coli* exotoxins, or the diphtheria and cholera toxins. Candidates for the ligand part could be the TGFa, (FGF or IL-2 receptors. The genetic complex of EGF and diphtheria toxin has been administered in outgrowth of human atherosclerotic plaque and managed to inhibit proliferation markedly.[96]

Local or systemic dministration of inactive substances that are selectively activation at the target site has been used as well, e.g. the photo-dynamic therapy for restenosis[97], with light excitable photosensitizers like hematoporphyrin derivatives.

More recently, ί-particle emmitting stents have been tried with encouraging initial results, as well as local radioactivity with Iridium at the time of stent implantation. In the latter study (SCRIPPS), ionizing radiation appeared to remarkably reduce the in-stent restenosis rate as assessed by repeat IVUS and angiography (P. Teirstein, personal communication). Reservations about these agents are the potential for the necrosed cells to produce mitogens with second wave of cell proliferation, and also their cutaneous photosensitivity which is dose limiting.

Targets for molecular therapy exist in all the pathogenetic pathways of restenosis. Endothelial cells, platelet adhesion and aggregation, intimal hyperplasia[98] and extracellular matrix formation can all be experimentally attenuated. Such inhibition can apply any of the basic strategies discussed above.[99]

Conclusions

Recent data from early platelet inhibition and anti-proliferative therapy may offer a new insight to the successful prevention of restenosis. At the same time intracoronary stents improve late patency and provide the means for more effective anti-restenotic strategies. Molecular options for the prevention of restenosis are attractive but still include many concepts to be clarified. If restenosis is indeed analogous to wound healing, then by inhibiting a protective vessel reaction after injury we may cause a deleterious outcome.

Restenosis prediction remains still crucial as it appears unreasonable to expose all angioplasty patients to the potential risks of these costly new approaches. Pre-procedural clinical characteristics, timely assessment of early elastic recoil and IVUS imaging may better define predictors of restenosis and clarify the time course of the contributing mechanisms. This will allow for more optimal targeting of the anti-restenotic strategies.

REFERENCES

1. Mueller RL, Sanborn TA. The history of interventional cardiology: Cardiac catheterization, angioplasty, and related interventions. Am Heart J 1995;129:146.

2. Waller BF, et al. Restenosis 1 to 24 Months after clinically successful coronary balloon angioplasty: a necropsy study of 20 patients. J Am Coll Cardiol 1991;17:58B.

3. Nobuyoshi M, et al. Restenosis after successful percutaneous transluminal coronary angioplasty: serial angiographic follow-up of 229 patients. J Am Coll Cardiol 1988;12:616.

4. Serruys PW, et al. Incidence of restenosis after successful coronary angioplasty: a time-related phenomenon. Circulation 1988;77: 361.

5. Kuntz RE, Baim DS. Defining coronary restenosis. Newer clinical and angiographic paradigms. Circulation 1993, 88(3):1310.

6. Beatt KJ, et al. Restenosis after coronary angioplasty: The paradox of increased lumen diameter and restenosis. J Am Coll Cardiol 1992;19:258.

7. Kuntz RE, et al. Generalized model of restenosis after conventional balloon angioplaty, stenting and directional atherectomy. J Am Coll Cardiol 1993; 21: 15.

8. Rodriguez A, et al. Early decrease in minimal luminal diameter after successful percutaneous transluminal coronary angioplasty predicts late restenosis. Am J Cardiol 1993;71:1391.

9. Rodriguez A, et al. Time course and mechanism of early luminal diameter loss after percutaneous transluminal coronary angioplasty. Am J Cardiol 1995;76:1131.

10. Rodriguez A, et al. Coronary stenting decreases restenosis in lesions with early loss in luminal diameter 24 hours after successful PTCA. Circulation 1995;91:1397.

11. Chesebro JH, et al. Restenosis after arterial angioplasty: A hemorrheologic response to injury. Am J Cardiol 1987;60:10B.

12. Willerson JT, et al. Frequency and severity of cyclic flow alternations and platelet aggregation predict the severity of neointimal proliferation following experimental coronary stenosis and endothelial injury. Proc Nat Acad Sci 1991; 88:10624.

13. Ip JH, et al. The role of platelets, thrombin and hyperplasia in restenosis after coronary angioplasty. J Am Coll Cardiol 1991; 17:77B.

14. Moreno P, et al. Macrophage infiltration in acute coronary syndromes. implications for plaque rupture. Circulation 1995;90:775.

15. Servi SD, et al. Granulocyte activation after coronary angioplasty in humans. Circulation 1990;82:140.

16. Weitz JI, et al. Clot-bound thrombin is protected from inhibition by heparin-antithrombin iii but is susceptible to inactivation by antithrombin III-independent inhibitors. J Clin Invest 1990; 86: 385.

17. Bar-Shavit R, Eldor A, Vlodavsky I. Binding of thrombin to subendothelial extracellular matrix. protection and expression of functional properties. J Clin Invest 1989;84:1096.

18. McNamara CA, et al. Thrombin stimulates proliferation of cultured rat aortic smooth muscle cells by a proteolytically activated receptor. J Clin Invest 1993;91: 94.

19. Casscells W. Migration of smooth muscle and endothelial cells. Critical Events in Restenosis. Circulation 1992;86: 723.

20. Clowes AW, Reidy MA, Clowes MM. Mechanisms of stenosis after arterial injury. Lab Invest 1983; 49: 208.

21. Clowes AW, Reidy MA, Clowes MM. Kinetics of cellular pProliferation after arterial injury. Lab Invest 1987; 49:327.

22. Taubman MB. Gene induction in vessel wall injury. Thromb Haem 1993;70(1): 180-183.

23. Schwartz RS, et al. Smooth muscle cell proliferation in coronary restenosis is limited to a few generations: Cell kinetic model implications. J Am Coll Cardiol 1994;23: 484A.

24. Glagov S, et al. Compensatory enlargement of human atherosclerotic coronary arteries. N Engl J Med 1987;316: 1371.

25. Losordo DW, et al. Focal compensatory enlargement of human arteries in response to progressive atherosclerosis. Circulation 1994;89:2570.

26. Isner JM. Vascular Remodeling. Honey, I think I shrunk the artery. Circulation 1994; 89(6):2937.

27. Mintz GS, et al. Mechanisms of late arterial responses to transcatheter therapy: a serial quantitative angiographic and intravascular study.Circulation 1994;90 (4), pt. 2: I-24.

28. Glagov S. Intimal hyperplasia, vascular modeling, and the restenosis problem. Circulation 1994;89:2888.

29. Pompa JJ, Topol EJ. Factors influencing restenosis after coronary angioplasty. Am J Med 1990;88:1-16N.

30. Hillegass WB, Ohman EM, Califf RM. Restenosis: The clinical issues. In:Topol EJ editor. Textbook of Interventional Cardiology. 2nd ed. Philadelphia: Saunders, 1994: 415.

31. deGroote P, et al. Local lesion-related factors and restenosis after coronary angioplasty: evidence from a quantitative angiographic study in patients with unstable angina undergoing double-vessel angioplasty. Circulation 1995; 91: 968.

32. Desmarais RL, et al. Elevated serum lipoprotein(a) is a risk factor for clinical recurrence after coronary balloon angioplasty. Circulation 1995;91:1403.

33. Hirshfeld JW, et al. Restenosis after coronary angioplasty: a multivariate statistical model to relate lesion and procedure variables to restenosis. J Am Coll Cardiol 1991; 18: 647.

34. Violaris AG, Melkert R, Serruys PW. Long-term luminal renarrowing after successful elective coronary angioplasty of total occlusions. Circulation 1995;91:2140.

35. Topol EJ, et al. A comparison of directional atherectomy with coronary angioplasty in patients with coronary artery disease. N Engl J Med 1993; 329:221.

36. Boehrer JD, et al. Directional atherectomy versus balloon angioplasty for coronary ostial and nonostial left anterior descending coronary artery lesions: results from a randomized multicenter trial. J Am Coll Cardiol 1995;25:1380.

37. Elliot JM, Berdan LG,e al. One-year follow-up in the coronary angioplasty versus excisional atherectomy trial (CAVEAT I). Circulation. 1995;91:2158.

38. Adelman AG, et al. A comparison of directional atherectomy with balloon angioplasty for lesions of the left anterior descending coronary artery. N Engl J Med 1993;329: 228.

39. Holmes DR, et al. A multicenter, randomized trial of coronary angioplasty versus directional atherectomy for patients with saphenous vein bypass graft lesions. Circulation 1995;91(7):1966.

40. Umans V, et al. Optimal use of directional coronary atherectomy is required to ensure long-term angiographic benefit: A study with matched procedural outcome after atherectomy and angioplasty. J Am Coll Cardiol 1994; 24:1652.

41. Warth DC, et al. Rotational atherectomy multicenter registry: acute results, complications and 6-month angiographic follow-up in 709 patients. J Am Coll Cardiol 1994; 24:641.

42. Popma JJ, et al. Results of coronary angioplasty using the transluminal extraction catheter. Am J Cardiol 1992;70:1526.

43. Safian RD, et al. Clinical and angiographic results of transluminal extraction coronary atherectomy in saphenous vein bypass grafts. Circulation 1994;89:302.

44. Litvack F, et al. Percutaneous excimer laser coronary angioplasty: results in the first consecutive 3,000 patients. J Am Coll Cardiol 1994;23:323.

45. Eigler NL, et al. Excimer laser coronary angioplasty of aorto-ostial stenoses. results of the excimer laser coronary angioplasty (ELCA) registry in the first 200 patients. Circulation 1993;88[part 1]: 2049.

46. Bittl JA, et al. Analysis of late lumen narrowing after excimer laser-facilitated coronary angioplasty. J Am Coll Cardiol. 1994;23:1314.

47. deMarchena EJ, et al. Effectiveness of Holmium laser-assisted coronary angioplasty. Am J Cardiol 1994;73:117.

48. Serruys PW, et al. Angiographic follow-up after placement of a self-expanding coronary artery stent. N Engl J Med 1991;324:13.

49. Serruys PW, et al. A comparison of balloon-expandable-stent implantation with balloon angioplasty in patients with coronary artery disease. N Engl J Med 1994;331: 489.

50. Fishman DL, et al. A randomized comparison of coronary-stent placement and balloon angioplasty in the treatment of coronary artery disease. N Engl J Med 1994;331: 496.

51. Leon MB, Wong SCW. Intracoronary Stents. A Breakthrough Technology or Just Another Small Step? Circulation 1994;89(3): 1323.

52. Popma JJ, et al. The impact of intravascular ultrasound (ivus) on post-stent deployment balloon dilatation strategies. J Am Coll Cardiol 1995;Sp. Is. (Feb): 49A.

53. Mintz GS, et al. Endovascular stents reduce restenosis by eliminating geometric arterial remodelling: a serial intravascular ultrasound study. J Am Coll Cardiol 1995;Sp. Is. (Feb): 36A.

54. Colombo A, et al. Intracoronary stenting without anticoagulation accomplished with intravascular ultrasound guidance. Circulation 1995;91:1676.

55. van der Giessen WJ, Hardhammar PA, et al. Prevention of (sub)acute thrombosis using heparin-coated stents. Circulation 1994;90(4):I-650.

56. Mintz GS, et al. The final % cross sectional narrowing (residual plaque burden) is the strongest intravascular ultrasound predictor of angiographic restenosis. J Am Coll Cardiol 1995;Sp. Is. (Feb): 35A.

57. Lincoff AM, et al. Local drug delivery for the prevention of restenosis. fact, fancy, and future. Circulation 1994; 90(4): 2070.

58. Riessen R, Isner JM. Prospects for site-specific delivery of pharmacologic and molecular therapies. J Am Coll Cardiol 1994; 23 (5): 1234.

59. Fram DB, et al. Localized intramural drug delivery during balloon angioplasty using hydro-gel-coated balloons and pressure-augmented diffusion. J Am Coll Cardiol 1994;23: 1570.

60. Wolinsky H. Local delivery: Let's keep our eyes on the wall. J Am Coll Cardiol 1994;24:825.

61. Fernandez-Ortiz A, et al. a new approach for local intravascular drug delivery. Iontophoretic balloon. Circulation 1994;89:1518.

62. Mitchel JF, et al. Enhanced intracoronary thrombolysis with urokinase using a novel, local drug delivery system: in vitro, in vivo, and clinical studies. Circulation 1995; 91: 785.

63. Laird JR, et al. Inhibition of neointimal proliferation with a beta particle emitting stent. J Am Coll Cardiol 1995;Sp. Is(Feb): 287A.

64. Schwartz RS, et al. Effect of external beam irradiation on neointimal hyperplasia after ex-perimental coronary artery injury. J Am Coll Cardiol 1992;19: 1106.

65. Wiedermann JG, et al. Intracoronary irradiation markedly reduces neointimal proliferation after balloon angioplasty in swine: persistent benefit at 6-month follow-up. J Am Coll Car-diol 1995;25: 1451.

66. Simons M, et al. Antisense c-myb oligonucleotides inhibit intimal arterial smooth muscle cell accumulation in vivo. Nature 1992; 359: 67.

67. Raizner AE, et al. Ciprostene for restenosis revisited: Quantitative analysis of angiograms. J Am Coll Cardiol 1993;21: 321A.

68. Popma JJ, Califf RM, Topol EJ. Clinical trials of restenosis after coronary angioplasty. Cir-culation 1991; 84: 1426.

69. Coller BS. New murine monoclonal antibody reports an activation-dependent change the conformation and/or microenvironment of the platelet glycoprotein IIb/IIIa complex. J Clin Invest1985; 78: 101.

70. Tcheng JE, et al. Pharmacodynamics of chimeric glycoprotein IIb/IIIa integrin antiplatelet antibody 7E3 Fab in high-risk coronary angioplasty. Circulation 1994;90: 1757.

71. The EPIC Investigators. Use of monoclonal antibody directed against the platelet glycopro-tein IIb/IIIa receptor in high-risk coronary angioplasty. N Engl J Med 1994;290: 956.

72. Harrington RA, et al. Bleeding associated with use of a platelet glycoprotein IIb/IIIa inhib-itor during routine coronary angioplasty: Is too much heparin the culprit? J Am Coll Cardiol 1994: 89:106A.

73. Topol EJ, et al. Randomised trial of coronary intervention with antibody against platelet IIb/IIIa integrin for reduction of clinical restenosis: results at six months. Lancet 1994;343:881.

74. Lefkovits J, Topol E. Direct thrombin inhibitors in cardiovascular medicine. Circulation 1994;90:1522.

75. Ellis SG, et al. Effect of 18- to 24-hour heparin administration for prevention of restenosis after uncomplicated coronary angioplasty. Am Heart J 1989;117:777.

76. Camenzind E, et al. Intracoronary Heparin Delivery in Humans. Acute Feasibility and Long-Term Results. Circulation 1995; 92: 2463.

77. van denBos A, et al. Safety and efficacy of recombinant hirudin vs heparin in patients with stable angina undergoing coronary angioplasty. Circulation 1993; 88: 2058.

78. Topol E, et al. Use of direct antithrombin, hirulog, in place of heparin during coronary angioplasty. Circulation 1993;87:1622.

79. Faxon DP, et al. Low molecular weight heparin in prevention of restenosis after angioplasty. Results of enoxaparin restenosis (ERA) trial. Circulation 1994;90:908.

80. Nunes GL, et al. Local delivery of a synthetic antithrombin with a hydrogel-coated angioplasty balloon catheter inhibits platelet-dependent thrombosis. J Am Coll Cardiol 1994;23:1578.

81. Bock LC, et al. Selection of single-stranded DNA molecules that bind and inhibit human thrombin. Nature 1992; 355: 564.

82. Serruys PW, et al. Evaluation of ketanserin in the prevention of restenosis after percutaneous transluminal coronary angioplasty. A multicenter randomized double-blind palcebo-controlled trial. Circulation 1993; 88: 1588.

83. Weintraub, WS, et al. Lack of effect of lovastatin on restenosis after coronary angioplasty. N Engl J Med 1994;331:1331.

84. Maresta A, et al. Trapidil (triazolopyrimidine), a platelet-derived growth factor antagonist, reduces restenosis after percutaneous transluminal coronary angioplasty. Results of the randomized, double-blind STARC study. Circulation 1994;90:2710.

85. Emanuelsson H, et al. Long-term effects of angiopeptin treatment in coronary angioplasty. reduction of clinical events but not angiographic restenosis. Circulation 1995;91:1689.

86. Powell JS, et al. Inhibitors of angiotensin-converting enzyme prevent myointimal proliferation after vascular injury. Science 1989; 245: 186.

87. Faxon DP. Effect of high dose angiotensin-converting enzyme inhibition on restenosis: final results of the MARCATOR study, a multicenter, double-blind, placebo-controlled trial of cilazapril. J Am Coll Cardiol 1995;25:362.

88. Nabel EG, Plautz G, Nabel GJ. Site-specific gene expression in vivo by direct gene transfer into the arterial wall. Science 1990; 249: 1285.

89. Takeshita S, et al. Increased gene expression after liposome-mediated arterial gene transfer associated with intimal smooth muscle cell proliferation. J Clin Invest 1994; 93: 652.

90. Nabel EG. Gene therapy for cardiovascular disease. Circulation 1995; 91: 541-47.

91. Mulligan R. The basic science of gene therapy. Science 1993; 260: 926.

92. Ohno T, et al. Gene therapy for vascular smooth muscle cell proliferation after arterial injury. Science 1994;265: 781.

93. Chang MW, t al. Cytostatic gene therapy for vascular proliferative disorders with a constitutively active form of the retinoblastoma gene product. Science 1995; 267 :518.

94. Stein CA, and Cheng YC. Antisense oligonucleotides as therapeutic agents- is the bullet really magical? Science 1993; 261: 1004.

95. Epstein SE, et al. Do antisense approaches to the problem of restenosis make sense? Circulation 1994; 88: 1351.

96. Pickering JG, et al. Prevention of smooth muscle cell outgrowth from human atherosclerotic plaque by a recombinant cytotoxin specific for the epidermal growth factor receptor. J Clin Invest 1993;91: 724.

97. Ortu P, et al. Photodynamic therapy of arteries. A novel approach for treatment of experimental intimal hyperplasia. Circulation 1992;85:1189.

98. Ferns GAA, et al. Inhibition of neointimal smooth muscle accumulation after angioplasty by an antibody to PDGF. Science 1991;253:1129.

99. Epstein SE, et al. The basis of molecular strategies for treating coronary restenosis after angioplasty. J Am Coll Cardiol 1994; 23: 1278.

33 BALLOON MITRAL VALVULOPLASTY

Christodoulos I. Stefanadis, Pavlos K. Toutouzas

History

As several balloon catheter intervention techniques were developing, the first report of balloon valvuloplasty as is performed today was by Kan and associates in 1982.[1] Two years later, Inoue[2] was the first to perform percutaneous mitral valvuloplasty (PMV) using his special balloon-catheter. Shortly thereafter, Lock et al[3] introduced PMV in the United States. As a variant to these transseptal techniques, Babic et al[4], employed a retrograde transarterial introduction of the balloon catheter and Al Zaibag[5] and Palacios[6] modified the transseptal technique by introducing the double balloon technique. All these variations involve transseptal catheterization. A purely retrograde approach for balloon mitral valvuloplasty, the retrograde nontransseptal balloon mitral valvuloplasty (RNBMV) was developed by Stefanadis et al[7-13] and first described in 1990.

Techniques

Transseptal

The transseptal *antegrade* approach employs standard transseptal technique to cross the atrial septum. A transfer guide wire is advanced through the atrial septum puncture and positioned either to the left atrium[14] or to the descending aortas.[3] A 14 F dilator[14] or 5- or 8-mm balloon dilating catheter[3,15] is used to dilate the atrial septum puncture and facilitate advancing the larger valvuloplasty balloon catheter. Thereafter, the valvuloplasty balloon catheter is advanced over the transfer guide wire and positioned across the mitral valve. Multiple dilations are performed to dilate the stenotic mitral valve. Variations of this technique include use of two balloons placed through either one[6] or two[8] separate transseptal punctures and use of a twin balloon catheter.[16]

In the transseptal _retrograde_ approach[4], after the guide wire has been advanced transseptally from the one femoral vein to the aorta, it is snared using a wire loop introduced from the opposite femoral artery, and drawn out the femoral artery. The balloon dilating catheter is introduced through the femoral artery and advanced over the guide wire to the mitral valve.

Nontransseptal

Attempts for purely retrograde approach employing conventional[17] or preshaped[18] catheters have had limited use, probably due to inconsistent entering to the left atrium. An effective technique for purely retrograde BMV has been described by Stefanadis et al.[7-13] This technique employs the use of a steerable cardiac catheter of which the tip may be configured into the desired form by external manipulations *(Figure 33.1).*[19] This catheter which was designed by Dr. Stefanadis and developed in the Department of Cardiology of the University of Athens, is a modification of commercially available standard catheters and accessories for coronary angiography and percutaneous coronary angioplasty. Modifications are made by the technical staff of our institution. The external diameter of the catheter is 7 to 9F, its usable length is 110cm, and the configuration of its tip may be altered by means of the external manipulations of a steering arm. The latter consists of a teflon coated, stainless steel wire, 0.014" in diameter, which passes along the lumen and emerges

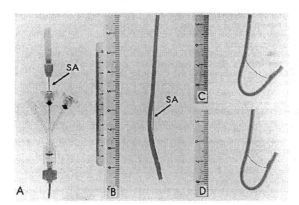

*Figure 33.1 The steerable guiding catheter used for retrograde left atrial catheterization. Manipulation of the steering arm enables the configuration of the distal part of the catheter to be altered by remote control. **Panel A:** Proximal part, showing the two hemostatic valves, the rotator, and the steering arm (SA). **Panel B:** Distal part in extended configuration. **Panel C:** Distal part in intermediate configuration. **Panel D:** Distal part in curved configuration. Reproduced from ref. 10 with permission.*

a short distance from the catheter tip. The wire is attached to the exterior of the catheter, close to its tip. The proximal end of the catheter is connected to a system of two hemostatic valves: the steering arm passes through one of these and the other may be used for the insertion of a guidewire into the catheter lumen. Of the three available sizes of this catheter (catheter tip: 1.7cm long in the small size; 2.2cm in the medium; 3cm in the large) that may be used, depending on the size of the left ventricle in individual patients, the medium and the small models have the advantage that they can be more easily curved and manipulated within the left ventricle. The medium model is effective in over 95 % of the cases.

All patients undergo right and left heart catheterization and left ventriculography before and immediately after valvuloplasty, and measurement of cardiac output, calculation of mitral valve orifice area, and grading of mitral regurgitation are performed. In all patients over 40 years elective coronary arteriography is performed routinely.

Under local anesthesia, two arterial sheaths are placed, a 9F in the right and a 6F in the left femoral artery; the latter is used for the continuous monitoring of arterial pressure. A pacing catheter is placed in the right ventricle via a sheath in the femoral vein. Following biplane left ventriculography in the RAO45° and LAO45° projections, two frames, one from each projection, are frozen to facilitate the manipulations of the steerable catheter toward the left atrium. A J tip exchange guidewire (0.035" or 0.038", 260cm in length) is advanced to the left ventricle with the aid of a pigtail catheter, using the right artery femoral route. The hemostatic valve that stabilizes the steering arm of the steerable left atrial catheter is released, and the catheter tip is straightened. The pigtail catheter is removed and the steerable left atrial catheter is then advanced to the left ventricle over the guidewire which passes through the second hemostatic valve. The tip of the guidewire is then withdrawn slightly into the catheter lumen and the steering arm is retracted, causing the catheter tip to form a curve close to the apex of the left ventricle. The curve is fixed in position by tightening the hemostatic valve, through which the steering arm passes. At the same time, heparin (100 IU/kg) is administered. Following counterclockwise rotation of the catheter, the plane of the curve is rotated so as the catheter tip to point toward the mitral valve. If necessary, the angle of the curvature is slightly readjusted, depending on the position of the mitral valve as determined from two frozen ventriculographic projections. The catheter is then retracted until its tip reaches a point immediately below the anterior mitral valve leaflet *(Figure 33.2)*. Either the recording of the left atrial pressures through the catheter, or the unobstructed movement of the J wire through the catheter lumen into the left atrial cavity, confirm the correct position of the catheter.

Difficulties may be encountered when the catheter tip is misplaced, towards either the outflow tract of the ventricle or the free ventricular wall. In the former case, the catheter is advanced a short distance towards the apex and rotated slightly clockwise, while the curve is opened. In the latter, the catheter is withdrawn slightly and rotated counterclockwise, and the curve is slightly tightened. Should these maneuvres be unsuccessful, the curve of the catheter is completely released, the catheter is moved toward the apex and the procedure is repeated from the beginning. All the above manipulations are performed under fluoroscopy using the same predetermined projections as in the left ventriculography.

Once the catheter has been placed correctly, the guidewire is inserted into the left atrium and is stabilized, either by forming spirals within the left atrial cavity, or by being introduced into a proximal branch of a pulmonary vein *(Figure 33.2)*. Both the hemostatic valves of the atrial catheter are then released and the atrial catheter is removed; a pigtail catheter is introduced over the guidewire into the atrium and atrial pressures are recorded.

After left atrial catheterization and recording of atrial pressures, a stiffer guide wire (0.035", J tip, heavy duty) is inserted into the atrium through the pigtail catheter and stabilized as above. The pigtail catheter is then removed.

As a final check on the route of the guidewire, a flow-directed catheter is introduced over this wire into the left ventricle. The balloon is inflated in the outflow tract of the left ventricle with a dilute dye solution and advanced toward the mitral valve. If this movement is unobstructed, it proves that the guidewire passes correctly through the inflow tract of the ventricle and has not become involved with the chordae tendineae *(Figure 33.3)*.

Thereafter, the right femoral arterial sheath is replaced with either a 14 F sheath or an adjustable introducer (Medina - Schneider, Europe) and the balloon catheter is advanced over the guide wire under fluoroscopy and positioned across the mitral valve. The balloon is then inflated by hand until the waist of the balloon at the level of the mitral valve disappears *(Figure 33.4)*. Although the same technique can be employed with two different balloon catheters using both femoral arteries, this bifemoral technique is not presently preferred because current balloon technology meets every demand.

After the removal of the balloon catheter, the hemodynamic measurements are repeated. Cine left ventriculography is also repeated in all patients to assess any change in mitral regurgitation severity.

On completion of the hemodynamic and ventriculographic measurements, protamine sulphate is administered; the patients are kept in the intensive care unit and the sheaths are removed. Hemostasis is performed by compression applied initially by hand for about 10 minutes and then by a controlled pressure device, so that the arterial pulse can be felt in the lower leg, until complete hemostasis is achieved. Most patients are discharged 24 hours after the procedure. If there are any arterial or other complications, the patients remains under observation; most are discharged 1 day later.

Selection of the size of the balloon catheters: For the *transseptal techniques* the most widely used balloon catheter worldwide is the Inoue balloon catheter. For this particular balloon catheter a stepwise dilatation technique is used.[14] The balloon is at first inflated to a diameter that depends on the quality of the valve and the body

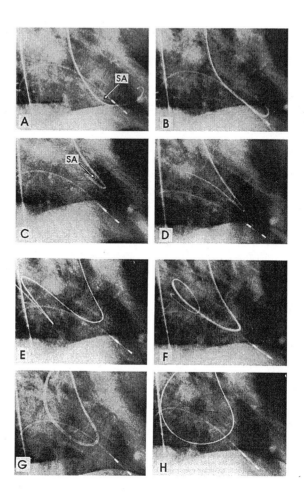

Figure 33.2 *Ventriculographic frames during retrograde left atrial catheterization (right anterior oblique projection).* **Panel A:** *Placement of the steerable left atrial catheter in the left ventricle.* **Panel B:** *The steering arm is retracted and the catheter tip is curved.* **Panel C:** *By counterclockwise rotation and retraction of the catheter, the plane of the curve is rotated until the catheter tip points toward the mitral valve; then, the catheter is retracted until its tip reaches a point immediately below the anterior mitral valve leaflet.* **Panel D:** *Introduction of a standard J guide wire into the left atrium.* **Panel E:** *The guidewire forms a spiral within the left atrium. The steerable left atrial catheter has been retracted.* **Panel F.** *A pigtail catheter is introduced into the left atrium over the guidewire.* **Panel G:** *The pigtail catheter within the left atrium. The guidewire has been retracted.* **Panel H:** *The long stiff guidewire is introduced and stabilized into the left atium. SA: steering arm. Reproduced from ref. 10 with permission.*

size of the patient. In subsequent inflations the balloon diameter is increased by 1 to 4 mm at a time, depending on conditions of the mitral valve, until satisfactory hemodynamic results are obtained or mild mitral regurgitation develops. For other balloon catheters it has been proposed that the choice of the balloon should be based upon the ratio: effective balloon dilating area / body surface area.[20] The optimal ratio for a given patient should be between 3.1 cm^2/m^2 and 4.0 cm^2/m^2.

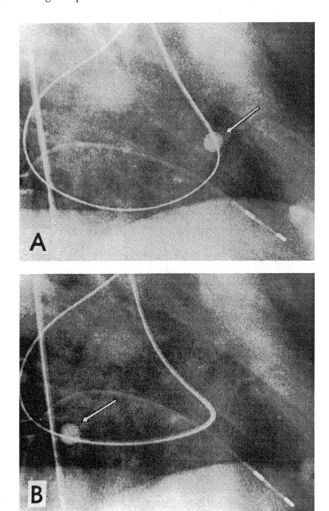

Figure 33.3 Ventriculographic projection shows test for correct insertion of the guidewire. Free movement of an inflated Swan-Ganz balloon shows that there is no involvement with the cordae tendineae (right anterior oblique projection). **Panel A:** *The baloon (arrow) is inflated in the outflow region of the left ventricle.* **Panel B:** *The balloon moves freely through the mitral valve into the left atrium. Reproduced from ref. 10 with permission.*

For the _retrograde nontransseptal technique_ the main factors taken into consideration are the diameter of the mitral valve annulus and the quality of the mitral valve. In general, balloon catheters of smaller diameter than those used in the transseptal techniques appear to be effective.[8,9] In case of a suboptimal result after the first dilation, and provided that there is no prohibiting mitral regurgitation, redilation is performed with a larger balloon catheter. However, in most cases the first dilation is adequate to achieve a successful result. In poor quality valves the first dilation is performed with a smaller balloon catheter than that used in good quality valves and the same stepwise approach is followed.

Mechanism

As demonstrated in pathologic and echocardiographic studies, the mechanism by which PMV relieves mitral stenosis is the same with that of surgical commissurotomy, that being the separation of the mitral leaflets along the fused commissures. In

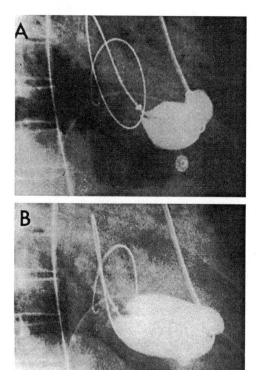

Figure 33.4 Ventriculographic projections of initial (panel A) and final (panel B) stages of a double valvuloplasty balloon in the stenotic mitral valve (right anterior oblique projection). Reproduced from ref. 8 with permission.

addition, fracturing of calcium deposits by the inflating balloon, may increase the flexibility of the mitral valve orifice. In this respect, the effectiveness of PMV is limited in cases with restricted valvular mobility caused by valve fibrosis or subvalvular disease. Complications such as leaflet tears, separation of the mitral valve leaflet and rupture of cordae, papillary muscle and mitral annulus may result from the inflation of oversized balloons.[15,21]

Effectiveness

Immediate results

In the majority of the patients a significant immediate hemodynamic and clinical improvement is accomplished with PMV. Mean mitral valve area (Figure 33.5) and cardiac output increase immediately after PMV, while transmitral gradient, mean left atrial pressure and mean pulmonary artery pressure decrease. Pulmonary vascular resistance also decreases after PMV and continues to fall gradually over the next 24 hours after the procedure.[4,8-14,22-28]

The increase in mitral valve area after PMV is inversely related to the echocardiographic score. In this score, valve rigidity, valve thickening, valve calcification, and subvalvular fibrosis are graded from 0 (least) to 4 (most) and summed.[29] Immediate outcome of PMV has been reported to be also directly related to balloon size

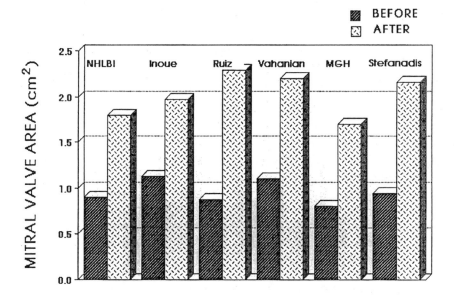

Figure 33.5 Mean mitral valve area before and after percutaneous mitral valvuloplasty in several series. (MGH: Massachussets General Hospital; NHLBI: National Heart, Lung and Blood Institute).

and inversely related to older age, evidence of calcium under fluoroscopy, valvular thickening, subvalvular fibrosis, presence of atrial fibrillation, presence of mitral regurgitation before the procedure and NYHA class before the procedure.[8-14,22-25,27]

Short-term results

Short-term clinical outcome reveals excellent symptomatic improvement in the majority of the patients.[23,25,27,30] Clinical and haemodynamic evidence of restenosis develops in a relatively low percentage of the patients undergoing the procedure. Restenosis is a time dependent event and it is better evaluated in long-term studies.

Long-term outcome

PBV provides an ongoing improvement in clinical status in the majority of the patients. Restenosis rates vary from 2.4% to 50% in follow-up studies ranging from 2 to 5 years in duration.[4,8-9,11-13,31-34] However, studies are not directly comparable because definition of restenosis and method of assessment vary among investigators. Besides, patient selection influences rates of restenosis as several risk factors for restenosis have been identified. Echocardiographic score (especially calcification and leaflet mobility), age, atrial fibrillation and smaller valve area after the procedure have been associated with higher rates of restenosis.[31-34]

The restenosis after closed or open surgical commissurotomy has been reported to be low.[34] Because of similarities in patient selection and mechanism of valve dilatation, it can be anticipated that PMV will share the same favorable long-term results with surgical comissurotommy.

Major event-free survival rates provide a more clear idea of the long-term outcome of PMV. Hung et al[35] showed a 100% cardiovascular event-free survival rate up to 42 months in patients with pliable, noncalcified valves, while the rate for patients with calcified valves and/or severe subvalvular lesions was 91 % at 12 months and held at 76% from 24 to 31 months. Pan et al[34] reported an overall five-year major event-free (death, restenosis and valve surgery) probability of 85%. The best results were obtained in patients with noncalcified valves and sinus rhythm (five-year major event-free probability: 95%), while the presence of atrial fibrillation and valve calcification before treatment determined an event-free probability of 60%. Cohen et al[26] demonstrated an estimated overall five-year survival rate of 76% and an estimated five-year event-free survival rate (absence of mitral valve replacement, repeat valvuloplasty, death from cardiac causes) of 51%. Analysis indentified as independent factors for predicting an unfavorable outcome mitral valve area after the procefure, mitral valve echocardiographic score, NYHA functional class and left ventricular end-diastolic pressure. Thus, long term outcome might be considered as a function of the adequacy of the initial balloon valvuloplasty, influenced by independent factors such as the progressive rennarrowing of the dilated valve (as predicted by the echocardiographic score) and progression of coexisting cardiovascular disease (as reflected by the left ventricular end-diastolic pressure and NYHA class).

Complications

The main complications of PMV are shown in *Table 33.1* with their incidence in several studies.[4,8-9,11,13-14,23-27,36]

Death

The main complication resulting in death is cardiac perforation and the development of cardiac tamponade, while other causes of death are systemic or cerebrovascular embolization, development of severe acute mitral regurgitation and right heart failure secondary to an increase in pulmonary hypertension during PMV in patients with severe pulmonary vascular obstructive disease. Mortality rates are comparable to that of surgical commissurotomy[36] and are related to patient selection and operator's experience.

Cardiac tamponade

This serious, albeit rare, complication may result from perforation of the heart as a complication of transseptal catheterization or from ventricular perforation caused by the guide wires or the dilating balloon catheters which may slip towards the apex of the left ventricle during inflation. Interestingly, in RNBMV incidence of haemopericardium or tamponade is zero. One reason for this is the avoidance of transseptal catheterization. In addition, the guide wire remains stabilized within the left atrium throughout the procedure, and therefore, it is difficult for the balloon to slip from the mitral orifice during dilation. However, even if this occurs, the balloon tends to move along the guidewire into the atrium rather than back into the left ventricle. Besides, the position of the guide wire within the left ventricle rules out the possibility of damage to the ventricular apex during insertion of the balloon catheter, because the catheter tip, constrained by the guidewire, never approaches this part of the heart.

Mitral regurgitation

Mild mitral regurgitation occurs in a large proportion of the patients undergoing PMV and it is well tolerated during follow-up. Severe mitral regurgitation is much less frequent *(Table 33.1)* and can be caused by tearing of the mitral leaflets and rupture of cordae or a papillary muscle. Severe mitral regurgitation has been reported to be higher with the Inoue technique compared to double balloon techniques[24]; however, stepwise dilatation and evaluation by color Doppler after each dilatation may reduce this incidence.

Table 33.1   SERIOUS COMPLICATIONS AFTER BALLON MITRAL VALVULOPLASTY

	Death (%)	Tamponade (%)	Mitral Regurgitation (severe %)	Lfet-to-right atrial shunt (%)	Embolic events (%)	Myocardial infarction (%)	Vascular (%)
NHLBI[36] (αρ.=738)	1,6	4	3	10[α]	3	1	1,2
M-Καρδιά[23] (αρ.=74)	2,7	9,3	13	7[β]	6,8	1,4	8
Inoue[14] (αρ.=527)	0	1,5	1,9	12,5[γ]	0,6	NR	0
Ruiz[24] (αρ.=407)	1,2	0,75	7,2	2,2[α]	1	NR	NR
Babic[4] (αρ.=294)	0,7	1,7	2,3	0	2,4	0,34	2,4
Vahanian[25] (αρ.=200)	0	0,25	6,5	4[α]	4	0	0,5
Cohen[26] (αρ.=146)	0,7	4,1	1,5	NR	2[ε]	NR	NR
ΓΝΜ[27] (αρ.=100)	1	2	1	4[δ]	2	NR	NR
Στεφανίδης (αρ.=200)	0,5	0	3,5	0	0	0	1,5

a = Q_p/Q_s >1,5; b = Q_p/Q_s >1,3; c = Q_p/Q_s >1,4; d = Q_p/Q_s >2; e = cerebrovascular only; MGH = Massachusetts General Hospital; NHLBI = National Heart, Lung and Blood Institute; NR = Not Reported

Atrial septal defect

Left-to-right atrial shunting is a very frequent finding immediately after transseptal PMV, detected in as much as 87%[37] of the cases if a sensitive method (such as transesophageal color flow echocardiography or green dye dilution curves) is used. However, the hemodynamically significant shunts are not as common *(Table 33.1)*. Factors predicting a shunt after valvuloplasty are smaller increases in valve area after valvuloplasty, absence of previous mitral commissurotomy, mitral valve calcification, smaller left atria and low cardiac output.[38-39] Mechanisms by which the tear in the interatrial septum is created, include dilatation of the interatrial seprum by the 5 or 8 mm balloon dilating catheters at the initial stage of the procedure, sawing motion of the balloon catheter shaft during inflation, excesive traction applied to the guide wire (retrograde transseptal technique)[4], inflation of the balloon catheter with the tail of the balloon across the atrial septum especially in small atria, and withdrawal of not fully deflated balloon catheters after valvuloplasty, the latter being perhaps the most important. Of course, when manipulations are prolonged and vigorous, the impact of these mechanisms is maximized. In a large number of patiens these shunts decrease in severity and in some they disappear at short term follow-up.[37-39] Considerations, however, remain about their clinical consequenses at a later stage. Mitral stenosis recurs eventually in a number of patients and, provided that the hole in the interatrial septum persists, this will lead either to the reappearance of shunts that had disappeard with time or to the deterioration of the existing ones. Besides, the clinical recognition of restenosis could be delayed in these patients because the presence of the atrial septal defect would tend to decompress the left atrium. Development of pulmonary hypertension remains always a possibility in these patients if recurrent mitral stenosis is not relieved.

Paradoxical embolization is also a potential complication.[40] Although no confirmed cases of this complication have been reported, the zero incidence of the purely retrograde techniques[8-13] compared to the considerable percentages of the other techniques[4,14,23-27,36] *(Table 33.1)* implies that paradoxical embolization may have occured in some patients.

The atrial septal defect may also affect the acuracy of the assessment of mitral valve area after valvuloplasty by hemodynamic measurements[40-42]

Some investigators envisaged in the use of "umbrellas" or other devices to close the atrial septal defect,[39] while others[40], when RNBMV was in an early stage, envisaged in the perfection of the retrograde approach.

Embolic events

Embolism may result from dislodgment of left atrial thrombus or debris from the mitral valve. Extreme care should be taken in the detection of left atrial thrombus before the procedure, especially in patients with atrial fibrillation. High risk patients should undergo meticulous anticoagulation. Gas embolism may also occur as a result of balloon rupture.

Vascular complications

Vasular complications related to the insertion of large sheaths and/or the introduction of the balloon catheters through the femoral vein (transseptal techniques) or artery (retrograde techniques) are infrequent and rarely surgical intervention is needed *(Table 33.1)*. The incidece of major injury to the femoral artery in the retrograde techniques is significantly lower compared to aortic valvuloplasty probably because patients are relatively young and mitral stenosis is not associated with generalized atherosclerosis as is aortic stenosis.

Learning curve

PMV is a procedure that demands adequate skills and experience on the part of the operator. Likelihood of a successful result is related to the experience of the operator. On the other hand, although PMV is effective in relieving the hemodynamic effects of rheumatic mitral stenosis, it does have important risks. The incidence of complications, including serious ones such as death, perforation and the development of cardiac tamponade, decrease with increasing experience.[36,43,44] It is of note that in the NHBLI registry where many centers participated, the incidence of death was significantly lower in high case volume centers compared to low volume ones (0.3% vs.2%).[36] Therefore, the performance of PMV should be limited in selected centers performing transseptal catheterization in sufficient volume to maintain adequate skills. RNBMV should also be performed by experienced operators. However, although there are no comparative studies, it appears that it has a fast learning curve[13] as it does not involve transseptal catheterization, and it can be performed in centers with no experience in the performance of atrial septum puncturing.

Cost

In countries where rheumatic mitral valve disease continues to be endemic and PMV could contribute significantly in the treatment by complementing the surgical approaches, important financial obstacles restrict considerably its application. In developing countries the cost of balloon mitral valvuloplasty is far greater than that of closed surgical commissurotomy, largely because of the cost of disposables. Conversely, in developed countries the cost of closed surgical commissurotomy is double that for PMV mainly due to physicians' fees and room charges.[45] RNBMV appears to have lower cost as it does not require the set for transseptal catheterization and the cost of the special catheter is expected to be low.

Which patient should undergo balloon mitral valvuloplasty?

All patients with symptomatic mitral stenosis are potential candidates for PMV. The two absolute contraindications for PMC are severe ($\geq 3+$) mitral regurgitation and the presence of a left atrial thrombus which should be ruled out by transesophageal echocardiography since transthoracic echocardiography is not very reliable. In case of left atrial thrombus and providing that the clinical and haemodynamic status of the patient does not warrant immediate surgery, a 2 to 3 months of anticoagulation therapy with warfarin is indicated with repeat echocardiographic examination thereafter. Anticoagulation therapy for 2 to 3 months should also receive patients with atrial fibrillation since they are very likely to have left atrial thrombus. A relative contraindication is a recent embolic event.

Even though predictors for immediate effectiveness consist a basis for selection of patients, a selection according to the long-term outcome appears to be a more appropriate approach. Accordingly, patients with mitral stenosis fall into the following categories:

1) Patients with low echocardiographic score. Patients with pliable noncalcified valves are the ideal candidates for PMV. The long-term outcome in this group of patients is excellent and PMV reflects the method of choice. In case of restenosis repeat BMV can still be performed with satisfactory results.

2) Patients with high echocardiographic score. Patients in this group with no or only one risk factor for an unfavorable outcome have a long-term outcome not as favorable as that of mitral valve replacement. However, PMV has several advantages over surgery, such as lower morbidity and procedure-related mortality, and avoidance of the risks of anticoagulation thromboembolism, infection and reoperation. Therefore, consideration of the individualized surgical risk will indentify these patients within this subgroup in whom PMV constitutes an appealing approach that defers mitral valve replacement for several years.[26]

3) Patients with multiple risk factors. As indicated by the poor long-term outcome, patients in this subgroup should be treated by mitral valve replacement. However, if these patients are deemed unsuitable candidates for surgery, PMV can still be performed as a palliative procedure.

4) Patients with restenosis after surgical commissurotomy. Incidence of restenosis after surgical commissurotomy varies from 10 to 30% over long-term follow-up.[46] Repeat surgical commissurotomy has been associated with greater mortality and morbidity than with the initial operation. PMV has shown to be an effective and safe procedure in this subgroup of patients.[46-47] Young patients in sinus rhythm, with less echocardiographic evidence of rheumatic mitral valve damage, are the ones that benefit most from the procedure.[47] Indentification of previous surgical commissurotomy as a predictor for unfavorable long-term outcome after PMV is controversial. Pan et al[34] reported a higher incidence of restenosis in patients with prior surgical commissurotomy, while Cohen et al[26] did not indentify this characteristic as as an unfavorable predictor for long-term outcome. However, even if restenosis is higher in these patients it remains to be answered if this implies an individual behavior or a more aggresive rheumatic disease that would influence unfavorably a reoperation as well.

5) Subclinical mitral stenosis. As previously noted, the anticipated benefits of PMV are far more beneficial if the quality of the valve is better and the age younger. Therefore, in experienced centers where the risks are minimized, an intervention at an earlier -even subclinical- stage of the disease, when the valve is pliable and non-calcific and there is no coexisting cardiovascular disease, appears justified. Provided that recurrent attacks of rheumatic fever are avoided, a future surgery would not only be defered but even overruled. This perspective applies most to very special subgroups of patients like young women who wish to become pregnant; PMV has been also applied to women that are already pregnant,[48] however, the benefit-to-risk ratio has not yet been determined.

6) Elderly patients. In developed countries elderly patients consist an important proportion of the patients who undergo PMV. In this group of patients PMV can be performed effectively with an acceptable risk in selected patients.[49-50] Elderly patients with low echocardiographic score and fluoroscopically invisible valvular calcification are the ones that benefit most, whereas it is better to refer patients with a high echocardiographic score and calcified valves for surgery. However, if the individualized surgical risk is high, PMV can still be a desirable palliative option in this latter subgroup of elderly patients.[50]

7) Concomitant valve disease. Combined aortic and mitral involvement is the most common pathologic finding in rheumatic heart disease and very often aortic regurgitation and mitral stenosis coexist in the same patient. Although there is debate on whether or not PMV has a beneficial effect in this subgroup of patients where the already volume-overloaded left ventricle might not tolerate an increase in inflow or a possible production or increase in mitral regurgitation, recent studies have shown that these patients are suitable candidates for PMV.[51]

Which technique?

Undoubtedly, PMV is an effective and safe procedure in experienced hands regardless of the technique used. However, there are certain cases where a particular technique has potential limitations. The *transseptal* techniques should not be preferred in cases where transseptal catheterization is difficult and risky, such as in patients that have undergone heart surgery and the anatomy of the heart may thus be changed or the interatrial septum may be thickened, or in patients with malformation of the chest where the usual landmarks are invalid. There are also concerns regarding the performance of the transseptal techniques in cases where the risk of embolism (paradoxical?) is high, such as in patients with a history of cerebrovascular, pulmonary or systemic embolism or in patients with pulmonary hypertension. On the other hand, the *retrograde* techniques are technically impossible in patients with an aortic mechanical prosthesis. These techniques have also the potential risk for arterial damage or may even be technically impossible in patients with severe atherosclerotic lesions in the femoral and the iliac arteries or in patients who have undergone vascular operation in the femoral or iliac arteries.

Conclusion

PMV is a nonsurgical treatment for mitral stenosis that has excellent short-and long-term results and low risk in experienced hands, being the treatment of choice in selected groups of patients. Future application of intracardiac imaging techniques, such as intracavitary echocardiography, will facilitate evaluation of risks and optimize the effectiveness and safety of this therapeutic modality. At present, it is anticipated that the nontransseptal retrograde approach will help broaden the application of PMV as it can be performed with excellent effectiveness and safety by interventional cardiologists who are not trained in the performance of transseptal catheterization.

Acknowledgement

The authors wish to express gratitude for the excellent assistance provided by Dr. Charalambos Vlachopoulos.

REFERENCES

1. Kan JS, et al. Percutaneous balloon valvuloplasty. A new method for treating pulmonary valve stenosis. New Engl J Med 1982:307:540.
2. Inoue K, et al. Clinical application of transvenous mitral commissurotomy by a new balloon catheter. J Thorac Cardiovasc Surg 1984:87:394.
3. Lock JE, et al. Percutaneous catheter commissurotomy in rheumatic mitral stenosis. N Engl J Med 1985:313:1515.
4. Babic UU, et al. Percutaneous transarterial balloon dilatation of the mitral valve: five year experience. Br Heart J 1992:67:185.
5. Al Zaibag M, et al. Percutaneous double balloon mitral valvotomy for rheumatic mitral valve stenosis. Lancet 1986:1:757.
6. Palacios I, et al. Percutaneous balloon valvotomy for patients with severe mitral stenosis. Circulation 1987:75:778.
7. Stefanadis C, et al. Percutaneous balloon mitral valvuloplasty by retrograde left atrial catheterization. Am J Cardiol 1990:65:650.
8. Stefanadis C, et al. Retrograde nontransseptal balloon mitral valvuloplasty. Immediate results and long-term follow-up. Circulation 1992:85:1760.
9. Stefanadis C, Toutouzas P. Retrograde nontransseptal mitral valvuloplasty. In Topol EJ (ed): Textbook of Interventional Cardiology, Philadelphia, WB. Saunders, 1994, 1253.
10. Stefanadis C, et al. Retrograde nontransseptal balloon mitral valvuloplasty using the Inoue balloon catheter. Catheterization and Cardiovascular Diagnosis 1994:33:224.
11. Stefanadis C, Toutouzas P, Balloon mitral valvuloplasty. A decade of experience. Eur Heart J 1995:16:1463.
12. Pitsavos C, et al. The accuracy of Doppler echocardiography for the estimation of mitral valve area after balloon mitral valvuloplasty. the role of iatrogenic atrial septal defect. Eur Heart J 1997 in press.
13. Stefanadis C, et al. Multicenter Experience with Retrograde Nontransseptal Balloon Mitral Valvuloplasty. Predictors for immediate and long-term outcome. Circulation 1996:94:1.

14. Inoue K, Hung JS. Percutaneous transvenou5 mitral commissurotomy (PTMC). The Far East experience, In Topol EJ (ed): Textbook of Interventional Cardiology, Philadelphia, WB. Saunders, 1990 , 887.

15. Block PC, Palacios IF. Aortic and mitral balloon valvuloplasty. The United States experience. In Topol EJ (ed): Textbook of Interventional Cardiology, Philadelphia, W B. Saunders, 1990, 831.

16. Berland J, et al. Balloon mitral valvotomy by using the twin-AT catheter. Immediate results and complications in 110 patients. Cathet Cardiovasc Diagn 1993:28:126.

17. Buchler JR, et al. Percutaneous mitral valvuloplasty in rheumatic stenosis by isolated transarterial approach : A new and feasible technique, Jpn Heart J 1987:28:790.

18. Orme EC, Wray RB, Mason JW. Balloon mitral valvuloplasty via retrograde left atrial catheterization. Am Heart J 1989:117:680.

19. Stefanadis C, et al. Retrograde left atrial catheterization with a new steerable cardiac catheter, Am Heart J 1990:119:375.

20. Roth RB , Block PC , Palacios IF. Predictors of increased mitral regurgitation after percutaneous mitral balloon valvotomy. Cathet Cardiovasc Diagn 1990:20:17.

21. Vahanian A, et al. Mitral valvuloplasty. The french experience. In Topol EJ (ed): Textbook of Interventional Cardiology, Philadelphia, WB. Saunders, 1990, 868.

22. The National Heart, Lung and Blood Institute Balloon Valvuloplasty Registry Participants: Multicenter experience with balloon mitral commissurotomy NHLBI balloon valvuloplasty registry report on immediate and 30-day follow-up results. Circulation 1992:85:448.

23. Herrmann HC, et al. The M-Heart percutaneous balloon mitral valvuloplasty registry. Initial results and early follow-up. J Am Coll Cardiol 1990:15:1221.

24. Ruiz CE, et al. Comparison of Inoue-single balloon versu5 double balloon techniques for percutaneous mitral valvotomy. Am Heart J 1992:123:942.

25. Vahanian A, et al. Results of percutaneous mitral commissurotomy in 200 patients. Am J Cardiol 1989:63:847.

26. Cohen DJ, et al. Predictors of long-term outcome after percutaneous balloon mitral valvuloplasty. N Engl J Med 1992:327:1329.

27. Palacios IF, et al: Follow-up of patients undergoing percutaneous mitral balloon valvotomy. Analysis of factors determining restenosis. Circulation 1989:79:573.

28. Levine MJ, et al. Progressive improvement in pulmonary vascular resistance after percutaneous mitral valvuloplasty Circulation 1989:79:1061.

29. Wilkins GT, et al. Percutaneous mitral valvotomy. An analysis of echocardiographic variables related to outcome and the mechanism of dilatation, Br Heart J 1988:60:299.

30. AI Zaibag M, et al. One-year follow-up after percutaneous double balloon mitral valvotomy Am J Cardiol 1989:63:126.

31. Block PC, et al. Late (two-year) follow up after percutaneous balloon mitral valvotomy, Am J Cardiol 1992:69:537.

32. Chen CR, et al. Long-term tesults of percutaneus mitral valvu loplasty with the 1 noue balloon catheter. Am J Cardiol 1992:70 :1445.

33. Desideri A, et al. Long-term (9 to 33 Month5) echocardiographic follow-up after successful percutaneous mitral commis5urotomy. Am J Cardiol 1992:69:1602.

34. Pan M, et al. Factors determining late success after mitral balloon valvotomy. Am J Cardiol 1993:71:1181.

35. Hung JS, et al. Short- and long- term results of catheter balloon percutaneous transvenous mitral commissurotomy. Am J Cardiol 1991:67:854.

36. The National Heart, Lung and Blood Institute balloon valvuloplasty registry. Complications and mortality of percutaneous balloon mitral commis5urotomy. Circulation 1992:85:2014.

37. Yoshida K, et al. Assessment of left-to-right atrial shunting following percutaneous mitral valvuloplasty by transesophageal color Doppler flow mapping, Circulation 1989:80:1521.

38. Cequier A, et al. Left-to-right atrial shunting after percutaneous mitral valvuloplasty. Incidence and long-term hemodynamic follow-up. Circulation 1990:81:1190.

39. Casale P, et al. Atrial septal defect after percutaneous mitral balloon valvuloplasty: Immediate results and follow-up. J Am Coll Cardiol 1990:15:1300.

40. Crawford MH. Iatrogenic Lutembacher's syndrome revisited. Circulation 1990:81:1422.

41. Otto CM, et al. Methodologic issues in clinical evaluation of stenosis severity in adults undergoing aortic or mitral balloon valvuloplasty. Am J Cardiol 1992:69:1607.

42. Manga P, et al. Mitral valve area calculations immediately after percutaneous balloon mitral valvuloplasty. Effect of the atrial septal defect. J Am Coll Cardiol 1993:21:1568.

43. Rihal CS, Nishimura RA, Holmes DR Jr. Percutaneous balloon mitral valvuloplasty'. the learning curve, Am Heart J 1991:122:1750.

44. Brandi-Pifano S, Palacios IF, Block PC, et al. Echophonocardiography in patients undergoing percutaneous mitral balloon valvotomy (PMV) : The learning curve of PMV, Am Heart J 1989:117:25.

45. Turi ZG, et al. Percutaneous balloon versus surgical closed commissurotomy for mitral stenosis. Circulation 1991:83:1179.

46. Serra A, et al. Balloon mitral commissurotomy for mitral restenosis after surgical commissurotomy. Am J Cardiol 1993:71:1311.

47. Rediker DE, et al. Mitral balloon valvuloplasty for mitral restenosis after surgical commissurotomy J Am Coll Cardiol 1988:11 :252.

48. Smith R, Brender D, McCredie M. Percutaneous transluminal balloon dilatation of the mitral valve in pregnancy, Br Heart J 1989:61:551.

49. Le Feuvre C, et al. Balloon mitral commissurotomy in patients aged > 70 years, Am J Cardiol 1993:71:233.

50. Tuzcu EM, et al. Immediate and long-term outcome of percutaneous mitral valvotomy in patients 65 years and older. Circulation 1992:85:963.

51. Chen CR, et al. Percutaneous balloon mitral valvuloplasty for mitral stenosis with and without associated aortic regurgitation. Am Heart J 1993:125:128.

Section G

ELECTROPHYSIOLOGY

34 PHARMACOLOGIC THERAPY OF ARRHYTHMIAS

John Kassotis, Roy Sauberman, James Coromilas

Disturbances of cardiac rhythm are often debilitating, recurrent and not uncommonly life threatening. The importance of an accurate diagnosis of arrhythmias and an understanding of the cellular mechanisms of arrhythmogenesis are crucial to successful treatment. Misdiagnosis of tachyarrhythmias can prove to be fatal. Over the last two decades we have refined our understanding of the mechanisms underlying cardiac arrhythmias. It no longer suffices to think of depolarization and repolarization of cardiac cells as a simple change in membrane resistance. The cardiac action potential is now understood in terms of the structural proteins which make up ion channels, which, in turn, control ion fluxes across the plasma membrane. Ideally, such a sophisticated understanding of arrhythmogenesis would lead to a more effective therapy. Unfortunately, our current knowledge of ion fluxes responsible for the cardiac action potential are based on normal tissue studies mostly in animal models. Correlating these results to abnormal tissue may not just be a simple extrapolation. Tissue abnormalities are essential for the initiation and propagation of various tachyarrhythmias. In addition, derangements in tissue structure, e.g. post infarction, alter the properties of the ion channels.

Suffice it to say that antiarrythmic drug therapy remains in a state of considerable flux. Despite a better understanding of the mechanisms of arrhythmias and an increased variety of therapeutic agents, treatment at the bedside is often empirical. With a more complex array of therapeutic agents, it has become apparent that a more precise classification system is necessary. The traditional Vaughan Williams classification system[1] has been increasingly scrutinized in favor of a more channel specific approach, as proposed by the Sicilian Gambit.[2] The Vaughan Williams classification highlights the most dominant action of each agent. However, since antiarrhythmic agents commonly act on multiple channels simultaneously, classification of an individual agent into a single class is both imprecise and misleading. In principle one should be able to select a specific drug to terminate an arrhythmia with a known mechanism. Unfortunately, this is not always the case in practice due to the non-specific action of these agents and lack of precise knowledge of arrhythmia mechanisms.

Tachyarrhythmias

In general, an arrhythmia may result from enhanced normal automaticity, abnormal automaticity, triggered activity (e.g. early afterdepolarizations (EAD) or delayed afterdepolarizations (DADs) reentry or less commonly, reflection and parasystole. Each of the above mechanisms can be reelated to an abnormality, in tissue substrate, on either an ion channel, cellular or macroscopic level. Theoretically arrhythmias are vulnerable to drug actions which specifically correct or modify one of these abnormalities in tissue substrate.

Tachycardias are conventionally classified as supraventricular or ventricular. The majority of sustained arrhythmias are reentrant in nature.[3] Supraventricular tachycardias are most commonly associated with narrow QRS complexes (QRS < 0.10 sec), except when they occur in the context of a preexisting bundle branch block.[4] Although rarely life threatening, they are a significant source of morbidity. Excluding atrial fibrillation and atrial flutter, most supraventricular tachycardias can be classified as either long RP or short RP tachycardias. In the case of the long RP tachycardias, the P wave precedes the QRS complex, as opposed to, the short RP tachycardias where the P wave can be buried within or is in the ST segment or T wave following the QRS complex. The differential diagnosis of the various long and short RP tachycardias is summarized in *Table 34.1*. The ventricular tachycardias are classified as nonsustained ventricular tachycardias (NSVT), polymorphic ventricular tachycardia including torsade de pointes (TdP), sustained monomorphic VT, and ventricular fibrillation (VF). *Table 34.2* summarizes the more common tachyarrhythmias, highlighting their presumptive mechanisms of initiation, the substrate required for their propagation, and distinguishing electrocardiographic characteristics.

Supraventricular tachycardias

Reentrant supraventricular tachycardias are characterized as rapid arrhythmias sustained within circuits propagated across atrioventricular bypass tracts, slow and fast AV nodal pathways, or within the atrial myocardium. After sinus tachycardia and atrial fibrillation, atrioventricular (AV) nodal reentrant tachycardia is the most common cause of paroxysmal supraventricular tachycardia (PSVT) and is believed to require two functionally distinct pathways.[5-7] The substrate for AVNRT consists of fast and slow pathways, with the fast pathway characterized by a rapid conduction velocity and a relatively long refractory period. The slow pathway is typically characterized by slow antegrade conduction and a short refractory period. Typical AVNRT

Table 34.1 *SUPRAVENTRICULAR TACHYCARDIAS: DIFFERENTIAL DIAGNOSIS*

Short RP (RP < PR)	Long RP (RP > PR)
Typical AV nodal reentrant tachycardia	Sinus tachycardia
AV reentrant tachycardia	Sinus node rentrant tachycardia
Nonparoxysmal junctional tachycardia (NPJT)	Atrial tachycardia
	Permanent junctional reciprocating tachycardia (PJRT)
	Nonparoxysmal junctional tachycardia (NPJT)
	Atypical AV nodal reentrant tachycardia

is usually initiated by atrial premature depolarizations which block in the fast pathway and conduct slowly in the anterograde direction over the slow pathway. If anterograde conduction is sufficiently slow, recovery occurs in the fast pathway permitting retrograde conduction through a reentrant circuit resulting in tachycardia. Although such pathways may be present in aymptomatic individuals, only a small percentage of these individuals satisfy the necessary heterogeneity between pathways to support a reentrant tachycardia.[7] In atypical AVNRT the circuitry is reversed and the arrhythmia is usually initiated by a ventricular premature depolarization.[7] Of those individuals with AVNRT, 90 % present with the typical form, while the remaining 10 % of individuals present with the atypical variant.[7]

Unlike AVNRT, where both distinct pathways exhibit decremental conduction , atrioventricular reentrant tachycardia (AVRT) is characterized by rapid non-decremental conduction across accessory atrioventricular (AV) pathways. Of the patients presenting with AVRT 75 % of patients exhibit anterograde conduction down the accessory pathway allowing for ventricular preexcitation, characterized electrocardiographically by a short PR interval and a delta wave, thus satisfying criteria for the Wolff-Parkinson-White (WPW) syndrome. Approximately 25% of patients with AVRT will not show antegrade conduction over the bypass tract but will have AVRT maintained by retrograde conduction (concealed bypass tract). Patients with Wolff-Parkinson-White, usually present with an orthodromic tachycardia characterized by anterograde conduction down the AV node with fast retrograde conduction up the accessory pathway. Less commonly, patients with WPW exhibit antidromic AV reentry, with nondecremental anterograde conduction down the accessory pathway followed by retrograde conduction across the AV node. Antegrade conduction via a bypass tract may result in rapid ventricular responses in patients who develop atrial fibrillation or atrial flutter. Individuals with shortest RR interval between preexcited complexes of less than 250 msec characterizing the accessory pathway are considered at risk for sudden death, secondary to VF. [8,9] Therefore, in patients with WPW presenting with atrial fibrillation or flutter with a rapid ventricular response, catheter ablation of the pathway is recommended.

Table 34.2   *CHARACTERISTICS OF VARIOUS ARRHYTHMIAS*

Arrhythmia	Mechanism	Substrate	Distiguishing ECG Findings
Sinus Tachycardia	Automatic	Sinus Node	Upright P waves in II, III, aVF preceding each QRS difficult to discern above HR > 180 because of P waves fusing to preceding T wave
Sinus node reentrant tachycardia	Re-entry	Sinus node	P waves, RP > PR Same morphology as sinus
Atrial fibrillation	Random Re-entry	Atria Left > Right	Irregularly, irregular QRS pattern, no P waves
Atrial flutter	Re-entry	Atria Right Atria	Saw-toothed pattern, flutter waves at 300 bpm, 2:1 AV block
Atrial tachycardia	Atrial Re-entry Automatic Triggered (DADs)	Atria	Pure morphology depends on site of origin, with variable atrial rate
AV nodal re-entrant tachycardia	Re-entry	AV node and transitional atrial tissue	Typical - P waves hidden in QRS or just following the QRS providing a pseudo R' in VI, RP<PR Atypical-Inverted P waves in II, III, F RP>PR
AV re-entry	Re-entry	Bypass tracts	Orthodromic - (RP < PR) Antidromic - delta waves, wide QRS
Permanent Junctional Reciprocating Tachycardia	Re-entry	Decrementally Conducting Postero-Septal Bypass Tract	RP>PR, inverted p waves in II, III, AVF
Nonparoxysmal juctional tachycardia	Automatic	AV node	AV dissociation, gradual onset
Multifocal atrial tachycardia	Automatic ?DADs	Atria	Variable P-P, PR intervals > 3 distinct P wave morphologies
Ventricular tachycardia (sustained)	Re-entry	Ventricles	A-V dissociation, Fusion and/or Capture beats, RBBB>0.14 sec, LBBB>0.16 sec
Ventricular tachycardia (non-sustained)	?Automatic	Ventricles	**Monomorphic** - Uniform morphology of QRS complexes, >3 beats but <30 sec **Polymorphic** - Variable QRS morphology, > 3 beats but <30 sec
Ventricular fibrillation	Random Re-entry	Ventricles	Chaotic ventricular activity with no discernable QRS complexes
Torsade de pointes	Triggered (EADs) ? Re-entry	Ventricles	shifting of QRS axis about a a common baseline preceded by prolonged QTc

Less common forms of SVT include junctional tachycardia, sinus node reentry, as well as, unifocal and multifocal atrial tachycardia. Non-paroxysmal junctional tachycardia (NPJT) is caused by increased impulse generation within the AV junction.[10] Although a rare cause of SVT in adults, it is more commonly seen associated with valve surgery, inferior wall myocardial infarction, myocarditis, and digoxin toxicity.[11] Unlike AVNRT and AVRT, the onset and termination of junctional tachycardia (JT) is gradual. There is also an entity called the permanent form of junctional reciprocating tachycardia. This is an AVRT with retrograde conduction via a slow decrementally conducting posteroseptal accessory pathway. This arrhythmia is generally poorly controlled by drug therapy, incessant in nature, often producing a cardiomyopathy and is amenable to radiofrequency ablation.[12-14]

Sinus node reentry accounts for less than 5 % of patients who present with PSVT. The reentrant circuit incorporates the S-A node[15], and generates P waves which are typical for sinus rhythm. A distinguishing feature of such reentrant arrhythmia's is their abrupt onset and termination, as well as, a positive response to carotid sinus massage. This may be the only means of distinguishing this arrhythmia from sinus tachycardia.[7]

Atrial tachycardias include those supraventricular arrhythmias which find their origin outside the S-A node incorporating atrial muscle as the substrate for reentry. Sustained atrial tachycardia can occur because of increased automaticity, triggered mechanisms, or reentry. Atrial tachycardias are categorized as unifocal or multifocal. Unifocal atrial tachycardia is characterized by a single P wave morphology, the exact morphology depends on the site of origin. Individuals with reentry as the mechanism of unifocal atrial tachycardia typically have underlying structural heart disease, whereas in those individuals whose arrhythmia is due to enhanced automaticity may or may not have underlying heart disease. Atrial tachycardias due to increased automaticity are usually incessant predisposing the patient to the development of a tachycardia-induced cardiomyopathy. Reentrant atrial tachycardias are usually paroxysmal. Unifocal atrial tachycardia with AV block is a relatively uncommon rhythm disturbance, whose occurrence may serve as a marker of digitalis toxicity.[6]

In contrast, multifocal atrial tachycardia (MAT), an irregular rhythm, is characterized by at least three distinct P wave morphologies. Multifocal atrial tachycardias are more common in the elderly and in over 60 % of cases are associated with significant cardiopulmonary disease.[16] Multifocal atrial tachycardias are believed to be generated by enhanced automaticity, but, triggered activity due to delayed after depolarizations has also been postulated to be the mechanism of MAT.[17]

Atrial fibrillation (AF) is the most commonly encountered sustained tachycardia. Although rarely life threatening, it remains a significant source of morbidity, especially in the elderly. It is most commonly associated with the presence of valvular heart disease, hypertensive heart disease and LV dysfunction. At times the result of alcohol, toxic, and autonomic precipitants, it can also occur in the absence of structural heart disease (lone atrial fibrillation). Complications include embolic events, tachycardia-induced cardiomyopathy and syncope. Atrial fibrillation is usually symptomatic, with symptoms ranging from palpitations and dyspnea to sudden death in the setting of underlying WPW. The accepted mechanism is one of multiple reentrant wavefronts which randomly excite available non-refractory atrial tissue.[18] Alternatively a single dominant focus related to enhanced autonomic tone may yield random myocardial excitation due to alternating sites of refractoriness.[19]

Ventricular arrhythmias

Ventricular arrhythmias may be divided into categories of ventricular premature complexes (VPC), frequent monomorphic VPCs, polymorphic VPCs, non-sustained monomorphic ventricular tachycardia (NSVT), sustained ventricular tachycardias (VT), and ventricular fibrillation (VF).

Early emphasis focused on suppression of ventricular ectopy in patients hospitalized in intensive care units following a myocardial infarction (MI). The understanding of ventricular arrhythmias has advanced since it was initially proposed that the increased frequency of ventricular ectopy, in the acute MI setting, predicted progression to ventricular fibrillation.[20] It is now recognized that VPC frequency does not predict the progression to VF, within the first 24 to 48 hours following an acute myocardial infarction.[21] Lidocaine was often used routinely for arrhythmia prevention. It has now been recognized that lidocaine, although it suppresses VPCs and prevents VF in some patients, may increase the risk of conduction block and asystole in others.[22] As a result, routine lidocaine use has been abandoned in many centers, since it has been associated with an increased mortality in the acute MI setting [23,24] and is reserved for hemodynamically compromising rhythm abnormalities.

It was previously established that in the sub-acute phase of a myocardial infarction (pre-discharge), the frequency and complexity of VPCs was associated with an increased morbidity and mortality.[25] Frequent VPCs (> 10 /hr) were regarded as a continuum with more life-threatening VT or VF [26], thus, it seemed logical to institute drug therapy designed to suppress ventricular ectopy to prevent the progression to more serious life threatening tachycardias. However, this hypothesis was refuted with the results of the Cardiac Arrhythmia Suppression Trial (CAST), which established that suppressing ectopy, in those post-infarction atients with class IC therapeutic agents, resulted in an increase in both sudden death and cardiac death.[27,28]

At the present time, based on various factors including the presence or absence of structural heart disease, ventricular arrhythmias are classified as benign, those associated with increased risk and malignant. This classification system stratifies the rhythms in terms of their associated mortality. Of the many etiologic factors that predispose to ventricular arrhythmias, the two most commonly implicated are ischemia and organic heart disease. The presence of heart disease helps distinguish between benign arrhythmias and those with increased risk. In fact, the presence of frequent VPC's in patients with depressed LV function increases their mortality, as opposed to, the occurrence of NSVT in the absence of structural heart disease which does not adversely affect one's mortality.

Asymptomatic or minimally symptomatic VPCs in patients without structural heart disease are classified as benign, and most commonly occur as isolated complexes. Benign VPCs may occur in healthy individuals of all ages[29] with more frequent repetitive activity found in those individuals with coronary artery and valvular disease. Among Individuals with symptomatic VPCs, confirmed by Holter, treatment may be justified. In general, patients in this subset exhibit a good prognosis with long term follow-up and it remains to be seen if such arrhythmias are markers for future cardiovascular disease.

Higher risk ventricular arrhythmias, often referred to as potentially malignant, are observed in those patients who exhibit NSVT, defined as >3 successive VPCs but not exceeding 30 seconds . We avoid defining NSVT as potentially malignant since this phrase implies that the NSVTs are just shorter forms of the sustained VT which is usually not the case. These are usually found in patients with LV dysfunction secondary to CAD with prior MI or cardiomyopathy. At the present time one should view non-sustained VT as more than a self limited variant of sustained VT. This patient population has an increased risk of sudden cardiac death, and an overall increased mortality. Patients with NSVT in the context of CAD or CHF have a worsened prognosis.[30] There is no current evidence that morbidity or mortality is improved by suppressing these arrhythmias in asymptomatic individuals. This is the primary focus of the Multicenter Unsustained Tachycardia Trial (MUSTT), which is designed to identify those patients with NSVT that warrant therapy.[30]

Malignant ventricular arrhythmias include sustained ventricular tachycardia and ventricular fibrillation. It is now well established that usually the underlying mechanism responsible for ventricular tachycardia, in the context of CAD, and prior MI is re-entrant in nature.[3,31] The exact mechanism of VT in the context of dilated cardiomyopathy remains undetermined (? re-entrant). The stability of these circuits enables reproducible initiation of these arrhythmias by programmed electrical stimulation. Sustained VT is occasionally initiated by enhanced automaticity. Degeneration of VT to VF is a common cause of sudden cardiac death, second only to primary VF in the context of an acute MI. A history of sudden cardiac death (SCD) portends a significant risk of recurrence. The mortality rate increases as the LV systolic function worsens in these patients. Appropriate identification of such high risk patients and administration of prophylactic therapy may have an important impact on survival and decrease in the incidence of sudden cardiac death.

Torsade de pointes (TdP), a variant of polymorphic VT, is characterized by QRS complexes which alternate their axis around a common baseline. Although the exact mechanism remains elusive, current evidence points to triggered activity in the form of early afterdepolarizations (EADs), as the initiating mechanism [32-34]. Etiologic factors predisposing to this arrhythmia include: drug therapy (e.g. quinidine[35], procainamide[36], and sotalol[37]; electrolyte disturbances; subarachnoid hemorrhage[38], congenital Q-T prolongation[39]; as well as, a host of other associations.

Most important is the fact that many of our conventional therapeutic modalities exacerbate this arrhythmia.

Effective pharmacological therapy can be identified in 30 to 40 % of patients with sustained ventricular tachycardias, and a higher percentage of those patients with supraventricular tachycardia (SVT) respond to drug therapy. The primary focus of this chapter is to highlight the pharmacologic modalities available for antiarrhythmic therapy, and where appropriate comparing these to other therapeutic modalities. Most importantly we will highlight the role of pharmacologic therapy as a primary intervention or as adjunctive therapy.

Drugs with class I action: sodium channel antagonists

Class I agents represent the oldest and most extensively studied group of antiarrhythmic drugs. Despite individual differences in chemical structure and receptor binding kinetics, the major unifying feature of the class I agents is that they block the fast inward sodium current (I_{Na}) in both working cardiac muscle and in the specialized conducting system. This property accounts for a decrease in the maximum rate of depolarization and a slowing of conduction velocity. In addition, these drugs display use-dependence, exerting more inhibition of I_{Na} at more rapid rates of stimulation and following longer periods of increased excitation (e.g. during a sustained tachyarrhythmia).[40] The clinical consequences of sodium channel blockade include conduction slowing manifested as increased QRS duration.

The sodium channel antagonists have been divided into three subgroups, referred to as class IA, IB, and IC. This classification has been based upon the combination of the magnitude of sodium channel blockade and the effect on action potential duration.[41,41A] The magnitude of sodium channel blockade is determined by the kinetics of interaction of the drug with the sodium channel[1,2,42,42A,42B] and the effect on APD depends largely on associated potassium channel blockade.[43] Class IA agents prolong conduction velocity and APD in cardiac cells featuring normal resting membrane potentials. In contrast, class IB agents only depress conduction velocity in partially depolarized or ischemic myocardium while shortening the APD. Class IC agents depress the inward sodium current in both normal and depolarized myocardium without affecting the APD (see *Table 34.3*).

Class IA agents: quinidine, procainamide, and disopyramide

Class IA agents block I_{Na}, slowing Vmax and conduction velocity in Purkinje fibers at normal membrane resting potentials. Prolongation of the QRS is consistently observed with higher doses and plasma concentrations of the drugs. To varying degrees, these drugs possess anticholinergic activity, with disopyramide having the most and procainamide having the least atropine-like effects.[44,44A] The added anticholinergic effects may counter the negative chronotropic and dromotropic properties of sodium channel blockade in the sinus and AV nodes and may lead to a net increase in the sinus rate and/or AV nodal conduction. However, among atrial and

Table 34.3 SUBCLASSIFICATION OF CLASS 1 ANTIARRHYTHMIC DRUGS*

Subgroup	Drugs	Effects on Depolarization	Effects on Repolarization
Class 1A	Quinidine Procainamide Disopyramide	1. Moderate depression of Vmax 2. Moderate slowing of CV 3. QRS widening seen only at high doses	1. Prolongation of APD 2. Prolongation of refractory periods 3. Prolongation of QT interval independent of QRS widening
Class 1B	Lidocaine Mexiletine Tocainide	1. Selective depression of Vmax in ischemic myocardium 2. Selective slowing of CV in ischemic myocardium 3. Minimal QRS widening	1. No change or shortening of APD 2. No change or shortening of refractory periods 3. No change or shortening of QT interval
Class 1C	Flecainide Propafenone Moricizine**	1. Marked depression of Vmax 2. Marked slowing of CV 3. QRS widening	1. Minimal change in APD 2. Minimal change in refractory periods 3. Prolongation of QT interval due to QRS widening

* At therapeutic doses,
**Moricizine acts like a Class IC drug at high doses.

ventricular tissue which lack autonomic innervation, the primary sodium blocking properties of the drugs prevail, effectively suppressing abnormal automaticity and conduction. As a result, these agents remain useful in the treatment of atrial and ventricular premature depolarizations and reentrant tachycardias.

An additional property of the class IA drugs is that they block potassium channels responsible for the delayed rectifier current (I_{Kr}) in a manner similiar to the class III drugs.[43] By inhibiting the outward potassium current, these agents prolong the action potential duration, refractory periods, and the corrected QT interval on the surface EKG. As a result, these drugs are able to prolong refractoriness while slowing or preventing depolarized tissue from regaining excitability. This class III effect may complement the primary sodium channel blocking effects and enhance the antiarrhythmic efficacy of the class IA drugs.

The class IA compounds are useful in the treatment and prophylaxis of a variety of atrial and ventricular tachyarrhythmias. Most sustained regular tachyarrhythmias are believed reentrant in origin, requiring a triggering premature impulse, a site of unidirectional block through which the impulse might return, and an excitable gap exceeding the absolute refractory period of the tissue comprising the circuit. These drugs may theoretically abolish the substrate responsible for reentry either by suppressing premature depolarizations, impairing conduction so as to convert a region of unidirectional block to bidirectional block, or prolonging local refractoriness within a reentrant circuit beyond its excitable gap. These agents have also been found to increase mean refractoriness while decreasing dispersion of refractoriness across both atria by their class III and anticholinergic effects. Many common arrhythmias which are based upon a reentrant mechanism may be treated with class IA agents, including atrial flutter, atrial fibrillation, ectopic atrial tachycardia, AV nodal reentrant tachycardia, AV reciprocating tachycardia, and monomorphic ventricular tachycardia.

However, the combined actions of the class IA agents may lead to a temporary increase in the ventricular response prior to conversion of a supraventricular tachycardia to sinus rhythm. The anticholinergic properties of these drugs may promote acceleration of conduction through the AV node, while the sodium and potassium channel blocking effects lead to a reduction in the atrial rate, creating less concealed conduction and diminished refractoriness within the AV node. Consequently, when these drugs are used to treat a supraventricular tachyarrhythmia, it is recommended that they be given in conjunction with an AV nodal blocking agent, such as a beta-blocker, calcium channel blocker, or digoxin.

Quinidine. Quinidine is usually given orally to reduce the risk of dose-limiting side effects, including hypotension, observed with parenteral administration. Quinidine may be complexed with either sulfate, gluconate, or polygalacturonate to form short and long-acting oral compounds to provide near 70% absorption. However, there exist differences in the relative quinidine content between the various preparations with quinidine sulfate containing 83% active drug, quinidine gluconate containing 62% active drug, and quinidine polygalacturonate containing 60% active drug. Regardless of the preparation given, 70-80% of absorbed quinidine is metabolized in the liver with the remainder excreted unchanged in the urine. The elimination half-life is 5-8 hours, and the therapeutic plasma concentration is 3-8 µg/ml.[45] As with all antiarrhythmic therapy, it is often necessary to adjust the initial dosage according to therapeutic drug levels in order to maximize efficacy while minimizing toxicity (Table 34.4).

Potential cardiovascular side effects of quinidine include: hypotension, due to its α-adrenergic blocking action; exacerbation of preexisting heart failure, attributed to its negative inotropic properties; and proarrythmia (torsade de pointes), related to excessive prolongation of action potential duration and QT interval.[46A,46B,46C] Quinidine may increase digoxin levels in patients taking digoxin by reducing the clearance of digoxin, necessitating a reduction in their daily dose.[47] In addition, quinidine may enhance the effects of other negative dromotropic and hypotensive medications, including β-blocking and calcium channel blocking agents. Quinidine may potentiate the effects of coumadin therapy through hepatic interactions. Common noncardiac side effects include nausea, diarrhea, tinnitis, deafness, blurred vision, diplopia, headache, dizziness, confusional states, fever, drug-induced lupus, and autoimmune thrombocytopenia. Any drugs which induce the hepatic enzymes containing cytochrome P450, such as phenytoin, phenobarbital, and rifampin, will increase quinidine metabolism, reducing the plasma levels. In contrast, medications which suppress hepatic enzyme activity (e.g. cimetidine) decrease quinidine metabolism, increase plasma levels, and require reduction in the quinidine dose.[48]

Procainamide. Procainamide is available as either an intravenous or oral preparation. Intravenous procainamide is given as a bolus at a rate of 20-50 mg/min with careful monitoring for possible drug-induced hypotension or conduction block until termination of the arrhythmia is achieved or a total of 1.0-1.5 gm has been given. Following completion of the loading dose, a maintenance infusion rate between 20-80 µg/kg/min is started, later titrated according to plasma levels. Plasma levels should be obtained five elimination half-lives (15-25 hours) after initiation of drug and after each dosage change so as to insure achievement of steady-state levels.

When standard procainamide capsules and tablets are given orally, absorption is high and peak plasma levels are usually achieved within 2 hours of ingestion. Sustained-release tablets prolong the absorption rate, increase the duration of action, and allow for reduced dosing frequency. Procainamide undergoes acetylation within the liver, forming the active metabolite N-acetylprocainamide (NAPA). Both the parent and metabolic compounds are excreted by the kidneys.[49,50] Among patients with normal renal function, the elimination half-life is 3-5 hours with 60-70% of the procainamide dose being excreted unchanged in the urine. However, in patients with either renal insufficiency or hepatic enzymes capable of rapid acetylation, the concentrations of NAPA in the plasma may equal or exceed that of the parent compound.[51] NAPA possesses predominantly potassium channel blocking activity.[52]

Table 34.4   PHARMACOKINETICS AND DOSING REGIMENS OF CLASS 1A DRUGS

Class 1A Drugs	Half-Life (hours)	Main Routes Elimination	Recommended Doses	Therapeutic Range (μg/ml)
Quinidine sulfate	5-8	Hepatic		2-5
Immediate Release Tablets			300-400 mg every 6-8 hours	
Extended Release Tablets			300-600 mg every 8-12 hours	
Quinidine gluconate				
Sustained Release Tablets			324-648 mg every hours	
Quinidine polygalacturonate Tablets			275 mg every 6-8 hours	
Procainamide hydrochloride	3-5	Hepatic		5-15
Immediate Release Capsules & Tablets			250-500 mg (50 mg/kg/day) every 3 hrs	
Sustained Release Tablets			500-1000 mg (50 mg/kg/day) every 6 hrs	
Intravenous			10-20 mg/kg at 20-50 mg/min 20-80 mcg/kg/min infusion**	
Disopyramide phosphate	4-6	Renal		2-5
Immediate Release Capsules		Hepatic	100-150 mg po every 6-8 hrs	
Controlled Release Capsules			200-300 mg po every 12 hrs	
Intravenous			1.5-2.5 mg/kg bolus followed by 0.4 mg/kg/hr infusion	

**The initial infusion rate of procainamide may be calculated by multiplying the desired plasma concentration of procainamide (3- 10 mcg/ml) by the estimated total clearance rate (2.7(creatinine clearance) + 3.9)(11). Later, the infusion rate may be adjusted according to serum levels of procainamide and NAPA levels.

When converting from intravenous to chronic oral therapy, the infusion should be stopped and one elimination half-life (3-5 hours) allowed to elapse. The initial daily oral dose may be calculated from the daily intravenous requirements and subsequently adjusted in accordance with plasma levels. For long-term oral therapy, total daily doses approximating 50 mg/kg/day are often required to achieve therapeutic levels. Sustained release preparations may be advantageous by minimizing the dosing interval and enhancing patient compliance.

Potential cardiovascular side effects of procainamide are similiar to those described for quinidine. Noncardiac side effects include nausea, anorexia, vomiting, rashes, fevers, agranulocytosis, arthalgias, myalgias, Raynaud's phenomenom and drug-induced lupus. Concurrent use of cimetidine may lead to a reduction in renal clearance of procainamide and its metabolites, thereby increasing the elimination half-life and necessitating a reduction in the procainamide dose.

Disopyramide. Like procainamide, disopyramide is available in both intravenous and oral preparations. Intravenous treatment is initiated with a loading dose of 1.5-2.5 mg/kg followed by an infusion rate of 0.4 mg/kg/hr. Oral dosing ranges from 300-600 mg/day depending upon the preparation. Bioavailability is approximately 80%, and peak plasma levels are achieved within 2 hours prior to being excreted in the urine. Metabolites of disopyramide have no antiarrhythmic properties but may contribute to the anticholinergic side effects observed with the parent drug *(Table 34.4)*.

Potential adverse cardiovascular effects from disopyramide therapy include decompensated congestive heart failure, attributed to its negative inotropic effects, and hypotension. Depressed sinus node activity and conduction block, leading to prolongation of the RR, PR, QRS and QT intervals, have also been observed. The most common noncardiac side effects seen with disopyramide relate to the potent anticholinergic properties of its metabolites, including dryness of the mouth, glaucoma, prostatism, constipation, and impotence. Less common side effects include hypoglycemia, cholestatic jaundice, nausea, rashes, and confusional states.

Class IB agents: lidocaine, mexiletine, and tocainide

The class IB drugs inhibit I_{Na} in cardiac tissue featuring either a decreased resting membrane potential or an increased rate of excitation. Depolarization of normal myocytes remain unaffected by these agents. These agents reduce automaticity within Purkinje fibers by reducing the rate of phase 4 depolarization and shifting the threshold voltage away from the resting membrane potential. These agents also block the window sodium current, thereby shortening the action potential duration and refractory periods in Purkinje fibers.[53] These drugs do not significantly affect atrial issue, nor do they exert significant autonomic effects. The net effect of these actions is to reduce abnormal automaticity and excitability in diseased or ischemic ventricular myocardium and slow intraventricular conduction in a use-dependent manner.[54]

Lidocaine. Lidocaine is not available as an oral preparation due to extensive first-pass hepatic metabolism into compounds with little antiarrhythmic activity *(Table*

34.5). Intravenous administration includes a loading dose of 0.7-1.4 mg/kg followed by an infusion rate of 20-50 µg/kg/min. The elimination half-life is normally about 2 hours and inversely related to hepatic blood flow. If the infusion is to continue beyond 24 hours, plasma levels may be checked and the dose titrated to achieve a therapeutic concentration of 2-5 µg/ml.

Lidocaine remains standard first line treatment for ventricular tachycardia and ventricular fibrillation related to acute ischemia, acute infarction, and digitalis toxicity. However, recent studies show that lidocaine is less effective than procainamide in terminating hemodynamically tolerated sustained monomorphic ventricular tachycardia in the setting of a healed myocardial infarction.[55]

Lidocaine is generally free from significant cardiovascular side effects except for rare cases of sinus arrest when given in conjunction with other SA nodal depressants. In patients with congestive heart failure, lower infusion rates must be used and plasma levels followed closely. At higher infusion rates, central nervous system complications may be observed, especially amongst the elderly. The more common side effects include drowsiness, numbness, speech disturbances, and altered states of conciousness, all of which may be reversed by decreasing or discontinuing the infusion. Concurrent therapy with phenytoin, phenobarbital, and rifampin, and other drugs which induce hepatic enzymes may lead to decreased plasma levels and the need to increase the infusion rate.

Mexiletine. Mexiletine, unlike lidocaine, may be administered orally as it undergoes < 10% first pass hepatic metabolism. Readily absorbed following oral administration, bioavailability approaches 90% with peak plasma concentrations achieved within 2-4 hours following ingestion. The normal elimination half-life ranges between 6-12 hours as 85-90% of the drug is metabolized within the liver while the remainder is excreted unchanged in the urine.[56] The usual oral dosage is 200-400 mg every 8 hours, though it may be reduced in patients with hepatic insufficiency. Although not often utilized clinically, the therapeutic plasma concentration is 0.6-1.7 µg/ml *(Table 34.5)*.

Table 34.5   PHARMACOKINETICS AND DOSE OF CLASS IB DRUGS

Class IB Drugs	Half-Life (hours)	Main Routes Elimination	Recommended Doses	Therapeutic Range (µg/ml)
Lidocaine	1.5-2.5	Hepatic		2-6
Intravenous			0.7-1.4 mg/kg bolus followed by 20-50 µg/kg/min infusion	
Mexiletine	6-12	Hepatic>>Renal		0.7-2.0
Capsules			100-300 mg every 8 hrs	
Tocainide	12-20	Renal		4-10
Tablets			300-600 mg every 8 hrs	

Mexiletine is not effective in the treatment of sustained VT or VF. [57] However, mexiletine remains used as sole therapy in the treatment of frequent, symptomatic premature ventricular depolarizations, or in combination with class 1A or III drugs in patients with sustained ventricular tachycardia and/or ventricular fibrillation. [58-60]

Although mexiletine has been reported to have negative inotropic effects using invasive hemodynamic studies[61], such negative inotropic effects have not been observed in other non-invasive studies nor observed clinically.[61A] A majority of patients chronically taking mexiletine (particularly those with concurrent liver disease or those taking ≥ 1g per day) will experience reversible central nervous system and/ or gastrointestinal side effects, including dizziness, disorientation, diplopia, nystagmus, tremor, lightheadedness, confusion, nausea, and anorexia. Rarely, hypotension and bradycardia may occur. Mexiletine has been found to increase plasma levels of theophylline when taken together, while concomitant use of hepatic enzyme inducing medication, such as phenytoin, phenobarbital, and rifampin, may decrease plasma levels of mexiletine.

Tocainide. Tocainide, like mexiletine, is nearly 100% absorbed orally, void of significant first-pass metabolism, and produces peak plasma levels within an hour of oral ingestion. Only 30% of the drug is metabolized in the liver with the remainder excreted unchanged in the urine. There are no known active metabolites. The elimination half-life is in the range of 12-20 hours, depending upon hepatic and/or renal function.[62,63] The usual oral dose is 400-800 mg every eight hours, and the therapeutic plasma concentration is 4-10 µg/ml *(Table 34.5)*.

Tocainide is indicated for the chronic treatment of non-malignant ventricular tachyarrhythmias.[64-66] Although responsiveness to intravenous lidocaine is often predictive of a response to tocainide, there is no such correlation in efficacy between tocainide and mexiletine.[67]

Tocainide has no significant negative inotropic effects, rendering its use safe in patients with preexisting congestive heart failure. The drug, however, may cause adverse central nervous system and gastrointestinal effects, including dizziness, lightheadedness, tremor, nausea, and anorexia. In fact, the onset of tremulousness is often utilized as identifying the maximal dosage allowed for an individual patient. In addition, potentially serious blood dyscrasias, including agranulocytosis, anemia, and thrombocytopenia have virtually eliminated the use of tocainide in the U.S.[68,69] Since tocainide-induced cytopenias usually occur within the first 12 weeks of therapy, it is recommended that weekly blood counts be monitored for the first three months of treatment. Early signs of bone marrow toxicity should prompt immediate discontinuation of this agent with blood counts typically returning back to normal within one week.

Class IC agents: flecainide, propafenone, and moricizine

Of all class I agents, the class IC drugs have greater sodium channel blocking activity in both normal and abnormal cardiac tissue and over a wider range of plasma concentrations. By suppressing I_{Na}, these drugs slow conduction and prevent premature depolarizations. In addition, they increase refractoriness within atrial tissue, the AV node and atrioventricular accessory pathways.[70] These electrophysiologic properties account for a greater prolongation in the AH, PR, HV, and QRS intervals as compared with that observed with class IA and IB drugs. However, these drugs do not increase ventricular APD or refractoriness. As a result, any accompanying prolongation of the QT interval is attributed to decreased conduction and widening of the QRS interval.

Flecainide. Flecainide is almost completely absorbed orally with peak plasma concentrations occurring within three hours of ingestion. Approximately 60% of the absorbed drug is eventually metabolized by the liver with the remainder excreted unchanged in the urine. There are no known active metabolites.[71,72] The elimination half-life ranges between 7-15 hours although there may be a significant delay in patients with underlying renal or hepatic insufficiency. The usual starting oral dose is 50 mg twice daily, and the therapeutic plasma concentration is 0.2-0.9 µg/ml *(Table 34.6)*.

The indications for flecainide have been restricted to the treatment of supraventricular tachycardias, including atrioventricular nodal reentrant tachycardia, atrioventricular reciprocating tachycardia, atrial flutter, and atrial fibrillation, as well as life-threatening ventricular arrhythmias refractory to other agents in patients without evidence of structural heart disease.[73-76]

Flecainide has ventricular proarrhythmic effects in patients with structural heart disease.[27] Other adverse cardiac effects include the aggravation of preexisting sinus node dysfunction and conduction system disease as well as increased pacemaker thresholds.[77,78] Combination therapy with other negative inotropic or dromotropic drugs, including class IA agents, beta-adrenergic antagonists, calcium channel antagonists, and digoxin should be either avoided or begun with frequent monitoring for evidence of left ventricular failure, sinus or AV node dysfunction, and/or conduction disease. Concomitant use of amiodarone has been found to increase plasma levels of flecainide, requiring reduction of the dose of flecainide by approximately 30%.[79] Potential noncardiac toxicity includes visual disturbances, dizziness, headaches, nausea, and paresthesias.

Propafenone. Propafenone is a class IC sodium channel blocking agent with class II properties. Like flecainide, it is almost completely absorbed orally, achieving peak plasma concentrations within three hours of ingestion. However, unlike flecainide, it undergoes extensive hepatic metabolism, resulting in eleven different circulating metabolites. Two of these metabolites, 5-hydroxypropafenone and N-desalkylpropafenone, display similiar electrophysiologic properties as the parent drug but with longer plasma half-lives.[80] The elimination half-life of propafenone varies from 2-12 hours, depending upon the extent and rapidity of hepatic metabolism.[81] Only 10-20% of the drug is excreted unchanged in the urine while the majority is excreted through the hepatobiliary system in the feces. The usual starting oral dose of propafenone is 150 mg every eight hours *(Table 34.6)*.

Table 34.6   *PHARMACOKINETICS AND DOSE OF CLASS 1C DRUGS*

Class 1C Drugs	Half-Life (hours)	Main Routes Elimination	Recommended Doses	Therapeutic Range (μg/ml)
Flecainide Tablets	7-15	Renal & Hepatic	50-200mg every 12 hrs	0.2-1.0
Propafenone Tablets	2-12	Hepatic	150-300 mg every 8 hrs	0.1-2.0
Moricizine Tablets	1-6	Hepatic & Renal	200-300 mg every 8 hrs	0.1-3.5

Propafenone is currently indicated only for the treatment of life-threatening ventricular tachyarrhythmias. As with other class IC agents, extreme caution should be exercised in the use of this drug in patients with ventricular arrhythmias and evidence for structural heart disease. Propafenone has also been found effective in the treatment of atrial fibrillation, atrial flutter, and the Wolff-Parkinson-White syndrome.[82-84]

The most common cardiac side effects of propafenone include conduction abnormalities (new AV or bundle branch block), worsening congestive heart failure, and ventricular proarrhythmia, particularly in patients with moderate-severe left ventricular dysfunction. Consequently, concurrent use of drugs likely to depress either nodal function, intraventricular conduction, or contractility, should be either avoided or carefully monitored. In addition, propafenone will increase digoxin plasma levels and potentiate the actions of coumadin, necessitating reduction in the dosages of these agents.[85,86] Potential non-cardiac side effects include dizziness, taste disturbances, blurred vision, nausea, anorexia, bronchospasm, reversible granulocytopenia and a lupus-like syndrome.

Moricizine. Formerly known as ethmozine, moricizine is also rapidly aborbed orally, reaching peak plasma levels within two hours of administration. As a result of first-pass metabolism, bioavailability is approximately 40%, while the plasma elimination half-life ranges from one to six hours. The usual starting oral dose is 200 mg every eight hours, and the therapeutic concentration ranges between 0.1-3.5 μg/ml *(Table 34.6)*.

Moricizine's kinetics of interaction with the sodium channel are between those of fast (Class IB) drugs and intermediate (IA) drugs.[2,42B] Moricizine does not block potassium channels and the net effect of moricizines electrophysiologic actions are to prolong QRS duration without affecting APD [87-90] and to decrease automaticity.[91,92] There properties have caused confusion in trying to classify the drug and the drug is classified as a IC drug or a drug exhibiting features of all three Class I subgroups.[93,94] In fact moricizine's actions can be easily explained by its sodium channel blocking activity which produces QRS prolongation and conduction slowing similar to that produced by Class IA drugs or at high doses, slowing in the range produced by IC drugs. The confusion engendered by trying to fit a new drug such as moricizine in the descriptive Vaughan-Williams classification is a strong argument for a mechanistic classification such as that proposed in the Sicilian Gambit.[2]

Potential adverse cardiac effects of moricizine include proarrhythmia, conduction disturbances and worsening heart failure.[96,97] Noncardiac complications may include dizziness, nausea, hepatitis, and thrombocytopenia.[97,98]

Drugs with class II action: β-adrenergic antagonists

Several β-blocking drugs, including propanolol, acebutolol, and esmolol, are approved for use as antiarrhythmic agents. In addition, the use of propanolol, metoprolol, and timolol after myocardial infarction has been found to reduce the incidence of ventricular fibrillation and sudden cardiac death.[99] β-adrenergic antagonists exert their antiarrhythmic action by blocking currents that are activated by beta-adrenergic agonists. These currents include the pacemaker current I_f and the L type calcium current I_{Ca-L}. At supratherapeutic concentrations, inward sodium current is blocked by some β-blockers. The net effect is to decrease spontaneous automaticity in the sinus node and Purkinje fibers, slow conduction and increase refractoriness within the AV node, stabilize membrane potentials against adrenergic acceleration of depolarization and repolarization in both atrial and ventricular tissue, and suppress triggered activity in Purkinje fibers. In addition, beta-blockers may be especially effective in some ischemic mediated arrhythmias.[100,101] *(Table 34.7)*.

β-blockers antagonize catecholamine-induced increases in sinus node automaticity. By blocking I_f and I_{Ca-L}, these agents decrease the rate of phase 4 depolarization and slow sinus node firing rates. Similarly, in the presence of increased adrenergic tone, these drugs also decrease abnormal automaticity and spontaneous activity within the His-Purkinje system.[102,103]

β-adrenergic blocking drugs also slow conduction and increase refractoriness within the atrioventricular node which results in the prolongation of the PR interval observed on the surface electrocardiogram. In contrast, in the absence of increased adrenergic tone, conduction and refractoriness within the His-Purkinje system and ventricular muscle remain unaffected, as evidenced by a lack of change in QRS and QT intervals.

The beta-adrenergic antagonists exert cardioprotective effects to patients following acute myocardial infarction. As these drugs decrease excitability in Purkinje fibers, beta-blockers effectively suppress premature ventricular depolarizations, while preventing sympathetically induced shortening of ventricular refractoriness.[103,104] In addition, the voltage required for initiation of ventricular fibrillation may be increased by beta-adrenergic blockade.[105] Finally, these drugs slow conduction within ischemic myocardium without altering the overall HV interval or QRS duration.[106] These effects may serve to reduce tachycardic response to hyperadrenergic state following myocardial infarction while preventing ventricular fibrillation and sudden death. Indeed, at least part of the survival benefit observed with beta-adrenergic

Table 34.7 COMPARISON OF COMMONLY USED β-ADRENERGIC ANTAGONISTS

	Propanolol	Metoprolol	Nadolol	Timolol	Atenolol	Pindolol	Acebutolol
Cardioselectivity	0	+	0	0	+	0	+
Intrinsic sympatho-mimetic activity	0	0	0	0	0	++	+
GI absorption (%)	>90	>95	30	>90	50	>90	>95
Bioavailability (% dose)	30	50	30	75	40	90	90
Lipid solubility	high	mod	low	low	mod	mod	mod
Elimination half-life (hr)	3.5-6	3-4	14-24	3-4	6-9	3-4	3-4
Route of elimination*	H	H	R	C	R	C	R

*H=hepatic; R=renal; C=combined hepatic and renal

antagonist therapy following myocardial infarction may be related to the anti-fibrillatory properties of these drugs.[99]

Beta-adrenergic a-ntagonists are clinically used in the treatment and prevention of both supraventricular and ventricular tachycardias. The specific indications for class II antiarrhythmic therapy is further discussed later in this chapter.

Propanolol. Propanolol is well absorbed orally, but total bioavailability remains low due to extensive first-pass hepatic metabolism. The usual elimination half-life is 4 hours, although this value may rise in the setting of hepatic dysfunction. The usual starting daily dose is 80 to 160 mg split into 4 equal doses. The drug may also be administered intravenously with 0.1-0.2 mg/kg given over several minutes and repeated as needed. Although therapeutic plasma concentrations are reported to vary between 0.02-1.0 μg/ml with higher doses often required for ventricular arrhythmias, in practice doses may be titrated to a significant reduction in heart rate as the blood pressure permits.

Indications for propanolol therapy include ventricular rate control in the setting of atrial fibrillation, atrial flutter, and other supraventricular tachycardias. The drug is also effective against inappropriate sinus tachycardia as well as exercise-induced atrial and ventricular arrhythmias. By prolonging refractoriness within the AV node, the drug may abolish paroxysmal supraventricular tachycardias, including atrioventricular nodal reentrant tachycardias and atrioventricular reciprocating tachycardias utilizing the AV node as part of the reentrant circuit. Post-infarction patients are eligible for chronic β-blockade which has been found to reduce the risk of future sudden cardiac death, at least in part by an antiarrhythmic mechanism.[99] In addition, beta-adrenergic antagonists may be effective against nonischemic ventricular tachycardia and fibrillation in selected patients.[107,108] Finally, propanolol is first line treatment for patients with the long QT syndrome by eliminating pause-related early depolarizations and polymorphous ventricular tachycardia.[109]

Potential adverse cardiac effects from propanolol therapy include symptomatic bradycardia, significant hypotension, exacerbation of congestive heart failure, development of complete heart block or asystole. Noncardiac side effects reflect the noncardioselectivity of the drug's activity and include possible bronchospasm, worsening diabetic control, impotence, decreased exercise tolerance, fatigue, insomnia, cold extremities, increased hypertriglyceridemia, and decreased HDL cholesterol levels. These noncardiac complications may be reduced with the selection of a cardioselective beta-adrenergic blocking drug, such as atenolol, metoprolol, or acebutolol or a less lipid soluble beta-adrenergic blocking drug such as nadolol, timolol, atenolol or acebutolol.

Drugs with class III action: sotalol, amiodarone, bretylium, ibutilide

Since the results of the CAST trial [27] an aggressive campaign has been waged to find effective antiarrythmic agents with alternative class action. The superiority of sotalol to class I drugs in ESVEM and amiodarone to class I drugs in CASCADE has suggested class III drugs may be the most effective agents available. The class III agents represent a diverse group of antiarrhythmic drugs sharing in common the ability to increase the action potential duration (APD) and the effective refractory period (ERP) of all cardiac cells. However, most of the currently available agents are not pure class III drugs as they also possess properties characteristic of the other classes. This overlap has made the understanding of pure class III activity very difficult. The effectiveness of class III drugs is attributed to their aforementioned electrophysiologic properties. However, in clinical practice the currently available class III agents have been found to be less effective than earlier anticipated. At this time, amiodarone and bretylium are reserved for refractory ventricular tachyarrhythmias. Most recently, the FDA has approved the use of ibutilide for effective cardioversion of atrial fibrillation and atrial flutter in place of electrical cardioversion.

Sotalol. Sotalol is a racemic mixture of d and l optical isomers, with the d isomer exhibiting class III activity, while, the l isomer has both class III and β-blocking properties.[110] Both isomers exhibit equipotent class III action. As a result of these combined class II and III actions sotalol increases the myocardial refractory period, in a dose dependent fashion, while, decreasing automaticity. The drugs net effect is to prolong the sinus cycle length (SCL), PR, QT/QTc, PA and AH intervals.[110] Sotalol's β-blocking activity is 0.3 times as potent as propranolol on a mg for mg basis.[111-113] It has been observed that at low concentrations sotalol is primarily a β-blocker with increasing class III activity at higher doses [114,115]. Unlike class I agents, sotalol does not effect the maximum rate of depolarization of phase 0 of the action potential nor does it prolong the QRS duration. However, as a function of a decreasing cycle length the ability of sotalol to prolong the APD is diminished.[116] Since the drug does not prolong the QRS duration, the prolongation of the QTc is accounted for by the increased JT interval. The class III effect is monitored by the change in the QTc, since therapeutic plasma levels have not been well correlated to either drug efficacy or clinically apparent toxicity.[114,117] Various clinical trials have reported a reduction in the overall inducibility of ventricular arrhythmias by d,l sotalol.[118-120]

The side effect profile is similar to that seen with beta- adrenergic blocking agents, with the exception of the proarrythmia manifested as torsade de pointes ventricular tachycardia. Otherwise, the drug is better tolerated than most β-blocking agents, as the prolongation of the action potential duration (APD) minimizes the negative ionotropic effect of this agent, possibly by allowing increased time for calcium influx into the myocytes. However, careful monitoring is advised when administering this agent to patients with CHF, and renal failure. Improper dosing increases the risk of drug induced torsade de pointes in these patients.

Although, d- sotalol has virtually no β-blocking action it decreases the sinus cycle length (SCL), while, prolonging the AH, PR, and QTc. D-sotalol exerts no effect on the conduction velocity (CV), QRS duration or the HV interval. The effect on the SCL is probably a result of S-A nodal action potential prolongation, as opposed to, residual β-blocking activity of the d-enantiomer.[21] Potential advantages of d-sotalol may be attributed to its minimal impact on myocardial contractility and lack of non-specific β-adrenergic antagonism which may prove beneficial in patients with congestive heart failure and reactive airways disease. However, the clinical efficacy observed with d,l sotalol may be partially explained by its class II action. The β-blocking properties of d,1-sotalol may protect against reversal of potassium channel blockade of d-sotalol by catecholamines.[121] Most recently, the Survival With Oral d-Sotalol in patients with left ventricular dysfunction after myocardial infarction (SWORD) trial was terminated because of a higher mortality among post-infarction patients receiving d-sotalol than in the control group.[122] Currently, d - sotalol has been withdrawn from all clinical trials.

Oral sotalol is well absorbed, is virtually 100 % bioavailable, and remains relatively unbound in plasma. The drug is a hydrophilic compound and is excreted unchanged in the urine. The elimination half life of the drug ranges from 10 to 15 hours. This agent, by virtue of its hydrophilicity, does not penetrate the CNS and, hence, may have lesser incidence of CNS side effects, compared with other β-blockers.

As mentioned, the side effect profile of d,l sotalol parallels that of most common β-blockers. The major toxicity's of the drug can be classified as cardiac and non cardiac. The most serious cardiac complication is torsade de pointes, which occurs in 2 - 5 % of patients. Other cardiac side effects include: bradyarrhythmias, hypotension, sudden death and congestive heart failure. Whereas the Class IA drugs cause torsade at low doses, the incidence of torsade with sotalol increase with increasing doses. The incidence of polymorphic VT, meeting the criteria for torsade de pointes, increases in those individuals who have a prolonged baseline QTc.[123,124] In addition to patients with a prolonged QTc the proarrhythmic tendency is higher in those individuals with a history of sustained VT, preexisting LV dysfunction, and bradycardia.[110,46C,123,124] The major non cardiac side effects include dizziness, fatigue, dyspnea, headache, nausea, and vomiting.

Since the current indications for sotalol are for life-threatening ventricular arrhythmias, patients receiving the drug, by definition comprise a high risk group. It has been found that the majority of proarryhthmic events occur in the first week of therapy[123,124] and when the dose is increased above a level of 320 mg/day . It is therefore prudent to hospitalize these patients for drug loading and careful monitoring. It is customary to wait 3 to 4 days following each dosage adjustment to assess effect. Drug therapy should be carefully titrated in those patients with renal insufficiency and severe LV dysfunction.

Amiodarone. Amiodarone, an antiarrythmic agent with complex electrophysiologic properties, is one of the most frequently used agents for the termination of refractory ventricular arrythmias. Initially touted as an anti-anginal drug, amiodarone was later found to have promise as an effective antiarrhythmic agent. Amiodarone is a benzofuran , classified as a class III agent, yet it exhibits features from all four major classes of antiarrhythmic action, as well as, anti-thyroid properties.[46C,126] Desethylamiodarone is the major active hepatic metabolite of amiodarone. The complexity of this drug's electrophysiologic actions stem from its complex pharmacokinetics and pharmacodynamics.

Amiodarone is well absorbed orally, with a bioavailability ranging between 22 and 86 %. The drug is highly protein bound, extensively metabolized by the liver and excreted primarily by the biliary tract. Amiodarone exhibits a long elimination half life ($t_{1/2}$), with its primary metabolite desethylamiodarone exhibiting an even longer therapeutic $t_{1/2}$. The $t_{1/2}$ of this agent ranges from 15 to 110 days, with desethylamiodarone possessing an even longer elimination $t_{1/2}$. Clinically the therapeutic efficacy of amiodarone is delayed. The active metabolite has a similar electrophysiologic profile to the parent compound, exhibiting an even longer delay in its onset of action.

Plasma levels correlate linearly with the oral dosing regimen. Plasma levels are of little clinical utility[127,128], as the drug exhibits a highly variable and unpredictable toxic to therapeutic drug ratio. Toxicity is related to cumulative organ specific accumulation of the drug.

Amiodarone's electrophysiologic properties are a function of the duration of therapy. The major changes observed on the electrocardiogram and during electrophysiologic testing are observed after chronic administration of the agent. Recently, the intravenous administration of this agent received FDA approval for clinical use in ventricular arrhythmias. The features of this drug may be related to its overall metabolic effects after prolonged administration. In fact, many of the changes observed mimic those observed in hypothyroidism.

Amiodarone decreases heart rate by a noncompetitive blockade of β-adrenergic receptors without negative inotropic properties.[129] The drug does not depress the myocardium which explains why it is well tolerated by patients with congestive heart failure. It has been used effectively in patients with refractory ventricular tachycardias awaiting heart transplantation. The effects on heart rate appear to reach a steady state within a few months, however, prolongation of the QTc may take up to a year to stabilize.[130,131] Following the initiation of treatment, timing of electrophysiologic studies has yet to be established.

Currently, amiodarone is an empirically dosed agent, resulting in a 20% reduction of inducible VT.[132,133] In those patients who remain inducible after drug, the subsequent VT is slower and better tolerated.[134,134] A unique and puzzling feature of amiodarone stems from its ability to prolong APD, QTc, like the class IA drugs, but , with a decreased incidence of torsade de pointes.[136] Unlike sotalol, amiodarone maintains its effect on the APD even at faster heart rates, however, it does not enhance myocardial contractility despite a prolongation of the APD. In addition, only the AV nodal refractory period, AH,and PR intervals exhibit significant prolongation acutely. The AV nodal conduction delay is attributed to β-and calcium channel blockade, while the prolongation of the QRS, which reflects slowing of conduction in ventricular muscle, is attributed to the sodium channel blocking ability of this agent.

Clinically, because of the potential for serious, at times fatal, side effects the drug is reserved for life-threatening arrhythmias not responsive to other drug interventions. The most troubling side effects include pulmonary toxicity, with the potential to develop irreversible pulmonary fibrosis. Hepatotoxicity is most commonly characterized by transient elevations in liver function tests, although rarely more severe liver toxicity is observed. Results of liver biopsies, post -amiodarone, mimic the changes observed with alcoholic hepatitis. Thyroid toxicity has resulted in both hyper and hypothyroidism. Less commonly, bluish skin pigmentation, nausea, peripheral neuropathy, corneal depositions and photosensitivity is observed. Amiodarone interacts with a variety of agents metabolized in the liver, including: digoxin, coumadin, diphenylydantoin, quinidine, procainamide, NAPA and verapamil. Amiodarone interacts less significantly with propafenone and flecainide.[79]

Bretylium. Bretylium is an adrenergic neuronal blocking agent with class III properties. Bretylium, a charged ion, possessing a unique quaternary ammonium structure is highly water soluble, as a consequence, it is not well absorbed by the lipid rich plasma membranes. Initially, bretylium was to be used as a antihypertensive agent [137-139], however, the subsequent discovery of potent antiarrhythmic properties led to its use as an antiarrythmic agent.[140] Bretylium exhibits two important antiarrythmic actions, a direct effect attributed to its class III action[141] and an indirect effect attributed to its adrenergic blocking action.[142]

Bretylium accumulates in the sympathetic ganglionic and post-ganglionic neurons, eliciting a biphasic hemodynamic response. Initially, the concentration of drug in the terminal sympathetic neurons causes a transient release of norepinephrine, (15-20 min) leading to an increase in both blood pressure (BP) and heart rate (HR). This initial sympathomimetic effect is then followed by a decreased release of norepinephrine (NE), leading to a decreased heart rate, blood pressure and systemic vascular resistance (SVR). However, the initial surge of norepinephrine may provoke ventricular arrhythmias. In fact, the use of bretylium in patients with digitalis toxicity is a relative contraindication, since, catecholamines are known to enhance the arrhythmias associated with digitalis toxicity. Bretylium potentiates the action of catecholamine infusions which may potentiates its antiarrhythmic effect.

The electrophysiologic properties of bretylium exhibit a more pronounced class III effect on Purkinje cells compared to ventricular myocardium. The direct class III effects are apparent with chronic administration. Bretylium prolongs the action potential duration (APD), and effective refractory period (ERP) of atrial and ventricular tissue but does not prolong conduction through the AV node.[143]

The oral administration of bretylium results in plasma levels 1/10th of those achieved with intravenous administration due to widely variable bioavailability, ranging from 10 -40 %.[143] As a consequence, oral administration has been abandoned in favor of the parenteral route in order to insure adequate steady state drug levels. Less than 5 % of the drug is protein bound in plasma while its elimination $t_{1/2}$ ranges from 7 - 13 hours, and has no known active metabolites.[143] The drug is predominately excreted by active tubular secretion by the kidney, exhibiting no liver metabolism.

The drugs major side effect is orthostatic hypotension (> 60 %), while nausea and vomiting occur with rapid IV infusions in the conscious patient.

The indirect antiadrenergic effects of the drug include decreased automaticity. This indirect action may mediate the antifibrillatory effect of this agent in the acute setting. The antifibrillatory action of bretylium parallels that exhibited by β-blocking agents. At the lower doses bretylium increases the ventricular fibrillation threshold (VFT) in both normal and ischemic myocardium. At higher doses this effect is more rapid (2 min) and longer lasting (6 - 12 hours).[141] The antifibrillatory effects of bretylium, reflecting class II - like properties, are rapid while its antitachycardic properties, reflecting class III activity, require long term administration.

Bretylium is reserved for refractory VF and VT. Amiodarone, in its intravenous form, has recently become available for refractory ventricular arrhythmias and in our opinion is the agent of choice for refractory VT after lidocaine and procainamide have failed.

Ibutilide. Ibutilide fumarate is a newly available intravenous agent approved as an alternative to the electrical cardioversion of atrial fibrillation and atrial flutter. Consistent with the action of other class III agents ibutilide has been shown to prolong repolarization. It has been proposed that the mechanisms by which ibutilide increases repolarization by enhancing the slow inward sofium current again during the plateau phase of the action potential and by blocking repolarizing potassium currents.[144,145] The proposed mechanism by which ibutilide terminates reentrant atrial arrhythmias may be related to the prolongation of atrial refractoriness with little if any change in conduction velocity.

Ibutilide is 41% protein bound, exhibiting linear pharmacokinetics with rapid systemic clearance. The drug has a half-life of elimination in the range of 3-6 hours. Ibutilide is administered intravenously because of the reduced bioavailability of oral ibutilide due to extensive first pass hepatic metabolism. The drug is rapidly metabolized in the liver with one of 8 metabolites being slightly active. Thus far, in human studies dosing is independent of dose, age, sex, left ventricular function, renal, or hepatic function. Ibutilide upon infusion increases the QT interval. This QT prolongation is directly related to its plasma concentration. Both the plasma concentration and the rate of infusion influence the QT interval change, with a maximum QT prolongation observed with the highest plasma levels and most rapid rates of infusion. The QT prolongation and risks of proarrhythmia are most pronounced during the first 40 minutes following therapy, with complete resolution of the QT prolongation 4-6 hours following infusion. Ibutilide increases the risk of proarrhythmia, in the form of polymorphic ventricular tachycardia (non-sustained) and torsade de pointes, however, the major risk is greatest during the first 40 minutes following infusion. Intravenous ibutilide has not been shown to significantly affect hemodynamics, even in patients with significant reductions in left ventricular function (LVEF < 35 %). Intravenous ibutilide is administered as 1 mg over 10 minutes (0.01 mg/kg) with a repeat infusion in 10 minutes if necessary.

The efficacy of ibutilide in the rapid conversion of atrial flutter is in the range of 40-50% , while, exhibiting a cardioversion efficacy of 30 % in atrial fibrillation.[146,147] Of those atrial arrhythmias which respond to intravenous ibutilide 75-80 % will do so in the first 30 minutes of administration. In summary, ibutilide is a new highly effective agent in the conversion of atrial fibrillation and atrial flutter to sinus rhythm. Comparisons with other pharmacologic agents is still pending, as well as, its safety and utility in conjunction with such agents. Although in the majority of cases ibutilide safely and effectively converts these atrial arrhythmias to sinus rhythm it should be used with continuous ECG monitoring for at least 4 hours after infusion or until QT normalization. The drugs proarrhythmic tendencies should be recognized and only used under conditions where rapid recognition and treatment of proarrhythmia can be instituted. Under these circumstances ibutilide appears to be a safe and effective agent in the pharmacologic treatment of common atrial arrhythmias.

Class IV antiarrhythmic agents - verapamil, diltiazem, nifedipine

The class IV agents selectively inhibit the slow inward calcium current. Calcium channel antagonists act primarily on the L-type channel[148], which serves to prolong the action potential plateau; while indirectly increasing calcium ion release from the sarcoplasmic reticulum. The effective refractory period (ERP) and conduction velocity of fast channel dependent tissue, (e.g. atria, ventricle, His- Purkinje (H-P) remain unaffected. It should be noted that these agents block the slow calcium channel in a concentration or dose dependent manner. The major effect of the class IV drugs is to decrease the rate of rise of phase 4 depolarization in the S-A and A-V nodal tissue, with a more pronounced effect on the A-V node.[145,146] Both the A-V nodal effective and functional refractory periods are increased, subsequently decreasing conduction across the node in both the retrograde and anterograde directions.[149,150]

Verapamil, a first generation calcium antagonist is almost completely protonated; explaining the drugs tendency towards use dependent block, analogous to the sodium channel interaction of class IC agents.[151] Verapamil, as compared to nifedipine, exhibits slow kinetics of interaction with calcium channels. Nifedipines rapid kinetics of interaction and vasodilating effects limit its effectiveness as an AV nodal blocker at physiologic heart rates. Diltiazem exhibits both tonic and use-dependent block. All three agents slow the recovery of calcium channels from the inactivated state following repolarization. It is the use dependence at physiologic heart rates and slow kinetics of interaction for verapamil and diltiazem which make these agents effective anti-arrhythmic agents. Nifedipine exhibits potent vasodilatory effects at low concentrations resulting in a compensatory increase in adrenergic tone. This may explain why nifedipine and other dihydropyridines do not slow conduction across the AV node, while, both diltiazem and verapamil prolong the P-R interval.

Verapamil is well absorbed orally, but, is only 20 % bioavailable because of

extensive first pass hepatic metabolism (*Table 34.8*). Verapamil is primarily eliminated via the kidneys, with only one known active hepatic metabolite, norverapamil.
Diltiazem exhibits > 90 % oral absorption, and is 45-50 % bioavailable. The majority of the drug is eliminated via the GI tract (65%), with the remainder renally
excreted (35%). Both drugs exhibit significant protein binding properties, > 80 %.
Nifedipine is almost completely absorbed orally, with rapid sublingual absorption,
with high first pass metabolism resulting in a bioavailability of 50 %. The drug is
extensively protein bound , > 95 %, exhibits no known active metabolites, and is
predominately excreted via the gastrointestinal tract.

Both diltiazem and verapamil can produce cardiac conduction delay (e.g. S-A
block, sinus bradycardia, and A-V block), negative ionotropic effect on LV function, as well as, hypotension. Nifedipine rarely causes conduction delay, however,
profound hypotension can occur. The conduction disturbances observed with these
agents are worsened by superimposed β-blocker administration, especially in those
individuals with underlying disease. Major noncardiac side effects include dizziness,
edema, headache, nausea, and constipation. As a consequence of their extensive
protein binding several major drug interactions must be considered. Most importantly one must carefully reevaluate digoxin levels, since plasma levels are increased
with verapamil. Phenobarbital and dilantin increase metabolism of the Calcium
channel blockers, and higher doses may be required for drug effect. Rifampin significantly decreases drug bioavailability. Common side effects associated with the
first generation Calcium antagonist include: dizziness, pedal edema, headache, nausea, AV block, bradycardia, heart failure and palpitations. Dizziness, pedal edema
and headache are side effects most commonly associated with nifedipine, while, AV
block and bradycardia are more commonly seen with verapamil and diltiazem, respectively.

Digoxin. Digoxin, a cardiac glycoside, exerts both a direct action on myocardial
cells, as well as, an indirect effect via the autonomic nervous system. Digoxin acts to
directly inhibit the myocyte Na-K ATPase[152], resulting in an increase in intracellular
calcium and enhanced myocardial contractility.[153] The drug acts indirectly by enhancing vagal stimulation and inhibiting sympathetic discharge. Both actions result
in a decrease in sinus node discharge and prolongation of AV nodal refractori-

Table 34.8   *PHARMACOKINETIC PROPERTIES OF FIRST GENERATION
CALCIUM ANTAGONISTS*

Agent	Structure	Bioavailability (%)	Half-life $t_{1/2}$ (h)	Protein Binding
Verapamil*	Phenylalkylamine+	25	4.0	90
Diltiazem*	Benzothiazepine+	40	5.0	90
Nifedipine*	Dihydropyridine	50	3.0	> 95

* All drugs exhibit minimal renal excretion (<5%).
+ Active metabolite.

ness.[154] The increase in AV ERP acts to reduce impulse propagation across the AV node. These neurohumoral effects of the drug account for both its therapeutic and toxic actions.

The drug is well absorbed orally (> 75 %) and is primarily excreted unchanged in the urine. The remainder is eliminated in stool or via hepatic metabolism [155]. In approximately 10 % of patients beginning on oral digoxin, plasma drug levels are significantly lower than expected. This is a result of alterations in the gut flora resulting in a rapid uptake and metabolism of the drug and a reduction in absorption. These patients may require antecedent antibiotic therapy prior to drug treatment.[156]

Digoxin exhibits a narrow toxic to therapeutic ratio, with therapeutic levels in the range of 1 - 2 ng/ml. However, proarrhythmia, especially in the setting of electrolyte disturbances, can be seen even with a therapeutic level of digoxin.[157] The plasma half life is 1.5 days and is prolonged in the face of renal insufficiency and malnutrition.[158,159] Therefore, in the elderly who have reductions both in renal function and lean body mass the digoxin dosage schedules need to be reduced and frequently monitored to avoid toxicity. Despite a reduction in clearance of this agent and longer half life there is no alteration of myocardial sensitivity with increasing age.

Absolute contraindications to the use of digoxin include obstructive hypertrophic cardiomyopathy in the absence of atrial fibrillation, WPW, high grade AV block, and, diastolic dysfunction with severe LVH and a hyperdynamic ventricle. It has been suggested that digoxin may increase mortality early after a myocardial infarction [160], however, the data remains inconclusive. Relative contraindications include the treatment of hyperthyroidism induced atrial fibrillation, hypoxic states, sinus bradycardia, sick sinus syndrome and renal insufficiency. Of note digoxin is not as effective in controlling the ventricular response during exercise when compared to either β-blockers or verapamil.

Digoxin exhibits both cardiac and non-cardiac side effects. The most serious cardiac toxicity stems from the proarrhythmic tendencies of this agent. Any rhythm disturbance can be a manifestation of digoxin toxicity. However, the rhythm disturbances most commonly seen include frequent VPDs, accelerated junctional tachycardias, atrial tachycardia with block, ventricular tachycardias, as well as, sinus node arrest.

Non -cardiac side effects includes gastrointestinal upset manifested as, nausea, vomiting, anorexia, and diarrhea. Other side effects are malaise, fatigue,facial pain, insomnia, vertigo, and visual disturbances. In our discussion of the other anti-arrhythmic agents we have been careful to highlight those drugs which potentiate the actions of digoxin or are themselves influenced by concomitant dosing of digoxin. Quinidine increases the plasma levels of digoxin by competing for protein binding sites. Erythromycin also increases plasma levels of digoxin, while, cholestyramine binds digoxin in the gut reducing absorption of the drug. Rifampin acts to reduce the plasma levels of digoxin by increasing its hepatic metabolism.

Adenosine. Adenosine is an endogenous purine nucleotide which exerts significant cardiovascular effects, including the slowing of the sinus cycle length (SCL), AV nodal conduction, as well as, peripheral vasodilatation. This compound reduces the SCL by directly inhibiting SA nodal automaticity, reducing the rate of phase 4 depolarization, and increasing the maximum diastolic potential [161,162]. Adenosine also prolongs AV nodal conduction and lengthens the AH and PR intervals, but does not affect the HV interval. These electrophysiologic actions allow for significant slowing of impulses across the AV node, often leading to the termination of supraventricular tachycardias.

Adenosine's actions are mediated by its interaction with the A1 adenosine receptor system and the activation of GTP binding proteins. The inhibitory G-proteins both inhibit adenylate cyclase and activate the $I_{k\text{-}Ach}$ channel, the mechanisms responsible for the negative dromotropic effects on the A-V and S-A nodes.[163]

Adenosine exerts a negative ionotropic effect on atrial tissue with little if any effect on the contractility or electrical properties of ventricular myocytes. The rapid uptake and metabolism of adenosine, allows for a short $t_{1/2}$ of 10 to 30 sec, while, minimizing potential untoward effects.

Adenosine evokes a vasodilatory response in most vascular beds, including the coronary artery circulation. This vasodilatory response can be accompanied by angina. Other untoward effects of adenosine include transient dyspnea and flushing.

Despite a short half life the drug is contraindicated in patients with asthma, second or third degree A-V block and the sick sinus syndrome. It is recommended that the dose of adenosine be reduced in the presence of dipyridamole. Caffeine and theophylline antagonize the effects of this agent.

Treatment of arrhythmias

Appropriate therapy of the various tachycardias must be tailored to the needs of the individual patient. Currently, several therapeutic modalities are available for effective treatment of these rhythm disturbances, including, pharmacotherapy, catheter and surgical ablation, and implantable defibrillators with the capacity for antitachycardia pacing. Selection of the appropriate therapeutic modality is based on a risk-benefit evaluation between the morbidity and mortality of the arrhythmia and that of the intervention. This discussion will focus on the available pharmacologic therapy for the common tachyarrhythmias encountered in clinical practice. We will highlight the appropriate pharmacologic therapy for the acute and chronic management of these arrhythmias. *(Tables 34.9-34.11)*

In the acute management of wide complex tachycardias the distinction between supraventicular and ventricular rhythms is often difficult. A common pitfall, which can lead to potentially catastrophic results, is the premise that a well tolerated arrhythmia must be supraventricular in origin. Any arrhythmia whose origin is questionably from the ventricle should be treated as such. Most importantly one must not use verapamil, whose hemodynamic effects can result in rapid hemodynamic collapse.

Table 34.9   RECOMMENDED THERAPY FOR SUPRAVENTRICULAR
                          TACHYCARDIAS

Tachycardia	First Choice	Second Choice	Alternative
Atrial Fibrillation/ Flutter (rate control)	Beta-blocker	Digoxin* Verapamil Diltiazem	
Atrial Fibrillation/ Flutter (rhythm control)	Sotalol Propafenone Amiodarone	Quinidine Disopyramide Procainamide	Flecainide*
AVNRT/AVRT (termination)	Adenosine++ IV Verapamil		
AVNRT/AVRT (prevention)	Verapamil Beta-blocker	Flecainide+ Propafenone Quinidine Procainamide Disopyramide	Amiodarone
Wolff-Parkinson-White Syndrome (WPW)	Flecainide+ Propafanone Quinidine Procainamide Disopyramide	B-blockers** Ca-channel blockers**	Amiodarone Sotalol
Atrial Tachycardia			
Reentrant	Flecainide+Sotalol Propafenone Quinidine Procainamide Disopyramide	Amiodarone	
Automatic	β-blockers Ca-channel blockers Digoxin	Flecainide+ Moricizine	
Multifocal	Replete Electrolytes	Verapamil Metoprolol	

+   In patients with no evidence of structural heart disease
++ Agents serve to terminate arrhythmia as well as a diagnostic tool to distinguish the type
of supraventricular tachycardia
* Only atrial fibrillation
** Used in combination with first line agent, may be dangerous as solo drug in WPW

Tachycardias which utilize the AV node as part of their reentrant circuit may
be terminated by agents which block conduction across the AV node, including
adenosine, calcium channel antagonists, β-adrenergic antagonists and digoxin. Of
special note is the emergence of adenosine as both an important therapeutic and
diagnostic agent in the acute treatment of supraventricular tachycardias. The recommended starting dose of adenosine is 6 mg followed, if needed, by 12 mg, administered as an intravenous bolus. Adenosine will terminate over 90 % of supraventricular tachycardias. Sinus node reentry also responds to the actions of adenosine.
On the other hand atrial fibrillation, atrial flutter, and sinus tachycardia will not be

Table 34.10 RECOMMENDED ANTIARRHYTHMIC DRUG THERAPY FOR VENTRICULAR TACHYCARDIAS

Tachycardia	First Choice	Comments/Alternatives
Ventricular Premature Depolarizations (VPD's)	β-blockers*	No Therapy in asymptomatic patients
Non-sustained Ventricular Tachycardia	β-blockers*	EP Guided Therapy or ICD in rases of CAD+LV dysfunction pending results of MUSTT trial
Sustained Ventricular Tachycardia*	Lidocaine Procainamide Cardioversion	Cardioversion first if hemodynamic or ischemic compromise Amiodarone, Sotalol, Procainamide for chronic therapy
Ventricular Fibrillation	Defibrillation	Lidocaine, procainamide, bretylium, amiodarone may be used for prophylaxis
Torsade de Pointes	Magnesium Cardiac Pacing Isoproterenol	Correct causes

* Certain idiopathic monomorphic ventricular tachycardias (e.g. exercise induced LBBB type or idiopathic VT with RBBB, LAD axis) are verapamil responsive as well as amenable to radiofrequency ablation

Table 34.11   GUIDELINES FOR DOSAGE FOR THE COMMONLY USED
              ANTIARRHYTHMIC AGENTS

Drug	Usual Dosage and Schedule
Esmolol (Brevibloc)	IV loading dose of 500 ug/kg/min over 1 minute followed by 25 µg/kg/min; maintainence dose can be increased by 25-50 µg/kg/min ever 4 minutes until desired effect is achieved
Amiodarone (Cordarone)	PO loading ranges from 800-1600 mg/day for 1-3 weeks followed by 600-800 mg/day for 1 month; maintainence is continued with 200-400 mg/day
	IV loading: 1.5 mg/ml at a rate of 15 mg/min over 10 minutes, followed by 1.8 mg/ml at a rate of 1mg/min over the next 6 hours. Maintainence is continued at a rate of 0.5 mg/min (concentration 1.8 mg/ml) over the remaining 18 hours.
Sotalol (Betapace)	PO starting dose is 80-160 mg twice a day in divided doses and the dose doubled every 48 hours up to a maximum dose of 320 mg bid
Bretylium (Bretylol)	IV Loading: 5 mg/kg with additional doses of 10 mg/kg to a maximum dose of 30 mg/kg. Maintainence at 5-10 mg/kg every 6 hours or continuous infusion at 1-2 mg/min
Verapamil (Isoptin, Calan)	IV loading: 5-10 mg over 2-3 minutes; can be repeated in 30 minutes if necessary. Followed by an IV infusion at 0.375 mg/min for 30 min; maintainence 0.125 mg/min
Adenosine (Adenocard)	IV administration initially at 6 mg, may be repeated at a dose of 6-12 mg. Administered as a rapid IV bolus.
Digoxin (Lanoxin)	PO Loading: 1-1.5 mg over 24 hours in 3-4 divided doses
	IV Loading: 1 mg over 24 hours as above Maintainence usually PO 0.125-0.25 mg/day

terminated by this agent, although transient AV nodal block may reveal concealed flutter or P waves which can clarify the underlying rhythm when the diagnosis is in doubt. Lastly, atrial tachycardias, either unifocal or multifocal are nearly always resistant to the actions of this agent. Despite a favorable side effect profile one must exhibit caution in administering adenosine in certain specific circumstances. Although a theoretical consideration one must monitor carefully the effects in those patients with hyperresponsive airways disease, as well as, in cardiac transplant recipients who may exhibit an exaggerated response to the actions of adenosine.[164]

Supraventricular tachycardias

Atrial tachycardia. Reentrant atrial tachycardia can be treated in general as described beelow for atrial flutter. Automatic atrial tachycardias (unifocal) are resistant to pharmacotherapy. There has been limited success with class IA, IC, and III agents, with a higher response rate observed with the IC drugs. However, radiofrequency ablation remains the treatment of choice in patients, with no apparent contraindications and a mappable automatic focus.

In the treatment of multifocal atrial tachycardia, which usually occurs in the elderly with severe underlying cardiopulmonary disease the most important intervention is to treat identifiable precipitents, which, include digoxin toxicity, electrolyte disturbances (most importantly hypomagnesemia and hypokalemia), hypoxia, and theopylline toxicity. Success with verapamil and metoprolol have been reported.[17]

Atrial fibrillation and atrial flutter. In the acute and chronic management of these arrhythmias, digoxin, β-blockers, and calcium channel blockers are administered for the control of the ventricular response. However, β-blockers and calcium antagonists control the rate more effectively than digoxin.

The class IA and IC agents are the most effective drugs for the chemical cardioversion of these arrhythmias. Alternatively, class III or DC cardioversion may be employed. Class IC agents are safe in those individuals without underlying structural heart disease. Sotalol is avoided in patients with underlying sinus, AV nodal disease, or a prolonged QTc (0.55 sec) due to an increased risk of torsade de pointes. Low dose amiodarone has been used successfully for the treatment of these rhythm disturbances. Ablative techniques are available for the treatment of type I atrial flutter, refractory to pharmacotherapy. Radiofrequency modification or ablation of the AV node with or without pacemaker placement is reserved for symptomatic patients with drug refractory atrial fibrillation.

Atrioventricular (AV) nodal reentrant tachycardia and orthodromic AV reentrant tachycardia. These arrhythmias are promptly terminated with intravenous adenosine, verapamil. For the long term management of recurrent, symptomatic arrhythmias, radiofrequency ablation is the therapeutic intervention of choice. Radiofrequency ablation of the slow pathway in AVNRT and the bypass tract in AVRT has been successful in termination of these rhythm disturbances with low risk of complete AV block.

In those patients who are not candidates for ablation, class IC agents in combination with AV nodal blocking agents in the absence of structural heart disease is an alternative therapeutic option. Successful control of these arrhythmias with class IA and III agents has also been reported.

Wolff-Parkinson-White syndrome. In those patients with WPW who present with atrial fibrillation and a rapid ventricular response, with bizarre pre-excited QRS complexes, drugs which selectively inhibit AV nodal conduction are contraindicated. Digitalis, calcium channel blockers, and β-blockers affect conduction across the AV node with little if any effect on the accessory pathway. By selectively inhibiting AV nodal conduction these agents increase conduction across the accessory pathway, increasing the ventricular response, consequently increasing the risk of VF. Procainamide can be used in the acute and chronic treatment of WPW, in hemodynamically stable patients. In those individuals with hemodynamic compromise DC cardioversion is the recommended first line therapy. Class IA ,IC and III agents have been shown to be effective in the treatment of this rhythm disturbance. In young patients, with WPW, and a high risk of sudden death (shortest RR interval of pre-excited complexes <250 msec), radiofrequency ablation may be an effective alternative; reducing the morbidity associated with lifelong antiarrhythmic therapy.

Sustained ventricular tachycardia (VT). Hemodynamically stable sustained VT can be treated acutely with either lidocaine, procainamide or drug refractory cases DC cardioversion. Cardioversion is a safe and effective means of terminating hemody- namically compromising VT. It is recommended that these patients have a baseline electrophysiologic study and 24-hour Holter recording. A beneficial response to antiarrhythmic drug therapy includes both noninducibility by programmed electri- cal stimulation (PES) and elimination of nonsustained VT on Holter recording. The Electrophysiologic Study Versus Electrocardiographic Monitoring (ESVEM) trial has shown that d,l-sotalol is the most efficacious drug for the treatment of these arrhythmias. Therefore, unless β-blockers or class III agents are contraindicated sotalol is recommended as first line therapy. Alternatively, class IA agents, e.g qui- nidine, can be used if sotalol is ineffective. Monotherapyt with mexiletine has been found to be ineffective in treating these rhythms, but a combination with quinidine can be used. If above drug therapies prove ineffective a patient can be treated with amiodarone or an ICD.

Ventricular fibrillation (VF). For survivors of out-of-hospital sudden cardiac death it is recommended that these patients be evaluated by EPS. In patients with exten- sive but correctable coronary artery disease with preserved LV function ventricular fibrillation may be adequately treated by revascularization (e.g coronary artery by- pass surgery or PTCA). For those patients found to have inducible sustained VT and EPS guided therapeutic approach is applied. At the present time patients found noninducible at the time of EPS are treated with an implantable cardiac defibrilla- tor. The advantage of initial implantable defibrillator placement, as opposed to, drug therapy has yet to be established. The ongoing Antiarrhythmic Drug Versus Implantable Defibrillators (AVID) study has been designed to answer this question.

REFERENCES

1. Vaughan Williams EM. A classification of antiarrhythmic actions reassessed after a decade of new drugs. J Clin Pharmacol 1984:24:129.

2. Task force of the working group on arrhythmias of the European society of cardiology: The Sicilian Gambit. A new approach to the classification of antiarrhythmic drugs based on the actions on arrhythmogenic mechanisms. Circulation 1991:84:1831.

3. Josephson ME. Clinical cardiac electrophysiology: techniques and interpretation. Philadel- phia: Lea & Febiger, 1993.

4. Wellens HJJ, Bar FWHM, Lie KI. The value of the Electrocardiogram in the Differential Diagnosis of a Tachycardia with a Widened QRS Complex. Am J Med 1978: 64:27.

5. Rosen KM, Mehtra A, Miller RA. Demonstration of dual atrioventricular nodal pathways in man. Am J Cardiol 1974: 33:291.

6. Goldreyer BN, Bigger JT Jr. Site of reentry in paroxysmal supraventricular tachycardia in man. Circulation 1971:43:15.

7. Ganz LI, Friedman PL. Supraventricular tachycardia. N Engl J Med 1995:332:162.

8. Morady F, et al. Electrophysiologic testing in the management of patients with the Wolff-Parkinson-White syndrome and atrial fibrillation. Am J Cardiol 1983:51:1623.

9. Klein GJ, et al. Ventricular fibrillation in Wolff-Parkinson-White syndrome. N Engl J Med 1979:301:1080.

10. Rosen KM. Junctional tachycardia: mechanisms, diagnosis, differential diagnosis and management. Circulation 1973:47:654.

11. Kerr CR, Mason MA. Incidence and clinical significance of accelerated junctional rhythm following open heart surgery. Am Heart J 1985:110:966.

12. Coumel P. Junctional reciprocating tachycardias. The permanent and paroxysmal forms of A-V nodal reciprocating tachycardias. J Electrocardiology 1975:9:79.

13. Cruz FE, et al. Reversibility of tachycardia-induced cardiomyopathy after cure of incessant supraventricular tachycardia. J Am Coll Cardiol 1990:16:739.

14. Fiorenzo G, et al. Catheter ablation of permanent junctional reciprocating tachycardia with radiofrequency current. J Am Coll Cardiol 1995:25:648.

15. Sanders WE, et al. Catheter ablation of sinoatrial node reentrant tachycardia. J Am Coll Cardiol 1994:23:926.

16. Kastor JA. Multifocal atrial tachycardia. N Engl J Med 1990:322:1713.

17. Levine JH, Michael JR, Guarnieri. Treatment of multifocal atrial tachycardia with verapamil. N. Engl J Med 1985: 312:21.

18. Pritchett ELC. Management of atrial fibrillation. N Engl J Med 1992:326:1264.

19. Reiffel J. Atrial Fibrillation. Cardiology Special Edition 1995:1:53.

20. Calvert A, Lown B, Gorlin R. Ventricular premature beats and anatomically defined coronary heart disease. Am J Cardiol 1977:39:627.

21. Campbell RWF, Murray A, Julian DG. Ventricular arrhythmias in the first 12 hours of acute myocardial infarction: natural history study. Br Heart J 1981:46:351.

22. Koster RW, Dunning AJ. Intramuscular lidocaine for prevention of lethal arrhythmias in the prehospitalization phase of acute myocardial infarction. N Engl J Med 1985:313:1105.

23. Hine LK, et al. Meta-analytic evidence against prophylactic use of lidocaine in acute myocardial infarction. Arch Intern Med 1989:149:2694.

24. MacMahon S, et al. Effects of prophylactic lidocaine in suspected acute myocardial infarction — an overview of results from randomized trials. JAMA 1988:260:1910.

25. Bigger JT Jr, et al. The relationships among ventricular arrhythmias, left ventricular dysfunction, and mortality in the two years after myocardial infarction. Circulation 1984:69:250.

26. Campbell RWF. Ventricular ectopic beats and non-sustained ventricular tachycardia. Lancet 1993:341:1454.

27. The Cardiac Arrhythmia Suppression Trial (CAST) Investigators. Preliminary report: effect of encainide and flecainide on mortality in a randomized trial of arrhythmia suppression after myocardial infarction. N Engl J Med 1989:321:406.

28. The Cardiac Arrhythmia Suppression Trial II Investigators. Effect of the antiarrhythmic agent moricizine on survival after myocardial infarction. N Engl J Med 1992:327:227.

29. Kennedy HL, et al. Long term follow-up of asymptomatic healthy subjects with frequent and complex ventricular ectopy. N Engl J Med 1985:312:193.

30. Buxton AE, et al. Prevention of sudden death in patients with coronary artery diseas: the multicenter unsustained tachycardia trial (MUSTT). Progress Cardio Dis 1993:36:215.

31. Josephson ME, et al. Recurrent sustained ventricular tachycardia 1. Mechanisms. Circulation 1978:57:431.

32. El-Sherif N, et al. QTU prolongation and polymorphic VT due to bradycardia dependent early after-depolarizations. Circ Res 1988:63:286.

33. Patterson E, et al. Early and delayed afterdepolarizations associated with cesium chloride induced arrhytmias in the dog. J Cardiovasc Pharmacol 1990:15:323.

34. Vos MA, et al. Reproducible induction of early afterdepolarizations and torsade de pointes arrhythmias by d-sotalol and pacing in dogs with chronic atrioventricular block. Circulation 1995:91:864.

35. Roden DM, et al. Clinical features and basic mechanisms of quninidine-induced arrhythmias. J Am Coll Cardiol 1986:8:73A.

36. Strasberg B, et al. Procainamide-induced polymorphous ventricular tachycardia. Am J Cardiol 1981:47:1309.

37. Ruffy R: Sotalol. J Cardiovasc Electrophysiol 1993:4:81.

38. Carruth JE, Silverman ME. Torsade de pointe atypical ventricular tachycardia complicating subarachnoid hemorrhage. Chest 1980:78:886.

39. Jackman WM, et al. The long QT syndromes: a critical review, new clinical observations and a unifying hypothesis. Prog Cardiovasc Dis 1988:31:115.

40. Johnson EA, McKinnon MG. The differential effect of quinidine and pyralamine on the myocardial action potential at various rates of stimulation. J Pharm Exp Ther 1957:120:460.

41. Vaughan Williams EM. Subgroups of class 1 antiarrhythmic drugs. Eur Heart J 1984:5:96.

41A. Harrison DC. Antiarrhythmic drug classification: new science and practical applications. Am J Cardiol 1985:56:185.

42. Campbell TJ. Kinetics of onset of rate-dependent effects of class I antiarrhythmic drugs are important in determining their effects on refractoriness in guinea-pig ventricle, and provide a theoretical basis for their subclassification. Cardiovasc Res 1983:17:344.

42A. Nattel S. Antiarrhythmic drug classifications: A critical appraisal of their history, present status, and clinical relevance. Drugs 1991:41:672.

42B. Coromilas J. Classification of anti-arrhythmic agents: electropharmacologic basis and clinical relevance: Contemporary Management of Ventricular Arrhythmias 1992: A. Greenspan, H. Waxman (eds). Cardiovascular Clinics, FA Davis Co.: 97.

43. Roden DM, et al. Quinidine delays Ik activation in guinea pig ventricular myocytes. Circ Res 1988:62:1055.

44. Lucchesi BR, Lynch J. Pharmacology of antiarrhythmic drugs. In Modern Pharmacology (eds. Craig CR, Stitzel RE). Little, Brown and Company, Boston/Toronto 1986 388.

44A. Mirro MJ, et al. Anticholinergic effects of disopyramide and quinidine on guinea pig myocardium. Mediation by direct muscarinic receptor blockade. Circ Res 1980:47:855.

45. Solkolow M, Ball RE. Factors influencing conversion of chronic atrial fibrillation with special reference to serum quinidine concentration. Circulation 1956:14:569.

46. 46A. Motulsky HJ, et al.: Quinidine is a competitive antagonist at alpha 1- and alpha 2-adrenergic receptors. Circ Res 1984:55:376.

46B. Roden DM, Hoffman BF. Action potential prolongation and induction of abnormal automaticity by low quinidine concentrations in canine Purkinje fibers. Circ Res 1985:56:857.

46C. Stratmann HG, Kennedy Hl. Torsades de pointes assocated with drugs and toxins: Recognition and management. Am Heart J 1987:113:1470.

47. Leahy EB., et al. Interaction between quinidine and digoxin. JAMA 1978:240:533.

48. Farringer JA, McWay-Hess K, Clementi WA. Cimetidine-quinidine interation. Clin Pharm 1984:3:81.

49. Gibson TP, et al. Acetylation of procainamide in man and its relationship to isonicotinic acid hydrazide acetylation phenotype. Clin Pharmacol Ther 1975:17:395.

50. Giardina EGV, Stein RM, Bigger JT. The relationship between the metabolism of procainamide and sulfamethazine. Circulation 1977:55:388.

51. Reidenberg MM, et al. Polymorphic acetylation of procainamide in man. Clin Pharmacol Ther 1975:17:722.

52. Jaillon P, et al. Electrophysiologic effects of N-acetylprocainamide in human beings. Am J Cardiol 1981:47:1134.

53. Colatsky TJ. Mechanisms of action of lidocaine and quinidine on action potential duration in rabbit cardiac purkinje fibers: an effect on steady state sodium currents? Circ Res 1982:50:17.

54. Morady F, et al. Rate-dependent effects of intravenous lidocaine, procainamide, and amiodarone on intraventricular conduction. J Am Coll Cardiol 1985:6:179.

55. Gorgels APM, et al. Comparison of procainamide and lidocaine in terminating sustaned monomorphic ventricular tachycardia. Am J Cardiol 1996:78:43.

56. Campbell RW. Mexiletine. N Engl J Med 1987:316:29.

57. Mason JW, et al. A comparison of seven antiarrhythmic drugs in patients with ventricular tachyarrhythmias. N Engl J. Med 1993:329:452.

58. Podrid PJ, Lown B. Mexiletine for ventricular arrhythmias. Am J Cardiol 1981:47:895.

59. Duff HJ, et al. Mexiletine-quinidine combination: electrophysiologic correlates of favorable antiarrhythmic interaction in humans. J Am Coll Cardiol 1987:10:1149.

60. Chezalviel F, et al.: Antiarrhythmic effect of sotalol-mexiletine combination on induced ventricular tachycardia in dogs. J Cardiovas Pharmacol 1993:21:212.

61. Gottlieb SS, Weinbert M: Comparative hemodynamic effects of mexiletine and quinidine in patients with severe left ventricular dysfunction. Am Heart J 1991:122:1368.

61A. Stein J, Podrid P, Lown B. Effects of oral mexiletine on left and right ventricular function. Am J Cardiol 1984:54:575.

62. Meffin PJ, et al. Response optimization of drug dosage: antiarrhythmic studies with tocainide. Clin Pharmacol Ther 1977:22:42.

63. Roden DM, Woosley RL. Tocainide. N Engl J Med 1986:315:41.

64. Woosley RL, et al. Suppression of ventricular ectopic depolarizations by tocainide. Circulation 1977:56:980.

65. Klein MD, Levine PA, Ryan TJ. Antiarrhythmic efficacy, pharmacokinetics and clinical safety of tocainide in convalescent myocardial infarction patients. Chest 1980:7:726.

66. Holmes B, et al. Tocainide: a review of its pharmacological properties and therapeutic efficacy. Drugs 1983:26:93.

67. Hession M, et al. Mexiletine and tocainide: Does response to one predict response to the other? J Am Coll Cardiol 1986:7:338.

68. Volosin K, Greenberg RM, Greenspon AJ. Tocainide associated agranulocytosis. Am Heart J 1985:109:1392.

69. Soff GA, Kadin ME. Tocainide-induced reversible agranulocytosis and anemia. Arch Intern Med 1987:147:598.

70. O'Hara G, et al. Effects of flecainide on the rate-dependence of atrial refractoriness, atrial repolarization, and atrioventricular node conduction in anesthetized dogs. J Am Coll Cardiol 1992:19:1335.

71. Guehler J, et al. Electrophysiologic effects of flecainide acetate and its major metabolites in the canine heart. Am J Cardiol 1985:55:807.

72. Roden DM, Woosley RL. Flecainide. N Engl J Med 1986:315:36.

73. Echt DS, et al. Mortality and morbidity in patients receiving encainide, flecainide, or placebo. N Engl J Med 1991:324:781.

74. Camm AJ, et al. Clinical usefulness of flecainide acetate in the treatment of paroxysmal supraventricular arrhythmias. Drugs 1985:29(suppl 4):7.

75. Borgeat A, et al. Flecainide versus quinidine for conversion of atrial fibrillation to sinus rhythm. Am J Cardiol 1986:58:496.

76. Benditt DG. Flecainide acetate for long-term prevention of paroxysmal supraventricular tachycardia. Circulation 1991:83:345.

77. Vid-mo H, Ohm OJ, Lound-Johansen P: Electrophysiologic effects of flecainide acetate in patients with sinus nodal dysfunction. Am J Cardiol 1982: 50:1090.

78. Hellestrand KJ, et al. Electrophysiologic effects of flecainide acetate on sinus node function, anomalous atrioventricular connections and pacemaker thresholds. Am J Cardiol 1984:53:30B.

79. Shea S, et al. Flecainide and amiodarone interaction. J Am Coll Cardiol 1986:7:1127.

80. Thompson KA, et al. Potent electrophysiologic effects of the major metabolites of propafenone in canine purkinje fibers. J Pharmacol Exp Ther 1988:244:950.

81. Siddoway LA, et al. Polymorphism of propafenone metabolism and disposition in man: clinical and pharmacokinetic consequences. Circulation 1987:75:785.

82. Ludmer PL, et al. Efficacy of propafenone in Wolff-Parkinson-White Syndrome: electrophysiologic findings and long-term follow-up. J Am Coll Cardiol 1987:9:1357.

83. Connolly SJ, Hoffert DL. Usefulness of propafenone for recurrent paroxysmal atrial fibrillation. Am J Cardiol 1989:63:817.

84. Bianconi L, et al. Effectiveness of intravenous propafenone for conversion of atrial fibrillation and flutter of recent onset. Am J Cardiol 1989:64:335.

85. Hodges M, Salerno D, Granrud G. Double-blind placebo-controlled evaluation of propafenone in suppressing ventricular ectopic activity. Am J Cardiol 1984:54:45D.

86. Kates RE. Interaction between warfarin and propafenone in healthy volunteer subjects. Clin Pharmacol Ther 1987:42:305.

87. Mann DE, et al. Electrophysiologic effects of ethmozin in patients with ventricular tachycardia. Am Heart J 1984:107:674.

88. Rosenshtraukh LV, et al. Electrophysiologic effects of moricizine HCl. Am J Cardiol 1987:60:27F.

89. Bigger JT. Cardiac electrophysiologic effects of moricizine hydrochloride. Am J Cardiol 1990:65:15D.

90. Danilo P, et al. Effects of phenothiazine analog, EN-313, on ventricular arrhythmias in the dog. Eur J Pharmacol 1977:45:127.

91. Hewett K, Gessman L, Rosen MR. Effects of procainamide, quinidine and ethmozin on delayed afterdepolarizations. Eur J Pharmacol 1983:96:21.

92. Dangman KH, Hoffman BF. Antiarrhythmic effects of ethmozine in cardiac Purkinje fibers: suppresion of automaticity and abolition of triggering. J Pharmacol Exp Ther 1983:227:578.

93. Vaughan Williams EM. Classification of the antiarrhythmic action of moricizine. J Clin Pharmacol 1991:31:216.

94. Clyne CA, Estes NAM, Wang PJ. Moricizine. N Engl J Med 1992:327:255.

95. Evans VL, et al. Ethmozine (moricizine HCl): a promising drug for "automatic" atrial ectopic tachycardia. Am J Cardiol 1987:60:83F.

96. Tschaidse P, et al. The prevalence of life-threatening proarrhythmic events during moricizine therapy. Circulation 1991:84(Suppl II):II-125.

97. Olshansky B, Kall JG, Wilbur D. Efficacy and adverse effects of moricizine for ventricular tachycardia. Circulation 1991:84(Suppl II):II-713.

98. Kennedy HL. Noncardiac adverse effects and organ toxicity of moricizine during short- and long-term studies. Am J Cardiol 1990:65:47D-50D.

99. Friedman LM, et al. Effect of propanolol in patients with myocardial infarction and ventricular arrhythmia. J Am Coll Cardiol 1986:7:1.

100. Kinoshita K, et al. Ischemia-and reperfusion-induced arrhythmias in conscious rats — studies with prazosin and atenolol. Jpn Circ J 1988:52:1384.

101. Inoue H, Zipes DP. Results of sympathetic denervation in the canine heart: supersensitivity that may be arrhythmogenic. Circulation 1987:75:877.

102. Stagg AL, Wallace AG. The effect of propanolol on membrane conductance in canine cardiac purkinje fibers. Circulation 1974:50(suppl III):III.

103. Davis LD, Temte JV. Effects of propanolol on the transmembrane potentials of ventricular muscle and purkinje fibers of the dog. Circ Res 1968:22:661.

104. Chang MS, Zipes DP. Differential sensitivity of sinus node, atrioventricular node, atrium, and ventricle to propanolol. Am Heart J 1988:116:371.

105. Gang ES, Bigger JT, Uhl EW. Effects of timolol and propanolol on inducible sustained ventricular tachyarrhythmias in dogs with subacute myocardial infarction. Am J Cardiol 1984:53:275.

106. Kupersmith J, et al. Electrophysiological and antiarrhythmic effects of propanolol in canine acute myocardial ischemia. Circ Res 1976:38:302.

107. Brodsky MA, et al. Antiarrhythmic efficacy of solitary B-adrenergic blockade for patients with sustained ventricular tachyarrhythmias. Am Heart J 1989:118:272.

108. Steinbeck G, et al. A comparison of electrophysiologically guided antiarrhythmic drug therapy with beta-blocker therapy in patients with symptomatic, sustained ventricular arrhythmias. N Engl J Med 1992:327:987.

109. Moss AJ. Prolonged QT syndromes. JAMA 1986:256:2985.

110. Hohnloser SH, Woosley RL. Sotalol. N Engl J Med 1994:331:31.

111. Blinks JR. Evaluation of the cardiac effects of several β-adrenergic blocking agents. Ann NY Acad Sci 1967:139:673.

112. Aberg G, et al. A comparative study of some cardiovascular effects of sotalol (MJ 1999) and propanolol. Life Sci 1969:8:353.

113. Gomoll AW, Braunwald E. Comparative effects of sotalol and propanolol on myocardial contractility. Arch Int Pharmacodyn Ther 1973:205:338.

114. Nattel S, et al. Concentration dependence of class III and beta-adrenergic blocing effects of sotalol in anesthetized dogs. J Am Coll Cardiol 1989:13:1190.

115. Wang T, et al. Concentration-dependent pharmacologic properties of sotalol. Am J Cardiol 1986:57:1160.

116. Lathrop DA, Varro A, Schwartz A. Rate-dependent electrophysiological effects of OPC-8212: comparison to sotalol. Eur J Pharmacol 1989:164:487.

117. Krapf R, Kirsch M. Torsade de pointes induced by sotalol despite therapeutic concentrations. Br Med J 1985:290:1784.

118. Mason JW. A comparison of electrophysiologic testing with Holter monitoring to predict antiarrhythmic drug efficacy for ventricular tachyarrhythmias. N Engl J Med 1993:329:445.

119. Ruder MA, et al. Clinical experience with sotalol in patients with drug-refractory ventricular arrhythmias. J Am Coll Cardiol 1989:13:145.

120. Soyka LF, Wirtz C, Spangenberg RB. Clinical safety profile of sotalol in patients with arrhythmias. Am J Cardiol 1990:65:74A.

121. Groh WJ, et al. b-adrenergic property of d-sotalol maintains class III efficacy in guinea pig ventricular muscle after isoproterenol. Cirulation 1995:91:262.

122. Waldo AL, et al. Effect of β-sotalol on mortality in patients with left ventricular dysfunction after recent and rmote myocardial infarction. The SWORD investigators. Survival with oral d-sotalol. Lancet 1996:348:7.

123. Kontopopulos A, et al. Sotalol induced torsade de pointes. Postgrad Med J 1981:57:321.

124. Hohnloser SH, Arendts W, Quart B. Torsade de pointes during sotalol therapy. Eur Heart J 1992:13(suppl):305.

125. Hohnloser SH, Klingenheben T, Singh BN. Amiodarone-associated proarrhythmic effects: A review with special reference to torsade de pointes tachycardia. Ann Intern Med 1994:121:529.

126. Pritchard DA, Singh BN, Hurley PJ. Effects of amiodarone on the thyorid function in patients with ischaemic heart disease. Br Heart J 1975:37:856.

127. Holt DW, et al. Amiodarone pharmacokinetics. Am Heart J 1983:106:840.

128. Latini R, Togoni G, Kates RE. Clinical pharmacokinetics of amiodarone. Clin Pharmacokinet 1984:9:136.

129. Singh BN. Electropharmacology of amiodarone. In Vaughn Williams EM, Campbell TJ (eds): Anti-Arrhythmic Drugs. Berlin: Springer-Verlag (1988), p. 335.

130. Anderson KP, et al. Rate related electrophysiologic effects of long-term administration of amiodarone on canine ventricular myocardium in vivo. Circulation 1989:79:948.

131. Kadish AH, et al. Amiodarone: correlation of early and late electrophysiologic studies with outcome. Am Heart J 1986:112:1134.

132. Waxman HL, et al. Amiodarone for control of sustained ventricular tachyarrhythmia: clinical and electrophysiologic effects in 51 patients. Am J Cardiol 1982:50:1067.

133. Horowitz LN, et al. Usefulness of electrophysiologic testing in evaluation of amiodarone therapy for sustained ventricular tachyarrhythmias associated with coronary heart disease. Am J Cardiol 1985:55:367.

134. Nademanee K, et al. Antiarrhythmic efficacy and electrophysiologic actions of amiodarone in patients with life-threatening arrhythmias: potent suppression of spontaneously occurring tachyarrhythmias versus inconsistent abolition of induced ventricular tachycardia. Am Heart J 1982:103:950.

135. McGovern B, et al. Long-term clinical outcome of ventricular tachycardia or fibrillation treated with amiodarone. Am J Cardiol 1984:53:1558.

136. Stanton HS, et al. Arrhythmogenic effects of antiarrhythmic drugs: a study of 506 patients treated for ventricular tachycardia or fibrillation. J Am Coll Cardiol 1989:19:209.

137. Boura ALA, et al. Darenthin: hypotensive agent of new type. Lancet 1959:2:17.

138. Dollery CT, Emslie-Smith D, McMichael J. Bretylium tosylate in the treatment of hypertension. Lancet 1960:6:296.

139. Boura ALA, Green AF. The actions of bretylium: adrenergic neurone blocking and other effects. Br J Pharmacol 1959:14:536.

140. Bacaner MB. Treatment of ventricular fibrillation and other acute arryhthmias with bretylium tosylate. Am J Cardiol 1968:21:530.

141. Anderson JL. Adrenergic neuron blockers as class III antiarrhythmic agents: bretylium and its analogs. In Singh BN, et al. (eds): Cardiovascular Pharmacology and Therapeutics. New York: Churchill-Livingston (1994), p. 712.

142. Heissenbuttal RH, Bigger JT. Bretylium tosylate: a newly available antiarrhythmic drug for ventricular arrhythmias. Ann Intern Med 1979:90:229.

143. Bigger JT, Hoffman BF. Antiarrhythmic Drugs. In Goodman & Gillman, p.867.

144. Lee KS. Ibutilide, a new compound with potent class III antiarrhythmic activity, activates a slow inward Na+ current in guinea pig ventricular cells. J Pharma Experiment Therapeutics 1992: 262:99.

145. Yang T, Snyders DF, Roden DM. Ibutilide, a methanesulfonanilide antiarrhythmic, is a potent blocker of the rapidly activating delayed rectifier K+ current (Ikr) in AT-1 cells. Concentration-, time-, voltage-, and use-dependent effects. Circulation 1995: 91:1799.

146. Stambler BS, et al. Efficacy and safety of repeated intravenous doses of ibutilide for rapid conversion of atrial flutter of fibrillation. Circulation 1996: 94:1613.

147. Ellenbogen KA, et al. Efficacy of intravenous ibutilide for rapid termination of atrial fibrillation and atrial flutter: a dose-response study. JACC 1996: 28:130.

148. Slish DF, Schultz D, Schwartz A. Molecular biology of calcium antagonist receptor. Hypertension 1992:19:19.

149. Talajic H, Nattel S. Frequency dependent effects of calcium antagonists on atrioventricular conduction and refractoriness: demonstration and characterization in anesthetized dogs. Circulation 1986:74:1156.

150. Schwartz A. Calcium antagonists: review and perspective on mechanism of action. Am J Cardiol 1989:64(suppl I):31.

151. Kawai C, et al. Comparative effects of three calcium antagonists, diltiazem, verapamil, and nifedipine on the sinoatrial and atrioventricular nodes. Circulation 1981:63:1035.

152. Smith TW. Digitalis: mechanism of action and clinical use. N Engl J Med 1988:318:358.

153. Marcus FI, Kapadia GJ, Kapadia GG: The metabolism of digoxin in normal subjects. J Pharmacol Exp Therap 1964:145:203.

154. Hinderling PH, Hartmann D: Pharmacokinetics of digoxin and main metabolites/derivatives in healthy humans. Ther Drug Monit 1991:13:381.

155. Lindenbaum J, et al. Inactivation of digoxin by the gut flora: Reversal by antibiotic therapy. N Engl J Med 1981:305:789.

156. Dobbs RJ, et al. Serum concentration monitoring of cardiac glycosides. How helpful is it for adjusting dosage regimens? Clin Pharmakokinetic 1991:20:175.

157. Lee TH, Smith TW: Serum digoxin concentration and diagnosis of digitalis toxicity: Current concepts. Clin Pharmacokinet 1983:8:279.

158. Ewy GA, et al: Digoxin metabolism in obesity. Circulation 1971:44:810.

159. Gault MH. Digitalis in renal failure. Int J Artif Organs 1988:11:141.

160. Muller JE, et al. Digoxin therapy and mortality after myocardial infarction. Experience in the MILIS Study. N Engl J Med 1986:314:265.

161. Belardinelli L, Isenberg G. Isolated atrial myocytes:adenosine and acetylcholine increase potassium conductance. Am J Physiol. 1983:244:H734.

162. Kurachi Y, Nakajima T, Sugimoto T. On the mechanism of activation of muscarinic K+ channels by adenosine in isolated atrial cells: involvement of GTP-binding proteins. Pflugers Arch. 1986:407:264.

163. West GA, Belardinelli L. Sinus slowing and pacemaker shift caused by adenosine in rabbit SA node. Pflugers Arch. 1985:403:66.

164. Lerman BB, Belardinelli L. Cardiac electrophysiology of adenosine:basic and clinical concepts. Circulation 1991:83:1499.

35 ABLATIVE THERAPY FOR ARRHYTHMIAS

J. Anthony Gomes, Davendra Mehta

The last decade has seen considerable advances in the management of cardiac arrhythmias. The development of catheter technology and the introduction of radiofrequency current has revolutionized the approach to management of tachyarrhythmias. This chapter will discuss the techniques, indications and outcome of RF ablative therapy of supraventricular and ventricular tachyarrhythmias.

Supraventricular tachycardias

Supraventricular tachycardias (SVT) are the most common cardiac arrhythmias seen in clinical practice. They account for more than 60% of all cardiac arrhythmias. The commonest supraventricular tachycardia is atrial fibrillation, which accounts for more than 50% of all supraventricular tachycardias; tachyarrhythmias due to AV nodal reentry, those utilizing concealed bypass tracts in the reentrant process and tachyarrhythmias associated with Wolff-Parkinson-White (WPW) syndrome. These tachycardias together account for approximately 40% of all supraventricular tachycardias. The less common varieties of supraventricular arrhythmias such as sinus node reentrant tachycardia, atrial tachycardias and inappropriate sinus tachycardias account for less than 15% of all supraventricular tachycardias.

Table 35.1 lists the classification of supraventricular tachycardias on the basis of the site of origin and the mechanism of the tachycardia. Tachycardias that arise in the region of the sinus node include inappropriate sinus tachycardia and sinoatrial reentrant tachycardia. Those that arise in the atrium may be reentrant in mechanism or automatic (due to triggered automaticity or abnormal automaticity). The other arrhythmias that arise in the atrium include atrial flutter and atrial fibrillation. Tachycardias that arise in the AV junction can be divided into two categories, AV junctional reentrant tachycardia due to reentry in the region of the AV junction utilizing most commonly a slow pathway for antegrade conduction and a fast pathway for retrograde conduction. An atypical variety which utilizes the fast pathway in antegrade conduction and a slow pathway for retrograde conduction or two slow pathways for both antegrade and retrograde conduction have also been described. The second variety is junctional tachycardia. This tachycardia is automatic in mechanism and seen in acute conditions such as immediately post myocardial infarction or in patients with heart failure. Finally, tachycardias associated with bypass tracts either overt WPW syndrome or concealed bypass tracts include orthodromic, antidromic or a mixed variety, atrial flutter and atrial fibrillation as well as ventricular fibrillation which is secondary to a rapid ventricular response over an accessory pathway due to atrial fibrillation or atrial flutter.

Table 35.1   CLASSIFICATION OF SVT

Sinus Node	Atrium	AV Junction	Tach With WPW/Con. Bypass Tract
Inappropriate Sinus Tachy	Atrial Tachycardia Reentrant Ectopic Unifocal/Multifocal	AV Junctional Reentrant Tachycardia	Orthodromic Antidromic Mixed
Sino-Atrial Reentrant Tachycardia	Atrial Flutter Atrial Fibrillation	Junctional Tachycardia (Automatic)	Atrial Flutter A-Fibrillation Ventricular Fib.

Ablative therapy - general concepts

The concept that cardiac tissue could be ablated with catheter techniques was demonstrated by Scheinman et al[1] and Gallagher et al[2] with the use of alternating current (50-60MHz). However, the use of alternating current has significant disadvantages. The other sources of current that are available for ablative therapy included audible sound (20-2,000Hz) radiofrequency current (1-1.5MHz), ultrasound (1.5-10MHz) and microwave (1,000-3000MHz). Radiofrequency (RF) current was initially utilized by Huang et al[3-5] and today is the gold standard[7] of current source for catheter ablation of tachycardias. The advantages of radiofrequency current over direct current[5] are listed in Table 35.2. The most important advantages of radiofrequency current include the absence of barotrauma, the lack of need for general anesthesia, very low or non existent proarrhythmogenecity, a homogenous lesion with a sharp and narrow margin and a small lesion size relative to direct current. Radiofrequency (RF) utilizes alternating current between 1.0 MHz to 1.5MHz. RF current generates electrolyte effects, faradic effects and converts electrical energy into heat. Catheter delivered RF energy causes electrosurgical desiccation. This causes coagulation necrosis without sparking or barotrauma. Transmission of RF current causes heat to desicate and results in coagulation necrosis without destruction of normal tissue. With the electrode in good contact with the myocardium, there is deep coagulation which spreads radically, the heating producing dehydration of tissues in extracellular and intracellular space with formation of coagulation necrosis and a light brown eschar. These lesions effect conduction and automaticity in cardiac tissue so that cardiac arrhythmias cannot be induced.

In the human heart for RF ablation, a catheter with a large tip electrode is connected to an electrosurgical unit as a cathode with a transcutaneous thoracic conducting patch as the anode. The energy is delivered by monitoring the temperature by increasing the power (20-50 watts) for a total of $\leq$ one minute or until there is a rise in impedance and loss of power or the desired effect is achieved. If there is a rise in impedance the catheter is removed and the coagulum is wiped out and the procedure is repeated. A loss of temperature, current or impedance implies loss of contact with tissue. A sudden marked rise in temperature with loss of power may imply tissue avulsion and thrombus formation on the catheter tip. [6]

Table 35.2   COMPARISON OF DIRECT CURRENT VERSUS RADIOFREQUENCY (RF) CURRENT FOR CATHETER ABLATION

	Direct Current	**RF Current**
Waveform	Monoph Damped Sinusoid	Continuous Unmodulated Sinusoid
Peak Voltage	1000 - 3000 V	<100V
Barotrauma	Yes	No
Sparking	Yes	No
General Anesthesia	Yes	No
Arrthomogenecity	High	Low/None
Catheter Damage	Frequent	Infrequent
Energy Loss	Less Possible	Possible
Lesion Necrosis	Inhomogenous with Irregular and Wide Margins	Homogenous with a Sharp and Narrow Margins
Lesion Size	Large	Small

Radiofrequency ablative therapy *(Table 35.3)* is utilized primarily in patients who have symptomatic tachycardia associated with the WPW syndrome requiring the need for chronic antiarrhythmic therapy. Sometimes asymptomatic patients particularly those who are in high risk professions such as athletes, police officers, bus drivers, airline pilots, may be considered for ablation; all tachycardias associated with concealed bypass tracts; AV nodal reentrant tachycardia; atrial tachycardias; atrial flutter and atrial fibrillation. Currently there is no technique to ablate atrial fibrillation, however, for this arrhythmia the two available procedures include ablation of the AV junction to produce AV block and modification of the AV junction.

Radiofrequency ablation for tachycardias associated with Wolff-Parkinson-White syndrome

The WWP syndrome[7-12] is characterized by the presence of an insulated pathway which connects the atrium to the ventricular myocardium. These accessory pathways are typically localized in the AV groove, the commonest location being left lateral.

Table 35.3   RADIOFREQUENCY ABLATIVE THERAPY

---

* Tachycardias associated with the WPW Syndrome

- Asymptomatic patients (athletes, police officers, bus driver, airline pilots, etc.)

* Tachycardias associated with concealed bypass tracts

* A-V nodal reentrant tachycardias

* Inappropriate sinus tachycardia

* Atrial tachycardias

* Atrial flutter

* Atrial fibrillation - (CHB/slow-fast AVN path)

Pathways may be separated into right sided as well as left sided. Right sided pathways may be separated into anteroseptal, midseptal, posteroseptal and lateral positions namely antero and postero-lateral. These pathways can be fairly well localized today with EKG algorithms which have been recently developed by correlating ablative sites to EKG δ-wave polarity.[13,14]

In 1968, the first surgical ablation of an accessory pathway was performed resulting in the cure of the WPW syndrome and the associated tachyarrhythmias.[15] The selective recording of depolarization of the bypass tract and the use of RF current greatly stimulated interest in ablative therapy.[16,17]

For left sided pathways, the ablative procedure can be performed either through retrograde catheterization with the ablation done at the mitral annulus on the ventricular side or through transeptal catheterization wherein ablation is done at the atrial side of the mitral annulus. The success rate of the two techniques is quite equivalent, however some high lateral pathways may not be approachable through the retrograde route but easily ablated transeptally. An electrode catheter with a large distal tip is utilized and electro-surgical unit capable of delivering more than or equal to 50 volts at frequencies of 250KHz to 750KHz is used. The catheter is connected to the electro-surgical unit as the cathode. The accessory pathways are localized by performing a standard diagnostic electrophysiologic study with the induction of the tachycardias associated with WPW syndrome. The greatest challenge is to localize the accessory pathway. A variety of electrophysiologic criteria are utilized for localization -[16-18] these include recording of bypass potentials,[1,2] atrial and ventricular fusion during pre-exited QRS complexes[3], *(Figure 35.1)* pre-δ wave ventricular activity[4], *(Figure 35.2)* retrograde atrial activation during ventricular pacing and during supraventricular tachycardia *(Figure 35.3)*. After adequate localization, radiofrequency current to achieve temperatures of 50-65° C with energies of 20 to up to 50 watts is utilized for a period of 30-60 sec. The application of radiofrequency current at the site of bypass tract location is one of the most dramatic procedures in cardiovascular medicine and when the current is applied to the appropriate site, within a matter of a few beats the QRS complex normalizes with loss in preexcitation. Following loss of preexcitation the current is continued in our laboratory for a total of 60 sec. It is not unusual to give a "bonus lesion" before removal of the catheter. Retrograde conduction, the induction of tachycardia as well as atrial pacing is performed to assess the presence of preexcitation. The disappearance of the accessory pathway with normalization of the QRS complex results in non inducibility of supraventricular tachycardia, unless there is an additional pathway which may become manifest following the ablative procedure. It is not unusual to see multiple accessory pathways in about 15-30% of patients with WPW syndrome. These may become evident only after ablating the evident pathway. Sometime although antegrade conduction disappears retrograde conduction persists either through the same pathway or through an additional concealed accessory pathway. If the latter is true then both pathways should be mapped and ablated. It is the practice in our laboratory to attempt ablation of multiple pathways at the same sitting.

Intravenous heparin is utilized amply with measurement of activated clotting time. General anesthesia is usually not utilized except in children. Local anesthesia and sedation is given with the use of demerol, morphine, benadryl and Verset. An echocardiogram is obtained following the ablation procedure and usually the patient stays overnight and is discharged the following day. The ablative procedure initially took several hours but with increasing experience of the operator, procedure time has substantially decreased. In the last one year more than 90% of procedures have lasted for less than 4 hours with fluoro time of less than one hour in our laboratory.

The success rate for ablation of free wall accessory pathways ranges from 85-99%. Success rate for right sided accessory pathways is around 85-95%. Significant complications such as acute cardiac tamponade, valve damage, damage to the coronary arteries, and thromboembolic phenomena have been seen in left sided accessory pathway ablation. These complications in the best of centers are less than 2%. The complication rate for right sided pathways is less than 1%. The only possible significant complication in right sided accessory pathways is the development of AV block and the risk is obviously greatest in patients with anteroseptal pathways. Although, the success rate seemed to be lower in right sided compared to left sided pathways, with the development of newer catheter technology and experience of the electrophysiologist, the success rate at both locations is almost equivalent. In the last one year for right sided ablation in our laboratory the success rate approaches that of left sided accessory pathways.

AV nodal reentry [19-25]

AV nodal reentry[19-25] is one of the most common reentrant supraventricular tachycardia seen in clinical practice. Although a considerable amount of work has been done in this tachyarrhythmia, to date, the exact location of the slow and fast pathways of the reentrant circuit remain incompletely understood. From data obtained from surgery and ablative therapy, it seems that the slow pathway enters the AV node relatively posterior and adjacent to the region of the coronary sinus. On the other hand, the exit of the fast pathway is anteriorly near the bundle of His. It also seems that both pathways possibly use a rim of atrial tissue in the reentrant process. Initially the fast pathway of the reentrant circuit was ablated and this pathway was localized anterior to the His bundle. This pathway is ususally utilized as the retrograde limb of the reentrant process. Ablation of the fast pathway was done by localizing a site of earliest retrograde atrial activation during reentrant SVT as well as retrograde activation during ventricular pacing. Ablation of the fast pathway results in impairment of antegrade fast pathway conduction with prolongation of the AH interval and retrograde fast pathway conduction block. Studies in our laboratory

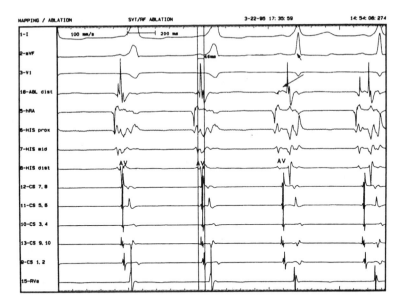

Figure 35.1 Atrial (A) and ventricular (V) fusion during pre-exited QRS complexes in a patient with an anteroseptal pathway. From top to bottom, are leads 1, AVF, V1, bipolar recording at the ablation site (abl. dist.), high right atrial recording (HRA), three His recordings (proximal, mid and distal), coronary sinus recordings (7-8; 5-6; 3-4; 9-10; 1-2) and right ventricular recording (RVA). Note that the A-V electrogram is fused on the ablation catheter. The third beat reveals block in the bypass tract due to bumping of the tract (bump normalization) with separation of A and V.

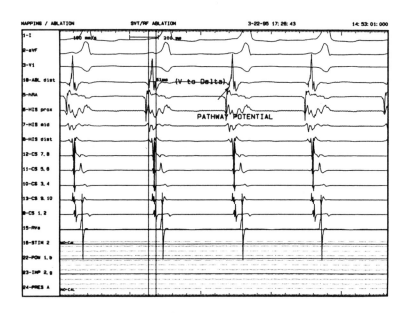

Figure 35.2 Demonstration of pathway potential and onset of the ventricular (V) electrogram before the onset of the δ-wave . Similar sequence of activation as in Figure 1. Note the presence of pathway potential in the ablation catheter recording shown by arrow (third QRS complex). Note that the local V electrogram precedes the delta wave by 51/msec (second QRS complex). For abbreviations see **Figure 35.1.**

have indicated that retrograde block during ventricular pacing following ablation in the only significant predictor for long term success. Fast pathway ablation however was given up because of the incidence of AV block of 6-11%. In our laboratory a modified technique was utilized to prevent AV block. In this method graded current was given until the appearance of junctional rhythm and current was not increased any further. Atrial pacing subsequently with monitoring of the PR interval virtually eliminated the risk of AV block.[25]

Today, however, slow pathway ablation is the method of choice for AV nodal reentry. Slow pathway ablation is done by utilizing the following techniques. Recording of slow pathway potentials or applying radiofrequency lesions starting below the os of the coronary sinus and progressing gradually upwards to about halfway in-between the area of the bundle of His and the coronary sinus at sites where the ventricular electrograms more than two times the voltage of the atrial electrogram. The higher one tends to ablate the slow pathway the higher the risk of AV block. There is no strict criteria to assess slow pathway ablation, however, we believe that the development of junctional rhythm has the best sensitivity for slow pathway ablation. In our laboratory, if junctional rhythm does not occur within about 20 seconds of the lesion then the ablation is aborted and the catheter position is changed. As soon as junctional rhythm develops the atrium is paced, and the PR interval is

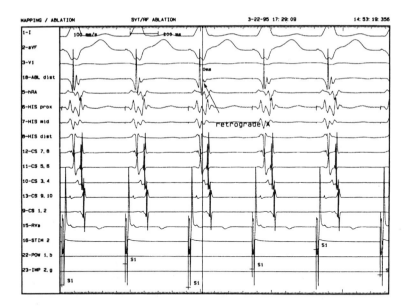

Figure 35.3 Retrograde activation sequence during ventricular pacing. Similar sequence arrangement as in Figure 35.1 *and 35.2. Note that during ventricular pacing the retrograde A on the distal ablation catheter precedes the A at the other sites. (third QRS complex). For abbreviations see* Figure 35.1.

continuously monitored. The absence of slow pathway conduction or the absence of discontinuous curves, *(Figure 35.4)* suggestive of dual pathway is also highly suggestive of slow pathway ablation. Nonetheless the non-induction following administration of Isoproterenol in a patient is in whom tachycardia was readily inducible prior to ablation also confirms a successful outcome.

Atrial tachycardia

Atrial tachycardias[26-31] accounts for less than 15% of all supraventricular tachycardias. These tachycardias are an inhomogenous entity. They are not unusually associated with congenital heart disease and cardiomyopathy particularly in the pediatric age group. In the adult population however, in more than 50% of patients there is no evidence of underlying myocardial disease. These tachycardias may be recalcitrant to a host of antiarrhythmic therapy. The mechanism of the tachycardias include: reentry, automaticity and triggered activity. It is difficult to characterize the exact mechanism but nonetheless the presence of entrainment, response to programmed stimulation, adenosine, vagal maneuvers and response to Isuprel can be used to assess the mechanism of these tachycardias.[30] Chen and co-workers found that the majority of tachycardias were due to reentry in the atrium. In the adult population there is a high prevalence of these tachycardias originating in the right

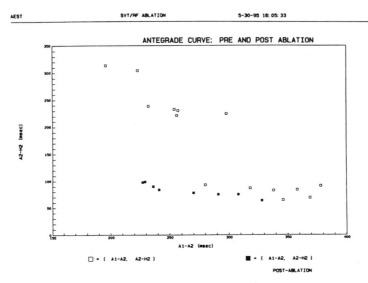

Figure 35.4 Antegrade AV nodal curves pre and post ablation On the abeissa are plotted the A1 and A2 intervals and on the ordinate the A2 H2 intervals pre (open square) and post (closed square) ablation. Note that as the A1 A2 interval is decreased, there is a sudden jump in A2 H2 due to block in fast pathway conduction with slow pathway conduction. There is no slow pathway conduction as suggested by the lack of jump in A2 H2 interval post ablation.

atrium whereas in children it is not unusual to see these tachycardias in the left atrium particularly in the region of the pulmonary veins. In a substantial proportion of children these tachycardias are incessant and may result in a cardiomyopathy. This is also true in adults but the incidence is much lower. Treatment of the tachy-cardia either with antiarrhythmic drugs or surgery or ablative therapy usually results in regression of the underlying cardiomyopathy. It has been suggested that these tachycardia arise in the region of the crista terminal in the adult. Studies in our laboratory have suggested that these tachycardias may originate any where in the right atrium with predominance in the area of coronary sinus and tricuspid annulus and the region of the inferoposterior right atrium. Of 23 patients who underwent attempted ablative therapy of atrial tachycardia, we found that the origin and the mechanism of the tachycardia was variable and not restrictive to any particular site. Radiofrequency ablation was successful in 76% of patients resulting in cure with a follow-up of approximately 1-2 years. On the basis of these observations and those of others we believe that radiofrequency ablation is the treatment of choice for these tachycardias.

Atrial flutter and fibrillation

Radiofrequency ablative therapy has been utilized in patients with atrial flutter[32-50], however, the best technique with the highest long term success is this arrhythmia is still evolving. Unlike other forms of tachycardia the success rate for atrial flutter is substantially lower ranging from anywhere from 60-80% with a recurrence of 20-50%. However in some failed patients previously ineffective antiarrhythmic therapy may become more effective. 15-30% of patient may subsequently develop atrial fibrillation. Whether the development of atrial fibrillation in these patients is related to the ablation of the flutter per se or rather to the prior presence of paroxysmal fibrillation or paroxysmal flutter fibrillation remains undefined at this time. Nonetheless we believe that radiofrequency ablation is primarily indicated for patients who have recurrent atrial flutter which does not respond to antiarrhythmic therapy, that the flutter is a Type I atrial flutter and there is no fibrillation at other times. However, flutter that transiently degenerates to fibrillation may be acceptable although there is no evident data to suggest that ablative therapy is successful on the long term in such patients. For atrial flutter three methods are used to guide ablation, one is mapping of flutter activity, the area which is the site of slow conduction (pre flutter activity of minus 40-80msec and the area of concealed entrainment) is chosen for ablation and this area corresponds to a site within the triangle composed of the inferior vena cava, the os of the coronary sinus and the posterior tricuspid annulus. We found initial good success at sites where the activation is minus 60-80ms before the flutter wave. The second method includes sequential anotomic lesions from the os of the coronary sinus to the inferior vena cava and from the os to the tricuspid annulus and from the tricuspid annulus to the inferior vena cava. Needless to say considerable advancement in this area is expected in the future particularly with the development of new sheathes and catheters which may make it easier to give linear lesions. The third method which has evolved more recently consists of giving a linear lesion between the inferior vena cava and the area of the posterior tricuspid annulus. Assessment of the route of exitation (unidirectional versus bidirectional) during pacing the area near the coronary sinus and lateral right atrium confirms anotomic block and is apparently associated with a high long term success rate.

Unlike atrial flutter, atrial fibrillation[38-50] is a much more complex arrhythmia the mechanism of which is poorly defined and therefore the treatment is undefined as well. Although a catheter maze has been attempted the complexity of this procedure makes it non applicable to the general population with either paroxysmal atrial fibrillation or sustained atrial fibrillation. Nonetheless in the future substantial advancement in this area is expected. Currently however, in patients who do not respond to antiarrhythmic therapy and require control of ventricular response, modification of the AV node or ablation of the AV node with the use of a permanent pacemaker is the approach that is universally used.

Ventricular tachycardias

Catheter ablation is being increasingly used for the management of ventricular arrhythmias although, the clinical utility is limited and related to the etiology of the
ventricular arrhythmia. The basic mechanism of the ventricular arrhythmia does not
seem to affect success or failure of catheter ablation since reentrant, automatic and
ventricular tachycardias related to triggered activity all seem to be amenable to
ablative therapy. However, the prerequisite for catheter ablation is localization of a
critical area which should be focal. In patients with structural heart disease, such as
coronary artery disease and cardiomyopathy, the substrate for reentrant ventricular
tachycardia (VT) is a diffuse area of scarring or fibrosis and thus cannot be always
eliminated by small lesions produced by radiofrequency current.[50-56] In 'idiopathic'
ventricular tachycardia on the other hand, the arrhythmia can be mapped to a focal
site usually in the right ventricle and thus can be successfully ablated in the majority
of patients.[57-60] The role, technique, results and complications of catheter ablation
in ventricular tachycardia of various etiologies is briefly discussed.

Ischemic cardiomyopathy

The role of catheter ablation of VT in patients with coronary artery disease is limited due to the diffuse and widespread nature of the substrate for the arrhythmia
and the presence of multiple 'forms' of VT. Conventional treatment for VT associated with coronary artery disease is anti-arrhythmic drugs, defibrillator implantation or both. Catheter ablation is considered as an adjunctive therapy to previously
ineffective or partially effective drug therapy.[54-56] It is also considered in patients
with implantable defibrillators who have frequent shocks due to 1 or 2 morphologies of VT which cannot be managed by drugs, either due to failure or intolerance.[61]
Reproducible induction and hemodynamic stability during VT are critical as endocardial mapping is performed while the patient is in VT. Fast VTs and those
associated with low blood pressure are thus not amenable. Slow VT is best suited
for ablation in patients with partially effective drug therapy.[56,57] Approximately 10%
of patients referred for management of VT associated with coronary disease are
suitable candidates for ablation.[55]

Mapping to find the site of VT origin and the site of ablation is performed
using a combination of techniques including pace mapping, activation-sequence
mapping, recordings of mid-diastolic potentials and application of the entrainment
principle. During pacemapping, multiple sites are paced at a rate identical to the
clinical ventricular tachycardia and 12-lead electrocardiograms are performed *(Figure 35.5)* to compare VT and paced rhythm morphologies.[62,63] Endocardial activation sequence mapping *(Figure 35.6)* involves sampling multiple endocardial sites
during VT to locate the endocardial electrocardiograms that precede the onset of
QRS complex. An electrogram 40 msec or more earlier than the onset of QRS
complex is presumed to be originating from the exit site of the reentrant circuit.[63]
However, there is a poor correlation between successful site of ablation and area of

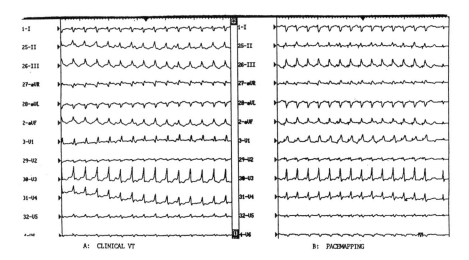

Figure 35.5 *12 lead EKG of ventricular tachycardia (panel A) and during pacing at site of VT origin. Note that the QRS complexes are identical in 11/12 leads.*

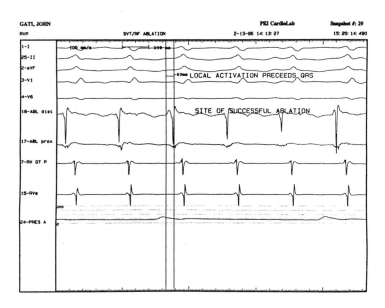

Figure 35.6 **Endocardial activation sequence mapping in ventricular tachycardia.**
From top to bottom are lead I, II, AVF, V_p, V_6 bipolar recordings from distal ablation site and proximal ablation site, RV outflow proximal recording, right ventricular apex (RVA), pressure recording. At the ablation site, the electrogram occurred 60msec before the QRS complex.

earliest activation which seems to be a more useful technique for surgical mapping.[52] Mid-diastolic potentials originate from the area of slow conduction and thus originate from VT site before the exit from the circuit.[64,65] These are low amplitude and fractionated electrograms. It has been further suggested that ablation is more likely to be successful when targeting areas in which isolated mid-diastolic potentials cannot be dissociated from the tachycardia by pacing and changes in tachycardia cycle length follow changes in cycle length of these potentials thereby separating active circuits from bystander pathways.[64,65] The most specific method for localizing active reentrant circuits in the ventricular myocardium is by concealed entrainment.[66,67] This is characterized by entrainment without evidence of fusion during incremental ventricular pacing. The paced QRS complexes are identical in morphology to clinical VT with a longer stimulus to QRS duration.

The results of ablation in patients with coronary disease have been very variable. In 4 recent studies, acute success was achieved in 56%, 80%, 80% and 100% patients.[53-55,58] Immediate complications include pericardial rub and exacerbation of heart failure. In hospital mortality has been in the range of 7% to 10% with a recurrence rate of 12-16% for a follow up in the range of 9-13 months.[53-55,58] Recurrence rate has been reported to be higher in patients with multiple morphologies of VT.[69] Surgical ablation, when feasible, on the other hand leads to a higher success rate.[70] Thus only a small proportion of patients with coronary artery disease are suitable candidates for radiofrequency ablation. Despite the acute success following ablation,recurrence rate is high and the majority of the patients require anti-arrhythmic drugs and implantable defibrillator.

Idiopathic VT associated with no structural heart disease

VT in this group of patients is usually focal and seen in younger patients, thus radiofrequency catheter ablation is being increasingly used to treat and attain a permanent cure in these patients.[57-60] Idiopathic ventricular tachycardia can be classified in two distinct groups: Right ventricular outflow tract VT which presents with a left bundle branch block morphology and right-axis and the so called 'fascicular' tachycardia which has a right bundle branch block like morphology with a left-axis suggesting origin from the left posterior fascicle.[71] The latter VT has negative or short HV interval.[72] As there is no structural disease of the ventricle, areas of slow conduction are not present. Localization of VT focus is done by pace mapping and identification of early local endocardial potentials. As compared to patients with VT related to coronary artery disease VTs with no structural heart disease are primarily localized by these methods with success rates of catheter ablation in the range of 95-100%. [57-60, 73] In a recent study, ablation at sites 39± 14 msec prior to QRS complex resulted in success.[57] Mid-diastolic potentials and fractionated electrograms are usually not recorded. In 'fascicular' tachycardia a 'P' or Purkinje potential is used to identify the site of reentry in the conduction system of the ventricle.[60] During tachycardia this potential precedes the local electrogram and is a very specific marker for a successful site. Furthermore in idiopathic VT success of ablation indicates that the mechanism of VT is related to a small focal site of abnormal tissue which is endocardial in location. Although these patients do not have any evidence of structural abnormality, catheter ablation has been associated with significant complications like myocardial perforation and aortic insufficiency.[57] The risk/benefit should be considered in each patient as the majority of patients with 'idiopathic' VT have good long term prognosis. A recent study reported symptomatic cure from catheter ablation in patents with non-sustained VT of right ventricular origin, mostly from the right ventricular outflow tract.[74]

Bundle branch reentry tachycardia

This is an unusual and rare type of ventricular tachycardia resulting from reentry within the bundle branches. It account for less than 5% of ventricular tachycardias.[75-76] It is postulated that the diagnosis might be often missed as:

1.   It commonly presents as syncope rather than palpitations.

2.   It might not be reproducibily induced by programmed stimulation.

3.   His bundle recordings are essential for the diagnosis of this VT. These are not always recorded in patients undergoing electrophysiology tests for VT. In patients in whom the anterograde limb is the right bundle, right ventricular stimulation might be inadequate and left ventricular stimulation might be needed to induce VT.

Bundle branch reentrant VT is invariably seen in patients with idiopathic dilated cardiomyopathy. At one center bundle-branch VT was responsible for 41% of VTs in patients with dilated cardiomyopathy.[76] Less often it is associated with ischemic cardiomyopathy and severe valvular regurgitation. The QRS morphology of the arrhythmia might be right or left bundle branch block like depending whether the left or right bundle is the anterograde limb of VT. Left bundle branch block like morphology is seen more frequently.

Sustained bundle-branch VT is typically associated with hemodynamic decompensation and presents as syncope or sudden death. For this reason 12-lead documentation of this tachycardia is rarely available. Electrophysiologic criteria for diagnosis as suggested by Caceras et al,[75] include 1) QRS morphology is typically left or right bundle branch block like 2) Onset of ventricular electrogram is preceded by a His bundle or a right bundle potential 3) Variation on ventricle -to-ventricle interval is preceded by variation in His-to-His interval. 4) Induction of VT during programmed stimulation is dependent on a critical His -purkinje delay 5) Pace induced block in the His-purkinje tissue terminates the tachycardia 6) Successful ablation of the right bundle abolishes bundle branch reentry. Multiple reports show that catheter ablation is the treatment of choice for this type of VT and is associated with permanent cure of this potentially life threatening condition.[77,78] Ablation of the right bundle branch abolishes VT with both right and left bundle branch block like morphology. Once diagnosed, ablation is relatively easy and is guided by the right bundle potential. During ablation right bundle potential is recorded by withdrawing the right ventricular catheter till a discrete potential is recorded with no atrial electrogram. This potential is seen about 20 msec after the distal His recording. The only risk associated with right bundle ablation is inadvertent damage to the His bundle leading to HV prolongation and complete heart block. Permanent pacemaker is implanted only if there is complete heart block or the HV interval is >100 msec.

Catheter ablation has been attempted in patients with VT caused by idiopathic dilated cardiomyopathy and arrhythogenic right ventricular dysplasia.[79,80] Acute success rate has been reported to be 50-80%. However, in view of the diffuse nature of these diseases recurrence rate is high (22-50%) for a follow-up ranging from 14-31 months. Most of the recurrent arrhythmias have different morphologies and may be related to progression of the disease rather than late failure of catheter ablation.[80]

Conclusions

Catheter ablation is the treatment of choice in patients with VT related to bundle branch reentry and idiopathic VT resistant to medical therapy. In these conditions catheter ablation is associated with a high success rate with long term cure. In patients with VT related to coronary artery disease, catheter ablation is considered as adjunctive therapy to drugs and implantable defibrillator as the success rate is low and ablation procedure relatively difficult due to the complex arrhythmia substrate. In patients with right ventricular dysplasia and dilated cardiomyopathy, catheter ablation of VT has limited value due to diffuse progressive disease and high recurrence rate.

REFERENCES

1. Scheinman MM, et al. Catheter induced ablation of the atrioventricular junction to control refractory supraventricular arrhythmias. JAMA 1982:248:851.

2. Gallagher JJ, et al. Catheter technique for closed chest ablation of the atrioventricular conduction system. N Engl J Med 1982:306:194.

3. Huang SKS, Bharati S, Graham AR. Closed chest catheter desiccation of the atrioventricular junction using radiofrequency energy: A new method of catheter ablation. J Am Coll Cardiol 1987:9:349.

4. Huang SKS: Radiofrequency catheter ablation of cardiac arrhythmias: Appraisal of an evolving therapeutic modality. Am Heart J 1989:118:1317.

5. Huang SKS, et al. Comparison of Catheter Ablation using Radiofrequency versus Direct Current Energy: Biophysical, Electro-physiologic and Pathologic observation. J Am Coll Cardiol 1991: 18:1091.

6. Haines DE, Veron AF. Observations on Eelctrode tissue interface temperature and effect on electrical impedance during Radiofrequency Ablation of ventricular myocardium. Circulation 1990: 82:1034.

7. Jackman WM, et al. Catheter ablation of accessory atrioventricular pathways (Wolff-Parkinson-White syndrome) by radiofrequency current. N Engl J Med 1991:324:1605.

8. Kuck KH, et al. Modification of a left-sided freewall accessory pathway by percutaneous catheter application of radiofrequency current in a patient with Wolff-Parkinson-White syndrome. PACE 1989: 12:1681.

9. Haissaguerre M, et al. Electrogram patterns predictive of successful catheter ablation of accessory pathways. Value of unipolar recording mode. Circulation. 1991:84:188.

10. Grogin HR, et al. Radiofrequency catheter ablation of atriofasicular and Nodoventricular Mahaim tracts: Cir. 1994: 90:272.

11. Lesh MD, Harevan GF. Comparison of the Retrograde and transseptal methods for ablation of left free wall accessory pathways. J Am Coll Cardiol 1993:22:542.

12. Manolis A, Wang PJ, Estes III NA. Radiofrequency ablation of left sided accessory pathway: Transaortic versus transseptal approach. Am Heart J 1994:128:896.

13. Gallagher JJ, et al. The preexcitation syndrome. Prog. Cardiovas. Dis. 1978: 20:285.

14. Fitzpatrick Al, et al. New algorithim for the localization of accessory atrioventricular connections using a baseline electrocardiogram. J Am Coll Cardiol in press.

15. Cobb FR, et al. Successful surgical interuption of the bundle of Kent in a patient with Wolff-Parkinson-White syndrome. Circulation 1968: 38:1018.

16. Jackman WM, et al. Direct endocardial recording from an accessory atrioventricular pathway: Investigation of the site of block, effect of anti-arrhythmic drugs, and attempt at nonsurgical ablation. Circulation 1983:68:906.

17. Winters S, Gomes JA. Intracardiac Electrode Catheter Recordings of atrioventricular Bypass tracts in Wolff-Parkinson-White syndrome: Techniques, Electrophysiologic characteristics and demonstration of concealed and decremental propagation. J Am Coll Cardiol 1986: 7:1392.

18. Haissaguerra M, et al. Electrogram patterns predictive of successful catheter ablation of accessory pathways. Value of unipolar recording mode. Circulation 1991:84:188.

19. Jackman WM, et al. Treatment of supraventricular tachycardia due to atrioventricular nodal reentry by radiofrequency catheter ablation of slow-pathway conduction. N. Engl J Med 1992:327:3:13.

20. Jazayeri MR, et al. Selective transcatheter ablation of the fast and slow pathways using radiofreqency energy in patients with atrioventricular nodal reentrant tachycardia. Circulation 1992:85:1318.

21. Langberg JJ, et al. A randomized prospective comparison of anterior and posterior approaches to radiofrequency catheter ablation of atrioventricular nodal reentry tachycardia. Circulation 1993:87:1551.

22. Hassaguerre M, et al. Elimination of atrioventricular nodal reentrant tachycardia using discrete slow potentials to guide application of radiofrequency energy. Circulation 1992:85:2162.

23. Kay GN, et al. Selective radiofrequency ablation of the slow pathway for the treatment of atrioventricular nodal reentrant tachycardia. Circulation 1992:85:1675.

24. Chen Shih-Ann, et al. Selective radiofrequency catheter ablation of tachycardia slow pathways in 100 patients with atrioventricular nodal reentrant tachycardia. Am HJ 1993:125:1.

25. Mehta D, Gomes JA. Long term results of fast pathway ablation in atrioventricular nodal reentry tachycardia using a modified technique. Br. HJ 1995:76:671.

26. Walch EP, et al. Transcatheter ablation of ectopic atrial tachycardia in young patients using radiofrequency current. Circ 1992:86:113.

27. Kay GN, et al. Radiofrequency ablation for treatment primary atrial tachycardia. J. Am Coll Cardial 1993:21:901.

28. Tracy CM, et al. Radiofrequency catheter ablation of ectopic atrial tachycardial using paced activation sequence mapping. J. Am Coll. Cardiol 1993:21:910.

29. Lesch MD, et al. Radiofrequency catheter ablation of atrial arrythmias. Results and mechanism. Cir. 1994:89:1076.

30. Chen SA, et al. Sustained atrial tachycardia in adult patients. Electrophysiological character-
    istics. Pharmalogical response, possible mechanisms and effects of radiofrequency ablation.
    Circ. 1996:90:1262.

31. Gomes JA, Mehta D, Langan MN: Sinus node reentrant tachycardia. PACE 1995:18:1045.

32. Feld GK, et al. Radiofrequency catheter ablation for the treament of human type 1 atrial
    flutter: identification of a critical zone in the reentrant circuit by endocardial mapping tech-
    niques. Circulation: 1992:86:1233.

33. Cosio FG, et al. Radiofrequency ablation of the inferior vena cava-tricuspid valve isthmus in
    common atrial flutter. Am J. Cardiol. 1993:71:705.

34. Lesh MD, et al. Radiofreqency catheter ablation of atrial arrhythmias: results and mecha-
    nisms. Circulation. 1994:89:1074.

35. Calkins H, et al. Catheter ablation of atrial flutter using radiofrequency energy. Am J Car-
    diol. 1994:73:353.

36. Kirkorian G, et al. Radiofrequency ablation of atrial flutter: efficacy of an anatomically
    guided approach. Circulation. 1994:90:2804.

37. Cancheng B, et al. Electrophysiologic effect of catheter ablation of inferior vana cava-tricus-
    pid annulus isthmus in common atrial flutter. Cir 1996:93:2471.

38. Huang SKS. Radiofrequency catheter ablation of cardiac arrhythmias: Appraisal of an evolv-
    ing therapeutic modality. Am Heart J 1989:118:1317.

39. Langberg JJ, et al. Catheter ablation of the atrioventricular junction with radiofrequency
    energy. Circulation 1989:80:1527.

40. Morady F, et al. A prospective randomized comparison of direct current and radiofrequency
    ablation of the atrioventricular junction. J am Coll Cardiol 1993:21:102.

41. Yeung-Lai-Wah JA, et al. High success rate of atrioventricular node ablation with radiofre-
    quency energy. J Am Coll Cardiol 1991:18:1753.

42. Lanberg JJ, et al. Catheter ablation of atrioventricular junction with radiofrequency energy
    using a new electrode catheter. Am J. Cardiol 1991:67:142.

43. Jackman WM, et al. Catheter ablation of atrioventricular junction using radiofrequency cur-
    rent in 17 patients: comparison of standard and large-tip catheter electrodes. Circulation
    1991:83:1562.

44. Scheinman MM. NASPE Policy Statement: Catheter ablation of cardiac arrhythmias, per-
    sonel and facilities. PACE 1992:15:715.

45. Fleck RP, et al. Radiofrequency modification of atrioventricular conduction by selective
    ablation of the low posterior septal right atrium in a patient with atrial fibrillation and a
    rapid ventricular response. PACE in press.

46. Williamson BD, et al. Radiofrequency catheter modification of atrioventricular conduction
    to control the ventricular rate during atrial fibrillation. N Engl J Med. 1994:331:910.

47. Feld GK, et al. Control of rapid ventricular response by radiofrequency catheter modication
    of the atrioventricular node in patients with medically refractory atrial fibrillation. Circula-
    tion 1994:90:2299.

48. Della Bella P, et al. Modulation of atrioventricular conduction by ablation of the 'slow'
    atrioventricular node pathway in patients with drug-refractory atrial fibrillation or flutter. J
    am Coll Cardiol 1995:25:39.

49. Kreiner G, et al. Effect of slow pathway ablation on ventricular rate during atrial fibrillation.
    Dependence in electrophysiological properties of fast pathway. Cir. 1996:93:277.

50. Wellens HJJ. Atrial fibrillation - the last big hurdle in treating supraventricular tachycardia.
    N Engl. J of Med. 1996:14:944.

51. Hartzler GO. Electrode catheter ablation of refractory focal ventricular tachycardia. J Am
    Coll Cardiol 1983:2:1107.

52. Morady F, et al. Catheter ablation of ventricular tachcyardia with intracardiac shocks: results
    in 33 patients. Circulation 1987:75:319.

53. Borggrefe M, et al. Catheter ablation of venticular tachycardia using defibrillator pulses: Electrophysiologic findings and long term results. Eur Heart J 1989:10:591.

54. Stevenson WG, et al. Identification of reentry circuit sites during catheter mapping and radiofrequency ablation of ventricular tachycardia late after myocardial infarction. Circulation 1993:88:1647.

55. Kim YH, et al. Treatment of ventricular tachycardia by transcatheter radiofrequency ablation in patients with ischemic heart disease. Circulation 1994:89:1094.

56. Morady F, et al. Radiofrequency ablation of ventricular tachycardia in patients with coronary artery disease. Circulation 1993:87:363.

57. Coggins DL, et al. Radiofrequency ablation as a cure for idiopathic ventricular tachcyardia of both left and right ventricular origin. J Am Coll Cardiol 1994:23:1333.

58. Wen MS, et al. Radiofrequency abaltion therapy in idiopathic left ventricular tachycardia with no obvious structural heart disease. Circulation 1994:89: 1690.

59. Wellens HJ, Smeets J. Idiopathic ventricular tachcyardia cured by radiofrequency ablation. Circulation 1993:88:2978.

60. Nakagawa H, et al. Radiofrequency catheter ablation of idiopathic ventricular tachycardia guided by Purkinje potential. Circulation 1993:88:2607.

61. Willems S, et al. Radiofrequency catheter ablation of ventricular tachycardia following implantation of an cardioverter defibrillator. PACE 1993:16:1684.

62. Josephson ME, et al. Ventricular activation during ventricular endocardial pacing. II role of pace-mapping to localize origin of ventricular tachycardia. Am J Cardiol 1982:50:11.

63. Marchlinski FE, et al. Localization of endocardial sites for catheter ablation of ventricular tachycardia. In: Fontaine G, Scheinman MM Eds. Ablation of Cardiac Arrhythmias. Mount Kisco, NY: Futura, 1987:289.

64. Fitzgerald DM, et al. Electrogram patterns predicting successful catheter ablation of ventricular tachycardia. Circulation 1988:77:806.

65. El-Sherif N, et al. Reentrant ventricular arrhythmias in the late myocardial infarction period: interruption of reentrant circuits by cryothermal techniques. Circulation 1983:68:644.

66. Morady F, et al. Concealed entrainment as a guide for catheter ablation of ventricular tachycardia in patients with prior myocardial infarction. J Am Coll Cardiol 1991:17:678.

67. Waldo AL, Henthorn RW. Use of transient entrainment during ventricular tachycardia to localize a critical area in the reentry circuit for ablation. PACE 1989:12:231.

68. Gursoy S, Chiladakis I, Kuck KH. First lessons from radiofrequency catheter ablation in patients with ventricular tachycardia. PACE 1993:16:324.

69. Blanck Z, et al. Catheter ablation of ventricular tachycardia. Am Heart J 1994:127:1126.

70. Blanchard SM, et al. Why is catheter ablation less successful than surgery for treating ventricular tachycardia that results from coronary artery disease. Pacing Clin Electrophysiol 1994:17:2315.

71. Mehta D, et al. Significance of signal-averaged electrocardiography in relation to endomyocardial biopsy and ventricular stimulation studies in patients with ventricular tachycardia without clinically apparent heart disease. J Am Coll Cardiol 1989:14:372.

72. Balhassen B, et al. Transcatheter electrical shock ablation of ventricular tachycardia. J Am Coll Cardiol 1986:7:1347.

73. Wilber D, et al. Adenosine sensitive ventricular tachycardia: clinical characteristics and response to catheter ablation. Circulation 1993:26:843.

74. Zhu D, et al. Radiofrequency catheter ablation for management of symptomatic ventricular ectopic activity. J Am Col Cardiol 1995:26:843.

75. Caceres J, et al. Sustained bundle branch reentry as a mechanism for clinical tachycardia. Circulation 1988:79:256.

76. Akhtar M, et al. Demonstration of reentry within the His-Purkinje system in man. Circulation 1974:50:1150.

77. Tchou P, et al. Transcatheter electrical ablation of right bundle branch : a method of treating macroreentrant ventricular tachcyardia due to bundle branch reentry. Circulation 1988:78:246.

78. Langberg JJ, et al. Treatment of macroreentrant ventricular tachycardia with radiofrequency ablation of the right bundle branch. Am J Cardiol 1989:62:220.

79. Leclerq JF, et al. Results of electrical fulgration in arrhythmogenic right ventricular disease. Am J Cardiol 1988:62:220.

80. Shoda M, et al. Recurrence of new ventricular tachycardia after successful catheter ablation in patients with arrhythmogenic right ventricular dysplasia. Circulation 1992:86 (Suppl):580.

36 IMPLANTABLE CARDIOVERTER-DEFIBRILLATORS

Leslie J. Lipka, James Coromilas

In those patients whose malignant ventricular arrhythmia are not controlled by medications, an implanted device capable of detecting and treating VT or VF is the remaining therapeutic option. Such a device is also often used as primary therapy for malignant ventricular arrhythmias.

The initial implantable cardioverter defibrillator (ICD) began clinical trials in 1980 after a decade of development by Dr. Michel Mirowski and his colleagues. Dr. Mirowski's vision was to miniaturize a defibrillator and make it the size of a pacemaker. In 1985, the device, manufactured by Intec Systems (Pittsburgh, PA) and then licensed to Cardiac Pacemakers Incorporated (CPI;St. Paul, MN), was FDA approved for widespread use. Since that time, the ICD has gained increasing acceptance and its technical evolution has been rapid. In 1993, ICDs manufactured by Medtronic (Minneapolis, MN) and Ventritex (Sunnyvale, CA) received FDA approval. Recently, an ICD by Intermedics (Angleton, TX) was approved as well. Other ICDs are under development. The FDA approved devices will be discussed in greater detail in this chapter.

Evolution

Initially, ICDs were designed to recognize and treat ventricular fibrillation only. These devices revolutionized therapy of lethal arrhythmias; however, they were relatively large, nonprogrammable, and their batteries had relatively short lives. These early devices were either nonprogrammable or only modifiable noninvasively in that placement of a magnet on the device could switch the device to a standby mode. The first device to be implanted in humans was the AID (Automatic Implantable Defibrillator); the initial implant in a patient occurred in February of 1980. Its weight was 250 grams and it delivered shocks of 25 or 30 joules. Its total discharge capability was 100 shocks. This device used a probability density function (PDF; see below) to sense arrhythmia. It possessed no heart rate detection criteria. The PDF detected ventricular fibrillation (VF) well and the device proved clinically effective.[1]

The next series of devices developed was also relatively simple. Although they are no longer manufactured, some are still in clinical use. This generation of ICD is exemplified by the CPI Ventak P 1500 series as well as the Ventak P 1600. Programmability is limited in these devices. Their energy output is fixed at 28 to 37 joules. The detection rate for ventricular tachycardia (VT) can be programmed between 110 and 200 bpm. The delay between tachycardia sensing and capacitor charging can be programmed from 2.5 to 10 seconds. This feature is useful in patients who have nonsustained VT. In these devices, a separate rate counting circuit is employed. These devices store some information which includes the number of shocks delivered, capacitor charge time, and lead impedance of the shocking leads. More advanced devices may also provide backup pacing for bradycardia, have some programmability, and may have telemetry (i.e. they are capable of disclosing and/or recording electrograms sensed by their electrodes).

The latest generation ICDs can deliver antitachycardia pacing in addition to bradycardia backup pacing, are extensively programmable, and store electrograms of events for which therapy was delivered. These ICDs are also capable of performing electrophysiologic testing noninvasively; this is done in a special EPS mode by programming the device to perform programmed electrical stimulation. In addition, these devices possess waveform pulse programmability. These devices can be programmed to deliver standard (monophasic) or biphasic shocks as therapy *(Figure 36.1)*. The importance of this feature is discussed below.

In addition, tiered therapy is a feature of newer ICDs. Tiered therapy refers to the ability to program an ICD to provide different responses to a specific arrhythmia. For example, VT at a relatively slow rate may be treated with antitachycardia pacing and if accelerated, treated with defibrillation.

Other features of the latest generation ICDs are discussed later in this chapter.

Hardware

The basic ICD consists of three elements *(Figure 36.2)*. These include electrodes for rhythm sensing, electrodes for defibrillating the myocardium, and the pulse generator. Ideally, rhythm sensing is accomplished by a closely spaced, bipolar pair of electrodes which is able to provide high amplitude, narrow electrograms with minimal farfield (electrical activity from distant tissue) activity. Rhythm sensing may be performed by a combination of rate and morphology sensing electrodes. The defibrillating electrodes are designed to have a large surface area and are positioned to deliver current density as uniformly as possible to the heart. Initially, the defibrillating electrodes were patches sewn directly to the pericardium or epicardium. However, the technology has advanced to the extent that defibrillation can be provided via an endocardially placed electrode which is introduced into the right ventricle

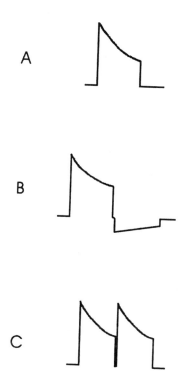

*Figure 36.1 **Defibrillation shock waveform morphology**. A) Monophasic exponentially decaying pulse and B) biphasic pulse, which is composed of two phases of opposite polarity. This is accomplished by the device changing its output polarity while it discharges. C) Sequential monophasic waveform in which two monophasic pulses are delivered sequentially. The pulses are delivered across two different electrode pairs.*

transvenously, similar to the manner in which a permanent transvenous pacemaker lead is placed.

The pulse generator consists of an integrated circuit based logic system and one or two lithium silver vanadium oxide or pentoxide batteries. The logic system monitors the heart rhythm via the signal recorded by the sensing electrodes. When the generator detects an arrhythmia, it follows its programmed algorithm and delivers therapy for the arrhythmia. All pulse generators are capable of delivering high energy countershock (which may be as high as 35 joules). They do this by transferring charge from the batteries to the capacitor, then discharging the capacitor via the shock electrodes, thereby delivering a shock to the patient. In addition, depending on the pulse generator model, therapy may include ventricular pacing for bradycardia or antitachycardia pacing for VT. Newer pulse generators are also capable of telemetry, which may be stored in the form of RR intervals or electrograms *(Figure 36.3)*.

Pulse generators

Available pulse generators weigh between 115 and 240 grams *(Table 36.I)*. The external case of the generator is made of titanium. Generator headers are now made

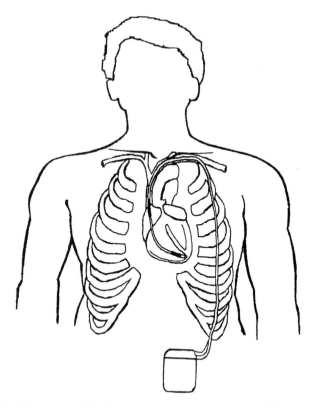

Figure 36.2 **The basic ICD**. *Representation of a transvenous ICD implanted in a patient. The device lead is implanted transvenously via the subclavian vein. The lead is then tunneled to connect with the header of the ICD pulse generator, which is implanted in the abdomen. The distal spring electrode is in the right ventricle and the proximal spring electrode is in the SVC/RA junction. The tip of the lead is the sensing electrode.*

to accept leads of several sizes. ICD pulse generators contain one or two lithium silver vanadium oxide batteries to supply 6.4 V. The devices are capable of delivering 100 to 200 shocks. The longevity of the device is generally three to four years. These devices are now programmable via radiofrequency links in a manner similar to permanent pacemakers. Thus, devices are programmed by the electrophysiologist using menu driven software which is part of the ICD microcomputer-based programmer. The programmer interacts with the ICD via a wand which sends and receives information in the form of radiofrequency energy.

Epicardial patches

Prior to August, 1993, all FDA approved device implantations used epi-myocardial defibrillating patches *(Figure 36.4)*. These patches are manufactured in several sizes.

Table 36.1 ICD PULSE GENERATOR FEATURES COMPARISON

Manufacturer/Model	Biphasic Waveform	Stored Electrogram	Bradycardia Pacing	ATP	Committed Shock	Weight (gms)	Pectoral Implant	Unipolar Technology	FDA Approved
Angeion Corporation Sentinel 2000	Yes	No	Yes	Yes	No	110	Yes	Yes	No
Biotronik, Inc. Phylax 06	Yes	Yes	Yes	Yes	No	109	Yes	Yes	No
Cardiac Pacemakers, Inc. (CPI) Ventak P1600	No	No	No	No	Yes	250	No	No	Yes
Ventak PRx	No	No; R-R intervals	Yes	Yes	No	228	No	No	Yes
Ventak P2	Yes	Yes	Yes	No	No	228	No	No	Yes
Ventak PRx III	Yes	Yes	Yes	Yes	No	179	No	No	Yes
Ventak MINI	Yes	Yes*	Yes	Yes*	No	139	Yes	No	Yes
Ventak MINI II	Yes	Yes	Yes	Yes	No	115	Yes	Yes	Yes
Intermedics, Inc. Res-Q 101-01	Yes	No	Yes	Yes	Yes	240	No	No	Yes
Res-Q II	Yes	Yes	Yes	Yes	No	147	Yes	Yes; Sep	No
Res-Q Micron	Yes	Yes	Yes	Yes	No	125	Yes	Yes; Pro	No
Medtronic, Inc. PCD	No	No; R-R intervals	Yes	Yes	No	196	No	No	Yes
Jewel	Yes	Yes	Yes	Yes	No	129	Yes	Yes; Sep	Yes

Table 36.1 ICD PULSE GENERATOR FEATURES COMPARISON

Manufacturer/ Model	Biphasic Waveform	Stored Electrogram	Bradycardia Pacing	ATP	Committed Shock	Weight (gms)	Pectoral Implant	Unipolar Technology	FDA Approved
Jewel Plus	Yes	Yes	Yes	Yes	No	131	Yes	Yes; Sep	Yes
Micro Jewel	Yes	Yes	Yes	Yes	No	118	Yes	Yes; Sep	Yes
Telectronics Pacing Systems									
Guardian ATP III	Yes	Yes	Yes	Yes	No	169	No	No	No
Sentry 4310	Yes	Yes	Yes	Yes	No	142	Yes	No	No
Sentry 4310 Hot Can	Yes	Yes	Yes	Yes	No	142	Yes	Yes	No
Ventritex, Inc.									
Cadence V-100	Yes	Yes	Yes	Yes	No	240	No	No	Yes
Cadence V-110	Yes	Yes	Yes	Yes	No	198	No	No	Yes
Cadet V-115	Yes	Yes	Yes	Yes	No	133	Yes	No	Yes

*All models except MINI+S
Sep = separate unipolar defibrillation system model is manufactured
Pro = programmable to unipolar defibrillation system mode

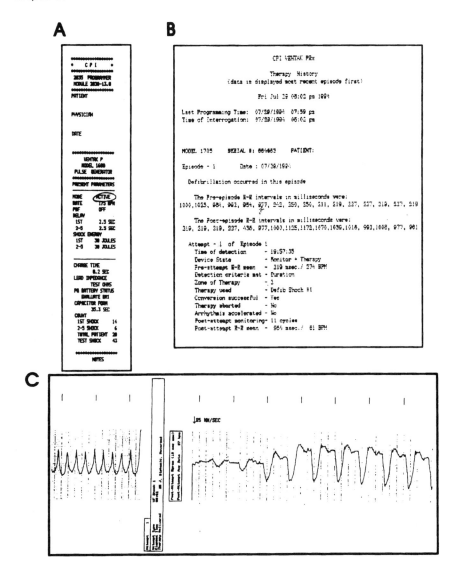

Figure 36.3 *Evolution of ICD data storage.* A) Report from CPI Ventak P 1600. B) Report from CPI Ventak PRx. The stored R-R intervals are displayed. C) Stored electrograms from CPI PRX III. The remainder of the report printout, which includes R-R intervals is not shown.

Larger patch systems have been associated with lower energy requirements to defibrillate the heart.[2] Defibrillators at the present time use two or three defibrillation patches or leads. Most ICDs can be attached to three defibrillating leads or patches by connecting two leads in parallel via a Y connector, thus forming a common anode or cathode. This technique is effective in reducing defibrillation thresholds to acceptable levels in patients with otherwise unacceptably high defibrillation thresholds.[3] The defibrillation threshold (DFT) is defined as the minimum energy required to successfully terminate ventricular fibrillation.

Nonthoracotomy lead systems

At present, there are two nonthoracotomy lead systems available in the U.S. The CPI Endotak was FDA approved for release in August of 1993. The Medtronic PCDT Transvene endocardial lead system was approved shortly afterwards. The Transvene system uses three leads, at least two of which are endocardially placed *(Figure 36.5)*. With the newer Medtronic ICD generators, only two leads are needed.

The CPI Endotak C series of lead systems consists of 70 to 100 cm long, tined endocardial leads that combine bipolar sensing, pacing, and defibrillation in one lead *(Figure 36.6)*. Because it performs both rate sensing and defibrillation, it is considered an integrated lead. The distal electrode, which consists of a porous tip, serves as the rate sensing cathode, which is the electrode which senses the ventricular electrogram. The distal spring electrode, so named due to its coiled configuration, is the anode for rate sensing and part of the system for morphology sensing and defibrillating. The proximal spring electrode is also a morphology sensing and defibrillating electrode. The lead body contains one rate sensing conductor and two morphology sensing/defibrillating conductors. Multiple configurations for the defibrillating electrodes are available, however, when the lead is used in conjunction with an Endotak subcutaneous patch or subcutaneous array, called the Endotak SQ Array. The CPI SQ lead array features three electrically common, multifilar coil elements that comprise one electrode.

Not surprisingly, implantation of the CPI Endotak lead system was associated with a learning curve.[4] In the CPI database, which includes data on all implantations of their devices, overall success rate with an Endotak lead system was 86%, while phase II clinical trials revealed a 91% success rate with the lead system. Overall, 57% of the implants in the CPI database were able to achieve acceptable results using only the endocardial lead. In one study of 37 Italian centers,[5] 306 of 307 implants were successfully performed using transvenous ICD implantation. 53% of the implants used the lead alone, the remainder received a subcutaneous patch or array. The DFT was 16.9 ± 5.7 joules.

The first single lead unipolar electrode system to gain FDA approval employs a Medtronic PCD 7219C (Jewel) pulse generator implanted in the left infraclavicular pocket. This system uses the ICD generator as the cathode for defibrillation, while the anode is the right ventricular lead. Because the pulse generator or 'Can'

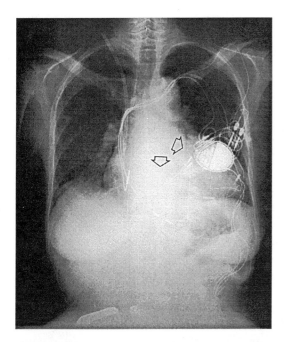

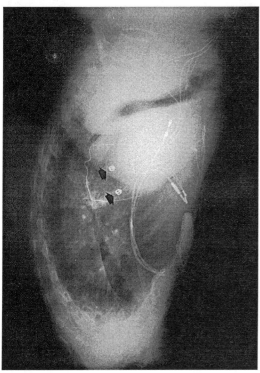

Figure 36.4 Chest radiograph in posteroanterior and lateral views of a patient with CPI epicardial patches. The epicardial patches are indicated in the posteroanterior view by the open arrows. Epicardial screw-in leads (solid arrows in the lateral view) are used for rate sensing. The patient also has a permanent pacemaker with several sets of leads as well as a central venous line.

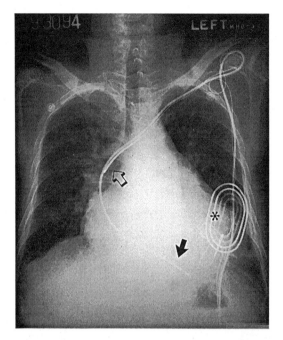

Figure 36.5 Chest radiograph in posteroanterior and lateral views of the Medtronic Transvene system. In this patient, a subcutaneous patch, as well as endocardially placed leads in the SVC and RV apex were used. These are indicated in A) by the asterisk (*), and the open and solid arrows, respectively. In addition, this patient has a bioprosthetic aortic valve, which is indicated by the solid arrow in the lateral view.

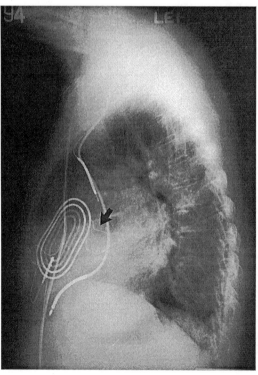

is an electrode in this system, this type of arrangement has been called a 'Hot' or 'Active Can' system. The advantage of this type of system is that it decreases the energy required to defibrillate the heart. Thus, Bardy et al reported a mean DFT of only 9.3±6 joules for the Medtronic system.[6] The CPI MINI II, which is another 'Active Can' device, recently gained FDA approval as well. The MINI II has been approved for left abdominal or left pectoral implantation. As shown in Table I, most ICD manufacturers are developing devices which employ unipolar defibrillation technology.

Sensing

Detection algorithms

At present, the basic feature for arrhythmia detection used in all devices is the rate cutoff. Other features and algorithms have been developed to increase the specificity of arrhythmia detection.

The onset criterion is another feature that is used to distinguish sinus tachycardia from VT. Thus, the ICD examines the RR intervals prior to the onset of tachycardia. A tachycardia which is sinus in origin would have a gradually increasing rate, while VT would have an abrupt change in RR interval at its start. This feature, however, may be unable to detect an exercise-induced VT.

An algorithm to distinguish atrial fibrillation from VT examines the regularity of successive RR intervals. This feature may be called a 'stability' feature as it determines the stability of the R-R interval. Stability obviously cannot be used in patients whose VT is grossly irregular. In addition, this feature cannot distinguish atrial fibrillation from VF. However, when used, stability is programmed with a rate cutoff well below those of VF.

PDF is an algorithm used by the CPI AICD to differentiate VT or VF from supraventricular tachycardia (SVT). This function assesses the amount of time that the electrogram is isoelectric. A narrow complex SVT is predominantly isoelectric, while VT theoretically is not. A limitation to this algorithm is that a VT with a relatively narrow QRS may not meet PDF detection criteria and would thus go undetected.

Some ICDs incorporate an automatic gain control (AGC) feature in the sensing circuit in order to avoid problems with under or oversensing. The AGC changes the amplification of the amplifier or the detection threshold of a signal based on the amplitude of recently sampled signals. The system filters the signals, thus rejecting slow-moving and accepting fast-moving intracardiac signals. During a refractory period lasting 140 msec, the ICD measures the amplitude of the cycle; the sensitivity is then automatically adjusted based on the amplitude of the last sensed event. If an R wave is absent, sensitivity is increased; once another R wave is detected, the sensitivity is readjusted. In the presence of normal rhythms, when an R wave is present, the sensitivity is adjusted once per second.

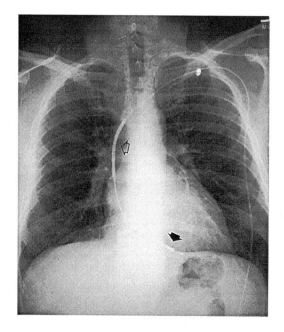

Figure 36.6 Chest radiograph in posteroanterior and lateral views of the CPI Endotak lead system. Using a single lead, spring electrodes are positioned in the superior vena cava and the right ventricular apex. The spring electrodes are indicated by the open and solid arrows respectively.

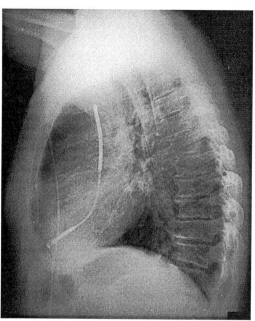

Other features and algorithms are presently in use. It is important to remember that any feature required to be fulfilled concurrently with the rate cutoff for the tachycardia detection will increase specificity but decrease the sensitivity for VT detection.

Zones of detection

In most of the current devices, up to three zones of tachycardia detection are available and can provide distinct therapy for slow VT, fast VT, and VF.

Each level or zone is defined by a range of tachycardia rates. This is used to distinguish different arrhythmias in a patient. Each zone has programmed rate criteria for tachycardia detection as well as a programmed therapy algorithm defined by the treating electrophysiologist. Generally, algorithms deliver more aggressive therapy with increasing duration of an episode of tachycardia. Thus, treatment of an episode of tachycardia may begin with several attempts at antitachycardia pacing at increasingly faster pacing rates, followed by low energy cardioversion and finally, high energy cardioversion. As a safety feature, if tachycardia persists, all ICDs will eventually deliver high energy shocks at the final point in the algorithm. However, the tachycardia duration prior to the first high energy (30 plus joules) shock will depend on the algorithm programmed into the ICD by the treating electrophysiologist.

The optional tachycardia detection features mentioned above can be used only for VT. VF is detected if a predetermined number of intervals have exceeded the VF detection rate. Most defibrillators use only a rate cutoff algorithm to detect VF because of the consequence of VF nondetection.

Committed/uncommitted devices

Another feature of the newer devices is the ability to reassess the tachycardia prior to initiating therapy. Older devices were considered 'committed' as once the tachycardia detection criteria were met, the capacitors of the device charged and a shock was delivered after the delay involved in charging the capacitors occurred. If the patient's tachycardia terminated prior to the shock delivery (i.e., the patient's VT was nonsustained), the shock was still delivered *(Figure 36.7)*. Current ICDs have the ability to reassess the tachycardia and abort, or divert, the shock if tachycardia criteria are no longer met even after the capacitors have been charged. Devices that possess this feature have been termed 'uncommitted'.

Therapy

Antitachycardia pacing

Pace termination of VT is based on the ability of a pacing pulse to capture excitable tissue within a reentrant circuit[7-9] *(Figure 36.8)*. The latest generation ICDs may be

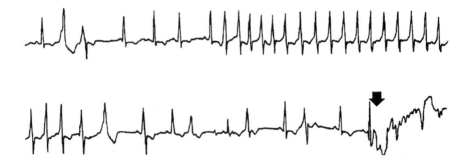

Figure 36.7 **Committed device firing during sinus rhythm**. *A patient with an early ICD develops VT which then terminates spontaneously to sinus rhythm with ventricular premature depolarizations (ECG strips are continuous; horizontal axis scale 25 mm/sec). However, the VT has met the detection criterion for the ICD and has persisted through the programmed delay; it thus causes the ICD to charge. While the ICD is charging, the patient's rhythm reverts to sinus rhythm with ventricular premature depolarizations. As the device does not reexamine the patient's rhythm prior to firing (i.e., the device is 'committed' to firing), the ICD fires (arrow) although the patient's VT has spontaneously terminated.*

programmed to deliver antitachycardia pacing via the pace/sense electrodes. These devices offer programmable options to optimize the antitachycardia pacing proto-col. After the VT has been detected, the programmed antitachycardia therapy is delivered. The device then detects the patient's rhythm following therapy and deter-mines whether further treatment is necessary. If no arrhythmia is detected, the device then ceases to deliver further therapy. If it detects a bradycardia, antibrady-cardia pacing is performed. If the tachycardia persists, additional ATP therapy may be delivered or cardioversion may be administered depending on the manner in which the ICD has been programmed. Generally, these programmed algorithms are tested in the electrophysiology (EP) laboratory, although algorithms effective in the EP lab may not be effective in the ambulatory patient for many reasons, including alterations in autonomic tone. Theoretically, in the upright or ambulatory patient, autonomic tone may change the conduction times and refractory periods within a reentrant loop, thus making pace termination of VT more difficult.[10] In addition, the VT induced in the EP laboratory may differ from the patient's clinical VT.

In general, pacing algorithms using bursts or extrastimuli as a percentage of the sensed tachycardia rate, known as rate adaptive modes, are probably more effi-cacious in terminating VT than modes that do not adapt to the VT rate.[7] Any type of pacing algorithm, however, may produce an acceleration of the VT[11] which may degenerate to VF. Because of this, some ICDs will advance therapy to a more ag-gressive level of therapy (i.e. cardioversion or high energy defibrillation) when ac-celeration is detected. This is also the rationale for implantation of an ICD rather

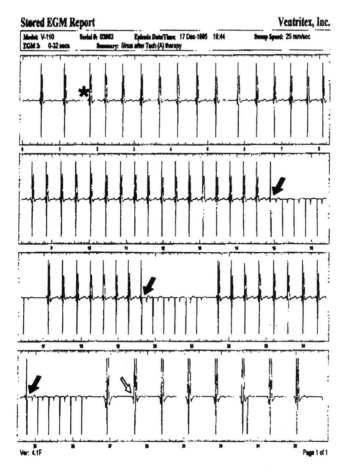

Stored EGM Report   **Ventritex, Inc.**

| Model: V-110 | Serial #: 03003 | Episode Date/Time: 17 Dec 1995 10:44 | Sweep Speed: 25 mm/sec |
| EGM 3: 0-32 secs | | Summary: Sinus after Tech (A) therapy | |

Ver: 4.1F   Page 1 of 1

*Figure 36.8 Ventritex Cadence electrogram printout. The patient develops VT, indicated
by the asterisk (*). The device detects the VT and attempts ATP three times, as indicated
by the solid arrows. The third ATP attempt successfully terminates the VT and sinus
rhythm resumes, as indicated by the open arrow. (Sweep speed 25 mm/sec.)*

than merely an antitachycardia pacemaker in patients whose VT is paceterminable
and who have never had VF.

ATP has been shown to be effective in termination of VT. For the Ventritex
Cadence, 93.5% of antitachycardia protocols for spontaneous VT were successful.[12]
Similar data were reported by Medtronic during the clinical trials of their PCDT
epicardial systems.[13] The PCD Transvene system had an efficacy rate of 89% in
terminating VT.

Most patients who receive a tiered therapy device ATP programmed into their
therapy algorithm by their treating electrophysiologist. In one study of patients re-

ceiving a CPI PRx device, ATP was successful as first therapy 92% of the time; acceleration of the VT occurred 8.5% of the time. ATP was most likely to be successful (94%) at rates of tachycardia between 131 and 160 bpm. It was 85% effective at rates between 191 and 220 bpm.[4]

ATP schemes. In general, pacing schemes available are: burst, ramp, scan, and ramp/ scan (*Figure 36.9 and 36.10*). A burst sequence consists of a programmed number of critically timed pulses in which the timing of all pacing intervals within the burst train are equal. In a scan pacing scheme, the cycle length of each burst in a scheme is decremented by a given amount of time between successive bursts. Thus, the interval between each pulse in a burst is the same, but the interval between each pulse in the successive burst is smaller. In a ramp sequence, each paced-to-paced interval within the burst is shortened, or decremented by a programmed length of time. With each additional pacing pulse in the sequence, the interval between pulses is shortened by the programmed ramp decrement amount until the last pulse is

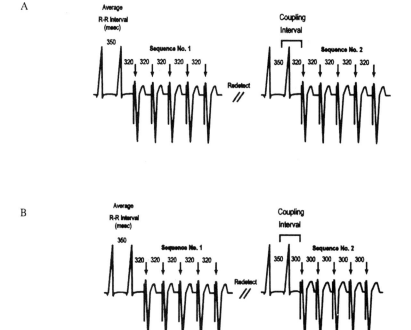

Figure 36.9 ATP pacing schemes. A) ATP burst therapy. The device has detected the average R-R interval to be 350 msec, which falls within the programmed VT range. A burst of ATP at 320 msec ensues. As shown, a burst sequence is one in which the cycle length between paced pulses remains constant. B) ATP scan therapy. Here, each ATP attempt is a burst; between each subsequent ATP burst, the cycle length between paced pulses is decremented by a programmed amount (20 msec in this example).

A ATP Ramp Therapy

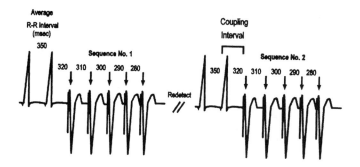

B ATP Ramp/Scan Therapy

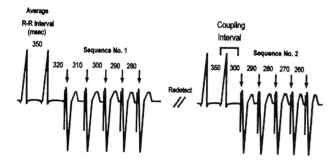

*Figure 36.10 **ATP pacing schemes**. A) ATP ramp sequence. The cycle length between paced pulses decreases by a programmed amount (10 msec in this example). B) ATP ramp/scan therapy. Each ATP attempt is a ramp; between each subsequent ATP ramp attempt, the initial paced coupling interval is decremented by a programmed amount (here, 20 msec); in addition, there is a 10 msec decrement between each pulse in the train.*

delivered. In the ramp/scan scheme, the first burst is a ramp scheme. Subsequent bursts consist of scan schemes in which each burst is a ramp.

Cardioversion

Cardioversion refers to the ability of a low energy shock to convert VT to sinus rhythm. Shocks for cardioversion of VT are synchronized to the onset of the ventricular depolarization which is sensed by the rate sensing leads. Shocks less than 0.5 joules generally cause minimal discomfort to the patient.[14] When compared with VT termination using high energy shock, low energy cardioversion also conserves battery life. Low energy cardioversion has been shown to have similar efficacy with that of pace termination of VT.[15, 16] The risk of accelerating the VT is still present, however. Siebels et al reported termination of 69% of episodes of induced mono-morphic VT by ICD cardioversion with ≤4 joules; ten of the 32 VT episodes were accelerated by the low energy cardioversion.[17]

In clinical trials using the Ventritex Cadence device, 90% of episodes of spontaneous VT were successfully treated with the first programmed cardioversion. Similar data were obtained using the Medtronic PCD epicardial or Transvene systems.[12]

Defibrillation

The mechanism of cardioversion of VT probably differs from that of defibrillation of VF. To defibrillate the heart, it is thought that a critical mass of ventricular myocardium must be depolarized. [18, 19] A critical threshold energy is also necessary [20] and it is thought by some that a sufficient current density must be achieved throughout the heart in order to avoid reinitiation of fibrillation by a subthreshold current density.[21] In general, newer systems using transvenous leads are associated with higher defibrillation thresholds in comparison with systems using epicardial patches.[2] Thus, the manner in which to optimize energy delivery is being studied. While monophasic waveform defibrillation *(Figure 36.1)* was present in the original ICDs, sequential or biphasic waveforms are present in newer ICDs. Sequential capacitor discharge patterns, using a three patch electrode system is available in the Medtronic PCD system; biphasic waveforms are available in most of the latest generation devices. The use of simultaneous defibrillation via two pathways using three electrodes reduces DFTs in patients with elevated DFTs.[3] Using a Y adapter, which connects two electrodes in parallel with one another to one pole of the generator, three electrodes are connected to the generator; this type of defibrillation can be used with any ICD. The Ventritex systems have also incorporated a programmable 'tilt' feature whereby the slope of the capacitor discharge can be altered to optimize defibrillation. Other devices in which the shape of the waveform cannot be programmed use a truncated waveform with a fixed tilt of 60%.[22]

Biphasic waveforms have generally produced lower DFTs than monophasic waveforms.[23-27] Although the mechanism remains unknown, the reduction in DFT energy was 26% using an epicardial system[28] and 40% using an endocardial system.[23, 24] Although endocardial systems have higher DFTs than do epicardial systems, the availability of biphasic waveforms should enable most patients to have satisfactory DFTs with an endocardial lead system.

Bradycardia pacing

Backup bradycardia pacing *(Figure 36.11)* is available in most ICDs, except the CPI Ventak P1550, 1555, and 1600 generators, which are no longer manufactured. The available bradycardia pacing is in the VVI mode. It is advantageous to incorporate pacing capabilities in ICDs as it avoids pacemaker-defibrillator interactions, which are discussed later in this chapter. In some devices such as the Medtronic PCD 7216, the programmable output for VVI pacing is the same output as that used for

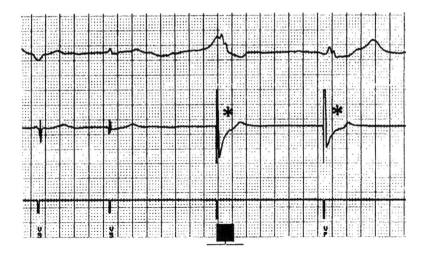

Figure 36.11 Report printout from a Medtronic Jewel with backup bradycardia pacing. In this segment of a recorded electrogram, the device markers display ventricular sensing (VS) followed by ventricular pacing (VP). The asterisks have been added by the authors to indicate the paced ventricular beats.

antitachycardia pacing. In order to ensure reliable pacing for VT, higher pacing outputs are needed for antitachycardia pacing. Thus, battery drain may occur in patients who are pacemaker dependent. In the Medtronic Jewel PCD 7219, Ventritex Cadence, and the CPI PRx II, III, and MINI ICDs, pacing outputs for bradycardia and antitachycardia pacing are distinct and programmable. By limiting the bradycardia pacing output, battery drain should be decreased. In addition, separate pacing parameters for postshock bradycardia pacing are useful as higher outputs are needed postdefibrillation as well. Defibrillators with backup bradycardia pacing are useful as, for example, in the Medtronic database, 17.3% of the patients who received the PCD' had a history of bradycardia.[13] With the Medtronic PCD, backup bradycardia pacing was used after one or more episodes of VT in 49%. More than 20% of the patients required long term bradycardia support.

Special features

Many additional features are available in the newer ICDs. Noninvasive programmed electrical stimulation is available in all of the new devices. This is useful for VT and VF induction to test ATP algorithms and defibrillation efficacy in the EP laboratory. Generally, VF can be induced by burst (fast) pacing of the RV as well as with low energy shocks into the T wave, a feature of the Medtronic PCD 7219. Programmed electrical stimulation is performed to induce VT and test the efficacy of antitachycardia pacing algorithms.

Many ICDs possess algorithms to check pacing and sensing thresholds. Functions are also available to check battery function and pacing lead impedance. In some ICDs, capacitor reformation occurs automatically and thus decreases the number of follow up visits necessary. Latest generation ICDs are also capable of real time telemetry. This allows the electrophysiologist to examine the electrogram as recorded via the rate sensing or shocking leads. This is helpful in troubleshooting problems and ascertaining proper function of the ICD.

Data history and stored electrograms

Knowledge of rhythms that trigger ICD therapy in a given patient is important for patient management. ICDs incorporate algorithms that distinguish pathological tachycardias from physiological or benign tachycardias. Thus, when patients report having received defibrillator shocks, it is important for the electrophysiologist to be able to decide whether these shocks were appropriate. Further management of the patient receiving appropriate shocks may include a change in antiarrhythmic drug regimen, further therapy for underlying conditions, or changes in detection algorithms or antitachycardia pacing protocols.

Early devices such as the CPI Ventak P 1550 and 1600 AICDs have very limited capabilities for data recall. This is limited to a counter that records the number of shocks delivered either as a first shock, or as a so called 'rescue' shock (shocks 2 through 5). These counters cannot be erased from the device memory. The number of episodes for which a first shock was unsuccessful at treatment of the arrhythmia can be deduced. However, it cannot be determined whether the rhythm treated was VT, VF, SVT, or sinus tachycardia (ST). Patient history must be relied on to make the best determination of the nature of the tachycardia. Unfortunately, data from some of the ongoing ICDs trials are limited by the fact that the ICDs implanted are older models and thus lack the ability to store electrograms. Thus, shocks are used as surrogate endpoints for malignant arrhythmia,

Data recall has improved with the newer ICDs. Some ICDs store R-R intervals during the episodes of detected VT or VF. The Medtronic PCD 7216 stores the R-R intervals preceding the onset of the last detected tachycardia and the R-R intervals following the last successful treatment. Another ICD which stores R-R intervals only is the CPI PRx. This device is no longer being manufactured as more sophisticated devices manufactured by CPI have been approved by the FDA.

Overall, stored electrograms provide a more accurate depiction of a patient's rhythm prior to receiving therapy from the ICD. None of the approved devices store electrograms prior to or during bradycardia pacing. All devices incorporate a simple counter that records therapy delivery. However, devices vary as to the amount of data they can store in memory. In general, the most recent events will overwrite older events. Thus, devices should be interrogated to download or replay recorded events before they are overwritten. Events recorded will also include nonsustained episodes that meet programmed detection criteria.

The CPI Ventak P2 1625 and later CPI devices have electrogram storage capabilities. In the CPI devices, the electrograms are recorded from the shocking electrodes and thus may better enable distinctions between narrow and wide complexes as well as provide P waves on the electrogram. In general, these electrograms tend to resemble the surface ECG *(Figure 36.12)*. Ventritex devices record electrograms from their rate sensing leads which have a smaller surface area; these electrograms resemble intracardiac electrograms and may be less helpful in determining whether the tachycardia is supraventricular or ventricular in origin.

Stored electrograms have been shown to alter patient management in a positive manner. In one study, the number of inappropriate therapies for non VT rhythms was decreased once stored electrograms were interpreted and therapy algorithms were changed or antiarrhythmic drugs were added to the patient's regimen. In this series, the stored electrograms that affected patient therapy were interpreted as atrial fibrillation (AF), SVT, artifact and T wave oversensing.[29] Another study showed that stored electrograms were valuable in detecting nonsustained arrhythmias that received no therapy. These episodes included nonsustained VT, AF, SVT, and artifact. Again, these stored electrograms produced changes in patient management in many cases.[30]

Specific devices

Medtronic, Inc.

Medtronic PCD models 7216A and 7217B were *(Table 36.1)* the initial devices produced by this company the two devices are similar. While the 7216A uses integrated bipolar sensing (i.e. between one myocardial pacemaker electrode and the negative defibrillation electrode), the 7217B uses conventional bipolar sensing. These devic-

Surface ECG

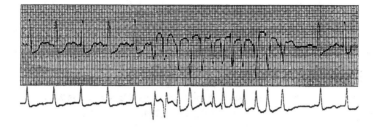

Stored Intracardiac Electrogram

Figure 36.12 Surface ECG (upper panel) and stored intracardiac electrogram (lower panel) of an episode of nonsustained VT from a patient with a CPI Ventak P2.

es contain no stored electrograms. However, 20 R-R intervals prior to the last detected VT/VF episode and 10 intervals after the last VT/VF episode are stored. Up to three high voltage defibrillating leads (two form an anode) can be attached to the header for the Medtronic PCD devices. The PCD can be programmed to deliver sequential or simultaneous shocks.

The latest generation Medtronic devices that have received FDA approval belong to the Jewelώ family of devices. With these devices, up to four therapies for VT (specified below) can be delivered after VT is detected. Faster VT can also receive up to four therapies. The three therapies for VT or 'Faster VT' include three methods of antitachycardia pacing and synchronized cardioversion. In addition, up to four shocks can be delivered for an episode of VF.

The three methods of antitachycardia pacing available in the Jewel 7219 series include ramp-plus, ramp pacing, and burst pacing. The ramp and burst pacing sequences are similar to those described previously under ATP schemes. Ramp-plus pacing consists of two VOO pulses programmed at separate intervals, followed by a set of VOO pulses at a third interval. This is a rate adaptive mode of therapy. The number of pulses in the first sequence, the R-S1(native sensed to first beat paced) interval, the S1-S2 and S2-n intervals, and the number of sequences to be delivered are programmable.

For the newer Medtronic devices, the longevity projection is 6 years if no bradycardia pacing is used and only quarterly shocks are delivered. The projection is reduced to 3.5 years is the patient is 100% paced with monthly shocks or 4.4 years if the patient is 100% paced and receives quarterly shocks. For the Micro Jewel ICD, which received FDA approval in July, 1996, the battery longevity is 8 years if the bradycardia pacing is not used and only biannual shocks are delivered. In addition, the pulse width and amplitude for the antitachycardia pacing pulse are the same for all antitachycardia pacing therapies, but are programmed separately from the bradycardia amplitude and pulse width. This feature saves on battery life compared to prior Medtronic devices.

CPI

The term, AICD, which stands for Automatic Implantable Cardioverter Defibrillator is a registered trademark of CPI; ICD is the generic term for the device. The first device to gain FDA approval was a device that was licensed from Intec Systems by CPI. Since that time, CPI has developed several generations of AICDs. Along the way, newer ICDs have replaced the older models. Only models 1720 and greater in addition to model 1645 are currently manufactured by CPI.

The CPI Ventak P 1500 and 1600 series, as mentioned previously, feature minimal programmability (Table 36.1). The CPI Ventakώ P 1600, which is not a tiered therapy device, will be discussed in greater detail as it is still in use and its features illustrate the detection algorithm of a simple device. In the 1600, features that are programmable include the rate (from 110 to 200 bpm in 5 bpm increments), morphology (on or off), the magnitude of the first shock (0.1 to 30 joules), and the delay period between detection and shock delivery. In this device, heart rate is monitored by an RR interval detector which counts the number of consecutive cycles that are short enough to meet the programmed rate criterion. If a long cycle occurs, the counter subtracts the cycle from the tally. When the tally reaches 8, a programmable delay period of 2.5, 5, 7.5, or 10 seconds ensues. During this delay, the tally may vary between 0 and 15, but at the end of the delay period, the tally must be at 8 or higher for the ICD to deliver a shock. If the tally is greater or equal to 8, the device is committed to delivering a shock even if the rhythm reverts to sinus. The device batteries charge the capacitor, which may require several seconds, and a shock is delivered. Several seconds after the first shock is delivered, sensing resumes. If the rate criterion is again met, a subsequent shock may be delivered. Delay between shocks may be approximately 15 seconds.

The morphology function in this device is a probability density function, discussed previously in this chapter. Because it may increase the time to tachyarrhythmia detection, it is frequently programmed off by the treating electrophysiologist.

The CPI Ventak P2 and P3 (Models 1625 and 1635) incorporate backup bradycardia pacing as well as stored electrograms. They do not have antitachycardia pacing capabilities, but are capable of delivering biphasic shocks. The CPI Ventak PRx (Models 1700 and 1705) possesses ATP capability. Therapy history provides information regarding zone of therapy, date and time of therapy occurrence and delivered therapy and its success. It does not store electrograms, but retains R-R intervals pre and post episode. It is capable of storing up to 128 therapy attempts in its memory. In addition, the device can display real time rate and morphology electrograms. However, it is only capable of delivering monophasic shocks.

The PRx II (model 1715) incorporates features of the PRx and the P2 1625, which stores electrograms. It weighs 233 grams and is 144 cc in volume. This device and those described previously have been replaced by the MINI and the PRxIII. The PRx III (models 1720 and 1725) is essentially the same pulse generator as the PRx II except that it is substantially smaller. These devices are capable of storing up to 2.5 minutes of intracardiac electrograms and up to 2000 annotated RR intervals. They are capable of delivering shocks of up to 34 joules. The 1720 and 1725 weigh 179 and 182 grams, respectively, with volumes of 97 and 105 cc. These devices, as well as the PRxII, provide the ability to program the characteristics of the ATP, bradycardia, and postshock bradycardia pacing pulses independently.

The Ventak MINI family of AICDs (1645, 1740's series) is the latest group of CPI devices to gain FDA approval. These devices contain only one lithium-silver vanadium oxide cell. They range in weight from 125 to 139 grams; their volumes range from 68 to 78 cc. For the sake of comparison, a permanent pacemaker pulse generator may weigh on the order of 28 grams and have a volume of 13 cc. The MINI family may be implanted in the pectoral subcutaneous or submuscular space based on the activity level of the patient, as well as the patient's size. These devices use the same detection, therapies, diagnostic and electrophysiology features as the

PRxII. In addition to providing tiered therapy and bradycardia backup pacing, the device life expectancy is up to six years. The life expectancy for the MINI+ and the MINI+S (extended longevity) is up to 8.4 years, depending on the therapy delivered. In addition, these devices can store more than 5 minutes of intracardiac electrograms which are recorded from the shocking electrodes. The MINI+S (Model 1645) does not provide antitachycardia pacing capabilities. In this AICD family, maximum delivered energy is 29 joules. However, the DFTs produced by these devices are on average 10 joules, which is lower than most other devices; thus, a similar margin of safety to other devices exists. The MINI II device has recently received FDA approval. It is an 'Active Can' device and is approved for pectoral or left abdominal implantation. It weighs 115 grams.

Antitachycardia pacing. In the CPI AICDs, several modes of antitachycardia pacing are available. These include burst, ramp, scan, and ramp/scan. Within an antitachycardia scheme, the following can be programmed: the number of bursts delivered, the number of pulses within each burst, the coupling interval, the burst cycle length and its characteristics, and a minimum pacing interval.

Magnet Mode. In all CPI devices, two functions can be performed when a magnet is applied to the pulse generator. First, tones that indicate the current tachycardia mode of the device become audible. Second, tachyarrhythmia therapy and induction modes are inhibited. If R-wave synchronous tones are emitted by the pulse generator when the magnet is applied, then the tachycardia mode is currently programmed to monitor plus therapy, which indicates that tachyarrhythmia therapy can be delivered, if the detection criteria are met, once the magnet is removed from the pulse generator. If a continuous tone is emitted, then the tachycardia mode is programmed to storage, off, or monitor only. This indicates that tachyarrhythmia therapy is not available even when the magnet is removed. In addition, most of the CPI devices have a feature called 'change tachy mode with magnet'. If this has been programmed on, then applying the magnet for more than 30 seconds will allow the programmer to change the 'tachy mode' from off to on, from on to off, or from monitor only to monitor plus therapy.

Ventritex, Inc.

The Ventritex Cadence V-100 pulse generator was the first device to incorporate antitachycardia pacing, biphasic waveforms, and stored electrograms to receive FDA approval. These devices can store up to 112 seconds of electrograms, depending on the number of episodes programmed to be recorded. Thus, the device can be programmed to store one 64 second, three 32 second, or seven 16 second events that exceeded the programmed rate cutoff *(Table 36.1)*.

The EHR or Extended High Rate algorithm is available in the Ventritex Cadence ICD. This involves a programmable timer that begins once the device's counters reach 'VT' level. If the VT has not terminated by the elapsed time programmed into the EHR feature, the Cadence abandons its less aggressive VT therapy and delivers its more aggressive therapy programmed for VF.

Ventritex manufactures an endocardial lead system that received FDA approval in May, 1996. In addition, Ventritex manufactures the V-110C pulse generator, which is a smaller device than the V-100. They also recently received FDA approval for their Cadet series of pulse generators. These devices are were approved for pectoral implantation in May, 1996. Other pulse generators, including models that employ unipolar lead technology are investigational.

Intermedics, Inc.

The Intermedics Res-QT 101-01 ACD (arrhythmia control device) system has been approved for market release. The device weighs 240 grams, can deliver tiered therapy, but does not store electrograms. Intermedics also manufactures epicardial patches to be used with the Res-QT device. An endocardial lead system has been approved for use in this country; smaller pulse generators (Res-QT II and Res-QT Micron) with additional features such as stored electrograms and active can models are currently investigational in the U.S. *(Table 36.1).*

Angeion Corporation

All devices produced by this company are currently investigational in the U.S. Their SentinelT 2000 is designed for pectoral implantation; its weight is 110 gms. It can be programmed to an active can configuration. This ICD contains backup bradycardia and ATP features. However, it does not store electrograms.

ICD implantation

Originally, ICDs were implanted by surgeons in the operating room, with the assistance of cardiologists whose interest was in electrophysiology. While the surgeons implanted the device, the cardiologist tested it to assure proper function. With the advent of transvenous lead systems, cardiologists, many of whom are trained in the implantation of permanent transvenous pacemakers, are also implanting ICDs. These devices may be implanted in the operating room by the cardiologist, or they may be implanted in an electrophysiology laboratory which has been built to operating room specifications.

Preoperative evaluation

Apart from routine presurgical evaluation, several items are addressed. It is important to establish whether the patient has myocardial ischemia preoperatively as concomitant CABG surgery might be indicated if the coronary anatomy warrants it. Because the patient's heart is fibrillated in the operating room during intraoperative ICD testing, ischemic myocardium may make defibrillation difficult. Revascularization has been shown to increase survival in patients following ICD implantation.[31, 32] It is also important to ascertain the patient's maximum heart rate, preferably by exercise treadmill test, in order to program the rate cutoff for the ICD therapy to be initiated. In this way, ICD therapy for sinus tachycardia is avoided.

Surgical approaches

Surgical implantation of the ICD leads can be performed via several different approaches. Originally, the epicardial patches were placed via an anterolateral thoracotomy. This approach can be used to implant a two patch defibrillating electrode system or a system involving a single large patch and an SVC electrode. This approach is considered to be less invasive than a median sternotomy, yet provides good exposure; this approach is favored by some surgeons in patients with previous surgery. Median sternotomy, subcostal thoracotomy, and subxyphoid approaches have also been used. Currently, transvenous placement of endocardial leads is the preferred approach to electrode placement. If the DFTs are elevated, addition of a subcutaneous patch or array is performed in order to increase the surface area of the shock electrodes. At present, even if a patient is undergoing concomitant open heart surgery, epicardial patches are generally no longer employed. Usually, endocardial lead systems are implanted and tested in the operating room or EP laboratory later during the postoperative hospitalization. However, in general, there is always the possibility that a thoracotomy will be needed if satisfactory DFTs are not achieved using the endocardial approach. In this case, epicardial patches are used.

Implantation of pulse generators is generally in the subrectus or subcutaneous tissue of the upper abdomen due to the large size of the devices. Some of the smaller devices may be implanted in the upper chest as with permanent pacemakers in patients who are sufficiently large. Implantation in the upper chest has been termed 'pectoral implantation'. Only certain devices have been approved for pectoral implantation *(Table 36.1)*.

Intraoperative electrophysiological testing

Intraoperative evaluation of the pacing/sensing as well as the defibrillation leads is performed during ICD implantation. An analyzer used to assess pacemaker systems is used to determine the amplitude of the R wave (ventricular depolarization) sensed on the leads in addition to pacing thresholds. Acceptable values include an R wave on the pace/sense lead of greater than 5 mV, an endocardial pacing threshold of less than 1.0 V, pacing lead impedance of 200-800 ohms, and morphology lead R wave of greater than 1 mV. In addition, a low energy shock (1-3 joules) is delivered to the defibrillation leads to determine shocking lead impedance as well as connection integrity.

Because R wave changes can occur after induction of ventricular fibrillation, the R wave should be examined during sinus rhythm, VT and VF. The cardioversion energy requirement (CER) is defined as the least amount of energy required to convert VT to SR. As the CER is lower than the DFT, the DFT is determined in the operating room during ICD testing. VF is induced with rapid pacing or by delivery of a shock on the T wave. It is desirable to obtain a 100% safety factor in the DFT value. However, a 10 joule safety margin between the DFT and maximal device output is acceptable.[33] At present, ICDs have a maximal output of at least 27 joules, depending on the device make and model; it is thus uncommon not to achieve an acceptable margin of safety. In general, DFT testing is begun at 20 joules and decremented by 5 joules per test until defibrillation is unsuccessful. A DFT of 10 or 15 joules is desirable; two to three defibrillations at an energy 10 joules less than the maximal output are needed to confirm the proper lead configuration and positioning during ICD implantation. Three to five minutes should be allowed between DFT tests in order to allow hemodynamic stabilization of the patient prior to the next defibrillation. In patients who are potentially unstable, DFT evaluation should be minimized; thus, only testing necessary to ensure an adequate safety margin and proper device function should be performed.[34]

Following defibrillator testing, the leads are tunneled to the ICD pocket and are connected to the device. The pulse generator is programmed to the desired parameters and is activated. VF is induced via the pace/sense leads and the generator senses and terminates the arrhythmia. After wound closure, defibrillation and bradycardia pacing functions are activated. ATP may be left off until predischarge testing is performed.

In general, the ICD is reevaluated 1 to 2 days post implantation prior to discharge of the patient to home. Again, lead function and integrity are checked. VF is induced, usually while the patient is sedated and unconscious and the ICD is allowed to defibrillate the patient (Figure 36.13). If applicable, VT is induced and the pacing algorithm programmed into the ICD by the electrophysiologist is tested.

Complications of ICD therapy

Operative morbidity and mortality

Operative morbidity and mortality of the implantation of the ICD via a thoracotomy approach is nearly 3% while that of a nonthoracotomy implantation is 1%.[31, 35] Several factors have been shown to contribute to operative risk. These include the surgical approach (i.e. thoracotomy greater surgical risk than nonthoracotomy), advanced age, concomitant cardiac surgery, comorbid disease, poor left ventricular function, class IV NYHA congestive heart failure (CHF). Joye et al [36] reported a 0% operative mortality in patients with an LVEF of >30% and 5.1% in patients with an LVEF <30%. Levine et al[37] reported a 42% operative mortality in patients with class IV CHF, thus highlighting the importance of the functional status of the patient.

One of the most serious postoperative complications is infection, which may occur with a frequency of 1-6%. Although immediate postoperative infections may occur, in general there is a delay of weeks to months following implantation. Presentation of infection includes local erythema, tenderness, or a draining sinus at the site of the ICD pocket; there may be fever or leukocytosis. Staphylococcus aureus

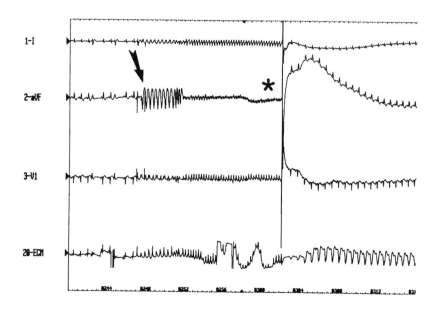

Figure 36.13 Noninvasive VF induction in the electrophysiology laboratory. Thirty-six seconds of data are shown. VF is induced by the defibrillator at the arrow. The device defibrillates (*) the patient and converts the rhythm to sinus. Shown are surface leads I, aVF, and V1 as well as an intracardiac electrogram (EGM). The horizontal scale represents time in seconds.

or epidermidis are commonly cultured; aureus from early presentation while epidermidis is associated with infections that present later. Subcutaneous tracking via the leads is common and may lead to sepsis as well as the seeding of distant organs. Complete removal of the ICD and lead system in conjunction with antibiotic treatment is usually required to eradicate the infection.

Postoperative complications associated with the thoracotomy approach to ICD implantation include pericarditis, atelectasis, paroxysmal atrial fibrillation, DVT, lead migration/dislodgement, or pneumonia. Rare complications include cardiac tamponade, CVA, or MI. A late complication associated with epicardial patches is the production of constrictive physiology.[38]

Technical issues

There are other complications of ICD therapy related to technical issues. The ICD batteries have a finite lifespan, requiring generator replacement approximately every three years, depending on the model and the number of discharges. Lead fractures may occur and cause either device failure or inappropriate shocks. Spurious ICD discharges are those that occur in the absence of sustained VT or VF. Without telemetry, it may be impossible to define the exact cause of the discharge which may include device malfunction or sensing of an SVT or AF, ST, oversensing of myopotentials or electrical noise from electrocautery systems. Other sources of electromagnetic interference which may impede proper ICD function include cellular telephones, diathermy, external defibrillation, therapeutic radiation, MRI, lithotripsy, home appliances, and store security systems.

Interactions of ICDs and pacemakers

Initial interactions noted between ICDs and permanent pacemakers included inappropriate ICD discharges due to ICD sensing of pacemaker artifact. In general, unipolar pacemakers can cause an ICD to discharge due to double sensing of the unipolar stimulus artifact and the QRS electrogram. Thus, by 'double counting,' the device might sense that the tachyarrhythmia rate cutoff has been exceeded and erroneously deliver tachyarrhythmia therapy. Because unipolar pacemakers have larger pacemaker artifacts than do bipolar devices, this problem occurs more commonly with unipolar pacemakers; it has been reported with bipolar devices, however.

In addition, there may be inappropriate inhibition of defibrillator discharge due to unipolar pacemaker discharge. In this case, the pacemaker may not sense the ventricular arrhythmia and thus it delivers a pulse to the ventricle. The pulse is sensed by the ICD as regular cardiac activity and thus does not detect the ventricular arrhythmia. During implantation of the ICD, placement of the ICD sensing electrodes and the permanent pacemaker leads are optimized to avoid farfield sensing of the pacemaker pulses.[39] In general, this potential interaction must be evaluated during device implantation, with the pacemaker programmed at maximal pacing outputs in the asynchronous mode. Also, unipolar pacemakers are not used in patients requiring ICD implantation.

Other interactions involve alteration of the ICD generator by inadvertent influence of a magnetic field during noninvasive evaluation of the pacemaker. This can result in defibrillator deactivation, inappropriate defibrillator discharge, or generator reprogramming. CPI devices can be inactivated with application of a magnet for thirty seconds. Because of this, the status of the ICD must be assessed after pacemaker reprogramming. In addition, pacemaker programming can result in ICD discharge; it is recommended that the ICD be temporarily inactivated while the pacemaker is reprogrammed. Pacemakers may also change their status to ERI (elective replacement indication) or POR (power on reset) after an ICD discharge. In these cases, the pacemaker may revert to a backup pacing mode which may be unipolar VVI. To avoid the possibility of unipolar pacing, it is recommended that only committed bipolar pacemakers (i.e., pacemakers that do not have a unipolar mode) be implanted in patients with ICDs.

Interactions of ICDs and antiarrhythmic agents

In clinical practice, antiarrhythmic drugs are a leading cause of elevated DFTs.[40, 41] In general, type Ia agents tend to increase the DFT.[42-44] Lidocaine has been shown to produce an increase in DFT as well, but only at concentrations greater than 5 ug/ml, i.v.[45, 46] Mexiletine has also been reported to increase the DFT.[47] In addition, class Ic agents increase DFTs. B-blockers[48] as well as amiodarone[44, 49, 50] may increase the DFT. Class III agents such as clofilium, d-sotalol and d,l-sotalol decrease the DFT.[51-53] The class IV agent, verapamil, increases the DFT.[54] In addition, anesthetic agents may alter the DFT. Fentanyl has been associated with decreased DFT when it was compared with anesthesia with enflurane, halothane, or sedation with pentobarbital.[55]

Generally, following initial ICD implant, patients are not administered antiarrhythmic drugs. They are discharged to home and on follow-up, the status of their arrhythmia is assessed. If the patient is receiving frequent shocks, then the addition of antiarrhythmic therapy may be considered. Because of the potential for increasing the DFT, the ability of the ICD to defibrillate the patient should be evaluated in any patient receiving long-term antiarrhythmic therapy. Antiarrhythmic agents may also alter the cycle length of clinical arrhythmias. Thus, the zones of therapy delivered by the ICD may need to be reprogrammed if the patient requires concomitant antiarrhythmic therapy.

ICD follow up

ICDs require periodic maintenance. For example, the dielectric material within the capacitors may deform over time if an extended period elapses between charges. This could produce prolongation of the time for the first charge after extensive disuse. To avoid this, ICD capacitors are reformed periodically either by manual or automatic programming. To reform the capacitors, the capacitors are charged and the charge is allowed to dissipate over time. Older devices necessitated office visits every two months in order to interrogate the ICD and reform its capacitors. Manufacturers of most newer devices recommend follow up every three months. Newer devices generally reform the capacitors automatically. The charge time of the capacitors increases over time. The elective replacement time of the device is indicated by an increase in the charge time to a time specified for the particular device.

Patients with an ICD in place should be monitored closely. At a follow up visit, the patient relates any arrhythmic symptoms and whether he or she detected any ICD therapy delivery. The device is interrogated via a radiofrequency link using a proprietary microcomputer with software designed for the specific ICD. Therapy history and any new stored electrograms are examined. Battery status and capacitor charge time are evaluated. In addition, the integrity of the system is checked by evaluation of the lead impedance and real time electrograms. The need for additional antiarrhythmic therapy or device malfunction is addressed. Alterations in therapy algorithms can be performed as needed.

When the elective replacement time occurs, the patient is scheduled for explantation of the old and implantation of a new generator. The generator used is usually a newer model; often no lead modification is necessary. ICD manufacturers have attempted to standardize the connections between the leads and pulse generators so that leads and generators can be mixed and matched to a certain extent. However, FDA approval is generally given for a device implanted with a particular set of leads.

In general, hospitalization following shocks is not necessary unless there is suspicion that the device delivered therapy when it was unnecessary. Hospitalization may also be required if there is a suspicion that the device did not deliver therapy when it should have. In addition, multiple shocks generally require hospitalization for further investigation. Electrolyte imbalance or worsening of heart disease may increase the occurrence of VT and thus precipitate ICD discharge. If the VT is recurrent despite treatment of underlying causes, antiarrhythmic agents may need to be added to the patient's medical regimen. Because many antiarrhythmic agents tend to increase the DFT of the ICD, the device should be retested with the patient on the antiarrhythmic agent in order to assure the ability of the ICD to defibrillate the patient while on the drug. With the latest generation ICDs, stored electrograms are often helpful in determining whether the device has malfunctioned.

Patient acceptance

Although lifesaving, the ICD may be psychologically problematic to the patient. Understandably, patients dislike the sensation of the ICD shock, which is painful, and may be delivered while the patient is still conscious. Some patients find the possibility of receiving a shock to be very anxiety provoking. Others find the possibility of not receiving a shock when required to be devastating. These problems may require psychotherapy. A small study suggested a 50% prevalence of psychological problems following ICD implantation.[56] Rarely, a device must be explanted at the patient's insistence because the patient is psychologically unable to tolerate the ICD.[57, 58]

Alteration in lifestyle, which is generally a consequence of the malignant arrhythmia and not that of the ICD implantation, may be an issue. Driving is often the focus of attention. Individual states have laws concerning whether and in what timeframe the patient may continue to drive after an episode of syncope. The states also regulate whether physicians must notify the department of motor vehicles when a patient that they are caring for develops syncope or has an ICD implanted.

ICD indications

Original indications

While it was an investigational device, the indications for ICD implantation were extremely rigorous in order that the devices be used only in patients at greatest risk for sudden cardiac death. To be a candidate for an ICD, the patient was required to have had documented VT or VF associated with loss of consciousness as well as recurrent VT or VF in spite of antiarrhythmic drug therapy, inducible VT or VF associated with loss of consciousness during EPS and a life expectancy of greater than or equal to six months. In addition, the patient was expected to have the emotional maturity and availability for long-term follow-up.

FDA indications

In 1985, the FDA approved the ICD for prevention of sudden cardiac death. The FDA approval is for ICD implantation in patients who 1) are survivors of at least one cardiac arrest, presumably due to hemodynamically unstable VT or VF, not associated with acute myocardial infarction and/or 2) have persistently inducible, hemodynamically unstable VT/VF in spite of conventional antiarrhythmic drug therapy. The recent results of the MADIT trial (see below) may also allow prophylactic use of the ICD.

Consensus guidelines

In addition, two consensus groups have published similar guidelines [59, 60] in order to further guide physicians in selecting patients who would benefit from ICD therapy. One guideline was organized by the AHA and ACC jointly; the second was published by NASPE. In essence, the two sets of guidelines are similar. The indications are divided into three categories: Class I: ICD is indicated by general consensus; Class II: ICD therapy is a reasonable option, but there is no consensus; Class III: ICD therapy is not justifiable.

The Class I indications for ICD therapy are the following:

1.   In treatment of a patient with VT or VF in whom EP testing or Holter monitoring cannot be used to predict the efficacy of antiarrhythmic therapy. This indication includes patients who are not inducible at EP study.

2.   In treatment of a patient with recurrent VT or VF despite antiarrhythmic drug therapy as guided by EP testing or Holter monitoring. This indication includes treatment of patients who failed an antiarrhythmic drug that was predicted to be effective by EPS or Holter monitoring.

3.   In treatment of the patient with spontaneous VT or VF in whom antiarrhythmic drugs are not tolerated. This indication includes treatment of patients who have an adverse drug effect or are poorly compliant with the drug regimen.

4.   In treatment of the patient with VT or VF who remains inducible (with a

clinically relevant VT or VF) at EP study despite optimal medical therapy. There are no qualifiers specified in terms of the number of drug trials, the rate of the drug slowed VT or the hemodynamic stability of the patient during the VT.

The class II indication for ICD therapy is in the treatment of the patient with syncope of unknown etiology and with inducible, sustained VT or VF at EPS in whom antiarrhythmic drugs are not tolerated, or are ineffective, or in whom the antiarrhythmic drug regimen is not adhered to.

The class III contraindications to ICD therapy include the following:

1. The patient with sustained VT or VF due to acute myocardial ischemia, acute MI, or reversible, toxic/metabolic disarray.

2. The patient with recurrent syncope of unknown etiology who has no inducible ventricular arrhythmia.

3. The patient with incessant VT or VF that is uncontrollable with antiarrhythmic drug therapy such that device firing may be unreasonably frequent.

4. The patient with VF secondary to the WPW syndrome.

5. The patient with medical, surgical, or psychiatric contraindications. This includes patients whose lifespans are limited by cardiac or other diseases.

Clinical outcome and impact on survival

Data published by Mirowski et al in 1983 showed decreased 1 year mortality in patients who had received an ICD.[61] In 1985, the ICD was approved for widespread use by the FDA based on Mirowski's data. Given the ethical concerns about conducting randomized, controlled trials in patients at high risk for sudden death, the FDA approved the device for clinical use without the use of such trials.

The success of the ICD in reducing sudden cardiac death has been reported in nonrandomized studies.[25, 62-67] However, it is not clear if total mortality will be reduced by ICD therapy. A recent, small, randomized study of patients with coronary artery disease who survived a cardiac arrest has indicated that patients treated with an ICD had increased survival compared with those who received conventional therapy.[68] Preliminary data from the Cardiac Arrest Study (Hamburg) of survivors of sudden cardiac death with documented VT or VF showed the propafenone arm to have an increased mortality when compared to the ICD arm.[69] However, there has been no difference in total mortality in the remaining treatment limbs of the study (ICD, metoprolol, or amiodarone therapy), although there has been a decrease in sudden cardiac death in those patients randomized to ICD therapy. In order to assess the impact of the ICD vs. antiarrhythmic drugs on total mortality, the NHLBI has sponsored a prospective, randomized controlled study named AVID (antiarrhythmic drugs versus implantable devices). This study, which is currently underway, randomly assigns patients with documented VF, or sustained VT associated with syncope, or hemodynamically unstable VT with near syncope and an LVEF less than or equal to 40% to therapy with antiarrhythmic drugs (d,l-sotalol or amiodarone) or a nonthoracotomy ICD. A Canadian study, the Canadian Implantable Defibrillator Study (CIDS), is also ongoing. This study randomized patients with prior cardiac arrest or hemodynamically unstable VT to ICD or amiodarone therapy.[70]

The broad nature of the guidelines for ICD implantation have made possible the initiation of studies of primary prevention of sudden cardiac death. The CABG Patch Trial randomizes patients who are undergoing coronary artery bypass grafting (CABG) who have an LVEF less than 36% and have a positive signal averaged ECG to either ICD or conventional therapy. The Multicenter Automatic Defibrillator Implantable Trial (MADIT) randomized patients with LVEF less than 36%, prior myocardial infarction, and sustained VT which was inducible in the electrophysiology laboratory to either ICD or conventional therapy. The VT in these patients was also required to be unsuppressable by procainamide administration during the EP study. This study was terminated early by the data safety monitoring committee due to a survival benefit of the ICD in this patient population (unpublished data). MUSTT (Multicenter Unsustained Tachycardia Trial) randomizes patients with nonsustained VT, reduced ejection fraction, coronary artery disease, and inducible monomorphic VT to therapy of the VT, including ICD if needed, or no therapy. The Sudden Cardiac Death in Heart Failure Trial (SCDHeFT) , an NHLBI sponsored trial of patients with congestive heart failure and ventricular ectopy will randomize patients to placebo (standard heart failure therapy), amiodarone, or Medtronic Jewel ICD therapy.

In addition, several studies have examined the efficacy of ICD implantation as a bridge to cardiac transplantation. In one small prospective study [71] of 15 high risk patients accepted for cardiac transplantation, no postoperative complications occurred in the eight patients who received endocardial ICD implantation. The patients who received epicardial ICD implantation did so because endocardial leads were not available at the time of implantation. In all patients, defibrillation thresholds were acceptable and 60% of the patients had an appropriate shock during mean follow-up of 11 months. In a retrospective, nonrandomized study[72] of 291 patients evaluated for cardiac transplantation, sudden death rates were lowest in those patients treated with ICDs compared with those treated with antiarrhythmic drug therapy or no antiarrhythmic therapy. Total mortality was not different and patients with an ICD had a higher nonsudden death rate. In another nonrandomized study of patients listed for cardiac transplantation, mortality was 4.7% in patients with an ICD, while mortality was 23.2% in patients without an ICD.[73] The multicenter DEFIBRILAT (Defibrillator as Bridge to Later Transplantation) trial was organized to examine the hypothesis that empiric use of ICDs reduces the sudden death rate in heart transplantation candidates. However, this trial was disbanded prior to enrollment of patients due to a lack of funding.[72]

The expense of ICD technology has also come under scrutiny. Several cost analyses have been performed.[74-76] A recent analysis[77] showed that in patients with an ejection fraction of less than 25%, the cost-effectiveness was $44,000 per year of life saved. In patients with an ejection fraction of greater than or equal to 25%, the cost-effectiveness was $27,200 per year of life saved. Regardless of ejection fraction, this was reduced to $18,100 per year of life saved without preimplantation electrophysiology testing. The savings were a result of decreased hospitalization. Cost-effectiveness of the endocardial ICD implantation was $25,700 per year of life saved in preliminary analysis. In patients with EF greater than or equal to 25%, the cost-effectiveness of an endocardial ICD was $22,400 per year of life saved. In patients with an endocardial ICD implantation who had no preceding electrophysiology study, the cost per year of life saved was $14,200. It is difficult to determine the appropriateness of ICD therapy in many of the patients included in this study. A randomized study by Wever et al [78] also found ICD therapy to be more cost effective than EP guided drug therapy in postinfarction survivors of cardiac arrest.

Developmental goals for the ICD

ICD technology has made great strides in the past few years. Device development is no doubt focusing on the following issues which have not yet been optimized.

Pulse generator size

Current pulse generators are large, in part due to the size of the batteries needed. In general, two batteries are used per pulse generator. These batteries are of a standard size at present. The size of the pulse generator generally necessitates implantation in the abdomen. As devices become smaller, a pectoral implant, as with a pacemaker, becomes possible. The Medtronic Jewel and the CPI MINI are currently approved for pectoral implantation. These devices are still larger than a pacemaker pulse generator and are generally implanted in the abdomen unless the patient is large.

Battery longevity

As the batteries are an integral part of the pulse generator, the pulse generator must be replaced when the batteries begin to lose their charge. The latest generation of pulse generators at present cost in excess of $15,000. As battery technology improves, devices will have increased longevity. This will enhance patient acceptance and will decrease the cost of long-term therapy with ICDs.

Defibrillation efficacy

Optimization of the defibrillation discharge and improved electrode design will lower the energy requirements for defibrillation. This, in turn, should increase battery longevity.

Bradycardia pacing

The newest ICDs offer backup VVI pacing. It is anticipated that rate responsive and dual chamber pacing will be incorporated in future devices. Ideally, a separate pacemaker, apart from that incorporated into the ICD, should not be necessary even in patients who are pacemaker dependent.

Sensing algorithms

Sensing devices to be used in conjunction with present technology are being developed. For example, sensors to monitor the patient's hemodynamic status are under development. In this way, the nature of the cardiac arrhythmia can better be determined, thus increasing the specificity of therapy. In addition, the urgency of reversion to sinus rhythm based on the patient's hemodynamic status can be determined and therapy can then be adjusted. Thus, if the patient becomes hemodynamically unstable, more aggressive therapy can be instituted. In addition, incorporation of atrial sensors in lead systems will help define the tachyarrhythmia and thus avoid defibrillator therapy during an atrial arrhythmia.

Conclusions

Since its inception less than two decades ago, the ICD has revolutionized the therapy of malignant ventricular arrhythmias. However, in today's cost conscious medical environment, the expense of ICD technology is an important issue, as it has been since the inception of the device. The results of randomized, controlled trials of ICD versus antiarrhythmic drug therapy are awaited so that it can be determined whether the cost of the ICD is justified.

REFERENCES

1. Mirowski M. The implantable cardioverter-defibrillator: an update. J Cardiovasc Med 1984: 9:191.
2. Mitrani R, et al. Current trends in the implantable cardioverter-defibrillator. In: D. Zipes and J. Jalife, eds. Cardiac Electrophysiology From Cell to Bedside. Philadelphia: W.B. Saunders Co., 1995:1393.
3. Brooks R, et al. Successful implantation of cardioverter-defibrillator systems in patients with elevated defibrillation thresholds. J Am Coll Cardiol 1993: 22:569.
4. CPI. data on file.
5. Raviele A, Gasparini G. Italian multicenter clinical experience with endocardial defibrillation: acute and long-term results in 307 patients. PACE 1995: 18:599.
6. Bardy G, et al. A simplified, single-lead unipolar transvenous cardioversion-defibrillation system. Circulation 1993: 88:543.
7. Fisher J, et al. Comparative effectiveness of pacing techniques for termination of well-tolerated sustained ventricular tachycardia. PACE 1983: 6:915.
8. Dillon SM, et al. Effects of overdrive stimulation on functional reentrant circuits causing ventricular tachycardia in the canine heart: mechanisms for resumption or alteration of tachycardia. J Cardiovasc Electrophysiol 1993: 4:393.

9. Waldecker B, et al. Overdrive stimulation of functional reentrant circuits causing ventricular tachycardia in the infarcted canine heart. Resetting and entrainment. Circulation 1993: 87:1286.

10. Schmidinger H, Sowten E. Physiological variation in the termination window of reentry tachycardia studied by non-invasive programmed stimulation. European Heart Journal 1988: 9:997.

11. Waldecker B, et al. Importance of modes of electrical termination of ventricular tachycardia for the selection of implantable antitachycardia devices. Am J Cardiol 1986: 57:150.

12. Ventritex. data on file.

13. Medtronic. data on file.

14. Zipes D, et al. Clinical transvenous cardioversion of recurrent life-threatening ventricular arrhythmias: low energy synchronized cardioversion of ventricular tachycardia and termination of ventricular fibrillation in patients using a catheter electrode. Am Heart J 1982: 103:789.

15. Waspe L, et al. Role of a catheter lead system for transvenous countershock and pacing during electrophysiologic tests: An assessment of the usefulness of catheter shocks for terminating ventricular tachyarrhythmias. Am J Cardiol 1983: 52:477.

16. Saksena S, et al. Comparative efficacy of transvenous cardioversion and pacing in patients with sustained ventricular tachycardia: A prospective, randomized, crossover study. Circulation 1985: 72:153.

17. Siebels J, Schneider M, Kuck K. Low energy cardioversion with the implantable cardioversion defibrillator devices for treatment of vetnricular tachycardia and ventricular fibrillation. Zeitschrift fuer Kardiologie 1993: 82:683.

18. Zipes D, et al. Termination of ventricular fibrillation in dogs by depolarizing a critical amount of myocardium. Am J Cardiol 1975: 36:37.

19. Pruente HM, et al. Animated images of cardiac membrane voltage during defibrillation. J Electrocardiol 1995: 28 (Suppl):7.

20. Chen P-S, et al. Comparison of defibrillation threshold and the upper limit of ventricular vulnerability. Circulation 1986: 73:1022.

21. Shibata N, et al. Epicardial activation after unsuccessful defibrillation in dogs. Am J Physiol 1988: 255:H902.

22. Troup P. Implantable cardioverters and defibrillators. Curr Probl in Cardiol. Vol. IV(12). Chicago: Med Publishers, 1989:675.

23. Saksena S, et al. Prospective comparison of biphasic and monophasic shocks for implantable cardioverter-defibrillators using endocardial leads. Am J Cardiol 1992: 70:304.

24. Wyse D, et al. Comparison of biphasic and monophasic shocks for defibrillation using a nonthoracotomy system. Am J Cardiol 1993: 71:197.

25. Winkle R, et al. Improved low energy defibrillation efficacy in man with the use of a biphasic truncated exponential waveform. Am Heart J 1989: 117:122.

26. Bardy G, et al. A prospective randomized evaluation of biphasic versus monophasic waveform pulses on defibrillation efficacy in humans. J Am Coll Cardiol 1989: 14:728.

27. Bardy G, et al. Electrode system influence on biphasic waveform defibrillation efficacy in humans. Circulation 1991: 84:665.

28. Bardy G, et al. Prospective comparison of sequential pulse and single pulse defibrillation with use of two different clinically available systems. J Am Coll Cardiol 1989: 14:165.

29. Hook B, et al. Implantable cardioverter-defibrillator therapy in the absence of significant symptoms. Circulation 1993: 87:1897.

30. Hurwitz J, et al. Importance of abortive shock capability with electrogram storage in cardioverter-defibrillator devices. J Am Coll Cardiol 1993: 21:895.

31. Mosteller R, et al. Operative mortality with implantation of the automatic cardioverter-defibrillator. Am J Cardiol 1991: 68:1340.

32. Autschbach R, et al. The effect of coronary bypass graft surgery for the prevention of sudden cardiac death: recurrent episodes after ICD implantation and review of literature. PACE 1994: 17:552.

33. Singer I, Lang D. Defibrillation threshold: clinical utility and therapeutic implications. PACE 1992: 15:923.

34. Singer I, et al. Is defibrillation testing safe? Pacing and Cardiac Electrophysiology 1991: 14:1899.

35. Cardiac Pacemakers I. Endotak, Clinical Summary Report. St. Paul, MN: Cardiac Pacemakers, Inc., 1993.

36. Joye J, et al. Perioperative morbidity and mortality after ICD implantation in 150 consecutive patients. Circulation 1991: 84:II-608.

37. Levine J, et al. Predictors of first discharge and subsequent survival in patients with automatic implantable cardioverter defibrillators. Circulation 1991: 84:558.

38. Goodman L, et al. Complications of automatic implantable cardioverter-defibrillators: Radiographic, CT and echocardiographic evaluation. Radiology 1989: 170:447.

39. Spotnitz H, et al. Methods of ICD-pacemaker insertion to avoid interactions. Ann Thorac Surg 1992: 53:253.

40. Reiffel J, Coromilas J, Zimmerman J. Drug-device interactions: Clinical considerations. PACE 1985: 8:369.

41. Epstein A, et al. Clinical characteristics and outcome of patients with high defibrillation thresholds. A muti-center study. Circulation 1992: 86:1206.

42. Woolfolk D, et al. The effect of quinidine on electrical energy required for ventricular defibrillation. Am Heart J 1966: 72:659.

43. Dawson A, Steinberg M, Shapland J. Effect of class I and class III drugs on current and energy required for internal defibrillation. Circulation 1985: 72(Suppl III):384.

44. Manz M, Jung W, Luderitz B. Interactions between drugs and devices: experimental and clinical studies. Am Heart J 1994: 127:978.

45. Echt D, et al. Effect of lidocaine on defibrillation energy requirements in patients (abstract). Circulation 1989: 80:II224.

46. Echt D, Cato E ,Coxe D. pH-dependent effects of lidocaine on defibrillation energy requirements in dogs. Circulation 1989: 80:1003.

47. Marinchak R, et al. Effect of antiarrhythmic drugs on defibrillation threshold: Case report of an adverse effect of mexiletine and review of the literature. PACE 1988: 11:7.

48. Ruffy R, et al. Adrenergically mediated variations in the energy required to defibrillate the heart: observations in closed-chest, nonanesthetized dogs. Circulation 1986: 73:374.

49. Huang S, et al. Effects of long-term amiodarone therapy on the defibrillation threshold and the rate of shocks of the implantable cardioverter-defibrillator. Am Heart J 1991: 122:720.

50. Fain E, Lee J, Winkle R. Effects of acute intravenous and chronic oral amiodarone on defibrillation energy requirements. Am Heart J 1987: 114:8.

51. Dorian P, et al. Oral clofilium produces sustained lowering of defibrillation energy requirements in a canine model. Circulation 1991: 83:614.

52. Echt D, et al. Evaluation of antiarrhythmic drugs on defibrillation energy requirements in dogs: sodium channel block and action potential prolongation. Circulation 1989: 79:1106.

53. Wang M, Dorian P. DL and D sotalol decrease defibrillation energy requirements. PACE 1989: 12:1522.

54. Schrader R, et al. Verapamil increases the internal defibrillation energy requirements in anesthetized dogs. J Cardiovasc Pharmacol 1992: 19:839.

55. Pinski S, et al. Patients with a high defibrillation threshold: Clinical characteristics, management and outcome. Am Heart J 1991: 122:89.

56. Morris P, et al. Psychiatric morbidity following implantation of the automatic implantable cardioverter defibrillator. Psychosomatics 1991: 31:58.

57. Fricchione G, Olson L ,Vlay S. Psychiatric syndromes in patients with the automatic implantable cardioverter defibrillator: Anxiety, psychological dependence, abuse, and withdrawal. Am Heart J 1989: 117:1411.

58. Tchou P, et al. Psychological support and psychiatric management of patients with automatic implantable cardioverter defibrillator. Int J Psych Med 1989: 19:393.

59. Dreifus L, et al. Guidelines for implantation of cardiac pacemakers and antitachyarrhythmia devices: a report of the American College of Cardiology/American Heart Association Task Force on Assessment of Diagnostic and Therapeutic Cardiovascular Procedures. J Am Coll Cardiol 1992:18:1.

60. Lehmann M, Saksena S. Implantable cardioverter defibrillator in cardiovascular practice: report of the Policy Conference of the North American Society of Pacing and Electrophysiology. NASPE Policy Conference Committee. PACE 1991: 14:969.

61. Mirowski M, et al. Mortality in patients with implanted automatic defibrillators. Ann Intern Med 1983: 98:585.

62. Veltri E, et al. Followup of patients with ventricular tachyarrhythmia treated with the automatic implantable cardioverter-defibrillator: programmed electrical stimulation results do not predict clinical outcome. J Electrophysiol 1989: 3:467.

63. Tchou P, et al. Automatic implantable cardioverter defibrillators and survival of patients with left ventricular dysfunction and malignant ventricular arrhythmias. Ann Intern Med 1988: 109:529.

64. Marchlinski F, et al. The automatic implantable cardioverter-defibrillator: efficacy, complications, and device failures. Ann Intern Med 1986: 104:481.

65. Kelly P, et al. The automatic implantable cardioverter-defibrillator: efficacy, complications, and survival in patients with malignant ventricular arrhythmias. J Am Coll Cardiol 1988: 11:1278.

66. Forgoros R, Elson J, Bonnet C. Actuarial incidence and pattern of occurrence of shocks following implantation of the automatic implantable cardioverter defibrillator. J Am Coll Cardiol 1989: 14:508.

67. Myerburg R, et al. Time to first shock and clinical outcome in patients receiving an automatic implantable cardioverter-defibrillator. J Am Coll Cardiol 1989: 14:508.

68. Wever E, et al. Randomized study of implantable defibrillator as first-choice therapy versus conventional strategy in postinfarct sudden death survivors. Circulation 1995: 91:2195.

69. Siebels J, Kuck K. Implantable cardioverter defibrillator compared with antiarrhythmic drug treatment in cardiac arrest survivors (the Cardiac Arrest Study Hamburg). Am Heart J 1994: 127:1139.

70. Connolly S, et al. Canadian Implantable Defibrillator Study (CIDS): study design and organization. Am J Cardiol 1993: 72:103F.

71. Saxon L, et al. Implantable defibrillators for high-risk patients with heart failure who are awaiting cardiac transplantation. Am Heart J 1995: 130:501.

72. Sweeney M, et al. Influence of the implantable cardioverter/defibrillator on sudden death and total mortality in patients evaluated for cardiac transplantation. Circulation 1995: 92:3273.

73. Grimm M, et al. The impact of implantable cardioverter-defibrillators on mortality among patients on the waiting list for heart transplantation. J Thorac Cardiovasc Surg 1995: 110:532.

74. Kupperman M, et al. An analysis of the cost effectiveness of the implantable defibrillator. Circulation 1990: 81:91.

75. O'Donoghue S, et al. Automatic implantable cardioverter-defibrillator: Is early implantation cost-effective? J Am Coll Cardiol 1990: 16:1258.

76. Larsen G, et al. Cost-effectiveness of the implantable cardioverter-defibrillator: effect of improved battery life and comparison with amiodarone therapy. J Am Coll Cardiol 1992: 19:1323.

77. Kupersmith J, et al. Evaluating and improving the cost-effectiveness of the implantable defibrillator. Am Heart J 1995: 130:507.

78. Wever E, et al. Cost-effectiveness of implantable defibrillator as first-choice therapy versus electrophysiologically guided, tiered strategy in postinfarct sudden death survivors A randomized study. Circulation 1996: 93:489.

Index